# DIAGNOSTIC MEDICAL SONOGRAPHY

# The Vascular System

# DIAGNOSTIC MEDICAL SONOGRAPHY

# The Vascular System

## SECOND EDITION

**Ann Marie Kupinski,** PhD, RVT, RDMS, FSVU

Technical Director
North Country Vascular Diagnostics, Inc.
Clinical Professor of Radiology
Albany Medical College
Albany, New York

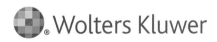
Wolters Kluwer

Philadelphia • Baltimore • New York • London
Buenos Aires • Hong Kong • Sydney • Tokyo

*Acquisitions Editor:* Jay Campbell
*Senior Product Development Editor:* Amy Millholen
*Development Editor:* Heidi Grauel
*Editorial Coordinator:* John Larkin
*Marketing Manager:* Shauna Kelley
*Production Project Manager:* Bridgett Dougherty
*Design Coordinator:* Joan Wendt
*Manufacturing Coordinator:* Margie Orzech
*Prepress Vendor:* S4Carlisle Publishing Services

Second Edition

9  8  7  6  5  4  3  2  1

Printed in China

**Library of Congress Cataloging-in-Publication Data**

Names: Kupinski, Ann Marie, editor.
Title: The vascular system / [edited by] Ann Marie Kupinski, PhD, RVT,
   RDMS, FSVU, Technical Director, North Country Vascular Diagnostics, Inc.,
   Clinical Associate Professor of Radiology, Albany Medical College, Albany,
   NY.
Description: Second edition. | Philadelphia: Wolters Kluwer Health, 2017. |
   Series: Diagnostic medical sonography
Identifiers: LCCN 2017027043 | ISBN 9781496380593 (hardback)
Subjects: LCSH: Blood-vessels—Ultrasonic imaging. | BISAC: MEDICAL / Allied
   Health Services / Radiological & Ultrasound Technology.
Classification: LCC RC691.6.U47 D43 2017 | DDC 616.1/307543—dc23 LC record available at https://lccn.loc.gov/2017027043

LWW.com

*To my husband, Mitchell for his ongoing love and support. To our son, Justin who helps in so many ways. You both show me what really matters in life. Accomplishments like this book are more rewarding because I can share them with you.*

To the readers of this book, I hope this book provides you valuable knowledge to light your way. Remember that "Science knows no country, because knowledge belongs to humanity, and is the torch which illuminates the world."

**LOUIS PASTEUR**

# CONTRIBUTORS

**Ali F. AbuRahma, MD, RVT, RPVI, FACS, FRCS (C)**
Professor of Surgery
Chief, Vascular & Endovascular Surgery
Director, Vascular Fellowship & Integrated Residency
   Programs
Medical Director, Vascular Laboratory
Co-Director, Vascular Center of Excellence
West Virginia University, Charleston Division
Charleston Area Medical Center
Charleston, West Virginia

**Olamide Alabi, MD**
Vascular Fellow
Oregon Health & Science University
Portland, Oregon

**Enrico Ascher, MD, FACS**
Professor of Surgery
Mount Sinai School of Medicine
Chief of Vascular Surgery
NYU Lutheran Medical Center
Brooklyn, New York

**Dennis F. Bandyk, MD, FACS, FSVU**
Professor of Surgery in Residence
University of California – San Diego School of Medicine
Chief, Division of Vascular & Endovascular Surgery
Sulpizio Cardiovascular Center
La Jolla, California

**Brian Burke, MD, RVT, FAIUM**
Assistant Professor of Radiology
Hofstra Northwell School of Medicine
Manhasset, New York

**Kari A. Campbell, BS, RVT**
Senior Vascular Technologist
D.E. Strandness Jr. Vascular Laboratory
University of Washington Medical Center
Seattle, Washington

**Kathleen A. Carter, BSN, RN, RVT, FSVU**
Norfolk, Virginia

**Terrence D. Case, MEd, RVT, FSVU**
Vascular Education Consultant
Hollywood Beach, Florida

**Michael J. Costanza, MD, FACS**
Associate Professor of Surgery
SUNY Upstate Medical University
Lead Physician, Vascular Surgery
VA Medical Center
Syracuse, New York

**M. Robert DeJong, RDMS, RDCS, RVT, FSDMS, FAIUM**
Radiology Technical Manager, Ultrasound
The Johns Hopkins Medical Institutions
Baltimore, Maryland

**Colleen Douville, BA, RVT, CPMM**
Director
Vascular Ultrasound and Neurophysiology
Swedish Health Services
Seattle, Washington

**Gail Egan, MS, ANP**
Nurse Practitioner
Interventional Radiology
Sutter Medical Group
Sacramento, California

**Scott G. Erpelding, MD**
University of Kentucky
Lexington, Kentucky

**Eileen French-Sherry, MA, RVT, FSVU**
Associate Chairperson
Department of Medical Physics and Advanced Imaging
Program Director, Vascular Ultrasound
College of Health Sciences, Rush University
Chicago, Illinois

**Traci B. Fox, EdD, RT(R), RDMS, RVT**
Assistant Professor
Diagnostic Medical Sonography Program
Department of Radiologic Sciences
Jefferson College of Health Professions
Research Assistant Professor
Department of Radiology
Sidney Kimmel Medical College at Thomas Jefferson
   University
Philadelphia, Pennsylvania

**Monica Fuller, RDMS, RVT, CTT+**
Product Application Specialist
Philips Ultrasound
Bothell, Washington

**Vicki M. Gatz, MSPH, RVT, FSVU**
Master Technologist
Gill Heart Institute Vascular Laboratory
University of Kentucky
Lexington, Kentucky

**Shubham Gupta, MD**
Assistant Professor of Urology
University of Kentucky
Lexington, Kentucky

**Anil P. Hingorani, MD, FACS**
Vascular Surgery Attending
NYU Lutheran Medical Center
Brooklyn, New York

**Jenifer F. Kidd, RN, RVT, DMU, FSVU**
Senior Vascular Sonographer
Macquarie Vascular Laboratory
Sydney, Australia

**Ann Marie Kupinski, PhD, RVT, RDMS, FSVU**
Technical Director
North Country Vascular Diagnostics, Inc.
Clinical Professor of Radiology
Albany Medical College
Albany, New York

**Steven A. Leers, MD, RVT, FSVU**
Associate Professor of Surgery
Medical Director UPMC Vascular Laboratories
Division of Vascular Surgery
University of Pittsburgh Medical Center
Pittsburgh, Pennsylvania

**Wayne C. Leonhardt, BA, RDMS, RVT**
Senior Clinical Vascular Instructor
Gurnick Academy of Medical Arts
Diagnostic Medical Sonography Program
San Mateo, California
Sonographer, Mission Imaging Services
Ashville, North Carolina

**Peter W. Leopold, MB, BCh, MCh, FRCS**
Chief of Vascular Surgery
Frimley Park Hospital
Surrey, England

**Natalie Marks, MD, FSVM, RPVI, RVT**
Vascular Medicine Attending
The Vascular Institute of New York
NYU Lutheran Medical Center
Brooklyn, New York

**Daniel A. Merton, BS, RDMS, FSDMS, FAIUM**
Diagnostic Medical Sonography Consultant
Laurel Springs, New Jersey

**Gregory L. Moneta, MD, FACS**
Professor and Chief, Vascular Surgery
Oregon Health & Science University
Knight Cardiovascular Institute
Portland, Oregon

**Susan Murphey, BS, RDMS, RDCS, CECD**
Certified Ergonomic Compliance Director
President
Essential Work Wellness
Jacksonville, Oregon

**Anne M. Musson, BS, RVT, FSVU**
Technical Director
Vascular Laboratory
Veterans Affairs Medical Center
White River Junction, Vermont

**Terry Needham, RVT, FSVU**
Chattanooga, Tennessee

**Diana L. Neuhardt, RVT, RPhS, FSVU**
CompuDiagnostics, Inc.
Phoenix, Arizona

**Marsha M. Neumyer, BS, RVT, FSVU, FSDMS, FAIUM**
International Director
Vascular Diagnostic Educational Services
Harrisburg, Pennsylvania

**Mark Oliver, MD, RVT, RPVI, FSVU**
Co-Director, Vascular Laboratory
Gagnon Cardiovascular Institute
Attending Physician
Morristown Medical Center
Morristown, New Jersey

**Kathryn L. Parker, MD**
General Surgery Resident
University of California
San Diego, California

**Karim Salem, MD**
Vascular Surgery Resident
University of Pittsburgh Medical Center
Pittsburgh, Pennsylvania

**Sergio X. Salles Cunha, PhD, RVT, FSVU**
Consultant
Angiolab – Noninvasive Vascular Laboratories
Curitiba, Paraná and Vitoria, Espirito Santo, Brazil

**William B. Schroedter, BS, RVT, RPhS, FSVU**
Co-Owner & Co-Technical Director
Quality Vascular Imaging, Inc.
Director of Education
Virtual Vein Center
Venice, Florida

**Leslie M. Scoutt, MD, FACR, FAIUM, FSRU**
Professor of Radiology and Surgery
Yale University School of Medicine
Vice Chair for Education
Department of Radiology & Biomedical Imaging
Associate Program Director
Diagnostic Radiology
Chief, Ultrasound Service
Medical Director
Non-invasive Vascular Laboratory
Yale-New Haven Hospital
New Haven, Connecticut

**Michael J. Singh, MD, FACS, RPVI**
Associate Professor of Surgery
Chief Vascular Surgery
UPMC Shadyside
Pittsburgh, Pennsylvania

**Gary Siskin, MD, FSIR**
Professor and Chairman
Department of Radiology
Albany Medical Center
Albany, New York

**S. Wayne Smith, MD, FACP, FSVM, RVT, RPVI**
Clinical Professor of Medicine
UNC Chapel Hill
Medical Director
Vascular Diagnostic Center
Rex UNC Healthcare
Raleigh, North Carolina

**Amy Steinmetz, RVT**
Director of Vascular Lab
UPMC St. Margarets
University of Pittsburgh Medical Center
Pittsburgh, Pennsylvania

**Steven R. Talbot, RVT, FSVU**
Technical Director
Vascular Laboratory
Research Associate
Division of Vascular Surgery
University of Utah Medical Center
Salt Lake City, Utah

**Patrick A. Washko, BSRT, RDMS, RVT, FSVU**
Technical Director
Vascular Diagnostic Center
Rex UNC Healthcare
Raleigh, North Carolina

**Jean M. White-Melendez, RVT, RPhS, FSVU**
Co-Owner & Co-Technical Director
Quality Vascular Imaging, Inc.
Director of Development
Virtual Vein Center
Venice, Florida

**R. Eugene Zierler, MD, RPVI, FACS**
Professor of Surgery
University of Washington School of Medicine
Medical Director
D.E. Strandness Jr. Vascular Laboratory
University of Washington Medical Center and Harborview
   Medical Center
Seattle, Washington

**Robert M. Zwolak, MD, PhD, FACS**
Professor of Surgery (Vascular)
Geisel School of Medicine
Dartmouth-Hitchcock Medical Center
Lebanon, New Hampshire
Chief of Surgery
White River Junction VA Medical Center
White River Junction, Vermont

# REVIEWERS

**Deanna Barymon**
Arkansas State University
Jonesboro, Arkansas

**Brenda Hoopingarner**
Fort Hays State University
Hays, Kansas

**Abigail Kurtz**
Baptist College of Health Sciences
Memphis, Tennessee

The second edition of *Diagnostic Medical Sonography: The Vascular System* has been updated to be sure that the content is current and reflects the standard of care in terms of noninvasive diagnostic vascular testing. Sonographic procedures, images, diagnostic criteria, and references have been revised as needed. This textbook contains both fundamental materials and advanced topics, hoping to appeal to readers with diverse educational backgrounds and experiences. This textbook is intended to be used as either an introduction to the profession or a comprehensive reference guide. The content provides groundwork for an essential understanding of anatomy, physiology, and pathophysiology. This material is expected to benefit sonographers, vascular technologists, students, practitioners, and physicians caring for patients with vascular disease.

Input from educators and colleagues was valuable in determining the addition of six new chapters. The first section of the textbook contains three new fundamental chapters discussing basic ultrasound scanning topics. These new chapters are "Orientation to Ultrasound Scanning," "Ultrasound Principles," and "Ergonomics: Avoiding Work-Related Injury." The second section presents basic vascular anatomy as well as arterial and venous physiology. The next four sections comprise chapters which focus on specific components of the vascular system, namely, the cerebrovascular, peripheral arterial, peripheral venous, and abdominal vascular systems. The peripheral arterial section has a chapter on nonimaging physiologic arterial testing which is essential in the diagnosis of vascular disease and often performed in conjunction with ultrasound testing. Within the peripheral venous section, a new chapter "Sonography in the Venous Treatment Room" was added. This chapter explores the ever-expanding role of the sonographer in the treatment of venous disease. The seventh and final section contains chapters with topics, including intraoperative sonography, hemodialysis access scanning, vascular applications of contrast agents, and quality assurance. This seventh section of the textbook includes the last two new chapters, "Evaluation of Penile Blood Flow" and "Complementary Vascular Imaging."

Every attempt was made to produce an up-to-date and factual textbook. The material is presented in an interesting and enjoyable format to capture the reader's attention and curiosity. The reader should find the chapters easy to follow, comprehensive, and thought-provoking. Descriptions of anatomy, physiology, pathology, normal, and abnormal sonographic findings are depicted in numerous illustrations and tables throughout the chapters. Several clinical case study examples are shown throughout the textbook to illustrate various sonographic findings.

The goal of this textbook was to be as complete as possible while recognizing that augmentation with ongoing supplemental information from peer-reviewed journals will be required. Learning is a lifelong process that can be a challenge but should be looked upon as a welcome exercise. The essential information contained within this textbook should establish a basis for those seeking to build their knowledge of vascular ultrasound.

**Ann Marie Kupinski**

# ACKNOWLEDGMENTS

I would first like to thank editors Diane Kawamura and Tanya Nolan (Abdomen and Superficial Structures) and Susan Raatz Stephenson and Julia Dmitrieva (Obstetrics and Gynecology) for their support throughout the completion of our three volumes of *Diagnostic Medical Sonography*. It was great to work with these talented individuals, and their ideas, encouragement, and knowledge were a tremendous help.

The team of individuals at Wolters Kluwer Health deserves my sincerest gratitude for all their hard work. Their expertise in all areas of development, editing, promotion, and production resulted in a wonderful final product. I'd like to especially thank Heidi Grauel, development editor, for all her patience, guidance, and technical assistance along the way. I would also like to thank Amy Millholen, development editor; Jay Campbell, acquisitions editor; and all the others who worked on this project and helped get this textbook completed. An additional "thank-you" goes out to Rachel Kendoll, Vascular Technology Program Director at Spokane Community College, for her help with some of the online ancillary materials and her excellent work on the companion workbook.

I am pleased that the second edition of this textbook contains contributions from so many recognized experts in the field. The contributors are from a broad range of backgrounds and experiences from across the United States as well as international contributors from Australia, Brazil, and England. The strength and thoroughness of this textbook is due to the fantastic authors who contributed to this project. I am so thankful to have their expertise and their wonderful chapters.

Images are a key component to any textbook. I'd like to thank the various authors within the book who helped contribute additional images for other chapters. There are several other individuals I would like to thank who contributed images found in this edition as well as the first: Phillip J. Bendick, PhD, RVT Royal Oak, MI; Karen Burns, RN RVT MBA, Chicago, IL; Michael Ciarmiello, Albany, NY; David Cosgrove, FRCR, London, England; Steven Feinstein, MD, Chicago, IL; Kimberly Gaydula, BS RVT, Chicago, IL; Damaris Gonzalez, RVT RDMS, Chicago IL; Kathleen Hannon, RN MS RVT RDMS, Boston, MA; John Hobby, RVT, Pueblo, CO; Debra Joly, RVT RDMS RDCS, Houston, TX; Steve Knight, BSc, RVT, RDCS, Half Moon Bay, CA; Kimberly Lopresti, RDCS, Philadelphia, PA; Daniel Matz, Frimley, Surrey, England; Antonio Sergio Marcelino, MD, Sao Paulo, Brazil; Jeff Powers, PhD, Bothell, WA; Besnike Ramadani, BS RVT, Chicago IL; Robert Scissons, RVT FSVU, Toledo, OH; Carlos Ventura, MD, Sao Paulo, Brazil; Hans-Peter Weskott, MD, Hannover, Germany. New image contributions to this second edition were provided by Derek Butler, BS, RVT, RDCS, RDMS, RT(R), Newburyport, MA; Aria Levitas, BS, Glens Falls, NY; and Richard Jackson, MD, Glens Falls, NY.

Lastly, I'd like to thank my family, friends, and colleagues who have personally helped me get to this point to function as an editor of a textbook. Thanks to my vascular friends across the country who have taught me so much. Special thanks goes to Sister Theresa Wysolmerski, CSJ, PhD of the College of Saint Rose, for getting me started with exploring science and for the friendship and guidance through the years. Thank you to Mr. Peter Leopold, MB BCh, MCh, FRCS Eng/Ed, for getting me started in ultrasound and for answering my countless questions on vascular disease. Finally, to my family and friends, especially my parents, son, and husband who have given me so much love and support through the years, thank you so very much!

**Ann Marie Kupinski**

The books in the *Diagnostic Medical Sonography* series will help you develop an understanding of specialty sonography topics. Key learning resources and tools throughout the textbook aim to increase your understanding of the topics provided and better prepare you for your professional career. This User's Guide will help you familiarize yourself with these exciting features designed to enhance your learning experience.

## Chapter Objectives

Measurable objectives listed at the beginning of each chapter help you understand the intended outcomes for the chapter, as well as recognize and study important concept within each chapter.

## Glossary

Key terms are listed at the beginning of each chapter and clearly defined, then highlighted in bold type throughout the chapter to help you to learn and recall important terminology.

## Pathology Boxes

Each chapter includes tables of relevant pathologies, which you can use as a quick reference for reviewing the material.

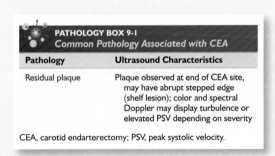

**PATHOLOGY BOX 9-1**
*Common Pathology Associated with CEA*

| Pathology | Ultrasound Characteristics |
| --- | --- |
| Residual plaque | Plaque observed at end of CEA site, may have abrupt stepped edge (shelf lesion); color and spectral Doppler may display turbulence or elevated PSV depending on severity |

CEA, carotid endarterectomy; PSV, peak systolic velocity.

## Critical Thinking Questions

Throughout the chapter are critical thinking questions to test your knowledge and help you develop analytical skills that you will need in your profession.

### CRITICAL THINKING QUESTIONS

1. You are scanning a 350-pound male for an aorta study. You notice you are having trouble visualizing the proximal aorta. What would be the best option to improve visualization of the aorta?

## Resources thePoint®

You will also find additional resources and exercises on thePoint, including a glossary with pronunciations, quiz bank, sonographic video clips, and weblinks. Use these interactive resources to test your knowledge, assess your progress, and review for quizzes and tests.

---

## Ultrasound Principles

TRACI B. FOX    **CHAPTER 2**

### OBJECTIVES

- List the parameters that describe the sound wave
- Describe the properties of sound propagation through soft-tissue
- Explain the principles of imaging with Doppler
- List the most common artifacts seen with ultrasound

### KEY TERMS

artifacts
bioeffects
Doppler
pulsed-wave
transducer

### GLOSSARY

**artifacts** Echoes on the image were not caused by actual reflectors in the body

**bioeffects** Ultrasound has the ability to cause changes to the tissue if proper settings are not used

**continuous-wave** Principle of constantly transmitting a sound wave into the patient to obtain a spectral Doppler waveform

**Doppler** Tool for measuring blood flow quantitatively or qualitatively using pulsed-wave or continuous-wave techniques

**pulsed-wave** Principle of sending in a small group of sound waves (a "pulse") and then waiting for that pulse to come back so an image can be displayed. Also used for spectral and color Doppler

**transducer** The part of the ultrasound machine that transmits and receives sound via an array of piezoelectric elements

### BASICS OF SOUND

In diagnostic ultrasound, sound waves are produced by piezoelectric elements within a device called a transducer. Sound waves are pressure waves, which are mechanical waves. When a piezoelectric element is shocked with electricity, a sound wave is generated that propagates into the medium (e.g., soft-tissue). When that sound wave encounters a tissue of a different acoustic impedance, the sound wave will be reflected back to the transducer. The ultrasound machine measures the time taken for the sound wave to travel to the reflector and return, and then it knows how far away the reflector is. With this information, a dot can be placed on the screen corresponding to the reflector depth and the strength (amplitude) of the return echo. A series of reflectors along one vertical line is called a scan line. After one scan line of information is obtained, the machine sends another pulse to create the next scan line. All the scan lines displayed on the screen form one complete image, called a frame.

#### Parameters of Sound

Sound waves are longitudinal waves, that is, the propagation of the wave is parallel to the movement of the molecules within the medium. As sound travels through the body, there are cyclic changes in pressure, density, and particle motion. The simplest unit of a wave is a cycle (Fig. 2-1). Cycles can be measured by their height, length, and other parameters. **Frequency** ($f$) is the number of cycles that occurs in 1 second. In a pulsed-wave ultrasound transducer, frequency is determined primarily by the thickness of the piezoelectric element. The unit of frequency, also called operating frequency, center frequency, and resonating frequency, is Hertz (Hz). In medical diagnostic ultrasound, the

9

# CONTENTS

# PART ONE

# FUNDAMENTALS OF ULTRASOUND SCANNING
## Orientation to Ultrasound Scanning

ANN MARIE KUPINSKI | M. ROBERT DE JONG

## CHAPTER 1

## OBJECTIVES

- Describe the anatomic planes
- Define the common terms used for vascular ultrasound orientation and direction
- Identify the common transducer orientations
- Describe the patient positions used in vascular ultrasound
- Define the appropriate presentation for a vascular ultrasound image

## GLOSSARY

**anechoic** A region of an ultrasound image free from echoes

**coronal plane** A vertical plane that divides the body into front (ventral) and back (dorsal) parts; also known as the frontal plane

**heterogeneous** A region of an ultrasound image having mixed or differing ultrasound echoes

**homogeneous** A region of an ultrasound image having a uniform appearance on ultrasound with echoes that appear similar

**hyperechoic** A region of an ultrasound image with echoes that are brighter than the surrounding tissue or brighter than normal

**hypoechoic** A region of an ultrasound image with echoes that are darker than the surrounding tissue or darker than normal.

**isoechoic** A region of an ultrasound image producing echoes that are the same as the surrounding tissue with equal brightness

**sagittal plane** A vertical plane that divides the body into right and left parts

**transverse plane** A plane that divides the body into superior and inferior parts; it is perpendicular to the coronal and sagittal planes

## KEY TERMS

**anechoic**

**coronal plane**

**echogenic**

**heterogeneous**

**homogeneous**

**hyperechoic**

**hypoechoic**

**isoechoic**

**sagittal plane**

**transverse plane**

To begin a study of ultrasound, including vascular ultrasound, one must be familiar with basic body anatomic planes, terminology, and orientations used. This chapter will review the commonly used terminology and abbreviations pertaining to scanning directions and image characteristics and describe various anatomic planes. Image orientation related to the transducer and scanning plane will also be described.

## ABBREVIATIONS

There are a host of abbreviations used in medicine and in vascular ultrasound. It is beyond the scope of this text to include all of them here. The specific abbreviations related to anatomy, testing areas, and ultrasound physics are included within the individual chapters. Table 1-1 presents a

| TABLE 1-1 | **Abbreviations** | | | |
|---|---|---|---|---|
| **Abbreviation** | **Meaning** | | **Abbreviation** | **Meaning** |
| AAA | Abdominal aortic aneurysm | | OP | Outpatient |
| ABD | Abdomen | | PAD | Peripheral arterial disease |
| ABI | Ankle brachial index (also known as ankle arm index [AAI]) | | PE | Pulmonary embolus |
| AI | Acceleration index | | PI | Pulsatility index |
| AVF | Arteriovenous fistula | | PPG | Photoplethysmography |
| AVM | Arteriovenous malformation | | PSV | Peak systolic velocity |
| BP | Blood pressure | | PTCA | Percutaneous transluminal coronary angioplasty |
| CABG | Coronary artery bypass graft | | PVD | Peripheral vascular disease |
| CAD | Coronary artery disease | | PVR | Pulse volume recording (also known as volume pulse recording [VPR]) |
| CDI | Color Doppler imaging | | Q | Flow (blood flow) |
| CVI | Chronic venous insufficiency | | RAR | Renal aortic ratio |
| CVA | Cerebrovascular accident | | RAS | Renal artery stenosis |
| DM | Diabetes mellitus | | RI | Resistance index (resistive index) |
| DVT | Deep venous thrombosis | | RT | Right |
| Dx | Diagnosis | | SAG | Sagittal |
| EDV | End-diastolic velocity | | TCD | Transcranial Doppler |
| HR | Heart rate | | TCI | Transcranial imaging |
| HTN | Hypertension | | TIA | Transient ischemic attack |
| Hx | History (history of compliant) | | TRV | Transverse |
| IDDM | Insulin-dependent diabetes mellitus | | UE | Upper extremity |
| IP | Inpatient | | US | Ultrasound |
| LE | Lower extremity | | VPR | Volume pulse recording (also known as pulse volume recording [PVR]) |
| LT | Left | | WNL | Within normal limits |

brief list of some abbreviations a vascular technologist or sonographer may encounter.

## ANATOMIC DESCRIPTIONS

Traditional nomenclature is used to convey anatomic direction and position. Table 1-2 summarizes the directional and locational terms used in ultrasound. Figure 1-1 depicts the directional terms on a drawing of a body. Note that this body is drawn in a standard anatomic position standing erect with arms at the side and the face and palms directed forward.

Ultrasound imaging is performed along various anatomic planes. These anatomic planes are produced by drawing an imaginary line through the body. Figure 1-2 illustrates a body in the standard anatomic position (erect) with the three scanning planes drawn in sagittal, coronal, and transverse.

The sagittal plane runs vertically along the long axis of the body. It separates the body into right and left sections.

Sagittal is sometimes referred to as longitudinal or a long-axis plane, but these terms are not always synonymous. A long-axis view implies a lengthwise view. Thus, a long-axis view of the subclavian artery is not in a sagittal plane of the body, but in the transverse plane of the body. The midline sagittal plane or median sagittal plane courses exactly through the midline of the body passing structures such as the spine and umbilicus. All other sagittal planes running vertically along the long axis of the body but not through the midline are parasagittal planes. In most cases when the term sagittal is used, it is implied to be in fact a parasagittal plane. It is important to note that in Figure 1-2 the sagittal plane is perpendicular to the ground. This orientation to the ground will change if the position of the subject is supine. If supine, as during an ultrasound examination, a sagittal plane will be parallel to the ground.

The coronal plane is perpendicular to the ground (in an erect subject) and splits the body into anterior and posterior

| TABLE 1-2   **Directional and Locational Terms Used in Ultrasound** | |
|---|---|
| **Term** | **Definition** |
| Anterior | Toward the front; a structure in front of another structure |
| Caudal (caudad) | Toward the feet |
| Cephalad (cranial) | Toward the head |
| Contralateral | A structure on the opposite side of the body |
| Deep | Away from the surface or skin |
| Distal | Farther away from the heart; farther away from the origin; farther away from the point of attachment |
| Dorsal | Related to the back of the body; toward the back of the body |
| Inferior | Toward the feet; a structure lower than another structure |
| Ipsilateral | A structure on the same side of the body |
| Lateral | Away from the center of the body or a structure; toward the side of the body |
| Medial | Toward the center of the body or a structure; toward the midline or middle of the body |
| Posterior | Toward the back of the body; a structure that is behind another structure |
| Proximal | Closer to the heart; closer to the origin; closer to the point of attachment |
| Superficial | Toward the surface or the skin |
| Superior | Toward the head; a structure higher than another structure |
| Ventral | Related to the front of the body |

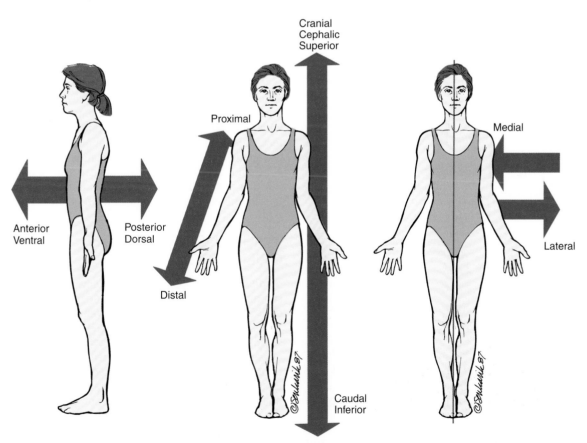

**FIGURE 1-1**  Directional terms used in ultrasound. The drawing illustrates a body in the standard anatomic position (standing erect with arms by the side, face and palms directed forward). (Adapted with permission from Kawamura DM, Lunsford BM. *Diagnostic Medical Sonography: Abdomen and Superficial Structures*. Philadelphia, PA: Lippincott Williams Wilkins; 2012.)

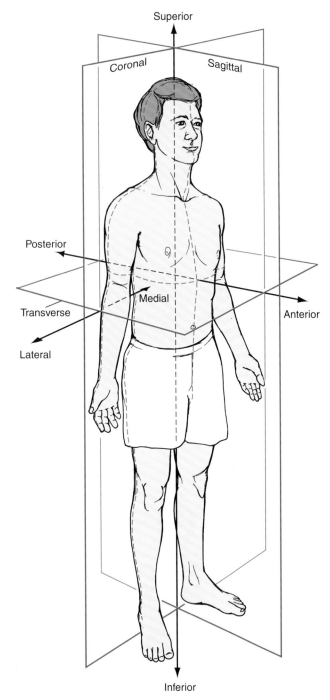

**FIGURE 1-2** The three anatomic planes, sagittal, transverse, and coronal (frontal), depicted as imaginary flat surface drawn through the body. (Adapted with permission from Kawamura DM, Lunsford BM. *Diagnostic Medical Sonography: Abdomen and Superficial Structures*. Philadelphia, PA: Lippincott Williams Wilkins; 2012.)

(or front and back) sections. It also courses vertically through the long axis of the body and is perpendicular to the sagittal plane. It is also known as the frontal plane.

The transverse plane passes through the body in a plane that is parallel to the ground (while erect) and perpendicular to the sagittal and frontal planes. The transverse plane separates the body into superior and inferior (or top and bottom) sections. The transverse plane is sometimes referred to as the short-axis, transverse or horizontal view. Again, a

transverse view of an organ or vessel may be in a sagittal plane depending on how the structure is positioned within the body. For example, a transverse view of the main renal artery is in a sagittal plane of the body. A long-axis view of the main renal artery is obtained in a transverse body plane.

Any plane that is not a true sagittal, coronal, or transverse plane, is considered to be an oblique plane. It is at an angle to the reference plane. There are several structures in the body that do not lie exactly in a sagittal or transverse plane, such as the kidneys and the pancreas. Imaging of the kidney in a long-axis view, with respect to the organ itself, requires the transducer to be in an oblique body plane.

## PATIENT POSITION DESCRIPTIONS

There are several positions in which a patient can be placed in order to perform an ultrasound examination. Positioning the patient correctly will enhance the visualization of the region of interest. Positions used for ultrasound scanning include the following and are depicted in Figure 1-3.

*Supine*: Lying on the back

*Prone*: Lying face down

*Right lateral decubitus (RLD)*: Lying on the right side; sometimes also called left side up (LSU)

*Left lateral decubitus (LLD)*: Lying on the left side; sometimes also called right side up (RSU)

*Right anterior oblique (RAO)*: Lying prone with the left side elevated

*Left anterior oblique (LAO)*: Lying prone with the right side elevated

*Right posterior oblique (RPO)*: Lying supine with the left side elevated

*Left posterior oblique (LPO)*: Lying supine with the right side elevated

Additional patient positions are required for certain vascular ultrasound examinations. Reverse Trendenberg position has the patient lying supine, but the body is tilted with the head elevated between 15 and 30 degrees above the feet. This position can facilitate venous filling in the lower extremities thus improving visualization of lower extremity veins. Sitting upright and standing can also be used during vascular examinations, including examinations of the aorta, mesenteric vessels, and venous insufficiency testing.

## IMAGE AND TRANSDUCER ORIENTATION

Medical images are typically displayed as if a patient is standing facing an observer with the patient's right side of their body aligned with the observer's left and vice versa. This same orientation will hold true if the patient is lying supine and the observer is viewing the patient from the feet upward. Appropriate transducer orientation must be followed to produce images that are oriented correctly per standard imaging policies. Correct presentation of the ultrasound image on the screen begins with appropriate orientation of the ultrasound transducer. Holding the transducer incorrectly can cause the image to be backward, causing right left, medial lateral, and superior inferior to be reversed. For example, if the transducer orientation is incorrect, the interpreting physician may report pathology in the upper

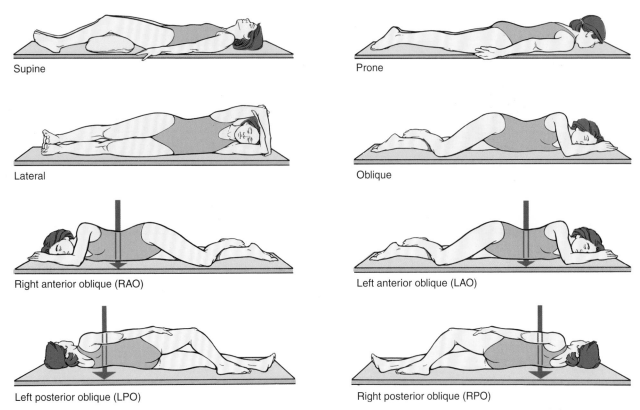

**FIGURE I-3** Patient positions used in ultrasound scanning. (Adapted with permission from Kawamura DM, Lunsford BM. *Diagnostic Medical Sonography: Abdomen and Superficial Structures*. Philadelphia, PA: Lippincott Williams Wilkins; 2012.)

pole of a kidney, when in fact it is really the lower pole, as now image orientation is not conventional and the upper pole is on the right aspect of the image as opposed to being properly displayed to the left aspect of the image. In vascular imaging, correct orientation is extremely important in determining antegrade or retrograde flow particularly with venous insufficiency testing.

All transducers have an indicator that is located along the narrow side of the transducer. This indicator may be a notch, a raised groove, or a light. When scanning in a transverse plane, the notch is placed closest to or pointing toward the right side of the patient (Fig. 1-4). On the ultrasound screen, each manufacturer will place a symbol or indicator corresponding to the position of the transducer indicator

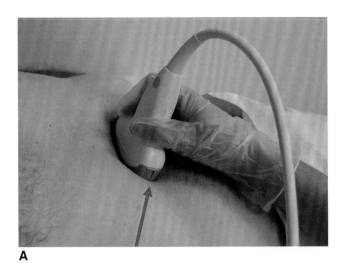

**A**

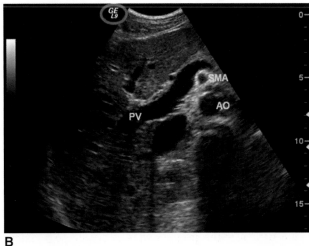

**B**

**FIGURE I-4** **A:** An ultrasound transducer positioned transverse on the abdomen with the position indicator noted by the red arrow. The transducer is oriented such that the indicator is pointing toward the right side of the patient. **B:** An ultrasound image taken in transverse orientation with the positional marker (in this case "GE L9") circled in red. This marker is placed on the screen to correspond to the position of the transducer indicator or notch on the patient. Note the red circle is at the patient's right side of the abdomen as it should be when following standard orientation techniques.

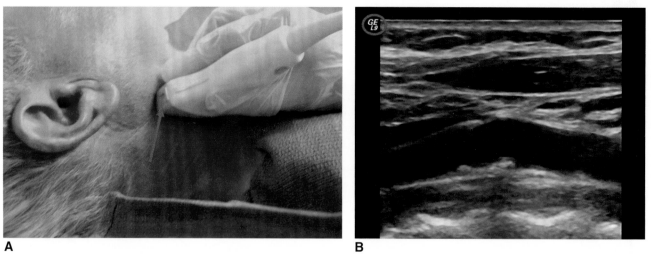

**A**                                                            **B**

**FIGURE 1-5 A:** An ultrasound transducer positioned sagittal along the neck with the position indicator noted by the red arrow. The transducer is oriented such that the indicator is pointing toward the head of the patient. **B:** An ultrasound image taken in sagittal orientation with the positional marker (in this case "GE L9") circled in red. This marker is placed on the screen to correspond to the position of the transducer indicator or notch on the patient. Note the red circle is closest to the patient's head as it should be when following standard orientation techniques.

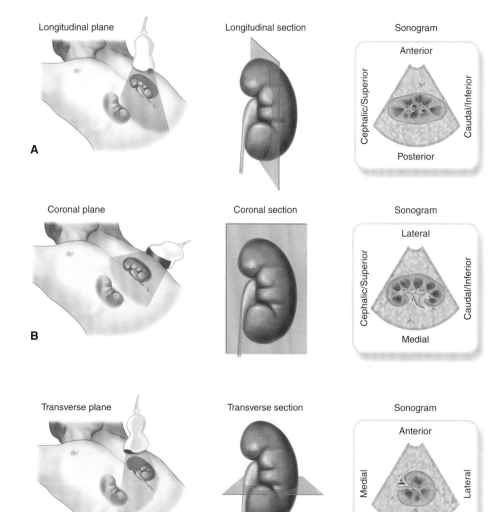

**FIGURE 1-6** Transducer orientation. **A:** This is a parasagittal anatomic plan providing a long-axis view of the left kidney. **B:** This is a coronal anatomic plane which also illustrates a view that is cutting the left kidney into a front and back (coronal) plane. **C:** A transverse anatomic plane providing a transverse view of the left kidney. (Adapted with permission from Kawamura DM, Lunsford BM. *Diagnostic Medical Sonography: Abdomen and Superficial Structures.* Philadelphia, PA: Lippincott Williams Wilkins; 2012.)

or notch (Fig. 1-4B). When scanning in a sagittal plane, the notch is placed closest to or pointing toward the head of the patient (Fig. 1-5). Again, on the ultrasound screen a symbol or indicator will be placed corresponding to the position of the transducer notch (Fig. 1-5B). In vascular imaging, this means that when in a sagittal or parasagittal plane, the head of the patient should always appear to the left of the screen. In a transverse plane with the patient supine, the right side of the patient should always appear on the left side of the screen.

Figure 1-6 provides a depiction of the body plane, transducer orientation, and ultrasound image appearance of the left kidney with three different approaches. Image labels should always be used to provide additional anatomic directional information and patient position, for example, "prone left kidney." Figure 1-7 depicts the image presentation with multiple scanning planes. These are the common image presentations that are recommended by imaging societies and academic programs. Individual laboratories may vary the image presentation based on certain applications. It is crucial to label all images if alternate presentations are used. It is the goal of standardization to allow any reader of the images to immediately understand the directionality of the structures within the image to allow for proper interpretation.

## IMAGING DESCRIPTIONS

Communicating through common terminology is essential when describing any medical finding but especially true for imaging. Ultrasound features have been defined with a

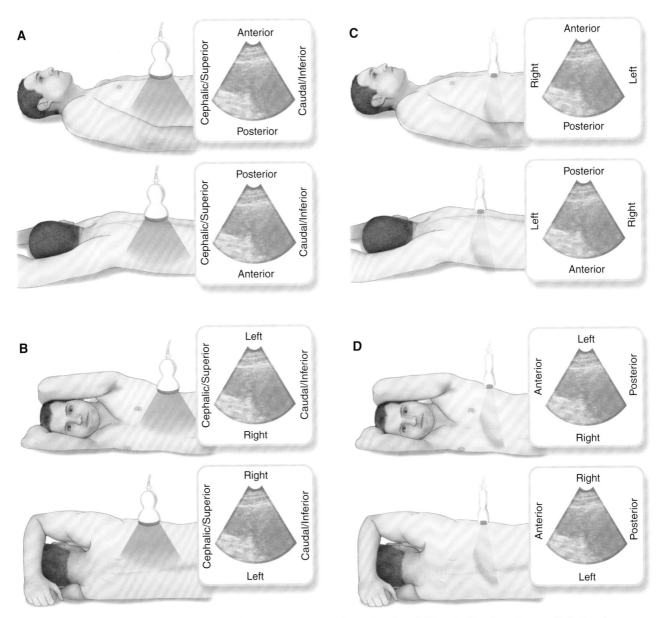

**FIGURE 1-7** Various image presentations using multiple patient positions and transducer orientations. **A:** The patient is supine and prone with the transducer orientated in a long-axis, sagittal plane. **B:** The patient is in left and right lateral decubitus positions to allow for a coronal image. **C:** The patient is supine and prone with the transducer in a transverse plane. **D:** The patient is in left and right lateral decubitus positions with the transducer in a transverse plane. (Adapted with permission from Kawamura DM, Lunsford BM. *Diagnostic Medical Sonography: Abdomen and Superficial Structures*. Philadelphia, PA: Lippincott Williams Wilkins; 2012.)

specific terminology relating to the appearance of an area of interest compared to the surrounding structures. Normal anatomy has been carefully characterized, and these detailed expressions help to identify abnormalities and pathology.

*Echogenic*: This term refers to a structure that produces ultrasound echoes. It does not further characterize those echoes but rather just states that they are present. The echogenicity of a structure will vary depending on the acoustic impedance between the structures. The appearance of returned echoes can also be changed with variations in equipment controls such as the overall image gain.

*Anechoic*: This describes a structure or region which does not return any echoes. It appears to be echo free on the image. The term *sonolucent* is a misnomer for anechoic. Sonolucent refers to the property of a medium that allows for the passage of ultrasound through the medium without reflecting the ultrasound back to its source. Anechoic usually refers to a fluid-filled or cystic structure although some solid masses may also be anechoic. Technical factors may also cause a structure to appear echo free.

*Hypoechoic*: This describes a structure or region which appears not as bright as the surrounding tissue.

*Hyperechoic*: This describes a structure or region which appears brighter than the surrounding tissue.

*Isoechoic*: This describes structures which are of equal echo brightness.

*Homogeneous*: This describes echoes which are uniform in appearance and of equal intensity

*Heterogeneous*: This describes echoes which are of different or mixed intensity. An example of this would be a region with both anechoic and hyperechoic portions.

## SUMMARY

- The use of appropriate abbreviations and terminology will facilitate better communication of ultrasound findings.
- Awareness of the various anatomic planes and orientation of structures within the body will aid in obtaining good quality ultrasound images with the aid of varying approaches.
- The patient's condition will often require multiple patient positions to be used. Different ultrasound applications will also necessitate multiple patient positions.
- Standard transducer orientations have been established which produce ultrasound images oriented in a standard fashion. These standard orientations assist with the communication of findings and proper interpretation.
- Description of ultrasound image characteristics with commonly accepted terminology is also valuable in producing a quality ultrasound examination.

## CRITICAL THINKING QUESTIONS

1. While attempting to visualize the aorta with a patient supine, bowel gas limits visualization. What can be done to aid in the completion of the examination?
2. In a sagittal view of the aortic bifurcation, how should the transducer be oriented and how should the image appear?

## MEDIA MENU

Student Resources available on the**Point**® include:
- Audio glossary
- Interactive question bank
- Videos
- Internet resources

# Ultrasound Principles

TRACI B. FOX **CHAPTER 2**

## OBJECTIVES

- List the parameters that describe the sound wave
- Describe the properties of sound propagation through soft-tissue
- Explain the principles of imaging with Doppler
- List the most common artifacts seen with ultrasound

## KEY TERMS

**artifacts**

**bioeffects**

**Doppler**

**pulsed-wave**

**transducer**

## GLOSSARY

**artifacts** Echoes on the image were not caused by actual reflectors in the body

**bioeffects** Ultrasound has the ability to cause changes to the tissue if proper settings are not used

**continuous-wave** Principle of constantly transmitting a sound wave into the patient to obtain a spectral Doppler waveform

**Doppler** Tool for measuring blood flow quantitatively or qualitatively using pulsed-wave or continuous-wave techniques

**pulsed-wave** Principle of sending in a small group of sound waves (a "pulse") and then waiting for that pulse to come back so an image can be displayed. Also used for spectral and color Doppler

**transducer** The part of the ultrasound machine that transmits and receives sound via an array of piezoelectric elements

## BASICS OF SOUND

In diagnostic ultrasound, sound waves are produced by piezoelectric elements within a device called a transducer. Sound waves are pressure waves, which are mechanical waves. When a piezoelectric element is shocked with electricity, a sound wave is generated that propagates into the medium (e.g., soft-tissue). When that sound wave encounters a tissue of a different acoustic impedance, the sound wave will be reflected back to the transducer. The ultrasound machine measures the time taken for the sound wave to travel to the reflector and return, and then it knows how far away the reflector is. With this information, a dot can be placed on the screen corresponding to the reflector depth and the strength (amplitude) of the return echo. A series of reflectors along one vertical line is called a scan line. After one scan line of information is obtained, the machine sends another pulse to create the next scan line. All the scan lines displayed on the screen form one complete image, called a frame.

### Parameters of Sound

Sound waves are longitudinal waves, that is, the propagation of the wave is parallel to the movement of the molecules within the medium. As sound travels through the body, there are cyclic changes in pressure, density, and particle motion. The simplest unit of a wave is a cycle (Fig. 2-1). Cycles can be measured by their height, length, and other parameters. **Frequency** ($f$) is the number of cycles that occurs in 1 second. In a pulsed-wave ultrasound transducer, frequency is determined primarily by the thickness of the piezoelectric element. The unit of frequency, also called operating frequency, center frequency, and resonating frequency, is Hertz (Hz). In medical diagnostic ultrasound, the

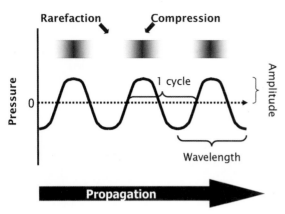

**FIGURE 2-1** Depiction of wave. One cycle of sound showing wavelength and amplitude parameters. (Adapted with permission from Penny S, Fox T, Godwin CH. *Examination Review for Ultrasound: Sonographic Principles & Instrumentation.* Philadelphia, PA: Lippincott Williams Wilkins; 2011.)

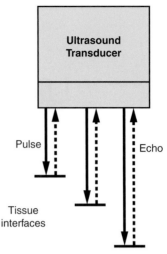

**FIGURE 2-2** Pulse-echo ultrasound. The deeper the reflector, the longer the round-trip time of the pulse. (Adapted with permission from Penny S, Fox T, Godwin CH. *Examination Review for Ultrasound: Sonographic Principles & Instrumentation.* Philadelphia, PA: Lippincott Williams Wilkins; 2011.)

frequency is typically in the range of 2 to 20 MHz. **Period** ($T$) is the time taken for one cycle to occur, in milliseconds (ms). **Propagation speed** ($c$) is the speed at which sound moves through the medium, in m/s or cm/s. Propagation speed is determined only by the medium through which the sound is traveling, and not by the transducer. Although different media have different propagation speeds, almost all ultrasound machines use the average of all the propagation speeds found within the tissues of the body, which is approximately 1,540 m/s. Therefore, ultrasound machines are programmed to use a propagation speed of 1,540 m/s, even if the sound is traveling through a tissue whose speed is not 1,540 m/s. **Wavelength** ($\lambda$) is the length (in mm) of one cycle of sound, from the beginning of the wave to the end of the wave. The wavelength is determined by the propagation speed divided by the operating frequency. **Amplitude** is the height of a cycle, from the baseline to the peak of the cycle. The units of amplitude depend on what the cycle of sound represents: pressure (Pascals), density (kg/m$^3$), or particle motion (mm). **Acoustic impedance** (Z, in rayls) is a property of the medium and is determined by the product of the density ($\rho$) and propagation speed ($c$). Acoustic impedance is an important factor in determining reflection of the echoes. Without a difference in impedances between adjacent tissues, no reflection is generated. The larger the difference in impedances, the larger the return echo.

When imaging the body, sound is sent into the body in groups of cycles, called pulses. With **pulsed-wave** (PW) ultrasound, a pulse is sent into the body by the transducer, and the machine waits for that pulse to return before transmitting the next pulse. This waiting period, called dead time or listening time, is essential so the machine can time the pulse travel and determine the depth of the reflector. Pulses have their own descriptive terminology. **Pulse repetition frequency** (PRF) is the number of pulses per second, in Hz or kHz. PRF is inversely related to the depth of the reflector and unrelated to operating frequency. Every time the transducer shocks the transducer, a pulse is generated. If the transducer is shocked 1,500 times in 1 second, then 1,500 pulses per second are generated. This would represent a PRF of 1,500 Hz. A PW transducer cannot send a new pulse without waiting for the return of the previous

pulse. When a deeper depth is desired, it takes longer for the pulse to reach the reflector and return to the transducer, decreasing the rate at which pulses can be sent (Fig. 2-2).

The length of the pulse is the **spatial pulse length** (SPL). Spatial pulse length is equal to the wavelength ($\lambda$) multiplied by the number of cycles in a pulse (n). For imaging applications, a short pulse is desired for improved resolution, usually 2 to 3 cycles per pulse, but Doppler applications may have as many as 30 cycles in a pulse. There are two measurements for the time it takes for a pulse to occur: pulse repetition period and pulse duration. **Pulse repetition period** (PRP) is the time it takes for a pulse to occur including the dead time. **Pulse duration** (PD) is a measurement of only the transmission part of the pulse and does not include dead time (Fig. 2-3). In PW ultrasound, the machine spends 99% of the time waiting for a previously transmitted pulse to return. In other words, only 1% of the time is the machine actively transmitting sound into the patient. Most of the time the machine is just waiting. The percentage of time the machine is transmitting sound into the patient is called the **duty factor** (DF) and is equal to the PD/PRP. Another type of ultrasound is when sound is transmitted continuously, called **continuous-wave** (CW) ultrasound. With CW ultrasound, a minimum of two piezoelectric elements are needed because piezoelectric elements can transmit and receive sound, but not at the same time.

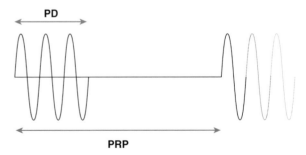

**FIGURE 2-3** Pulse duration (PD) and pulse repetition period (PRP). Both measurements depict the time it takes for a pulse to occur, but PRP includes the listening (dead) time.

Therefore, with CW ultrasound, one element is constantly transmitting, and the other is constantly receiving. CW transducers have a 100% transmission time, which means the duty factor is 100%. CW transducers cannot generate an image because the machine never stops to time how far away the reflectors are, and therefore CW probes are used only for spectral Doppler.

## INTERACTION OF SOUND WITH TISSUE

### Attenuation

As sound travels through tissue, some of its energy is lost as a result of attenuation. Attenuation may result from absorption of the beam, which is the conversion of sound to heat, from scattering of the beam, and from reflection of the beam. Attenuation varies by medium, and in order from lowest attenuation to highest attenuation are water, fluids, fat, soft-tissue, muscle, bone, and air. Air attenuates (by reflection) approximately 100% of the beam, leaving little to no energy to propagate through the tissue. Bone is also a significant attenuator, reflecting 50% of the sound and causing enough absorption of the beam so that sound cannot return to the transducer, causing a shadow to appear deep to the bone. For this reason, air and bone are best avoided during an ultrasound examination.

Although attenuation varies by tissue, the average rate of attenuation through soft-tissue is 0.5 dB/cm/MHz. In other words, for every MHz the transducer is and for every centimeter the sound travels, the beam will lose approximately 0.5 dB of intensity or power. Attenuation increases with frequency. The higher the frequency, the higher the rate of attenuation, and, therefore, the worse the ability to penetrate. Ultrasound imaging is the paradox of wanting the highest frequency to have the best spatial resolution but also needing the ability to penetrate into the tissue. With Doppler studies, lower frequency transducers (5 to 7 MHz) tend to be used because of penetration and aliasing, although a higher frequency transducer should be considered for the B-mode (grayscale) part of the examination if spatial resolution is critical.

### Reflection and Refraction

The two types of reflectors are specular and nonspecular. A **specular reflector** is larger than the wavelength of the transmitted beam, and includes broad structures such as the diaphragm and organ capsules. When sound strikes a specular reflector perpendicularly, the reflectors show up on ultrasound as a bright white line. Sound that strikes a specular reflector at an angle other than 90 degrees is not reflected back to the transducer, and is not displayed.

When sound encounters a structure that is smaller than the transmitted beam's wavelength, it is called a **nonspecular reflector**. At nonspecular reflectors, there is scattering of the sound wave, and the beam is spread out over many directions. Unlike specular reflectors, nonspecular reflectors are not angle dependent; scatter occurs regardless of the angle of incidence (Fig. 2-4). As a result of the scattering of sound, some echoes return to the transducer, called **backscatter**. Nonspecular reflectors make up the parenchyma of the

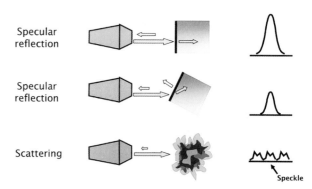

**FIGURE 2-4** Reflector types. Specular reflectors are usually large, smooth surfaces and are angle dependent. Nonspecular cause scattering of the sound and are not angle dependent because of backscatter. (Adapted with permission from Penny S, Fox T, Godwin CH. *Examination Review for Ultrasound: Sonographic Principles & Instrumentation.* Philadelphia, PA: Lippincott Williams Wilkins; 2011.)

organs and appear as tiny dots of varying shades of gray. Nonspecular reflectors are not as bright as specular reflectors because the amplitude of nonspecular reflectors is much weaker. There is a special type of nonspecular reflector that occurs when the reflector is very small compared with the beam's wavelength, called a Rayleigh scatterer. Red blood cells, which measure 6 to 8 microns, are an example of a Rayleigh scatterer. The hallmark of Rayleigh scattering is that the amount of scatter is proportional to the frequency to the fourth power ($f^4$). Therefore, as transducer frequency goes up, scatter increases dramatically, limiting penetration. This is one of the reasons lower frequency transducers are used for Doppler studies.

An interface is the boundary of two tissues adjacent to one another. **Reflection** of sound at an interface occurs when two conditions are met: an angle of incidence perpendicular to the interface and a difference in the acoustic impedances of the two media. The amount of reflection that occurs is proportional to the impedance mismatch, or difference in impedances between the two media. The farther apart the two impedances are, the stronger the reflection. The greater the reflection, the less sound there is to propagate deeper into the tissue. This is why reflection is a type of attenuation. For example, if 60% of sound is reflected at an interface, only 40% is available to be transmitted. At a soft-tissue to air interface, approximately 100% of sound is reflected, leaving nothing to be transmitted. **Refraction** at an interface may occur if two different conditions are met: a nonperpendicular, or oblique angle of incidence, and a difference in propagation speeds between the two media. Refraction is a change in direction of the transmitted beam at the interface. With perpendicular incidence, sound will be transmitted into the tissue at the same angle with no change in direction at the interface. With oblique incidence and assuming disparate propagation speeds, the transmitted sound will change in direction. If the propagation speed of the second medium is greater than 1,540 m/s, the angle of the transmitted angle will be greater than the incident angle. If the propagation speed of the second medium is less than 1,540 m/s, the angle of the transmitted angle will be less than the incident angle (Fig. 2-5).

The **range equation** is used by the machine to determine the travel time of the pulse. For echoes to appear on the

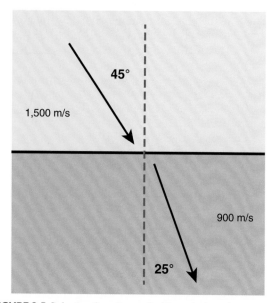
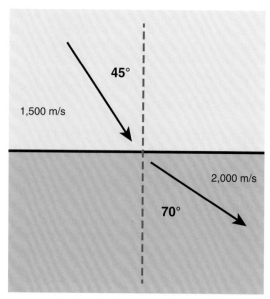

**FIGURE 2-5** Refraction. Sound transmitted through a boundary at a nonperpendicular angle will change direction on the basis of the differences in propagation speed.

screen with B-mode imaging, the location of the reflectors must be known. The machine measures the time taken for a transmitted pulse of sound to return to the transducer and calculates the distance to the reflector ($d$) using the equation $d = ct/2$, where $c$ is the propagation speed, assumed to be soft-tissue at 1,540 m/s, and $t$ is the round-trip travel time of the sound. Assuming soft-tissue, it takes 13 μs for sound to reach a depth of 1 cm and return to the transducer. This is often called the **13 μs rule** and is possible because ultrasound machines assume a soft-tissue medium. However, it is possible for reflectors to be displayed in the wrong location if the actual propagation speed is not exactly 1,540 m/s. The fact that not all tissues have propagation speeds of exactly 1,540 m/s produces an artifact in which the reflectors are displayed at the wrong location on the display (Fig. 2-6).

## TRANSDUCERS

The sonographer needs to have a proper transducer for the studies performed. In some examinations, it is possible that

more than one transducer will be needed, depending on the indication or patient's body habitus. The three most common transducer types are the curvilinear array, the linear array, and the phased array. All of today's modern transducers are broadband, that is, they have the ability to use the different frequencies that are present in the beam. A 5.0 MHz transducer, therefore, may have the ability to image at frequencies between 3 and 7 MHz. The **curvilinear array** transducer (Fig. 2-7), sometimes called a "curved" or "convex" array, is a transducer most commonly used for abdominal work. This transducer may also be used for vascular studies, such as lower extremity venous examinations in a patient with a large body habitus. The **linear sequential array** transducer (Fig. 2-8), commonly called a linear array, is the workhorse of the vascular department, used for most peripheral arterial and venous examinations and extracranial cerebrovascular studies. The **phased array** (Fig. 2-9) transducer is typically a small rectangular or square footprint transducer used for cardiac or abdominal applications. This transducer is also used for transcranial Doppler studies.

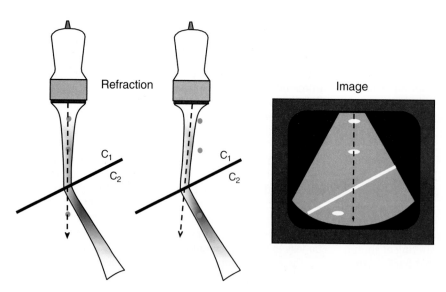

**FIGURE 2-6** Propagation speed error. When sound travels through a medium whose propagation speed is not 1,540 m/s, the echoes may appear in the wrong locations. (Adapted with permission from Bushberg JT, Seibert JA, Leidholdt EM, et al. *The Essential Physics of Medical Imaging*. 3rd ed. Philadelphia, PA: Wolters Kluwer; 2011.)

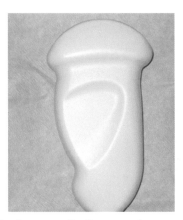

**FIGURE 2-7** Curvilinear array. Curvilinear, curved, or convex array transducer. Used in abdominal and obstetric/gynecologic examinations as well as some vascular examinations. (Adapted with permission from Penny S, Fox T, Godwin CH. *Examination Review for Ultrasound: Sonographic Principles & Instrumentation*. Philadelphia, PA: Lippincott Williams Wilkins; 2011.)

The shape of the image is determined by the transducer. The curvilinear transducer has a curved near field with sloped sides. The width of the near field is determined by the face of the transducer, with smaller footprint probes having a narrow near field and larger transducers having a wider near field (Fig. 2-10). Linear array transducers have the ability to be displayed as two image shapes: rectangular or vector (trapezoidal). The rectangular image shape is just that: a rectangle, with a flat top and bottom and straight sides (Fig. 2-11). The vector image shape slopes the sides of the rectangle to form a trapezoid, which is useful in vascular studies when a wider field of view is needed (Fig. 2-12). The vector image shape produced by a linear transducer is sometimes called a virtual convex. The phased array transducer may have a sector or vector image shape. Both are shaped like slices of pie, but the vector image shape has a flat top instead of a point (Fig. 2-13).

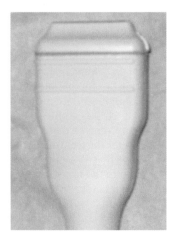

**FIGURE 2-8** Linear array. Also known as a linear sequential array, at higher frequencies may be used in small-parts examinations. At lower frequencies, used for vascular examinations. (Adapted with permission from Penny S, Fox T, Godwin CH. *Examination Review for Ultrasound: Sonographic Principles & Instrumentation*. Philadelphia, PA: Lippincott Williams Wilkins; 2011.)

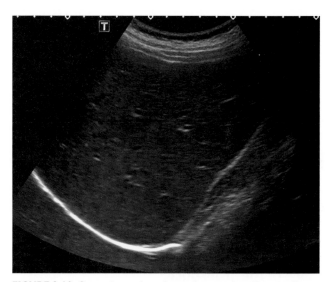

**FIGURE 2-10** Convex image shape. Image shape produced by a curvilinear (curved, convex) transducer. This image is a sagittal liver.

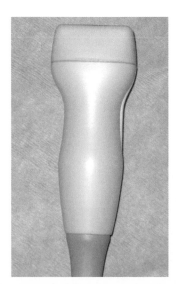

**FIGURE 2-9** Phased array. Small footprint sector/vector transducer. (Adapted with permission from Penny S, Fox T, Godwin CH. *Examination Review for Ultrasound: Sonographic Principles & Instrumentation*. Philadelphia, PA: Lippincott Williams Wilkins; 2011.)

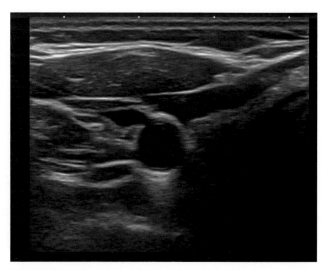

**FIGURE 2-11** Linear image shape. Rectangular image shape produced by a linear array transducer. This image is a carotid artery in transverse.

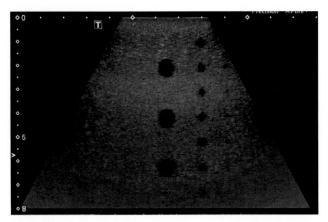

**FIGURE 2-12** Vector image shape. This vector image shape was created by a linear array transducer in virtual convex mode. Linear transducers may have their scan lines steered to form a vector image shape, effectively creating a wider field of view from a linear transducer.

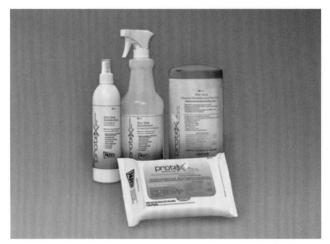

**FIGURE 2-14** Transducer disinfectant. Commercially available disinfectant sprays and wipes for ultrasound transducers. Check with manufacturer's cleaning recommendations before using. (Image courtesy of Parker Laboratories, Fairfield, NJ.)

Except for their shape, PW ultrasound transducers are constructed essentially the same way. All the transducers currently have piezoelectric elements made of **lead zirconate titanate** (PZT) to generate the sound waves, and a damping material to limit the number of cycles in the pulse. Transducers also have a matching layer to improve the transmission of sound into the patient, needed because of the impedance difference between the piezoelectric element and the patient's skin. The curvilinear and linear array transducers are often called sequenced, or sequential, transducers because their elements are energized in sequence, from one end of the transducer to the other. The linear array transducer may also be operated by phasing, which is when individual elements are energized in such a way that a specific beam shape is created. One use of phasing in a linear sequenced array is the creation of the vector image shape and color box steering.

## Care of the Transducer

The ultrasound transducer is a potential transmitter of infectious disease if not properly cleaned and disinfected.

The first step in cleaning an ultrasound transducer is the removal of all the gel and other fluids from the surface of the probe while wearing the appropriate **personal protective equipment** (PPE). Nonintracavitary ultrasound transducers may not be watertight, so be careful when cleaning these transducers, and never immerse them completely in water or cleaning solution. After the transducer has been cleaned, a low-level disinfectant that is approved by the manufacturer should be applied to the transducer (Fig. 2-14). If the transducer is to be used on broken skin or open wounds, the transducer should be covered with a sterile cover, and sterile gel should be used to avoid contaminating the wound. The transducer should be appropriately cleaned and disinfected after the completion of the examination.

## Power and Intensity

To generate sound, the piezoelectric elements within the transducer are shocked with electricity. The source of

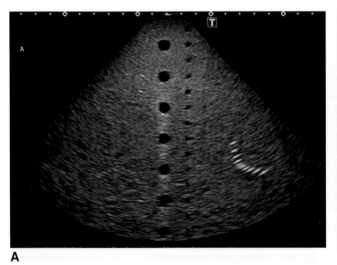

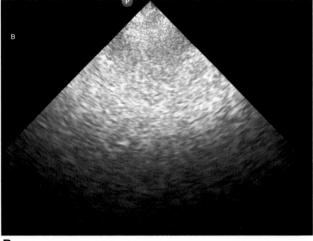

A    B

**FIGURE 2-13** Vector and sector image shapes. **A:** This image was produced by a phased array transducer designed to produce a vector image shape, which is like a sector but with a flat top. **B:** This image is a sector image, also produced by a phased array, but designed so the scan lines come from a common point of origin.

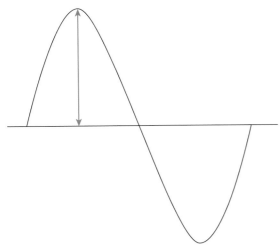

**FIGURE 2-15** Amplitude. Amplitude represents the height of the waveform, from baseline to peak. Units of amplitude depend on what is being represented by the waveform (e.g., pressure, density, particle motion).

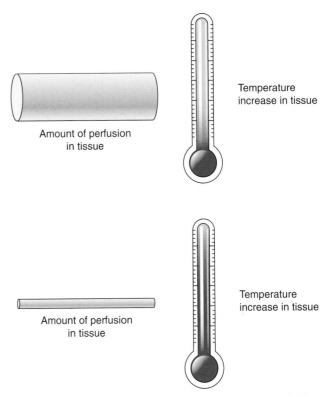

**FIGURE 2-16** Dissipation of heat. Heat is created as ultrasound travels. The more perfusion to a tissue bed, the faster that heat will be dissipated, reducing the potential for damage from thermal bioeffects.

electricity is from a part of the machine called the **pulser**. The initial amount of power used to shock the elements determines the amplitude, or strength of the sound wave (Fig. 2-15). The intensity of the sound is determined by the amount of power in the beam divided by the area of the beam. The beam area is ever changing—narrowing in the near field as it nears the focal zone and diverging in the far field. Intensity is equal to power divided by area, so assuming power stays the same, and ignoring attenuation for the time being, the intensity will increase as the beam narrows. Power and intensity are important because they relate to patient safety, and the operator of an ultrasound machine needs to be respectful of the principle of ALARA: as low as reasonably achievable. ALARA means to always use the lowest power and for the shortest amount of time as needed for an examination to reduce the potential for bioeffects.

Bioeffects that can occur as a result of ultrasound include thermal bioeffects, which is the production of heat in tissue as sound travels, and cavitation, which is the creation of bubbles in the tissue. Doppler studies tend to have an increased risk of bioeffects because of higher power and longer pulse durations compared to B-mode examinations. Two indices are used by manufacturers to provide information on the risk of bioeffects at given technical settings, the **mechanical index** (MI) and the **thermal index** (TI). The MI is the likelihood of mechanical bioeffects occurring. Below a level of 0.4 MPa, no cavitational bioeffects have been documented. The TI identifies the risk of thermal injury due to the tissue. The risk of thermal bioeffects varies depending on the type of tissue being insonated and the degree of perfusion of the tissue. In areas with a lot of blood flow, the heat is carried away from the tissue like a leaf in a rapidly flowing river. In this way, the heat is dissipated. In tissue with low perfusion, the heat may accumulate, and the tissue is at higher risk for damage from heat (Fig. 2-16).

The intensity of the beam varies depending on where the beam is sampled and whether the beam is pulsed or continuous. Therefore, different intensities can be used to describe the intensity of the beam. With relation to thermal bioeffects, the **spatial peak, temporal average intensity** (SPTA) is usually used. With an unfocused transducer, an intensity below 100 mW/cm² SPTA has never demonstrated thermal bioeffects. Thermal bioeffects have also never been demonstrated in a focused beam less than 1 W/cm² SPTA, or if the temperature increase in tissue remains below 1.5°C.

## SPATIAL AND TEMPORAL RESOLUTION

### Spatial Resolution

There are two broad categories of resolution: spatial and temporal resolution. Spatial resolution includes axial, lateral, elevational resolution. Temporal resolution is the same as frame rate. **Axial resolution** is the resolution of reflectors that are parallel to the beam. Axial resolution is dependent on SPL, with a shorter pulse equating to better axial resolution (Fig. 2-17). The higher the operating frequency of the transducer, the better the axial resolution. With an increase in operating frequency, though, there is a trade-off in penetration ability. The higher the operating frequency, the worse the ability to penetrate (Fig. 2-18). **Lateral resolution** involves reflectors perpendicular to the beam and is determined by the width of the beam. Unlike axial resolution, which does not change with depth, lateral resolution varies with depth because the beam gets narrower as it leaves the transducer until it gets to its narrowest point, the focal zone. Deep to the focal zone, the beam gets wider because of divergence of the beam. The best lateral resolution occurs where the beam is the narrowest, which is in the region of the focal

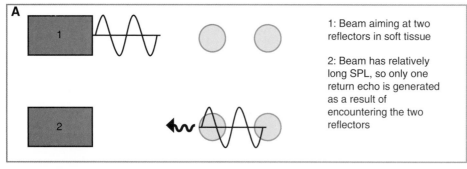

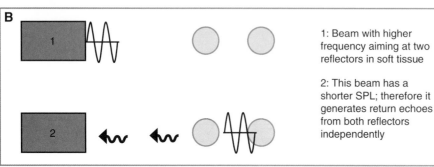

FIGURE 2-17 Axial resolution. Axial resolution is equal to one-half of the spatial pulse length (SPL). The best axial resolution is from short pulses. **A:** With a long pulse, the pulse is in both reflectors at the same time, so only one reflection is returned. **B:** With a shorter pulse, the reflector is able to strike both reflectors independently, so two reflections are returned. (Adapted with permission from Penny S, Fox T, Godwin CH. *Examination Review for Ultrasound: Sonographic Principles & Instrumentation.* Philadelphia, PA: Lippincott Williams Wilkins; 2011.)

zone. Figure 2-19 depicts the difference between axial and lateral resolution.

The width of the beam is called the slice-thickness or elevational plane. This plane has a discernible width and is the cause of slice-thickness or partial-volume thickness artifact, which occurs when there is poor **elevational resolution**. This artifact is a common artifact in vascular imaging (Fig. 2-20).

## Temporal Resolution

**Temporal resolution** is another way of saying **frame rate**, or the number of images (frames) produced per second.

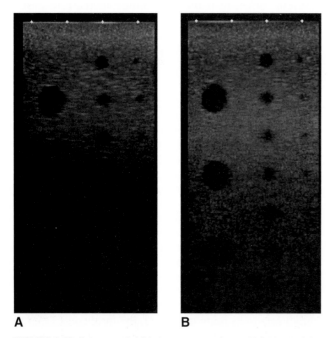

**A**         **B**

FIGURE 2-18 Frequency. **A:** High-frequency transducer with better spatial resolution but worse penetration. **B:** Lower-frequency transducer has better penetration but worse spatial resolution.

Several factors influence the frame rate, including depth of image, width of image, number of focal zones, and the use of color Doppler. A frame is completed when a series of scan lines have been created. The longer it takes to create the scan lines, the longer it takes to create a frame. The deeper the depth, the worse the frame rate because it takes longer for sound to complete its travel to and from the transducer. The more focal zones used, the worse the frame rate, because each focal zone requires its own pulse. So two focal zones would require two pulses per scan line, three focal zones would require three pulses per scan line, and so on. The image width, or number of scan lines per frame, also affects frame rate because the more scan lines that need to be displayed, the longer it takes to create a frame, and the worse the frame rate (Fig. 2-21). The way in which color Doppler affects frame rate will be discussed in the color Doppler section.

## DOPPLER

Doppler studies are possible because a reflector in motion, like a red blood cell, has a different reflected frequency compared to the transmitted frequency. The machine performs a calculation, explained in detail in what follows, and the velocity of the moving reflector is calculated.

## Doppler Effect

The Doppler shift is the difference between the transmitted frequency of the ultrasound transducer and the returned frequency of the reflector. If a reflector is stationary, the reflected frequency will be identical to the transmitted frequency, and the Doppler shift will be zero. If the reflector is moving in a direction that is toward the transducer, then the reflected frequency will be greater than the transmitted frequency, called a positive Doppler shift. Likewise, if the reflector is moving away from the transducer, the reflected

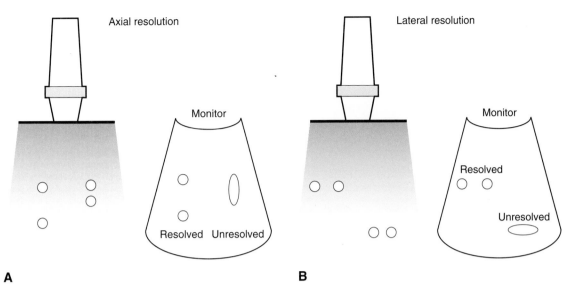

Axial resolution

Lateral resolution

Monitor

Monitor

Resolved

Resolved    Unresolved

Unresolved

**A**

**B**

**FIGURE 2-19** Axial and lateral resolution. **A:** Axial resolution relates to reflectors parallel to the transducer. **B:** Lateral resolution relates to reflectors perpendicular to the transducer. (Adapted with permission from Penny S, Fox T, Godwin CH. *Examination Review for Ultrasound: Sonographic Principles & Instrumentation.* Philadelphia, PA: Lippincott Williams Wilkins; 2011.)

**FIGURE 2-20** Elevational resolution. The elevational, or slice-thickness plane, is focused with a lens in most transducers. Artifacts may occur as a result of unwanted reflectors in the elevational plane. **A:** Depiction of axial, lateral, and elevation planes on an ultrasound beam. **B:** Slice thickness (elevation plane) of the beam. (Adapted with permission from Bushberg JT, Seibert JA, Leidholdt EM, et al. *The Essential Physics of Medical Imaging.* 3rd ed. Philadelphia, PA: Wolters Kluwer; 2011.)

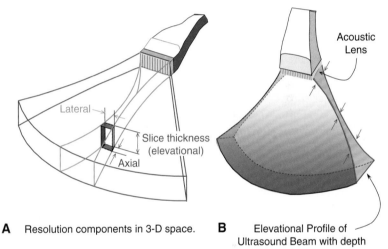

Acoustic Lens

Lateral

Slice thickness (elevational)

Axial

**A**    Resolution components in 3-D space.

**B**    Elevational Profile of Ultrasound Beam with depth

**FIGURE 2-21** Temporal resolution. Temporal resolution, or frame rate, is affected by depth (PRF), number of scan lines, line density, and (not pictured) number of focal zones. (Adapted with permission from Bushberg JT, Seibert JA, Leidholdt EM, et al. *The Essential Physics of Medical Imaging.* 3rd ed. Philadelphia, PA: Wolters Kluwer; 2011.)

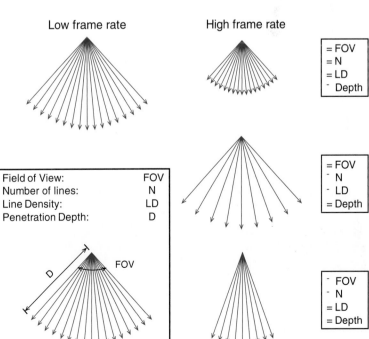

Low frame rate

High frame rate

| | |
|---|---|
| = | FOV |
| = | N |
| = | LD |
| ⁻ | Depth |

| | |
|---|---|
| = | FOV |
| ⁻ | N |
| ⁻ | LD |
| = | Depth |

| | |
|---|---|
| ⁻ | FOV |
| ⁻ | N |
| = | LD |
| = | Depth |

Field of View:         FOV
Number of lines:       N
Line Density:          LD
Penetration Depth:     D

D    FOV

Direction of flow

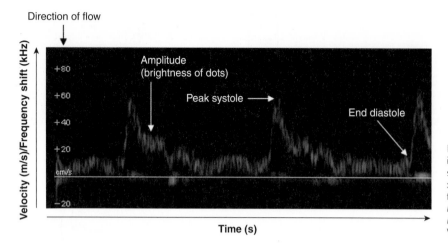

**FIGURE 2-22** Spectral graph. Frequency shift information is presented as velocities on a modern spectral display. The y-axis displays velocity and the x-axis represents time. (Adapted with permission from Penny S, Fox T, Godwin CH. *Examination Review for Ultrasound: Sonographic Principles & Instrumentation*. Philadelphia, PA: Lippincott Williams Wilkins; 2011.)

frequency will be lower than the transmitted frequency, called a negative shift. A Doppler device measures the Doppler shift in order to calculate the velocity using the equation

$$V = c(Fd)/2f(\cos\theta),$$

where $v$ is the velocity of the blood, $c$ is propagation speed, $Fd$ is the Doppler shift, $f$ is operating frequency, and $\cos\theta$ is the cosine of the Doppler angle. There are a few concepts that are critically important in the performance of Doppler examinations. These concepts relate to the fact that the Doppler equation does not use the Doppler angle itself but its cosine:

- The most accurate Doppler shift is zero degrees. The closer the Doppler angle is to zero, the more accurate the Doppler shift measurement.
- Zero degrees will also provide the highest Doppler shift.
- At 90 degrees the Doppler shift is zero. Therefore, no Doppler shift will be obtained at a 90 degrees angle.
- Angles greater than 60 degrees should not be used because the degree of error is too high.

## Spectral Doppler

Spectral Doppler, which includes PW and CW spectral Doppler, provides the familiar waveform with its audible component that is often used to help screen for vascular disease. Spectral Doppler displays the signal information on a graph in which the frequency shift (converted to velocity) is displayed on the y-axis and time on the x-axis (Fig. 2-22).

Pulsed-wave Doppler uses similar principles as B-mode imaging, in that a pulse is transmitted and must wait for the

previous pulse to return. This waiting period is the reason for the primary disadvantage with PW Doppler: **aliasing**, which is a wraparound of the spectral waveform causing positive shifts to be displayed as negative (Fig. 2-23). PW Doppler is limited by PRF. The maximum frequency shift that can be sampled is equal to the **Nyquist Limit**, which is one-half the PRF. If the Doppler shift exceeds the Nyquist limit, there will be aliasing, and the spectral waveform will appear to wrap around the spectral window. To eliminate aliasing, the PRF must be increased (to increase the Nyquist limit), or the Doppler shift must be decreased. How can the sonographer lower the Doppler shift? Either lower the frequency or increase the Doppler angle (which decreases the cosine of the Doppler angle). Another option, if all else fails and aliasing is still present, is to use a CW transducer. CW transducers do not have a limit on the measurable velocity, but also do not permit selecting a specific depth for sampling. Continuous-wave transducers send sound continuously instead of in pulses. One element sends sound, whereas a separate element receives. No image is generated with a dedicated CW probe, but only a spectral waveform, so a two-element CW probe is often called "blind" Doppler (Fig. 2-24). In cardiac imaging, the Pedoff probe is a dedicated CW probe.

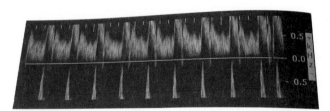

**FIGURE 2-23** Aliasing. If the frequency shift exceeds the Nyquist limit (½ PRF), a wraparound of the spectral waveform will occur, called aliasing. (Adapted with permission from Penny S, Fox T, Godwin CH. *Examination Review for Ultrasound: Sonographic Principles & Instrumentation*. Philadelphia, PA: Lippincott Williams Wilkins; 2011.)

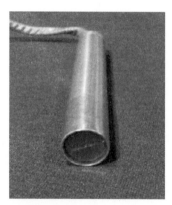

**FIGURE 2-24** Continuous-wave (CW) Doppler. Dedicated CW probe used in vascular examinations. Note the two-element transducer. (Adapted with permission from Penny S, Fox T, Godwin CH. *Examination Review for Ultrasound: Sonographic Principles & Instrumentation*. Philadelphia, PA: Lippincott Williams Wilkins; 2011.)

Pulsed-wave spectral Doppler permits selection of a sample volume at an operator-selected depth. The sonographer is able to not only pick the vessel to be insonated, but also determine how wide the sample volume should be. In addition, with PW spectral Doppler the sonographer can choose an appropriate angle correction to more accurately measure the velocities in that vessel. With CW spectral Doppler, the sample volume is large and is determined by the overlap of the transmitted and received frequencies. The sonographer does not get to select a particular vessel to sample; all vessels within the transducer's large sample volume will be included in the waveform. With CW spectral Doppler, a zero-degree angle is assumed because angle correction is not possible.

The creation of the spectral waveform is complex. Remember that the spectral waveform is made up of many different frequency shifts over time. A complex processing technique, called **Fast Fourier Transform (FFT),** converts this complex information into the spectral waveform with which sonographers are familiar. If there is a narrow range of velocities (frequency shifts) at a given point in time, then the envelope (Fig. 2-25) will be narrow. If there is a wide range of velocities at a given point of time, then the envelope will be thicker. The window, the area beneath the waveform, will be clear when there is a narrow range of velocities in a vessel, and filled in when there are many different velocities present. This filling in of the spectral window is called **spectral broadening** (Fig. 2-26).

## Color Doppler

Color Doppler imaging is a type of PW Doppler in which information regarding direction of flow and mean velocity is displayed as a color on top of the B-mode display. The hue of the color (e.g., red, blue) corresponds to either a positive or a negative Doppler shift. Some laboratories use BART, which stands for Blue Away, Red Toward. Other laboratories align the color by convention, with arteries red and veins blue (Fig. 2-27). The important thing is for the sonographer to know whether the direction of flow is correct.

Color Doppler images are created by sending multiple pulses of sound down the scan lines of a color gate to determine movement of the reflectors. Stationary reflectors remain a shade of gray, whereas moving reflectors are assigned

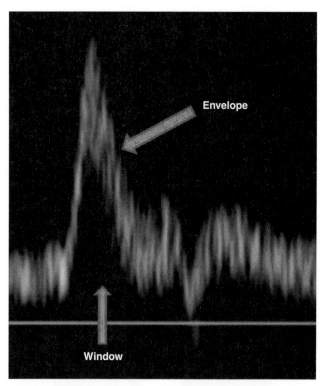

**FIGURE 2-25** Spectral envelope. The spectral waveform provides information beyond velocity measurements. The amplitude is the strength of the waveform, representing the number of red blood cells, and the presence or absence of a window provides information on how many different velocities are present at a given time. The appearance of the waveform is determined by the blood flow characteristics, as well as the technical factors set by the operator. (Adapted with permission from Penny S, Fox T, Godwin CH. *Examination Review for Ultrasound: Sonographic Principles & Instrumentation.* Philadelphia, PA: Lippincott Williams Wilkins; 2011.)

color pixels of a hue consistent with their Doppler shift direction. The color scale (Fig. 2-28) indicates which color (usually a shade of blue or red) is a positive shift (toward the transducer) and which is a negative shift (away from the transducer). The more often each scan line is sampled, called packet size or ensemble length, the more sensitive the machine is to slow flow. The process of obtaining the color Doppler information greatly decreases the frame rate. For this reason, small gates should be used when performing

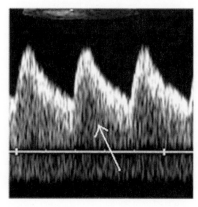

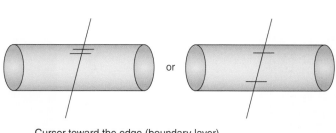

Cursor toward the edge (boundary layer) or gate to wide open results in broadening (no window)

**FIGURE 2-26** Spectral broadening. If the window *(arrow)* is filled in, spectral broadening is present. Spectral broadening does not always signify pathology, because it can be caused by certain technical settings, and is always seen in CW Doppler. (Adapted with permission from Penny S, Fox T, Godwin CH. *Examination Review for Ultrasound: Sonographic Principles & Instrumentation.* Philadelphia, PA: Lippincott Williams Wilkins; 2011.)

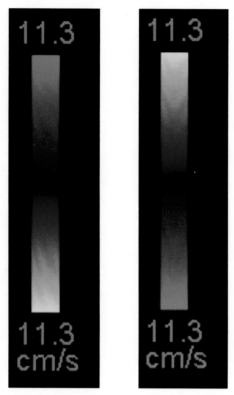

**FIGURE 2-27** Color scale: BART *(right)* versus RABT *(left)*. In most vascular examinations, the operator usually sets the color so that red represents arteries and blue represents veins. This depends on the lab and may vary, however. In echocardiography, BART is always assumed, in which red is always a positive shift (towards) and blue is always a negative shift (away).

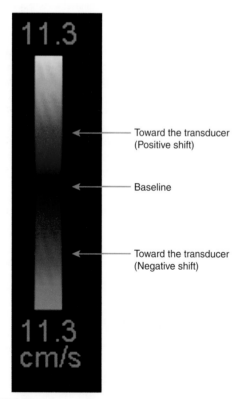

**FIGURE 2-28** Color scale. Standard velocity color scale. The numbers at the top and bottom only represent mean velocity information. The black in the middle is the baseline. Above the baseline is a positive shift. Below the baseline is a negative shift.

color Doppler examinations, especially if the vessel is deep. The processing algorithm used to process color Doppler, called **autocorrelation**, allows for identification of only mean velocity information, not the peak systolic and end diastolic information obtained by spectral Doppler.

Aliasing, the display of positive shift information as a negative shift, is also present in color Doppler because it is a PW technique, although in the case of color Doppler aliasing can be a useful tool to identify high-velocity flow jets. Another similar limitation is inability to acquire a signal at a 90 degrees angle because color Doppler relies on the Doppler shift to display color information.

Color Doppler does not have the sensitivity to flow that PW spectral Doppler has, so the sonographer should never assume that a vessel is occluded on the basis of color Doppler information alone. PW spectral Doppler with high sensitivity settings (e.g., low scale, large sample volume) should always be used in addition to color Doppler.

## Power Doppler

Power Doppler, also called amplitude Doppler and **color power angio** (CPA), provides flow information that relies on the amplitude of the Doppler shift, but not on the shift itself. This is important because there is no Doppler shift at a 90 degrees angle, but power Doppler does not need the shift, only the amplitude of the signal. The amplitude is determined by the number of red blood cells moving through the vessel, with higher amplitudes causing a stronger signal. Power Doppler is very sensitive to small vessels or vessels with slow flow, but is very susceptible to movement. Movement (breathing, coughing, and the heart) in the area of the vessel causes an artifact called flash, which obscures the image and makes it less or nondiagnostic (Fig. 2-29).

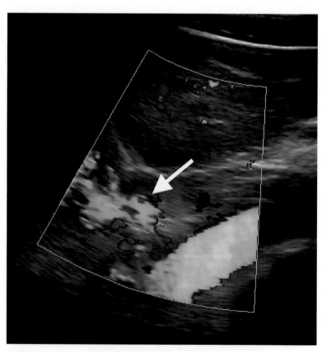

**FIGURE 2-29** Flash artifact with power Doppler. Power Doppler is very sensitive to motion. Any nonvascular motion will be displayed as a color signal. In this image, the nearby heart movement *(arrow)* is causing flash artifact near the proximal aorta.

# KNOBOLOGY AND IMAGE OPTIMIZATION

This section will review the basic knobology for B-mode and Doppler imaging. A good Doppler study begins with a good B-mode image, and it is critical that the image be optimized so that subtle plaque or other pathologies are not missed.

## B-mode Controls

- **Overall gain** – The overall gain (amplification) adjusts the brightness of all the dots on the screen equally. They all increase or they all decrease in brightness. This control is used when the overall appearance of the image is too bright or too dark.
- **Time gain compensation (TGC)** – TGC is adjusted when only part of the image is too bright or too dark. The individual slider controls are used to achieve a uniform level of brightness across the entire image. The TGC is needed because the echoes in the far field tend to be darker than the near-field echoes on account of attenuation. The TGC sliders adjust for this attenuation.
- **Focal zone** – Most machines allow the sonographer to set the number and location of the focal zones. Lateral resolution is best at the focal zone, which is where the beam area is most narrow. As technology advances, some machines are doing this automatically, but if the machine has a manual focal zone control, it is essential that it be adjusted so that the focal zone is at or below the area of interest.
- **Frequency** – The thickness of the element primarily determines the operating frequency of the transducer, but today's machines permit the operator to select from a range of frequencies that are present within the beam called the **bandwidth**. Although for B-mode imaging the general rule is to use the highest frequency that still permits adequate penetration of the beam, for Doppler studies high frequencies are not used because of aliasing and increased scatter.
- **Depth** – The imaging depth, which is controlled by the PRF, should be set so that area of interest is completely displayed, without a large amount of "wasted space" at the bottom of the image. However, pertinent anatomy should not be cut off, either.
- **Tissue harmonic imaging (THI)** – THI produces images using sound energy returning from the patient that is double the operating frequency. THI produces images with better lateral resolution and produces images with fewer artifacts, especially reverberation. As with all imaging settings, use THI when it improves the image, and turn it off if the image is worse or if anatomic structures are not displayed.
- **Spatial compounding** – With spatial compounding, the transducer sends the beam into the patient from different directions to minimize image artifacts and improve the appearance of soft-tissue. All manufacturers have different names for spatial compounding, such as SieClear (Siemens Healthcare, USA), CrossXBeam (GE Healthcare), Aplipure (Toshiba America Medical Systems), and SonoCT (Philips Healthcare).

## Spectral Doppler Controls

The next set of controls is specific to spectral Doppler. It is important to optimize the controls when performing spectral Doppler to ensure accurate velocity measurements.

- **PRF/Scale** – Depending on the manufacturer of the machine, this control may be labeled "scale" or "PRF." Increasing the scale permits measurement of higher velocities without aliasing. Lowering the scale allows for measurement of slower flow. The PRF should be optimized so that the spectral waveform should occupy about two-thirds of the spectral window without touching the top or bottom of the display.
- **Spectral gain** – Spectral gain controls the brightness of the spectral waveform. Gain that is too high may result in overmeasurement of the waveform, whereas gain that is too low may result in undermeasurement. The optimal gain results in a waveform that is readily visible without background echoes on the spectral display.
- **Sample volume/range gate** – In PW spectral Doppler, there is a controllable range gate to permit sample depth selection. The sample volume, the area within the range gate, can also be adjusted in size to permit for a small area of sampling or a large area of sampling.
- **Angle correction** – The greatest advantage of PW spectral Doppler is the ability to select a depth (via the range gate) and then angle correct to more accurately measure velocities. The Doppler equation needs this angle correction to compute the velocity. If the angle correction is wrong, the velocity is wrong. The velocity is most accurate when the angle correction is at 0 degrees, that is, the beam is parallel to the flow. At angles over 60 degrees, the velocity has too high a degree of error to be reliable.
- **Sweep speed** – For certain studies, the sonographer may wish to display more or fewer spectral waveforms on the screen at one time. For example, in renal artery studies a fast sweep speed is used to stretch out a waveform so that individual parts of the waveform can be more accurately measured.
- **Baseline** – The baseline represents the bottom most part of the spectral waveform. The baseline is adjustable and is usually so placed as to avoid the appearance of aliasing.
- **Invert** – The spectral waveform can be inverted to either display the waveforms above or below the baseline. Some sonographers prefer to keep waveforms above the baseline, even in the presence of a negative Doppler shift. The invert button flips the waveform so that negative shifts are displayed above the baseline and positive shifts below it.

## Color Doppler Controls

The controls for color Doppler are similar to those of spectral Doppler.

- **Gate** – The gate size and location in color Doppler are user-controllable. Optimally, the gate should be no larger than necessary because of the poor frame rates associated with color Doppler. From a frame rate perspective, it is better to have a long gate than a wide one because the wider the gate, the more scan lines are required. In addition to size and location of the gate, with the linear array the gate can also be steered. The proper steer angle is one in which the gate is not 90 degrees to the vessel.

- **PRF/Scale** – The color PRF/scale adjusts the sensitivity to flow, with lower PRF/scale settings used for slow flow and higher PRF/scale settings used for fast flow. Color Doppler is a PW technique, so it is subject to aliasing. Increase the PRF/scale in the presence of aliasing.
- **Color gain** – The color gain should be increased when a vessel is not filling well with color, and the scale/PRF is appropriately set. If there are color pixels "bleeding" outside of the vessel, then the color gain should be decreased.
- **Invert** – The color scale can be inverted so that negative shifts are displayed on top of the scale and positive shifts are displayed below on the scale—in other words, from BART (blue away, red toward) to RABT (red away, blue toward). As stated earlier, the color assignment is dependent on individual laboratory protocols.

## ARTIFACTS

Despite advances in technology, artifacts are still a part of ultrasound imaging. **Reverberation**, a common artifact consisting of linear repeating echoes that appear as a result of a strong specular reflector near the surface (Fig. 2-30). A type of reverberation artifact, called **comet tail,** is commonly caused by small bits of calcium or surgical clips (Fig. 2-31). **Shadowing**, which occurs as a result of the attenuation of sound, is seen in the presence of calcified plaque and overlying bone (Fig. 2-32). When sound travels through an area of decreased attenuation compared to the surrounding tissue, the tissue deep to the weak attenuator appears brighter, called **enhancement** (Fig. 2-33). Sometimes sound travels in the region of a strong specular reflector and causes a duplication of a reflector deep to the original structure.

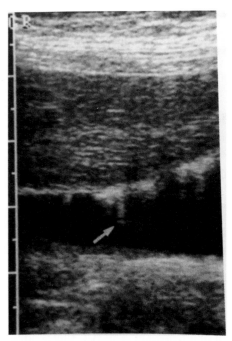

**FIGURE 2-31** Comet tail. Comet-tail artifacts *(arrow)* are small reverberations, commonly tiny calcifications or surgical clips. (Adapted with permission from Penny S, Fox T, Godwin CH. *Examination Review for Ultrasound: Sonographic Principles & Instrumentation*. Philadelphia, PA: Lippincott Williams Wilkins; 2011.)

Grating lobes are artifacts associated with array transducers. This artifact may have the appearance of thrombus in a vessel (Fig. 2-34), but is readily recognizable as artifact in real time. This **mirror-image** artifact can occur with B-mode, spectral, and color Doppler (Fig. 2-35). When mirror-image artifact occurs with spectral and color Doppler, it is usually because either the angle is too close to 90 degrees or the gain setting is too high. **Clutter** is an artifact caused by wall motion. Wall motion produces a high-amplitude, low-frequency noise along the baseline that is eliminated with the use of high-pass filters, also called a wall filter. In most vascular imaging, a low wall filter setting should be used, or useful diastolic information along the baseline may be eliminated (Fig. 2-36).

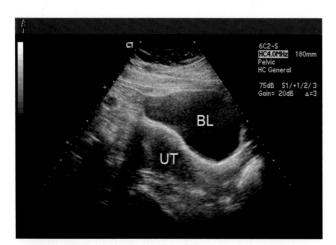

**FIGURE 2-30** Reverberation. Sagittal image of a urinary bladder with reverberation artifact. This artifact is commonly seen deep to a strong specular reflector, such as the bladder wall in this example. (Adapted with permission from Stephenson SR. *Diagnostic Medical Sonography: Obstetrics and Gynecology.* 3rd ed. Philadelphia, PA: Lippincott Williams Wilkins; 2012.)

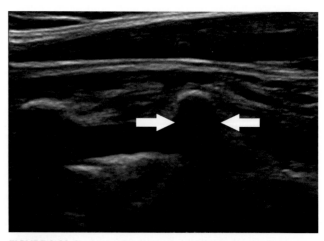

**FIGURE 2-32** Shadowing. Shadowing *(arrows)* occurs deep to strong attenuators, such as the bone of the spine anterior to the vertebral artery in this image.

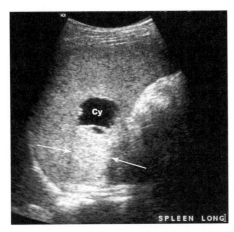

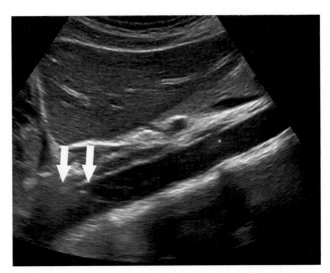

**FIGURE 2-33** Enhancement. Enhancement *(arrows)* occurs deep to tissue that weakly attenuates compared to the surrounding tissue. In this image, enhancement is seen deep to a liver cyst. (Adapted with permission from Penny S, Fox T, Godwin CH. *Examination Review for Ultrasound: Sonographic Principles & Instrumentation*. Philadelphia, PA: Lippincott Williams Wilkins; 2011.)

**FIGURE 2-34** Grating lobes. Grating lobes *(arrows)* occur from array transducers and are a result of extraneous sound energy getting picked up by the transducer. Arrows point to grating lobe artifact near the proximal aorta.

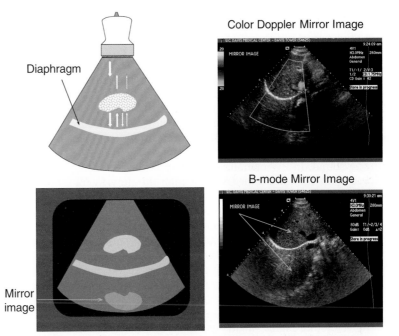

**FIGURE 2-35** Mirror-image artifact. Mirror-image artifact occurs deep to a strong specular reflector and causes a false image to appear deep to the real image. (Adapted with permission from Bushberg JT, Seibert JA, Leidholdt EM, et al. *The Essential Physics of Medical Imaging*. 3rd ed. Philadelphia, PA: Wolters Kluwer; 2011.)

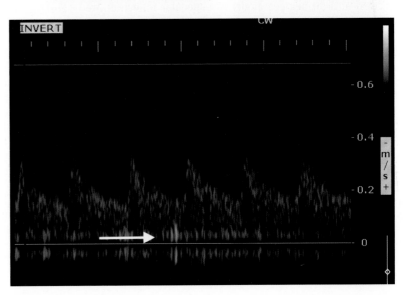

**FIGURE 2-36** Clutter. Clutter represents noise along the baseline *(arrow)*. Wall filters are used to remove clutter.

## SUMMARY

- Ultrasound is created when piezoelectric elements inside of a transducer are energized. The frequency of the sound, which is the number of cycles per second, is in the range of 2 to 20 MHz.
- Other parameters used to describe the sound waves are period (time it takes for one cycle to occur), wavelength (the length of one cycle of sound), and propagation speed (the speed of sound through the medium). Amplitude is a measure of the strength of the beam, and impedance is a property of the medium that describes acoustic resistance to sound.
- With pulsed-wave (PW) operation, a group of cycles, called a pulse, is sent into the patient, and the pulse returns to the transducer. By measuring how long it took for the sound to return, the machine is able to determine the depth of the reflector.
- Continuous-wave (CW) transducers have two elements so that sound can simultaneously be transmitted and received by the transducer. Although no image is generated by a CW probe, the machine is able to measure spectral Doppler waveforms at very high velocities.
- With pulsed-wave operation, new terminology is needed. The pulse repetition frequency (PRF) is the number of pulses per second, and the pulse repetition period is the time it takes for one pulse to occur, including the time spent waiting for the pulse to come back.
- Pulse duration is also the time it takes the pulse to occur, but does not include the listening time. Duty factor is the percentage of time the transducer is always transmitting sound. In PW operation, the duty factor is usually less than 1%, and with CW operation the duty factor is 100%.
- As sound travels through soft-tissue, some of its energy is given off in the form of heat, called absorption. Absorption is part of the process of attenuation, which causes the beam to weaken as it travels through tissue. Other forms of attenuation are reflection and scattering. Air and bone are two tissues that sound cannot penetrate effectively.
- Specular reflectors represent organ boundaries, vessel walls, and other large, bright, linear reflectors. Specular reflectors are highly angle dependent and must be imaged at a 90 degrees angle. Nonspecular reflectors are small reflectors that scatter sound and give parenchyma its appearance. Red blood cells are Rayleigh scatterers, which are nonspecular reflectors that are very, very small compared with the wavelength of the sound.
- Reflection at an interface occurs when sound strikes tissue of a different impedance. If the sound strikes the boundary at normal incidence (90 degrees), a reflection will be generated and picked up by the transducer.
- Refraction occurs at an interface when sound travels through tissues of differing propagation speeds. With refraction sound travels through the interface, but the transmission angle is different than the incident angle.
- It takes 13 µs for sound to travel into the patient a distance of 1 cm and return to the transducer.
- Curvilinear transducers have a wide near field of view and are commonly used for abdominal work and in patients with a larger body habitus.

- Sector and vector transducers are phased array transducers and are commonly used in echocardiography.
- Linear array transducers are used for vascular work in the lower frequency range and high resolution imaging in the higher frequency range.
- The piezoelectric elements found in the ultrasound transducer are a man-made ceramic called lead zirconate titanate (PZT).
- Ultrasound transducers must be cleaned properly to prevent the spread of infectious agents. Ultrasound transducers can never be heat sterilized.
- The intensity of the beam depends on the initial power and the area over which the power is applied. The higher the power, the higher the intensity. The greater the area, the lower the intensity.
- Ultrasound must be used according to the principle of ALARA: as low as reasonably achievable. The two types of bioeffects that can occur are mechanical (nonthermal) and thermal.
- Axial resolution describes the distance two reflectors can be parallel to the beam and still be resolved as two discrete echoes. Axial resolution is improved by using a shorter pulse.
- Lateral resolution describes the ability of the beam to pass between two reflectors perpendicular to the beam. A narrow beam offers better lateral resolution.
- Elevational resolution is related to the width of the beam or slice-thickness. Thinner beams in the elevation plane mean fewer artifacts inside vessels.
- Temporal resolution is the same as frame rate. Higher frame rates are more desirable. Temporal resolution is affected by the number of focal zones, the image depth, and the number of lines per frame (the line density and image width).
- The Doppler shift is the difference between the transmitted frequency and the reflected frequency. If the red blood cells are moving toward the transducer, the reflected frequency is higher than the transmitted frequency. If the red blood cells are moving away from the transducer, the reflected frequency is lower than the transmitted frequency.
- Zero degrees is the most accurate angle and has the highest Doppler shift. At 90 degrees no Doppler shift is generated, and this angle has a Doppler shift of zero. Never use a Doppler angle of greater than 60 degrees because of the increased degree of error above the angle.
- Spectral Doppler may be pulsed-wave or continuous-wave. Pulsed-wave Doppler is limited by an artifact called aliasing, which occurs with deeper vessels and/or higher velocities. Continuous-wave Doppler does not have that limitation.
- The Nyquist limit is the PRF above which aliasing occurs, and is equal to one-half the PRF.
- Spectral Doppler is processed using a technique called Fast Fourier Transform (FFT), and color Doppler is processed using autocorrelation.
- Power Doppler does not offer direction or velocity information, but helps with visualization when there is slow flow and/or small vessels.
- Some ultrasound controls are overall gain (overall image brightness), TGC (changed image brightness at different depths), focal zone (should be at or below area of interest), depth (structures should be adequately visualized

but without too much wasted space beneath the area of interest).

- Tissue harmonic imaging uses sound created by the patient's tissue and is double the frequency of the transmitted beam.
- Spatial compounding sends the sound into the patient in multiple directions, offering better coverage of the structures visualized.
- Spectral Doppler controls include scale (PRF) for setting the velocity range of the Doppler; gain, which determines the brightness of the spectral waveform; angle correction, which permits adjusting the angle for non-parallel flow; sweep speed, which determines how many heartbeats will be displayed on one strip; and baseline, which controls where the waveforms will begin.
- Color Doppler controls are similar to spectral Doppler, such as scale and gain, but in color Doppler there is a gate that is steerable with linear transducers.
- Common artifacts include reverberation, comet tail, shadowing, enhancement, mirror image, and clutter.

## CRITICAL THINKING QUESTIONS

1. You are scanning a 350-pound male for an aorta study. You notice you are having trouble visualizing the proximal aorta. What would be the best option to improve visualization of the aorta?
2. You are performing a carotid ultrasound, and you notice aliasing of the spectral waveform. What are some of your options to correct this artifact?
3. During the color Doppler part of a subclavian vein ultrasound for line placement, you notice another vessel deep to the one you are scanning. It has the same direction of flow as the more superficial vessel. What is going on here?

## MEDIA MENU

Student Resources available on thePoint® include:
- Audio glossary
- Interactive question bank
- Videos
- Internet resources

## SUGGESTED READINGS

AIUM. Guidelines for cleaning and preparing external- and internal-use ultrasound probes between patients. 2014. Available at http://www.aium.org/officialstatements/57. Accessed Sept 12th, 2016.

AIUM. Statement on mammalian biological effects in tissues with naturally occurring gas bodies. 2015. Available at http://www.aium.org/officialStatements/6. Accessed Sept 12th, 2016.

AIUM. Statement on mammalian biological effects of heat. 2015. Available at http://www.aium.org/officialStatements/17. Accessed Sept 12th, 2016.

AIUM. Statement on mammalian biological effects of ultrasound in vivo. 2015. Available at http://www.aium.org/officialStatements/9. Accessed Sept 12th, 2016.

Bushberg JT, Seibert JA, Leidholdt EM, et al. *The Essential Physics of Medical Imaging*. 3rd ed. Philadelphia, PA: Wolters Kluwer; 2011.

Kremkau F. *Sonography Principles and Instrumentation*. 9th ed. St. Louis, MO: Elsevier; 2016.

Penny S, Fox T, Herring Godwin C. *Examination Review for Ultrasound: Sonographic Principles & Instrumentation*. Philadelphia, PA: Lippincott Williams Wilkins; 2011.

Zierler RE, Dawson D. *Strandness's Duplex Scanning in Vascular Disorders*. 5th ed. Philadelphia, PA: Wolters Kluwer; 2015.

# Ergonomics: Avoiding Work-Related Injury

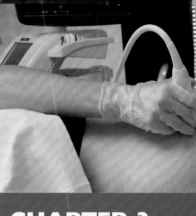

SUSAN MURPHEY

## CHAPTER 3

## OBJECTIVES

- Understand the impact of work-related musculoskeletal disorders in sonography
- Recognize the risk factors for work-related musculoskeletal disorders
- Understand the concept of neutral posture and its significance in reducing risk for injury
- Identify practical solutions for reducing risk factors

## GLOSSARY

**awkward postures** When body parts are positioned away from their neutral position. These postures can put stress on the joints and their associated muscles. The further from neutral and the longer the duration of awkward posture, the greater is the potential risk. Examples include flexion/extension of the wrist, abduction of the shoulders ("winged elbows"), flexion of the shoulders (reaching), bending/twisting at the waist, and bending the neck

**contact stress** Sustained contact between a body part and an external object. Examples include resting the wrist or forearm against a sharp edge

**duration** The period of time that a body part is exposed to an ergonomic risk factor. Longer durations of exposure increase the severity of the risk

**force** The exertion of physical effort applied by a body part to perform a task. Higher forces and/or longer durations of force application can increase the severity of the risk. Examples include pushing/pulling, lifting, gripping, and pinching

**load/loading** The force exerted by an object on a (contracted) muscle, as opposed to muscle *tension* which is the force exerted by the muscle on an object. Muscular activity increases in proportion to the force exerted upon it or the force exerted by the muscle on an object

**repetition** Repeated motions, often including other ergonomic risk factors such as force and/or awkward posture. Severity of the risk increases with higher repetition of motions and with the addition of other ergonomic risk factors

**static postures** A body part is held in a single position over a long period of time. The severity of risk of a static posture can increase if the posture is awkward, applies continual force, and/or is held for long durations. Examples include sitting or standing in single position for a long duration

## KEY TERMS

**awkward postures**

**ergonomics**

**neutral posture**

**scanning in pain**

**sonographer injury**

**WRMSD (work-related musculoskeletal disorders)**

Work-related musculoskeletal disorders (WRMSDs), also known as musculoskeletal disorders (MSDs), musculoskeletal strain injuries (MSIs), and cumulative trauma disorders (CTDs), are defined as painful conditions that are caused by or aggravated by workplace activities. These disorders, affecting the muscles, nerves, ligaments, and tendons, have been identified in a number of professions, including sonography. Unlike acute injuries that occur in the workplace, such as slips, trips, and falls, WRMSDs result from overuse, and develop over a period of time from repeated exposure to risk factors. WRMSDs are the leading cause of pain, suffering, and disability in American workplaces and among the most frequently reported cause of lost or restricted work time.[1] These painful conditions often impose a substantial personal toll on those affected, who may no longer be able to work or perform simple personal tasks or activities of daily living.[2] In the workplace, staffing shortages resulting from injuries to workers can affect patient access to care in addition to the morale, physical health, and well-being of staff. Table 3-1 summarizes the number of days lost from work based on the type of nonfatal occupational injury or illness in private industry in 2011.[3]

## CAUSES OF WRMSD

WRMSD result from repeated exposure to risk factors. The duration and frequency of exposure determines the onset of symptoms. Across all industries, repetitive strain injuries generally peak between 45 and 54 years of age because of the accumulation of exposure to risk factors. WRMSDs arise primarily from arm and hand movements such as gripping, holding, twisting, and reaching. These common movements are not particularly harmful in and of themselves, but repeated frequently, often in a forceful manner, along with a pace that lacks sufficient time for recovery can be injury producing. WRMSDs are associated with work patterns that include:

- **Exerting excessive force** including pushing, pulling, and lifting

- **Performing the same or similar tasks repetitively**, either continually or frequently for an extended period of time without adequate recovery time
- **Working in awkward postures or being in the same posture for long periods of time**, such as prolonged or repeated reaching above shoulder height, leaning/twisting the torso, awkward postures of the neck, and wrists
- **Contact pressure** of a localized body part against hard or sharp edges
- **Cold temperatures** in combination with any one of the above risk factors may also increase the potential for MSDs to develop
- **Vibration** both whole-body and hand-arm vibration can cause a number of health effects

With the exception of cold temperatures and vibrations, the practice of sonography generally includes exposure to one or more of these risk factors. All of these *physical* risks contribute to the likelihood of developing a WRMSD. However, there are also *psychosocial* factors that can contribute to risk. Psychosocial risk factors are related to how workers interact with the work environment and the demands of their job. They include[4]:

- Lack of influence or control over one's job
- Increased demands (e.g., to produce more)
- Lack of or poor communication
- Monotonous tasks
- Perception of low support (e.g., from manager or coworker)

These psychosocial risk factors can be a significant source of stress in the work environment. Workplace stress can influence the perception of pain as well as the development and persistence of WRMSDs. Combined exposure to several risk factors may place workers at a higher risk for MSDs than exposure to any one risk factor. Fortunately, understanding risk factors known to contribute to WRMSD can provide the tools for developing a proactive approach to preventing injury.

## WORK-RELATED MUSCULOSKELETAL DISORDERS IN SONOGRAPHY

Regardless of industry, most work requires the use of the arms and hands. Therefore, WRMSD often affects the hands, wrists, elbows, neck, and shoulders. Awkward postures of the trunk, neck, and upper extremities, as well as excess gripping and downward force applied with the transducer contribute to sonographer symptoms of discomfort and risk for injury. Symptoms most commonly reported by sonographers include pain or injury to the shoulder, neck, back, hand, and wrist.[5] Up to 90% of sonographers reported shoulder pain, with 69% reporting low back pain and more than half (54%) of sonographers surveyed reporting work-related symptoms of the hand and wrist.[5]

Much has been written about the ergonomic challenges faced by sonographers. The first published account of ergonomic concerns regarding "sonographer's shoulder" was reported by Craig in 1985.[6] A subsequent study by the Health Care Benefit Trust in 1997 reported data collected from nearly 1,000 sonographers practicing in the United States.[7] Their results showed that 84% of sonographers

| | | | Typical Parts |
|---|---|---|---|
| | | Percent | of Body |
| **Nature of Injury** | **Number** | **of Total** | **Affected** |
| Total | 908,310 | 100.0 | — |
| Sprains, strains, and tears | 340,870 | 37.5 | — |
| Sprains | 84,560 | 9.3 | Ankle, knee |
| Strains | 209,740 | 23.1 | Back, shoulder |
| Major tears to muscles, tendons, or ligaments | 17,150 | 1.9 | Shoulder, knee |
| Multiple strains, sprains, and tears | 7,130 | 0.8 | — |
| Sprains, strains, and tears, unspecified | 22,290 | 2.5 | — |

**TABLE 3-1   Nonfatal Occupational Injuries and Illnesses Resulting in Days Away from Work, by Nature of Injury, Private Industry, 2011[3]**

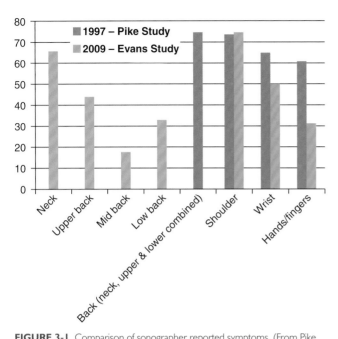

FIGURE 3-1 Comparison of sonographer reported symptoms. (From Pike I, Russo A, Berkowitz J, et al. The prevalence of musculoskeletal disorders among diagnostic medical sonographers. *J Diagn Med Sonogr* 1997;13(5): 219–227; Evans K, Roll S, Baker J. Work-related musculoskeletal disorders (WRMSD) among registered diagnostic medical sonorgraphers and vascular technologists. *J Diagn Med Sonogr* 2009;25(6):287–299.)

reported musculoskeletal pain related to scanning, with neck, shoulder, wrist, hands/fingers, and back as the most commonly affected sites. Professional organizations such as the Society of Diagnostic Medical Sonography (SDMS) have advocated on behalf of sonographers to provide education and resources for the prevention of WRMSDs. Industry Guidelines for the Prevention of Work-Related Musculoskeletal Disorders in Sonography have been established, and there have been significant ergonomic improvements to the design of sonographic workstation equipment.[8] Virtually all ultrasound systems now have some degree of adjustability and exam tables have been designed specifically for various ultrasound applications. In spite of these improvements, a 2009 study indicates that 90% of clinical sonographers experience symptoms of WRMSD, an increase from 81% in the initial study of 1997.[7,9] Figure 3-1 compares the injuries reported in these studies.

Tasks contributing to the increasing number of sonographers scanning in pain are likely to include physical, psychosocial, and workflow work practices. Workstation equipment plays an important role in the prevention of WRMSDs, yet not all scanning environments have access to ergonomic workstation equipment. Furthermore, technologic advances have led to an increasing interaction with computers, often with the same mechanical risk factors as scanning, which increase the exposure time to ergonomic hazards. Staff shortages and increased workload can result in job-related stress and insufficient rest periods, further increasing the rate of exposure to risk. In addition, there have been few changes to the clinical practice of ultrasound. Many sonographers are being taught the same scanning techniques as were used 30 years ago, several of which have known risk factors such as awkward posture, force, static posture, and repetition (Fig. 3-2).

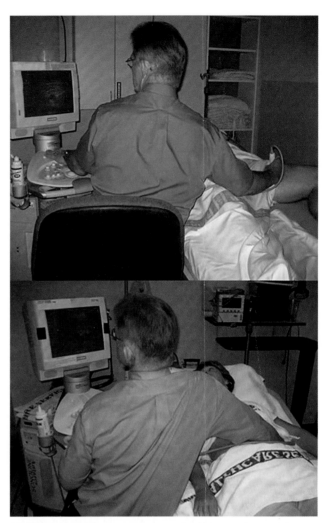

FIGURE 3-2 Traditional scan techniques often include risk factors such as excess abduction and awkward postures of the trunk (bottom) as well as excess reach and awkward neck postures (top).

## UNDERSTANDING THE RISKS

WRMSD are the result of the accumulation of damage from prolonged periods of exposure to risk factors. Unlike acute injuries, the risk factors for WRMSD may not be readily apparent because there is not a sudden onset of symptoms. The symptoms only occur after prolonged exposure. As a result, it's much harder to recognize the risk factors and be proactive in addressing them because by the time symptoms occur, there is already likely some degree of damage.

Repeated exposure to risk factors interferes with the ability of the body to recover, resulting in the accumulation of trauma to the muscles and tendons. The most common conditions among sonographers are carpal and cubital tunnel syndrome, epicondylitis of the elbow, shoulder capsulitis and tendonitis.[5] Under normal conditions, muscles and tendons are designed to be used regularly in order to maintain elasticity and function. They contract and relax during movement, allowing blood to circulate, supplying muscles with necessary nutrients, and removing toxins. However, when the frequency and duration of loading exceeds the ability of the muscles and tendons to adapt, inflammation occurs, followed by degeneration, microtears, and scar formation. Continued exposure can cause swelling, resulting in compression of the nerves and deterioration of tendons and ligaments, which further stresses the muscles and joints. This can lead to decreased range of motion and muscular dysfunction associated with various conditions of MSDs as a result of cumulative trauma.

## Muscle Injury

Muscle contraction utilizes chemical energy from metabolized carbohydrates and produces lactic acid as a by-product. Awkward postures can cause blood flow to contracted muscles to be restricted by compression on the blood vessels during prolonged muscular contraction. The muscles are unable to receive oxygenated blood flow to rid themselves of toxins, and there is a more rapid onset of fatigue caused by excess muscle firing. When muscles are contracted for long periods of time because of awkward or fixed postures, pain results, a sign that the muscles are overloaded and there is a buildup of lactic acid. The severity of pain depends on the duration of muscle contraction and the recovery time between exertions, which allows the muscles to relax and flush themselves of the irritating buildup of toxins. Repeated trauma from overuse to the muscles can result in chronic pain and injury. When a muscle is unable to meet the demands of a task, there is additional strain put on the tendons associated with that particular muscle.

## Tendon Injury

Tendons are fibrous connective tissues that attach muscles to bones. WRMSDs of the tendons result from repetitive or frequent work activities and awkward postures that put strain on the tendons. Tendon-related MSDs manifest in two major categories: tenosynovitis and tendonitis.

### Tenosynovitis

MSDs associated with tendon sheaths can occur in areas such as in the hand and wrist (Fig. 3-3). The sheath produces synovial fluid, which keeps the tendon lubricated, allowing it to elongate without adhering to the surrounding fascia. Repetitive or excessive movement of the hand can affect the lubricating properties of the tendon sheath, producing inadequate amounts of fluid or fluid with poor lubricating qualities. This creates friction between the tendon and its sheath, resulting in inflammation and swelling of the tendon, known as tenosynovitis. Examples include trigger finger and De Quervain's tenosynovitis. Similarly, Ganglion cysts result when an inflamed sheath fills with lubricating fluid and causes a bump under the skin. Repeated episodes of inflammation can result in the abnormal formation of fibrous tissue, hindering tendon movement.

### Tendonitis

Tendons without sheaths are generally found around the shoulder, elbow, and forearm and are vulnerable to repetitive motions and awkward postures. Repeated stress on the tendon from prolonged muscle contraction can cause tendon fibers to tear, resulting in inflammation (Fig. 3-4). Tendonitis is the general term used to describe inflammation of the tendon. In joints such as the shoulder where tendons pass through a narrow space between bones, there is a sac of

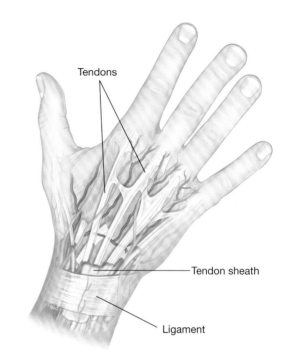

**FIGURE 3-3** Finger tendons and their sheaths.

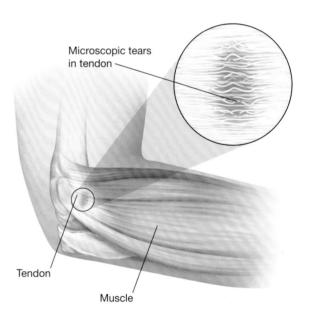

**FIGURE 3-4** Microscopic tears in tendon.

lubricating fluid called the bursa. As the tendons become increasingly thickened because of inflammation, the bursa can also become inflamed because of excess friction. Inflammation of the bursa is known as bursitis (Fig. 3-5).

## Nerve Injury

Nerves consist of bundles of fibers that carry signals between the brain and spinal cord or other parts of the body to control the activities of muscles and convey impulses of sensation such as temperature, pain, and touch. When muscles, tendons, or ligaments surrounding the nerves become swollen, there is increased pressure on the nerves.

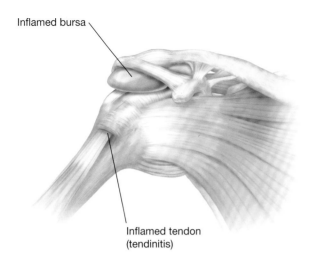

Shoulder with bursitis

**FIGURE 3-5** Tendonitis and bursitis.

Inflammation resulting from repetitive motions or awkward postures can cause nerve compression resulting to muscle weakness, tingling sensations, and numbness (Fig. 3-6).

## LARGE BEFORE SMALL

Keep in mind that muscles should support the tendons, not the other way around. Tendonitis can occur when the task performed exceeds the capacity of the muscle. As a result, the tendon attempts to bear the load, resulting in injury to the tendon. The same is true of smaller muscles. Utilizing large muscles before small helps assure that the capacity of the muscle is suitable for the load required by the task. For example, pushing rather than pulling the ultrasound system during transport uses the large gluteal and hamstring muscles of the legs rather than the smaller muscles of the arms and back as when pulling. Similarly, using a palmar (whole hand) grip on the transducer rather than a pinch grip uses the larger hand muscles rather than smaller muscles of the fingers.

- Utilize larger muscles before recruiting small ones
- Rely on muscle strength, not tendon strength
- Tendonitis results from tendons pushed beyond their capacity
- Muscle strength must support the activity of the tendon

## SYMPTOM RECOGNITION

Recognition of symptoms is important for early reporting and treatment of MSDs. Often the onset of symptoms is gradual, owing to repeated exposure to risks, making it difficult to recognize as a work-related disorder. Work activities or postures that cause these disorders may be painful during work or at rest. In fact, symptoms may be heightened at rest or in the evening after a long day of prolonged exposure to risks rather than while performing the work tasks. Pain is the most common symptom and may be accompanied by joint stiffness, redness or swelling, and/or muscle tightness. Numbness, tingling, and skin color changes may also occur.

Table 3-2 outlines occupational risk factors and symptoms of the most common disorders of the upper body associated with WRMSDs.[10]

The impact of WRMSD ranges from minor discomfort to career-ending injury. In the study by Pike et al., 20% of sonographers who were symptomatic suffered career-ending injuries.[7] The onset of WRMSD symptoms occurs as early as 6 months from the onset of employment (15% incidence), increasing to 45% after 3 years, with rates as much as 72% after 10 years of employment.[11] Successful treatment of WRMSDs can be difficult if reporting is delayed or the worker is sent back to the same work environment that produced the initial injury. Therefore, early reporting of symptoms and efforts to *prevent* injuries are critically important. Recognizing the signs of WRMSDs is vital to early reporting. Otherwise, an injury can become longstanding, and sometimes, irreversible. The first onset of pain is a signal that the muscles and tendons need to rest and recover.

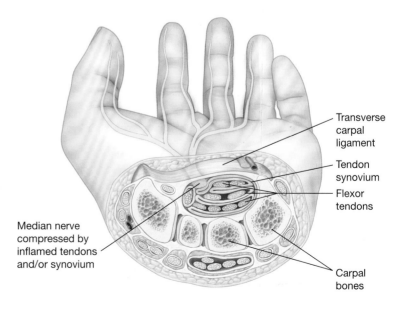

**FIGURE 3-6** Nerve Injury.

### TABLE 3-2    Common WRMSDs of the Upper Body[10]

| Disorders | Occupational Risk Factors | Symptoms |
| --- | --- | --- |
| Tendonitis/tenosynovitis | Repetitive wrist motions<br>Repetitive shoulder motions<br>Sustained hyperextension of arms<br>Prolonged load on shoulders | Pain, weakness, swelling, burning sensation or dull ache over affected area |
| Epicondylitis (tendonitis or the medial or lateral elbow tendons) | Repeated or forceful rotation of the forearm and bending of the wrist at the same time | Same symptoms as tendonitis |
| Carpal tunnel syndrome | Repetitive wrist motions | Pain, numbness, tingling, burning sensations, wasting of muscles at base of thumb, dry palm |
| De Quervain's disease | Repetitive hand twisting and forceful gripping | Pain at the base of thumb |
| Thoracic outlet syndrome | Prolonged shoulder flexion<br>Extending arms above shoulder height<br>Carrying loads on the shoulder | Pain, numbness, swelling of the hands |
| Tension neck syndrome | Prolonged restricted posture | Pain |

WRMSDs may progress according to the stages shown in Table 3-3. Not every individual has the same progression of symptoms, but this should not delay reporting.

## CONCEPT OF NEUTRAL POSTURE

Injury avoidance requires reducing the frequency and duration of exposure to risk factors. One of the most prevalent risk factors for sonographers is awkward posture, which requires excess muscle firing and, as a result, a quicker onset of fatigue. As described earlier, excess muscle firing can affect the integrity of the muscle through vascular interruptions and a buildup of waste products (lactic acid) from prolonged muscular contraction.

Regardless of the activity being performed, the goal is to be in neutral posture as much as possible. A neutral posture requires the least amount of muscular effort, protecting the muscles and tendons from overloading and the subsequent risk for injury. *Non-neutral* or awkward postures result in increased muscle firing, decreased endurance, and earlier onset of fatigue (Fig. 3-7). The further from neutral, the more muscular effort is required. Heavily loaded muscles, that is, those with significant muscular contraction, are more difficult to control, affecting fine motor control. Because hand–eye coordination and fine motor control is critical to

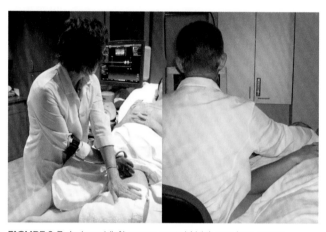

**FIGURE 3-7** Awkward (left) or non-neutral (right) scanning postures.

the ability to acquire an ultrasound image, neutral posture may improve image quality and decrease the struggle time to obtain the desired diagnostic information.

A neutral posture is balanced around the center of gravity of the human body, minimizing muscular effort. If one leans, bends, or reaches out of this balanced posture, postural imbalances occur, resulting in increased muscle strain and uneven loads on the bones and joints. Postural imbalances develop when prolonged periods of non-neutral postures are maintained, degrading muscle integrity and increasing the load on joints. The same is true of force, whether push/pull, lifting, or gripping; the excess muscle firing required results in a quicker onset of fatigue and increased risk for injury.

Frequent changes to workstation setup and scanning technique must be made while scanning in order to maintain a neutral posture as much as possible. A sonographer's postural relationship to the equipment should change during the course of the exam, depending on the area being scanned in order to maintain a neutral posture.

Neutral scanning posture includes the following:
- Facing forward without neck rotation or excess neck flexion/extension

### TABLE 3-3    Staging of Work-Related Musculoskeletal Disorder Symptoms[10]

| Early stage | Aching and tiredness of the affected limb occurs during the work shift but disappear at night and during days off work. No reduction of work performance. |
| --- | --- |
| Intermediate stage | Aching and tiredness occur early in the work shift and persist at night. Reduced capacity for repetitive work. |
| Late stage | Aching, fatigue, and weakness persist at rest. Inability to sleep and to perform light duties |

- Upright spine with no twisting or bending of the trunk
- Hands/arms in front of body during scanning with elbows close to trunk
- Avoid excess reaching with scanning and nonscanning arm
- Avoid awkward wrist positions, including excess flexion, extension, or rotation
- Forearms close to the body and approximately parallel to floor
- Feet well supported on floor, chair rung, or ultrasound system when seated
- Knees slightly lower than hips when sitting
- Weight evenly distributed over both feet when standing

Sonographers should make frequent adjustments to the height and position of the ultrasound system, exam table, and/or patient to keep their scanning arm in front of their mid-coronal line and with no more than 30 degrees abduction, whenever possible.

Adjustments of equipment and patient position include the following:

- Position the ultrasound system parallel to the exam table with no appreciable space between the two.
- Adjust the system monitor so that the top of the monitor is at eye level and the monitor is directly in front of the sonographer. Do not share the monitor with others.
- Adjust the system control panel to minimize reach and maintain elbow of nonscanning arm at side of body with 90 degrees or more elbow flexion. Reposition as needed throughout exam.
- Adjust the exam table height so that the angle of abduction of scanning arm is 30 degrees or less and elbow flexion 90 degrees or more.
- If sitting, adjust the chair height to maintain neutral trunk, neck, and arm posture and with knees slightly lower than hips.
- Position patient at nearest edge of exam table to reduce abduction and reach of scanning arm. Reposition as needed throughout exam to maintain neutral scanning posture.
- Scanning upper extremity and neck structures can often be done more ergonomically with the patient sitting in a chair or wheelchair to facilitate better positioning for the sonographer.

In addition, it is important to consider alternate scan techniques to encourage neutral posture while scanning, rather than relying solely on traditional scanning techniques. The goal is to adjust the equipment to support a neutral posture, rather than adjusting the sonographer's posture into a non-neutral configuration in order to fit the equipment (Figs. 3-8 and 3-9).

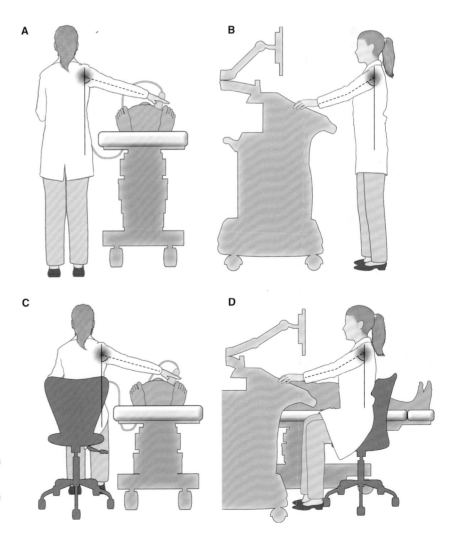

**FIGURE 3-8 A:** Non-neutral (awkward) standing scanning posture with abduction of scanning arm greater than 30 degrees. **B:** Non-neutral (awkward) standing scanning posture with excess forward reach of nonscanning arm. **C:** Non-neutral (awkward) seated posture with abduction of scanning arm greater than 30 degrees. **D:** Non-neutral (awkward) seated posture with excess forward reach of nonscanning arm.

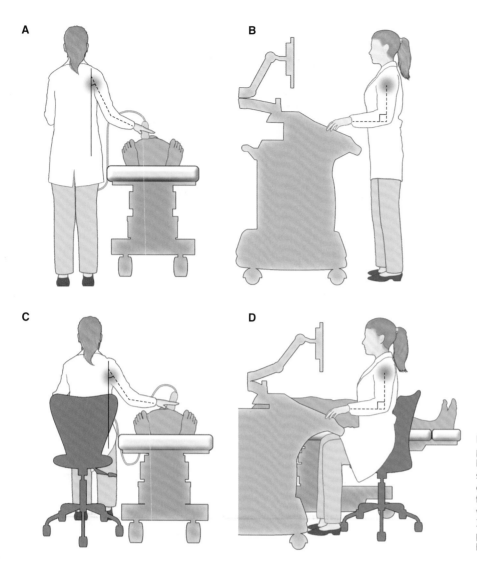

FIGURE 3-9 **A:** Neutral standing scanning posture with abduction of scanning arm limited to 30 degrees. **B:** Neutral standing scanning posture with nonscanning arm close to the body with 90 degrees elbow flexion.**C:** Neutral seated scanning posture with abduction of scanning arm limited to 30 degrees. **D:** Neutral seated scanning posture with nonscanning arm close to the body with 90 degrees elbow flexion.

## SONOGRAPHER RESPONSIBILITY

Early reporting, diagnosis, and intervention can limit the severity of injury. This can improve the effectiveness of treatment, minimizing the likelihood of disability or permanent damage. It is the responsibility of sonographers, students, and other users of ultrasound to follow current best practices to reduce the risk of developing MSDs. A sonographer can minimize the risk for injuries in a number of ways including the following practical considerations.

### Chair Position

Adjusting the chair height is critical in reducing arm abduction, which is a major risk for shoulder injury. The chair should be positioned high enough so that the scanning arm is close to the side of the sonographer's body, with an abduction angle of 30 degrees or less. For chairs whose height cannot be adjusted, add something to the chair to sit on, such as a folded towel, a lumbar support cushion, or a seat cushion. Alternatively, some may find that standing up while scanning gives the height needed to maintain a more neutral posture. A facility may have other chairs that

are not in use elsewhere and may be more appropriate for the ultrasound department.

### Exam Tables

A low table height is most important in order to reduce the abduction of the scanning arm. Having the patient move close to the sonographer will also help. This prevents unnecessary reaching and arm fatigue. Most sonographers are not in the habit of lowering the table sufficiently to minimize arm abduction. The table should be positioned low enough to allow the scanning arm to rest at the side of the sonographer, but not so low as to cause a sonographer to lean over to reach the patient. For tables that are not height adjustable, mattresses can be added or subtracted to obtain an optimal height or investigate having them retrofitted with a different size caster in order to achieve the most suitable height.

### Ultrasound System

Newer ultrasound system have adjustability and ergonomics incorporated into their platform designs. Taking advantage of this adjustability can significantly improve scanning posture. Many newer systems now have adjustment capabilities in the control panel or keyboard of the system. Optimize the position of the control panel to reduce reaching with the nonscanning arm.

## Monitors

Take advantage of adjustable height monitors by placing them in a position that allows a sonographer to be facing forward with the neck in a relaxed position and the chin tipped slightly downward. For equipment with stationary monitors, check with the facility's engineering department to see if modifications can be made to the monitor to make it height adjustable. Note that it is important to check with the ultrasound equipment manufacturer to make sure modifications will not void the warranty on the equipment.

If it is the practice of the department to allow the patients to observe the monitor, consider adding an external monitor just for the patient. Thus, the monitor with the ultrasound system is reserved for the sonographer. This prevents twisting of the neck and trunk to view the monitor. A small, second monitor added to the top of systems with fixed height monitors may be helpful for viewing while standing to scan.

## Computer Equipment

Configuration of computer equipment used for picture archive and communication systems (PACS) and/or electronic medical records can be as important as the scanning equipment in the exam rooms. Place the CPU tower so that there is leg room under the table where the sonographer will be sitting. Try to obtain a height-adjustable chair or make the adjustments to the chair as mentioned above. Place the monitor on something, if necessary, to raise it to eye level. Note the height of the keyboard and move it to a comfortable position.

## Other Scanning Tips

If the transducer is so narrow that it requires a "pinch grip" to hold it, try to use adaptive products that can be slipped over the transducer to widen it. This will result in less strain and tension on small muscle groups.

Inexpensive straps are available that can hold the transducer cable. These straps are worn around the forearm. They eliminate drag on the transducer from the weight of the cable and the need to grip it tightly to counteract the torque on the wrist.

The scanning arm should be supported on the patient or by placing support cushions or a rolled-up towel under the elbow. This simple modification can significantly reduce the strain and fatigue of the shoulder and neck muscles.

## Ongoing Education and Training

Ongoing education and training is encouraged and can be obtained from multiple sources. Resources include journals, textbooks, online webinars, and videos. Employer or academic program-sponsored in-services can also provide valuable information. Virtually all professional organizations have seminars, lectures, workshops, and conferences which deal with proper scanning techniques and avoiding work-related injuries. Manufacturers can also be a resource for education and training.

## Seeking Assistance

Workers have a right to a safe workplace. The key to prevention of WRMSDs is mutual ownership, where both the employer and employee accept a shared responsibility for safety. Sonographers and students are encouraged to work with their employers and clinical sites in a collaborative effort to address ergonomic concerns. If a sonographer still thinks a job is unsafe or if they have questions, they can contact Occupational Safety and Health Administration (OSHA). The law requires employers to provide their employees with safe and healthful workplaces. This means that if a feasible means of abating the recognized hazard exists, employers are expected to implement such measures. The OSHA law also prohibits employers from retaliating against employees for exercising their rights under the law (including the right to raise a health and safety concern or report an injury). OSHA can help answer questions or concerns from employers and workers. Information on regional OSHA offices can be accessed at https://www.osha.gov/html/RAmap.html or via 1-800-321-OSHA (6742).

## SUMMARY

- Avoid non-neutral and prolonged static postures.
- Take the time to optimize all equipment to suit individual postural requirements before beginning to scan; this includes the scanning chair, exam table, ultrasound system controls, and monitor.
- Take steps to minimize prolonged exposure to risk factors such as by accepting limitations of imaging capabilities with difficult to image patients with high body mass index (BMI), limited mobility, and/or monitoring or/intensive care equipment that restricts access to acoustic window.
- Use correct body mechanics when moving wheelchairs, beds, stretchers, and ultrasound equipment.
- Utilize patient positioning/lift devices instead of manually transferring or repositioning patients.
- Properly position patients and consider alternative positions depending on the area being examined.
- Organize desk area workspaces so that computer keyboard, monitors, and chairs are appropriately adjusted.
- Participate in ongoing education and training of safety and ergonomics specific to job tasks.
- Document and report ergonomic concerns, persistent pain, or injury to employer and seek competent medical advice.

## CRITICAL THINKING QUESTIONS

1. You are asked to perform a bedside exam, but upon arrival to the patient's room, you discover that there is equipment/furnishings in the way so there is not enough space to position your ultrasound system at the bedside without resulting in awkward postures to access the patient. What should you do?

2. A morbidly obese patient comes in for an abdominal Doppler examination. You begin to scan, but discover that the scanning chair doesn't go up high enough to allow you to access the region of interest without reaching/abducting your scanning arm above the height of your shoulder. What should you do?

3. The lab you're working in has height-adjustable chairs and exam tables, but the ultrasound system is fixed in height. How can you optimize you're postural alignment?

## MEDIA MENU

Student Resources available on the**Point**® include:

- Audio glossary
- Interactive question bank
- Videos
- Internet resources

### REFERENCES

1. Occupational Safety and Health Administration. Available at https://www.osha.gov/SLTC/ergonomics/. Accessed March 5, 2016.
2. Department of Labor. Available at https://www.osha.gov/pls/oshaweb/owadisp.show_document?p_table=UNIFIED_AGENDA&p_id=4481. Accessed June 6, 2016.
3. Bureau of Labor Statistics. Available at http://www.bls.gov/opub/mlr/2013/article/using-workplace-safety-data-for-prevention.htm. Accessed August 6, 2016.
4. Canadian Centre for Occupational Health and Safety; Work-related Musculoskeletal Disorders-Risk Factors. Available at https://www.ccohs.ca/oshanswers/ergonomics/risk.html. Accessed December 7, 2016.
5. Roll S, Selhorst L, Evans K. Contribution of positioning to work-related musculoskeletal discomfort in diagnostic medical sonographers. *Work* 2014;47(2):253–260. Available at http://www.ncbi.nlm.nih.gov/pmc/articles/PMC3840125/. Accessed August 6, 2016.
6. Craig M. Sonography: an occupational health hazard? *J Diagn Med Sonogr* 1985;1(3):121–126.
7. Pike I, Russo A, Berkowitz J, et al. The prevalence of musculoskeletal disorders among diagnostic medical sonographers. *J Diagn Med Sonogr* 1997;13(5):219–227.
8. Society of Diagnostic Medical Sonography. Industry standards for the prevention of work-related musculoskeletal disorders in sonography. Available at http://sdms.org/docs/default-source/Resources/industry-standards-for-prevention-of-work-related-msk-disorders.pdf. Accessed December 7, 2016.
9. Evans K, Roll S, Baker J. Work-related musculoskeletal disorders (WRMSD) among registered diagnostic medical sonorgraphers and vascular technologists. *J Diagn Med Sonogr* 2009;25(6):287–299.
10. Canadian Centre for Occupational Health and Safety; Work-related Musculoskeletal Disorders. Available at https://www.ccohs.ca/oshanswers/diseases/rmirsi.html. Accessed August 6, 2016.
11. Muir M, Hrynkow P, Chase R, et al. The nature, cause, and extent of occupational musculoskeletal injuries among sonographers. *J Diagn Med Sonogr* 2004;20(5):317–325.

# PART TWO

# Introduction to the Vascular System

# Vascular Anatomy

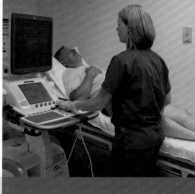

ANN MARIE KUPINSKI

## CHAPTER 4

## OBJECTIVES

- Define the major components of the vascular system
- Describe the arrangement of the blood vessel walls
- Identify the major vessels of the arterial system
- Identify the major vessels of the venous system

## KEY TERMS

**arteriole**

**artery**

**capillary**

**vein**

**venule**

## GLOSSARY

**arteriole** A small artery with a muscular wall; a terminal artery that continues into the capillary network

**artery** A blood vessel that carries blood away from the heart

**capillary** A small blood vessel with only endothelium and basement membrane through which exchange of nutrients and waste occurs

**vein** A blood vessel that carries blood toward the heart

**venule** A small vein that is continuous with a capillary

Ultrasound is a medical imaging modality used to define various structures as well as any pathology within the body. Sonographers and vascular technologists control the ultrasound equipment and the acquisition of the images, and thus are vital to obtaining accurate and adequate clinical information. To perform an ultrasound examination successfully, a thorough knowledge of anatomy is essential. This chapter will present the basic anatomic components of the vascular system. Additional detailed anatomic information pertaining to specific organs, regions, pathology, or disorders is contained within several of the subsequent chapters.

## VASCULAR ARCHITECTURE

Blood is circulated throughout the body by a network of arteries, veins, and capillaries. Arteries carry blood rich in nutrients and oxygen from the heart out to the various organs and tissue beds. Veins return the deoxygenated blood with waste materials back toward the heart. Capillaries are

part of the microvasculature where exchange of oxygen, nutrients, and waste occurs.

## Arteries

Arteries and veins have three layers of cells within their vessel walls (Fig. 4-1). These layers are called the tunica intima, tunica media, and tunica adventitia (Fig. 4-2). The word tunica refers to a distinctive layer of cells. Many simply refer to these blood vessel layers as the intima, media, and adventitia. The intima is the innermost layer consisting of an endothelial cell lining with connective tissue components beneath it. This is the layer of cells in contact with the blood. The media is the middle layer within a blood vessel and is a strong muscular layer. It is the thickest component of an arterial wall. It is composed mainly of smooth muscle cells circularly arranged around the vessel. There are varying amounts of elastic fibers and collagen present. The adventitia is the outermost layer of a blood vessel wall and

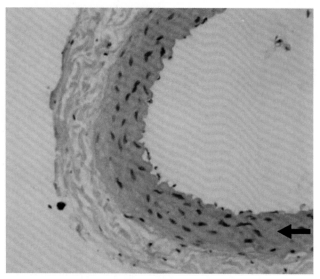

**FIGURE 4-1** Cross section of an arterial wall. The black arrow is indicating the thick layer of smooth muscle cells within the tunica media.

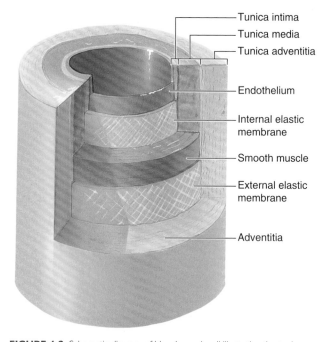

— Tunica intima
— Tunica media
— Tunica adventitia

— Endothelium

— Internal elastic membrane

— Smooth muscle

— External elastic membrane

— Adventitia

**FIGURE 4-2** Schematic diagram of blood vessel wall illustrating the tunica intima, tunica media, and tunica adventitia.

is in contact with the tissue surrounding the vessel. The adventitia is composed of collagen, nerve fibers, and small blood vessels. The small blood vessels in the walls of large arteries and veins are called the vaso vasorum. The term vaso vasorum translates from Latin as "the vessels of the vessels." There are different types of vaso vasorum, but all function to bring a blood supply with nutrients to the blood vessel walls. Some diseases are associated with changes in the vaso vasorum, and the role of the vaso vasorum in the development of atherosclerosis continues to be investigated.

Arteries are classified according to their size. Arterioles are about 100 microns or less in diameter. They have been called the "stopcocks" of the vascular system. They are the principal point of resistance to blood flow within the vascular

system. Circular smooth muscle layers control the degree of contraction of these vessels and thus alter vessel resistance. Small- and medium-sized arteries average approximately 4 mm in diameter and are mainly distributive vessels. This group of vessels includes all the arteries excluding the aorta and its largest branches. Small- and medium-sized arteries have well-developed smooth muscle layers. They also have more elastic and fibrous tissue than the arterioles but less than that of the large arteries. Large elastic arteries are the aorta and its largest branches (the brachiocephalic, left common carotid, left subclavian, and common iliac arteries). They have a large amount of elastic fibers in their walls and less smooth muscle cells. Their primary function is to provide a conduit for blood flow to the tissues.

## Veins

Veins have the same laminar structures as the arteries, although they tend not to be as muscular as the arteries. In some veins, they have more elastic fibers and collagen than muscle fibers. Their walls are thinner in comparison to arteries of similar size. Wall thickness does vary depending on the region of the body, with lower extremity veins having thicker walls than upper extremity veins.

Venules are the smallest component of the venous system and measure approximately 20 microns in diameter. Their walls are mainly connective tissue. Some venules are as permeable to certain substances as the capillaries, and some exchange occurs across these vessels. Small and medium-sized veins range in diameter from 1 to 10 mm. These include all the veins except the portal vein and the vena cavae and their main tributaries. The small and medium-sized veins have a thin media and a thicker adventitia. The large veins, namely the portal vein, inferior and superior vena cava and their main tributaries have a distinguishing characteristic of a large adventitia. The adventitia of large veins is their thickest layer and is made up of mostly collagen and some elastic tissue.

A unique feature of veins is the presence of valves (Fig. 4-3). Most veins have valves that prevent the retrograde movement of blood. Valves are formed by inward projections of the intima and are strengthened by the presence of collagen and elastic fibers. The valves are covered by endothelial cells. Valves are bicuspid, which means they have two leaflets that are shaped as semilunar cusps. They attach to the vein wall by their convex edges, and their free concave edges are oriented toward the heart. When blood flow reverses, the valves close and blood fills a slightly enlarged space between the wall of the vein and the valve called the sinus. Valves are numerous in the legs, where venous flow moves against the force of gravity. Valves are usually absent within the veins of the thorax and abdomen.

## Capillaries

The capillaries are the smallest vessel in the body, measuring approximately 8 microns in diameter, just big enough to let a red blood cell pass through. Their walls are composed primarily of a layer of endothelial cells and a small amount of basement membrane. This layer of endothelial cells is typically referred to as the intima. These thin walls are ideal for the diffusion of products across the capillaries. The capillaries are the primary place in the body where

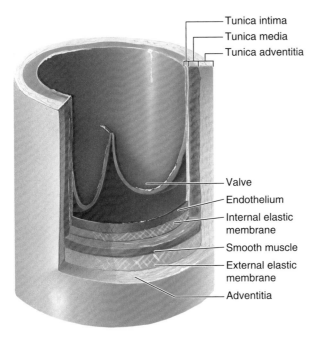

**FIGURE 4-3** Schematic diagram of a venous valve.

Tunica intima
Tunica media
Tunica adventitia
Valve
Endothelium
Internal elastic membrane
Smooth muscle
External elastic membrane
Adventitia

## CEREBROVASCULAR ANATOMY

The principal arteries supplying the head and neck are the right and left common carotid arteries (CCA). The left CCA is the second of three major vessels that arise from the aortic arch (Fig. 4-4). The right CCA originates from the brachiocephalic artery (formerly called the innominate artery). The CCA ascends the neck laterally and bifurcates into the internal carotid (ICA) and external carotid (ECA) arteries in the midcervical region at the superior border of the thyroid cartilage or at about the level of the fourth cervical vertebrae (Fig. 4-5). The right and left ICA supplies much of the circulation to the brain and eyes. They usually lie posterior and lateral to the ECAs and have no extracranial branches. With very rare exceptions, the ICA has no branches in the cervical region. The intracranial segment of the ICA consists of three portions, namely, the petrous, cavernous, and cerebral. The ophthalmic artery is the first branch of the cerebral portion of the ICA. The ophthalmic artery has several branches, including the supraorbital, frontal, and nasal arteries. The cerebral portion of the ICA terminates into four branches: the anterior cerebral, middle cerebral, posterior communicating, and anterior choroidal arteries.

The ECAs are usually medial and anterior to the ICAs. Eight major branches arise off the ECA. Anterior branches include the superior thyroid, lingual and facial. Posterior branches of the ECA are the occipital, posterior auricular, ascending pharyngeal, maxillary, and superficial temporal arteries (Fig. 4-6). The superficial thyroid is usually the first branch of the ECA. The ECA supplies blood flow to the face and neck.

The vertebral arteries arise off the subclavian arteries and ascend the neck (Fig. 4-7). The right and left vertebral arteries along with the right and left ICA are the four vessels that supply the brain with blood flow. The vertebral artery enters the transverse process of the sixth cervical vertebra and runs superiorly. The vertebral artery continues coursing through the foramina in the transverse process of the other five cervical vertebrae. It then bends medially before entering the cranial cavity through the foramen magnum.

nutrient exchange occurs. Oxygen and nutrients pass across the capillaries into the tissue while at the same time carbon dioxide and waste products leave the tissues and enter the blood of the capillary. Capillary permeability does vary somewhat depending on the tissue bed with efficient barriers in place to limit the diffusion of large molecules, particularly in the brain.

Blood enters into the capillary from the arterial side of the circulation via the arterioles. Blood leaves the capillary on the venous side of the circulation via the venules. There are different types of capillaries characterized by slightly different arrangements of the endothelial cells. There are also places in the body where an arteriole and venule are connected together without a true capillary between them.

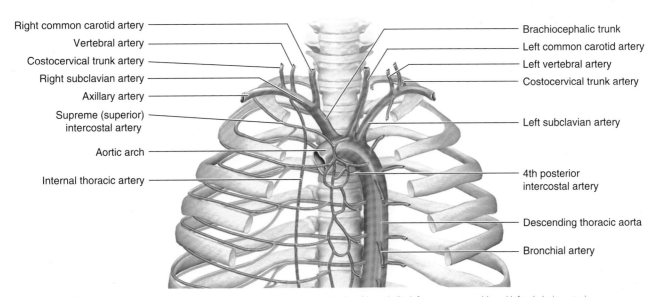

Right common carotid artery
Vertebral artery
Costocervical trunk artery
Right subclavian artery
Axillary artery
Supreme (superior) intercostal artery
Aortic arch
Internal thoracic artery
Brachiocephalic trunk
Left common carotid artery
Left vertebral artery
Costocervical trunk artery
Left subclavian artery
4th posterior intercostal artery
Descending thoracic aorta
Bronchial artery

**FIGURE 4-4** Illustration of the aortic arch and its major branches: the brachiocephalic, left common carotid, and left subclavian arteries.

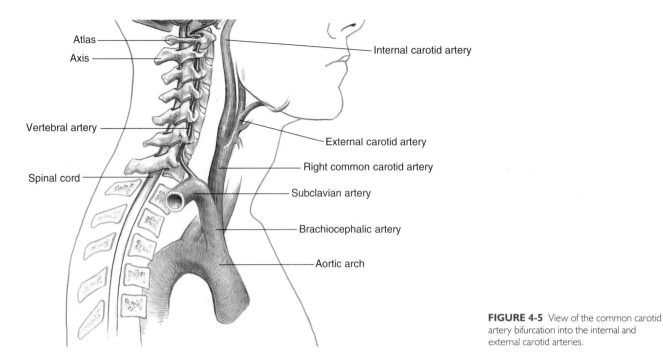

Atlas

Axis

Internal carotid artery

Vertebral artery

Spinal cord

External carotid artery

Right common carotid artery

Subclavian artery

Brachiocephalic artery

Aortic arch

**FIGURE 4-5** View of the common carotid artery bifurcation into the internal and external carotid arteries.

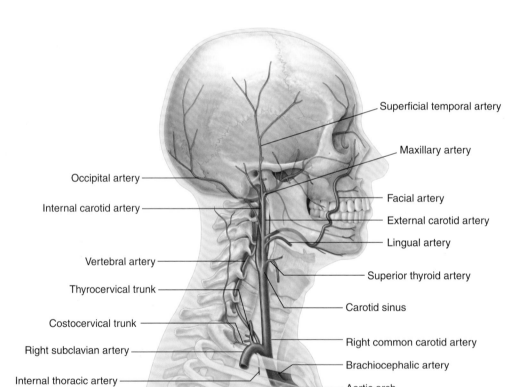

Occipital artery

Internal carotid artery

Vertebral artery

Thyrocervical trunk

Costocervical trunk

Right subclavian artery

Internal thoracic artery

Superficial temporal artery

Maxillary artery

Facial artery

External carotid artery

Lingual artery

Superior thyroid artery

Carotid sinus

Right common carotid artery

Brachiocephalic artery

Aortic arch

**FIGURE 4-6** Illustration of the external carotid artery and its branches.

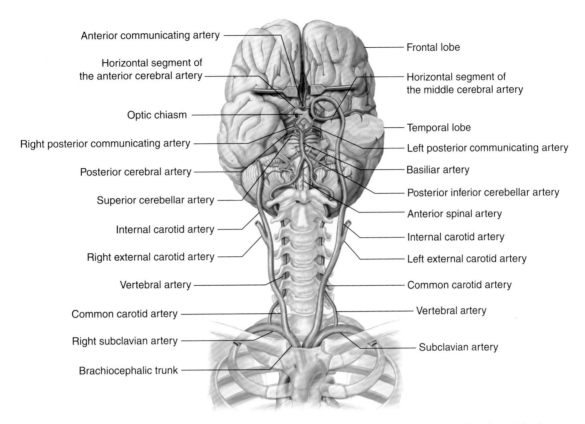

Anterior communicating artery

Horizontal segment of
the anterior cerebral artery

Optic chiasm

Right posterior communicating artery

Posterior cerebral artery

Superior cerebellar artery

Internal carotid artery

Right external carotid artery

Vertebral artery

Common carotid artery

Right subclavian artery

Brachiocephalic trunk

Frontal lobe

Horizontal segment of
the middle cerebral artery

Temporal lobe

Left posterior communicating artery

Basiliar artery

Posterior inferior cerebellar artery

Anterior spinal artery

Internal carotid artery

Left external carotid artery

Common carotid artery

Vertebral artery

Subclavian artery

**FIGURE 4-7** Diagram indicating the orientation of the vertebral arteries through the cervical vertebrae and into the cranial cavity.

After entering the skull, the two vertebral arteries join to form the basilar artery.

The circle of Willis is a unique arrangement of the branches of the ICAs and vertebral arteries. This arrangement of vessels provides a vital collateral network to maintain cerebral perfusion in the event of disease. The circle of Willis is formed by the right and left anterior cerebral arteries that are interconnected via the anterior communicating artery and by the right and left posterior cerebral arteries that are connected via the posterior communicating arteries (Fig. 4-8). Chapter 10 will further describe intracranial vascular anatomy.

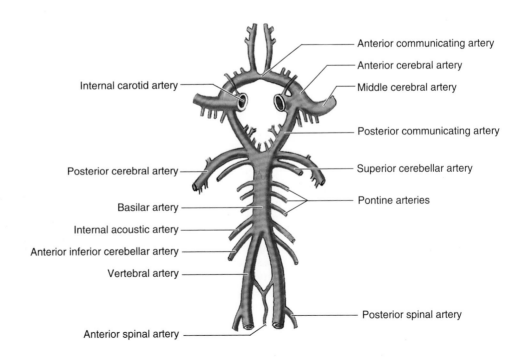

Internal carotid artery

Posterior cerebral artery

Basilar artery

Internal acoustic artery

Anterior inferior cerebellar artery

Vertebral artery

Anterior spinal artery

Anterior communicating artery

Anterior cerebral artery

Middle cerebral artery

Posterior communicating artery

Superior cerebellar artery

Pontine arteries

Posterior spinal artery

**FIGURE 4-8** Circle of Willis.

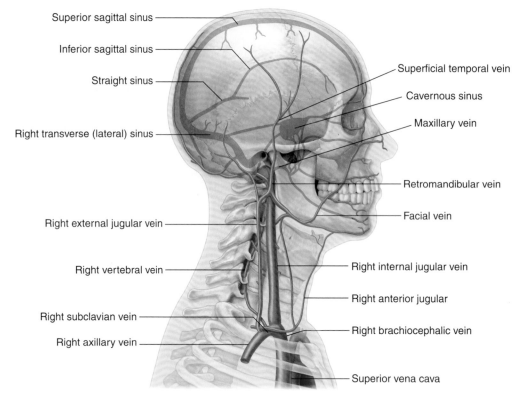

Superior sagittal sinus

Inferior sagittal sinus

Straight sinus

Right transverse (lateral) sinus

Right external jugular vein

Right vertebral vein

Right subclavian vein

Right axillary vein

Superficial temporal vein

Cavernous sinus

Maxillary vein

Retromandibular vein

Facial vein

Right internal jugular vein

Right anterior jugular

Right brachiocephalic vein

Superior vena cava

**FIGURE 4-9** Venous drainage of the brain, head, and neck.

Venous drainage of the head and neck includes the external jugular, internal jugular, and vertebral veins (Fig. 4-9). The external jugular courses through the neck and returns blood from portions of the cranial cavity, face, and neck. The external jugular vein flows into the subclavian vein. The internal jugular vein collects blood from the brain and superficial parts of the face and neck. The internal jugular vein courses along the anterolateral edge of the ICA and CCA. The internal jugular vein unites with the subclavian vein to form the brachiocephalic (innominate) veins. The vertebral vein is formed from numerous small tributaries of the internal vertebral venous plexuses. These vessels join with small veins from the muscles of the neck and form a dense plexus around the vertebral artery. These veins descend in the transverse foramina of the cervical vertebrae. This plexus ends in a single trunk, the vertebral vein, which emerges from the sixth cervical vertebra and empties into the brachiocephalic vein.

## Collateral Pathways

There are multiple collateral pathways within the cerebrovascular system, and the following describes a few of the more common pathways. Some involve only extracranial pathways that mainly arise off the ECA. The superior thyroid, lingual, ascending pharyngeal, and maxillary arteries will carry blood supplied from the ECA across the midline to the contralateral ECA. The occipital artery of the ECA can collateralize with the vertebral artery. There are other pathways that connect branches of the extracranial arteries with segments of the intracranial arteries. The ECA again serves as the main supplier of blood traveling through the

frontal and dorsal nasal arteries feeding into the ophthalmic artery. The circle of Willis is likely the best known and most important collateral pathway. This intracranial pathway will be discussed in detail in Chapter 10.

## THE AORTIC ARCH AND UPPER EXTREMITY ARTERIES

The ascending aorta is approximately 3 cm in diameter and begins at the aortic valve. It courses upward, becoming the aortic arch. It continues upward and backward, crossing the trachea. It then continues posteriorly on the left side of the trachea and curves downward, becoming the descending aorta.

The first and largest branch of the aortic arch is the brachiocephalic artery (see Fig. 4-4). The brachiocephalic artery is typically 4 to 5 cm in length. At the sternoclavicular joint, the artery divides into the right CCA and the right subclavian artery. The second branch of the aortic arch is the left CCA. The last branch of the aortic arch is the left subclavian artery.

The subclavian arteries give rise to branches that supply the brain, neck, thoracic wall, and shoulder, including the vertebral and internal mammary arteries (Fig. 4-10). Beyond the outer border of the first rib, the subclavian artery becomes the axillary artery. From the axilla to approximately 1 cm below the elbow joint, the artery is known as the brachial artery. The largest branch of the brachial artery is the deep brachial artery or profunda brachii. The brachial artery ends by dividing into the radial and ulnar arteries near the neck of the radius. The ulnar artery is usually slightly larger than the radial artery. The ulnar artery continues distally

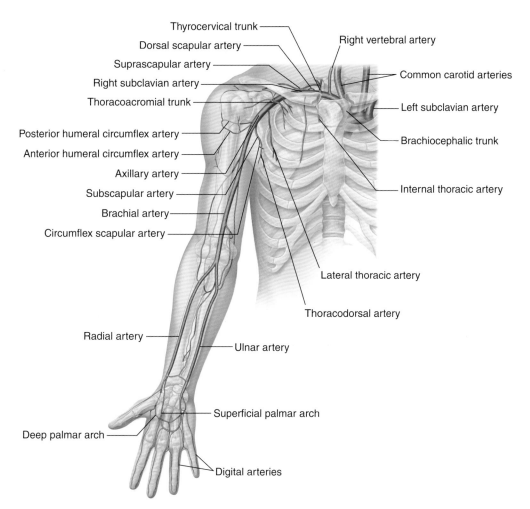

Thyrocervical trunk

Dorsal scapular artery

Suprascapular artery

Right subclavian artery

Thoracoacromial trunk

Posterior humeral circumflex artery

Anterior humeral circumflex artery

Axillary artery

Subscapular artery

Brachial artery

Circumflex scapular artery

Right vertebral artery

Common carotid arteries

Left subclavian artery

Brachiocephalic trunk

Internal thoracic artery

Lateral thoracic artery

Thoracodorsal artery

Radial artery

Ulnar artery

Superficial palmar arch

Deep palmar arch

Digital arteries

**FIGURE 4-10** Diagram of the upper extremity arterial system.

and courses along the ulnar border of the wrist. Beyond this point, the artery becomes the superficial palmar arch (Fig. 4-11). Major branches of the ulnar artery include the ulnar recurrent and interosseous arteries in the forearm, palmar and dorsal carpal branches at the wrist and deep palmar and superficial palmar arch of the hand. The radial artery passes along the radial aspect of the forearm to the wrist, and then winds around the lateral aspect of the wrist to the dorsum of the wrist. It continues distally to join the deep palmar branch of the ulnar artery to form the deep palmar arch (Fig. 4-12). Branches of the radial artery include the radial recurrent, muscular, palmar carpal, and superficial palmar arteries. The superficial and deep palmar arches of the hand are continuations of the ulnar and radial arteries, respectively. The superficial palmar arch is completed by a branch of the radial artery. The deep palmar arch is completed by a branch of the ulnar artery. Both systems supply the digital arteries.

## Collateral Pathways

Collateral pathways of the upper extremity arterial system involve several common routes. In the event of a brachiocephalic or subclavian artery occlusion, collateral flow can enter the distal subclavian artery via the vertebral artery. This pathology is referred to as "subclavian steal." It produces

variations in flow through the vertebral arteries, which are further described in Chapter 7. The superior and inferior ulnar collateral arteries and the posterior ulnar recurrent artery form a medial vascular arcade that will reenter into the distal ulnar artery. A lateral vascular arcade is formed by radial collateral artery (a branch of the profunda brachii) and the radial recurrent artery reentering the distal radial artery. Another pathway is the posterior vascular arcade formed by the middle collateral artery (a branch of the profunda brachii) and the interosseous recurrent artery that reenter into the anterior interosseous artery.

## THE SUPERIOR VENA CAVA AND UPPER EXTREMITY VENOUS SYSTEM

The dorsal digital veins unite to form the dorsal metacarpal veins, which end in a venous network on the back of the hand. The radial part of the network drains into the cephalic vein, whereas the ulnar part of the network drains into the basilic vein. The palmar digital veins flow over the palmar surface of the wrist and help form the medial antebrachial veins (Fig. 4-13).

The veins of the arm have both superficial and deep components similar to the lower extremities. The superficial veins of the arm include the cephalic, basilic, and medial

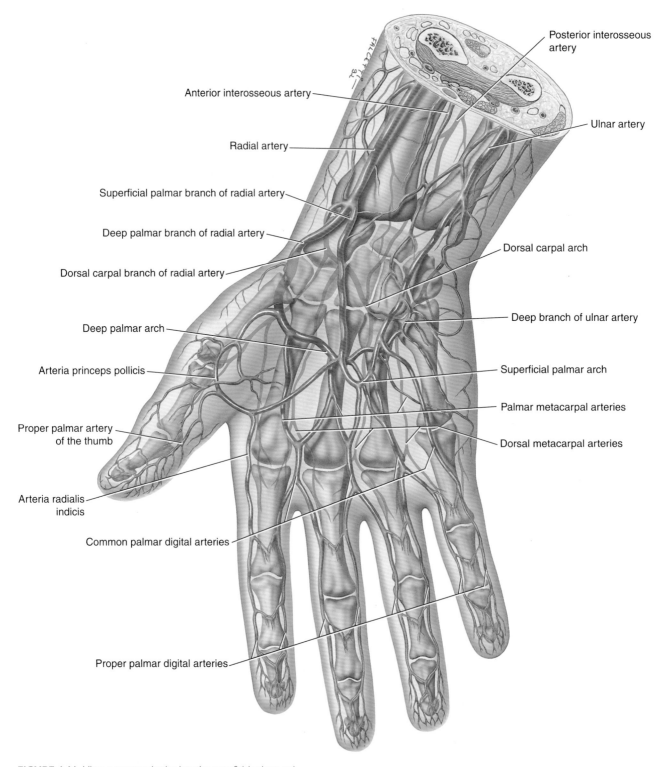

**FIGURE 4-11** Ulnar artery terminating into the superficial palmar arch.

antebrachial veins. The cephalic vein winds around the radial border of the forearm and continues along the lateral border of the biceps muscle. It then empties into the axillary vein just below the clavicle (Fig. 4-14). The basilic vein courses along the ulnar aspect of the forearm and continues proximally along the medial border of the biceps muscle. It joins the brachial vein to form the axillary vein.

Both the cephalic and basilic veins communicate with the median cubital vein at the antecubital fossa. The median antebrachial vein courses the forearm slightly toward the ulnar side of the arm. It ends into either the median cubital vein or the basilic vein.

The deep venous tributaries of the forearm are the venae comitantes of the radial, ulnar, and interosseous arteries.

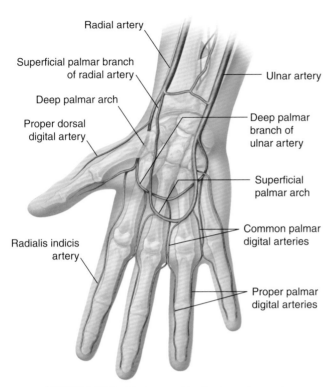

**FIGURE 4-12** Radial artery supplying the deep palmar arch.

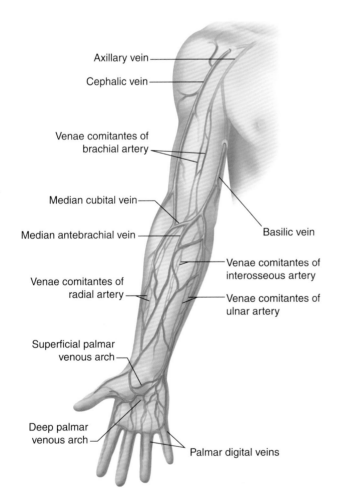

**FIGURE 4-13** Venous drainage of the hand and veins of the upper extremity.

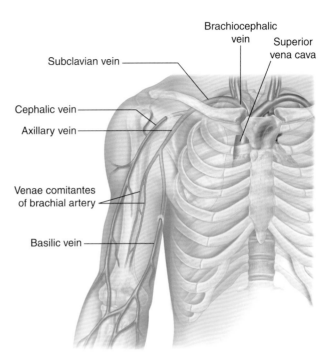

**FIGURE 4-14** View of the upper extremity veins crossing the axillary region.

They are paired veins, which follow the path of the arteries. These tributaries all unite at the elbow to form the brachial veins. There are usually two brachial veins that course along each side of the brachial artery. The axillary vein begins at the junction of the brachial and basilic veins. It becomes the subclavian vein just past the outer border of the first rib at the point of termination of the cephalic vein. The axillary vein lies medial to the axillary artery, which it partially overlaps. The brachiocephalic veins are formed at the junction of the internal jugular and subclavian veins at each side of the base of the neck. The superior vena cava is formed by the junction of the two brachiocephalic veins just behind the right side of the sternum.

## MAJOR VESSELS OF THE THORAX, ABDOMEN, AND PELVIS

The descending thoracic aorta is the continuation of the aorta beyond the aortic arch. Branches of the descending aorta include the bronchial, esophageal, phrenic, intercostal, and subcostal arteries. The abdominal aorta begins at the level of the 12th thoracic vertebra as it passes through the aortic hiatus of the diaphragm (Fig. 4-15). There are three major branches off the anterior aspect of the abdominal aorta. The first branch is the celiac artery. This is also known as the celiac trunk or celiac axis. It is a fairly short vessel, only 1-2 cm in length. It gives rise to the hepatic, splenic, and left gastric arteries (Fig. 4-16). The superior mesenteric artery is the next branch of the aorta, just below the celiac artery (Fig. 4-17). It supplies most of the small intestine and some of the large intestine. It courses inferiorly, running parallel with and anterior to the aorta. The last anterior branch of the aorta is the inferior mesenteric artery. It arises about 3 or 4 cm above the aortic bifurcation. It supplies mainly the large intestine.

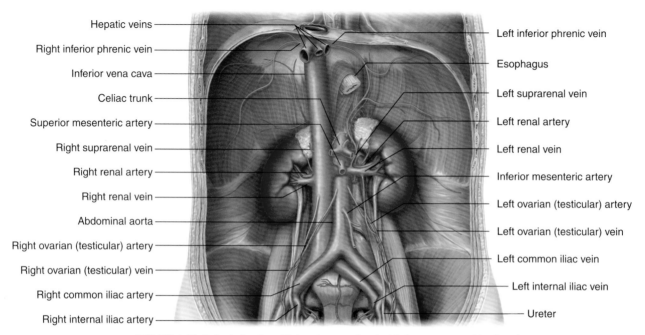

Hepatic veins

Right inferior phrenic vein

Inferior vena cava

Celiac trunk

Superior mesenteric artery

Right suprarenal vein

Right renal artery

Right renal vein

Abdominal aorta

Right ovarian (testicular) artery

Right ovarian (testicular) vein

Right common iliac artery

Right internal iliac artery

Left inferior phrenic vein

Esophagus

Left suprarenal vein

Left renal artery

Left renal vein

Inferior mesenteric artery

Left ovarian (testicular) artery

Left ovarian (testicular) vein

Left common iliac vein

Left internal iliac vein

Ureter

**FIGURE 4-15** Abdominal aorta and its branches as well as the inferior vena cava and its tributaries.

The renal arteries branch off the lateral aspect of the aorta just below the superior mesenteric artery (see Fig. 4-17). The right renal artery is longer and usually slightly higher than the left renal artery. The right renal artery courses posterior to the inferior vena cava as it continues to the right kidney. Both renal arteries approach the kidneys slightly posterior to the renal veins.

Just below the level of the renal arteries, two additional arteries branch off the anterolateral aspect of the aorta. These are the testicular arteries in the male and ovarian arteries in the female. Posteriorly off the aorta, there are four pairs of lumbar arteries that course laterally and posteriorly along the lumbar vertebrae. Occasionally, there is a fifth smaller pair. A single middle sacral artery is a small posterior branch of the aorta. It arises just above the bifurcation of the iliac vessels.

The aorta terminates at the level of the fourth lumbar vertebra into the right and left common iliac arteries (Fig. 4-18). The common iliac arteries each bifurcate into the external and internal iliac arteries. The internal iliac arteries, which are also known as the hypogastric arteries, supply the pelvic organs. The external iliac arteries continue distally to supply the lower extremities. At the inguinal ligament, these arteries are then known as the common femoral arteries.

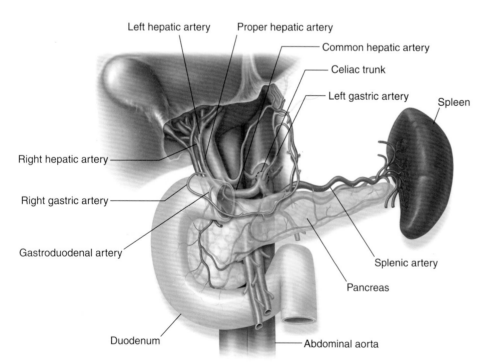

Left hepatic artery

Proper hepatic artery

Common hepatic artery

Celiac trunk

Left gastric artery

Spleen

Right hepatic artery

Right gastric artery

Gastroduodenal artery

Splenic artery

Pancreas

Duodenum

Abdominal aorta

**FIGURE 4-16** Celiac artery and its branches.

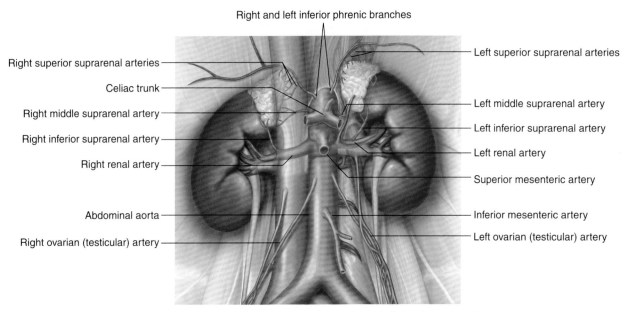

Right and left inferior phrenic branches

Right superior suprarenal arteries

Celiac trunk

Right middle suprarenal artery

Right inferior suprarenal artery

Right renal artery

Abdominal aorta

Right ovarian (testicular) artery

Left superior suprarenal arteries

Left middle suprarenal artery

Left inferior suprarenal artery

Left renal artery

Superior mesenteric artery

Inferior mesenteric artery

Left ovarian (testicular) artery

**FIGURE 4-17** View of the branches of the abdominal aorta, including the renal arteries.

The venous system of the pelvis is composed of the external iliac veins, which are the continuation of the common femoral veins above the inguinal ligament (Fig. 4-19). The internal iliac veins join the external iliac veins to form the common iliac veins. The left common iliac vein courses proximally, passing beneath the right common iliac artery at the level of the aortic bifurcation. The left and right common iliac veins join to form the inferior vena cava. The inferior vena cava travels through the abdomen along the right side of the aorta. The renal, hepatic, lumbar, ovarian, and testicular veins drain into the inferior vena cava.

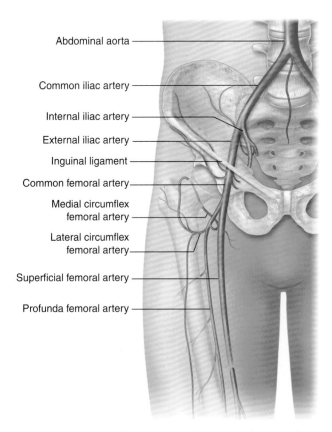

Abdominal aorta

Common iliac artery

Internal iliac artery

External iliac artery

Inguinal ligament

Common femoral artery

Medial circumflex femoral artery

Lateral circumflex femoral artery

Superficial femoral artery

Profunda femoral artery

**FIGURE 4-18** Diagram of the termination of the abdominal aorta into the iliac vessels.

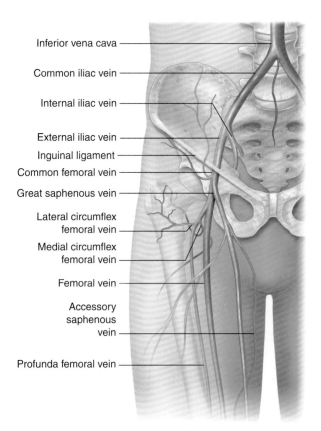

Inferior vena cava

Common iliac vein

Internal iliac vein

External iliac vein

Inguinal ligament

Common femoral vein

Great saphenous vein

Lateral circumflex femoral vein

Medial circumflex femoral vein

Femoral vein

Accessory saphenous vein

Profunda femoral vein

**FIGURE 4-19** Diagram of the venous system of the pelvis.

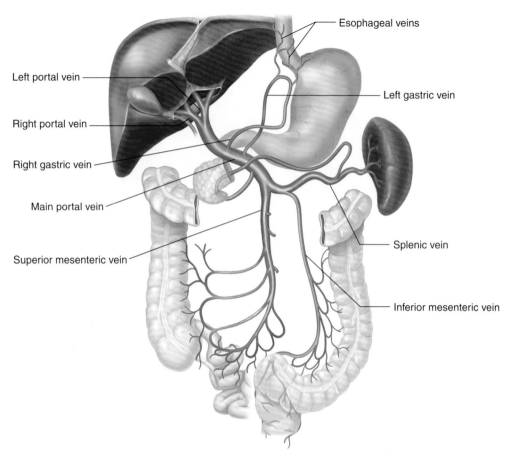

**FIGURE 4-20** Diagram illustrating the main portal vein and its tributaries.

The liver has a unique arrangement of vessels (Fig. 4-20). The hepatic artery (a branch of the celiac artery) carries fully oxygenated blood into the liver. It typically supplies 30% of the total blood flow into the liver. However, the liver receives the remaining 70% of its blood flow via the portal vein. The portal vein forms at the junction of the splenic and superior mesenteric veins posterior to the neck of the pancreas and anterior to the inferior vena cava. The drainage of the liver is accomplished by the hepatic venous system, which drains into three hepatic veins: the left, right, and middle hepatic veins. These three hepatic veins empty into the inferior vena cava. The middle and left hepatic veins join into a common trunk before entering the inferior vena cava in approximately 96% of individuals (Fig. 4-21).

## Collateral Pathways

Collateral pathways for the aortoiliac system vary depending on the level of occlusion. Branches of the superior and inferior mesenteric arteries can provide collateral blood flow that reenters via the internal iliac artery. In the event of a unilateral common iliac occlusion, collateral circulation can be provided by the contralateral iliac artery. More distal disease involving the external iliac arteries can be compensated for with collateral flow from gluteal, lumbar, and intercostal arteries reentering into the lateral circumflex artery or deep femoral artery.

The pancreaticoduodenal arcade is a primary collateral pathway between the celiac and superior mesenteric

arteries. The superior and inferior mesenteric arteries are linked via the marginal artery of Drummond and the arc of Riolan. The renal arteries have poor collateral pathways. With a slow progression of renal artery stenosis, adrenal,

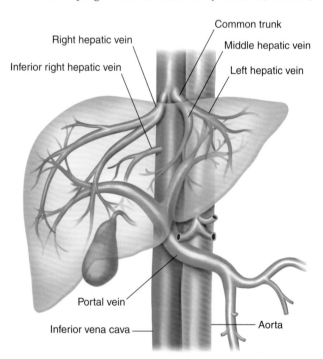

**FIGURE 4-21** Diagram of the hepatic veins of the liver.

ureteral, and renal capsular arteries may enlarge to provide some collateral flow. However, this flow is insufficient to keep the kidneys functioning normally.

## THE ARTERIES AND VEINS OF THE LOWER EXTREMITIES

The common femoral artery is the continuation of the external iliac artery below the inguinal ligament (Fig. 4-22). The common femoral artery divides into the superficial femoral and profunda femoris arteries. The profunda femoris artery is also known as the deep femoral artery. The profunda femoris artery is posterior and lateral to the superficial femoral artery. Branches of the profunda femoris artery include numerous perforators and the medial and lateral circumflex arteries. The superficial femoral artery courses distally, passing through the adductor canal. The popliteal artery is the continuation of the superficial femoral artery and courses behind the knee in the popliteal fossa. Branches of the popliteal artery include the sural (also known as the gastrocnemius artery) and genicular arteries. Terminal branches of the popliteal artery include the anterior tibial, posterior tibial and peroneal arteries (Fig. 4-23). Initially, the popliteal artery bifurcates into the anterior tibial artery and the tibial-peroneal trunk. The tibial-peroneal trunk continues for a short distance and bifurcates again into the posterior tibial and peroneal arteries. The anterior tibial artery passes through an opening in the interosseous membrane, then proceeds distally in the anterior

compartment of the leg. It continues anterior to the ankle joint and becomes the dorsalis pedis artery. The posterior tibial artery courses medially in the posterior compartment of the leg. It continues posterior to the medial malleolus and terminates into the medial and lateral planter arteries. The peroneal artery is located deep within the leg and descends along the medial aspect of the fibula. It terminates into branches that communicate with the posterior and anterior tibial arteries. The arteries of the foot include the medial and lateral plantar and dorsalis pedis arteries, all of which help to give rise to the plantar arch. Arising off the plantar arch are the metatarsal arteries, which divide into the digital arteries.

The veins of the leg have both deep and superficial systems. The dorsal venous arch of the foot joins into the great saphenous vein (GSV) just anterior to the medial malleolus. The GSV is the longest vein in the body. It ascends the leg medially with several tributaries emptying into the GSV before it terminates into the common femoral vein at the saphenofemoral junction (Fig. 4-24). The small saphenous vein (SSV) begins as a continuation of the lateral segment of the dorsal venous arch of the foot. The SSV courses posteriorly up the calf, penetrating the deep fascia in the upper half of the calf. In approximately 70% of individuals, the SSV terminates into the popliteal vein at the saphenopopliteal junction. In the remainder of cases, the SSV continues above the knee as the vein of Giacomini.

The deep venous system begins with the deep plantar arch, which continues as the medial and lateral plantar veins.

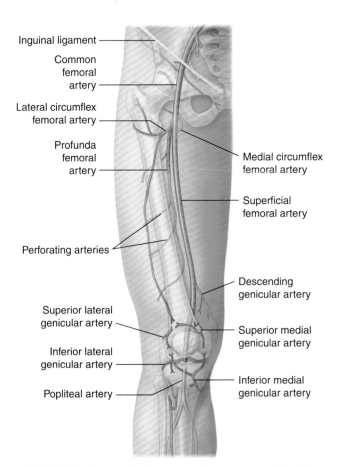

**FIGURE 4-22** Diagram of the lower extremity arteries through the thigh.

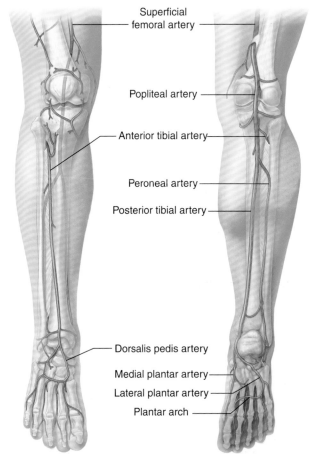

**FIGURE 4-23** Diagram of the lower extremity arteries through the calf.

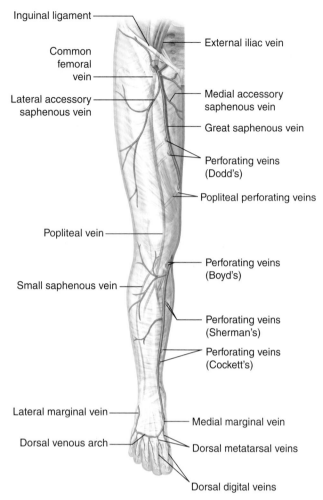

**FIGURE 4-24** Diagram of the superficial veins of the leg.

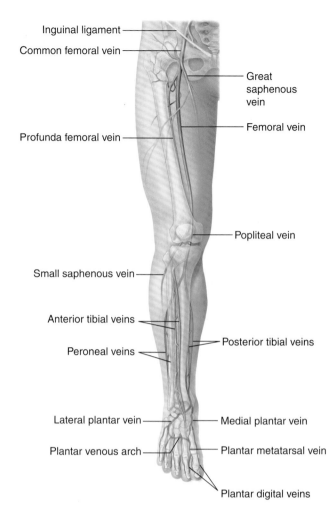

**FIGURE 4-26** Illustration of the lower extremity deep venous system.

These veins then unite to form the posterior tibial veins (Fig. 4-25). The paired posterior tibial veins accompany the posterior tibial artery. The paired peroneal veins ascend the calf in the same plane as the peroneal artery. Approximately two-thirds of the way up the calf, the peroneal veins join the posterior tibial veins to form the tibio-peroneal trunk veins. The anterior tibial veins are the continuation of the vena comitantes of the dorsalis pedis artery. The anterior

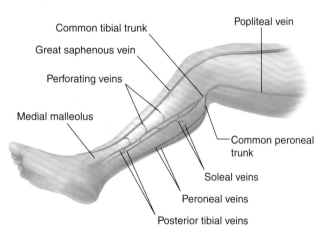

**FIGURE 4-25** Diagram of the orientation of the peroneal and posterior tibial veins of the calf.

tibial veins pass between the tibia and the fibula through the upper part of the interosseous membrane. The veins then unite with the tibio-peroneal trunk veins to form the popliteal vein. The popliteal vein is medial to the popliteal artery distally and moves lateral to the artery as it passes through the adductor canal. The femoral vein is the continuation of the popliteal vein and accompanies the superficial femoral artery to the groin (Fig. 4-26). The profunda femoral (deep femoral) vein courses the thigh along the profunda femoris artery. The profunda femoris and femoral veins unite to form the common femoral vein. The common femoral vein lies medial to the common femoral artery. The external iliac vein is the continuation of the common femoral vein above the inguinal ligament.

## Collateral Pathways

Many of the collaterals that bypass superficial femoral or popliteal artery occlusions arise from the profunda femoral artery. The lateral circumflex femoral artery can also act as a collateral. Blood flow can reenter the distal superficial femoral artery, the popliteal artery, and the proximal tibial arteries through a network of geniculate arteries and their branches. With more distal occlusion, branches of the anterior tibial, peroneal, and posterior tibial arteries can provide collateral circulation to the more distal portions of the leg and to the foot.

## SUMMARY

- The blood vessels of the body have the same basic microscopic arrangement of three layers: the intima, media, and adventitia.
- Varying combinations of muscle, collagen, elastic fibers, and connective tissue provide essential differences between the arteries and the veins to allow for their specific functions.
- Arteries and veins of differing sizes are oriented to provide for the efficient delivery of nutrients to the organs and tissue beds as well as to return the blood back to the heart to complete the cycle.
- The network of arteries and veins is complex but if examined by region (arm, leg, abdomen, etc.) can be easier to understand.
- Proper knowledge of vascular anatomy will aid the vascular technologist or sonographer to achieve a technically adequate vascular ultrasound examination.

## CRITICAL THINKING QUESTIONS

1. When examining the carotid system, the physician asks you to be sure to document the origin of the superficial thyroid artery. Normally, in which direction should you focus your examination to visualize this vessel?

2. In your department, part of the documentation includes tapping over the superficial temporal artery and observing the ECA Doppler signal for oscillations in the waveform produced by the tapping. This is done to confirm the vessel being insonated is the ECA. Why are there no oscillations within the ICA?

3. If a patient presents with an abdominal aortic aneurysm that is present from just below the renal arteries to the bifurcation of the common iliac arteries, what branches of the aorta may be involved in the aneurysmal dilation?

4. You are asked to examine a patient with a penetrating injury to the medial aspect of the midthigh. What vessels may have sustained an injury and thus should be thoroughly examined?

## MEDIA MENU

Student Resources available on thePoint® include:
- Audio glossary
- Interactive question bank
- Videos
- Internet resources

### SUGGESTED READINGS

Cronenwett JL, Johnston KW. *Rutherford's Vascular Surgery*. 8th ed. Philadelphia, PA: Saunders-Elsevier; 2014.

Gilroy AM, MacPherson BR, Ross LM. *Atlas of Anatomy*. New York, NY: Thieme; 2008.

Kadir S, ed. *Diagnostic Angiography*. Philadelphia, PA: W.B. Saunders; 1986.

Krstić RV. *Human Microscopic Anatomy: An Atlas for Students of Medicine and Biology*. Berlin, Germany: Springer-Verlag; 1991.

Netter FH. *Atlas of Human Anatomy*. 4th ed. Philadelphia, PA: Saunders-Elsevier; 2006.

Standring S, ed. *Gray's Anatomy: The Anatomical Basis of Clinical Practice*. 40th ed. Edinburgh, Scotland: Churchill-Livingstone; 2008.

# Arterial Physiology

ANN MARIE KUPINSKI **CHAPTER 5**

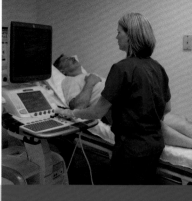

## OBJECTIVES

- List the various hemodynamic forces acting upon the arterial system
- Describe the relationship between pressure, flow, and resistance
- Identify the factors that control peripheral blood flow
- Define physiologic changes associated with arterial disease

## GLOSSARY

**inertia** The tendency of a body at rest to stay at rest or a body in motion to stay in motion

**kinetic energy** The energy of work or motion; in the vascular system, it is in part represented by the velocity of blood flow

**laminar flow** Flow of a liquid in which it travels smoothly in parallel layers

**Poiseuille Law** The law that states the volume of a liquid flowing through a vessel is directly proportional to the pressure of the liquid and the fourth power of the radius and is inversely proportional to the viscosity of the liquid and the length of the vessel

**potential energy** The stored or resting energy; in the vascular system, it is the intravascular pressure

**viscosity** The property of a fluid that resists the force tending to cause fluid to flow

## KEY TERMS

**inertia**

**kinetic energy**

**laminar flow**

**potential energy**

**pressure**

**resistance**

**turbulence**

**velocity**

**viscosity**

A general understanding of the physiology of the vascular system is important when performing ultrasounds on the circulatory system. Although anatomy provides information on the structures being scanned, one must understand function too. There are numerous factors that impact the arterial system. Relationships that govern blood flow result in spectral waveforms that can vary depending on the system being scanned. This chapter reviews the basics of normal arterial physiology and pathophysiology.

## FLUID ENERGY

Blood, like any other fluid, will move from one point to another in response to differences in total energy. The total energy of a system is made up of both potential and kinetic energy. Potential energy is also known as stored or resting energy. In the vascular system, it is represented primarily by the intravascular pressure, which distends the vessels. This pressure is supplied by the contraction of the heart.

Kinetic energy is the energy of work or motion. The velocity of moving blood represents the kinetic energy component of the vascular system. Blood will move from an area of high energy (pressure) to an area of lower energy (pressure). The highest pressure in the vascular system occurs in the left ventricle of the heart where the pressure is approximately 120 mm Hg. The blood leaves the left ventricle, flowing down an energy (pressure) gradient until it returns to the right atrium. The lowest pressure is found at the right atrium where pressure is 2 to 6 mm Hg.

There is another component to the energy of the vascular system related to differences in the level of body parts. Gravitational potential energy is the potential for doing work related to the force of gravity. If blood is positioned above a reference point (which is usually the right atrium), it has the ability to do work because gravity will act on the blood to move it downward. The gravitational potential energy is reduced in dependent parts of the body (below the reference point). Hydrostatic pressure is also pressure within the vessels related to the reference point of the right atrium. Hydrostatic pressure increases in the lower portions of the body because of the weight of the column of blood within the vessels. The farther below the reference point the greater the hydrostatic pressure. The formula for gravitational potential energy is the same as that for hydrostatic pressure but with an opposite sign. Thus, gravitational potential energy and hydrostatic pressure tend to cancel each other. More about hydrostatic pressure will be discussed in Chapter 6.

## The Bernoulli Principle

The Bernoulli principle states that when a fluid flows without a change in velocity from one point to another, the total energy content remains constant, providing no frictional losses. However, in reality, there is always some energy "lost." Of course, energy cannot be "lost" but is merely transferred to a different form. In the vascular system, energy is almost all dissipated in the form of heat because of friction.

The total energy in the vascular system is a balance between potential energy (pressure) and kinetic energy (velocity). If the velocity of blood goes up, there must be a pressure decrease. One can think of this as taking energy from one form (the blood pressure) in order to increase another form of energy (the blood velocity). This principle is used in cardiac imaging. By measuring the velocity at stenotic valve, one can determine the pressure drop across a valve and thus the clinical significance (Fig. 5-1).

## Viscosity and Inertia

In the vascular system, energy "losses" are the result of viscosity and inertia. Viscosity is the property of a fluid that resists the force tending to cause fluid to flow. It can be defined as the friction existing between bordering layers of fluid. Imagine two open containers, one filled with water and one filled with honey. If both containers were tilted to allow the liquids to pour out, the water would flow more quickly than the honey. The honey is more viscous than the water, and more viscous fluids flow more slowly.

Blood viscosity increases with increases in hematocrit (the concentration of red blood cells). Hematocrit is the most important influence on blood viscosity. Hematocrit is an important consideration when performing transcranial Doppler evaluations as intracranial velocities vary significantly with variations in hematocrit.

Inertia is the tendency of a body at rest to stay at rest or a body in motion to stay in motion unless acted upon by an outside force. It is one of the fundamental principles of physics described by Sir Isaac Newton. A classic example of the force of inertia is, when the brakes are applied while riding in a car, an individual has the tendency to move forward. The seat belt is the outside force that stops this forward movement. Inertial losses in the vascular system occur whenever blood is forced to change direction or velocity. In order to change direction, a force needs to be applied and some energy is "lost." Inertial losses depend on the density and velocity of the blood flow. In blood vessels, energy losses because of viscosity effects are greater than those because of inertia.

## VELOCITY AND FLOW

Often the terms blood velocity and blood flow are used interchangeably, but they mean two different things. Velocity refers to the rate of movement (displacement) with respect to time. It has the units of distance per unit of time, such as cm/s or m/s. Blood flow is also referred to as volume flow. It represents the volume of something moved per unit of time. It has the units of mL/s, L/s, mL/min, or L/min.

Velocity and flow are related by the equation:

$$V = \frac{Q}{A}$$

where $V$ is velocity, $Q$ is volume flow, and $A$ is area. Given a constant flow, velocity will vary inversely with the cross-sectional area. Thus, if the flow is the same, the velocity must increase if the area of a blood vessel decreases (Fig. 5-2). This change in velocity allows one to estimate the degree of cross-sectional stenosis within an individual vessel such as the internal carotid artery.

Throughout the entire circulatory system, the cross-sectional area increases from the aorta moving through the arteries, then arterioles, and finally into the capillaries (Fig. 5-3). Blood velocity thus decreases as blood travels from the aorta, through the arteries, then the arterioles, and finally through the capillaries. This slowing down of blood flow

### Bernoulli's Principle

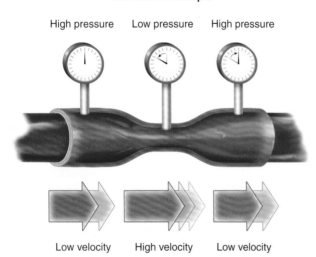

**FIGURE 5-1** Illustration of the Bernoulli principle. In a vessel where the area decreases and the blood velocity increases, the pressure must decrease.

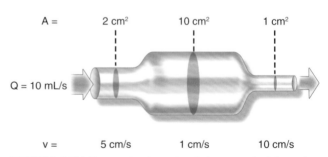

**FIGURE 5-2** This illustrates the changes in velocity as a result of changes in diameter. Note the steady rate of flow throughout the conduit.

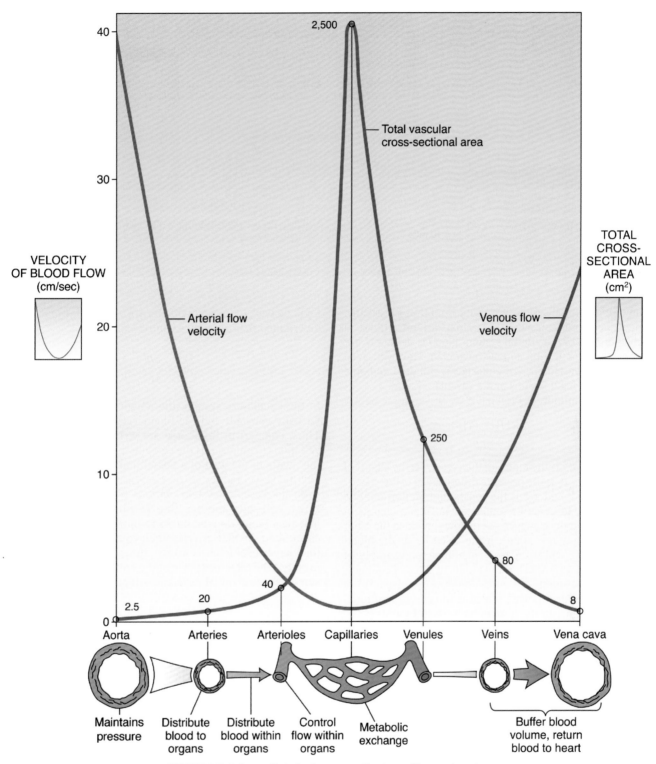

**FIGURE 5-3** A diagram illustrating the cross-sectional area of the vascular system.

at the capillary level is important in the proper exchange of nutrients and waste that occurs within the capillaries. The cross-sectional area of the vascular system then decreases from the capillary to the venules, then the veins, and lastly into the superior and inferior vena cavae. As the blood is returned to the heart via the venous system, the velocity increases.

## POISEUILLE LAW

Poiseuille law describes the steady laminar flow of Newtonian fluids. Steady flow refers to a system where flow is nonpulsatile. Laminar flow describes flow that moves in a series of layers (this will be discussed in more detail later in the chapter). A Newtonian fluid is a homogeneous fluid such as air or water.

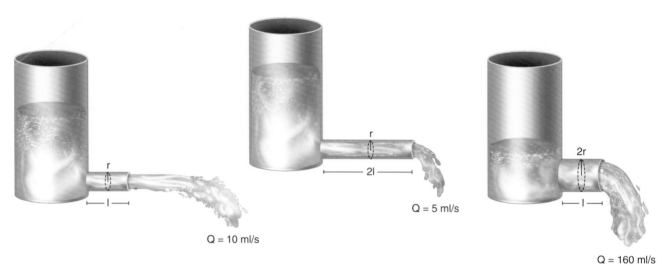

Q = 10 ml/s

Q = 5 ml/s

Q = 160 ml/s

**FIGURE 5-4** Effects of radius and length on flow.

Flow in the arterial system is pulsatile and thus not steady. Blood does tend to move in a laminar fashion at least in some portions of the arterial system. Blood is definitely not homogeneous and thus is non-Newtonian. However, even with all these variations, Poiseuille law is still used to define pressure/flow relationships in the vascular system.

The full definition of Poiseuille law is:

$$Q = \frac{\pi(P_1 - P_2)r^4}{8\eta l}$$

where $Q$ is flow, $r$ is the radius of the vessel, $l$ is the length of the vessel, $P_1 - P_2$ is the pressure difference, $\eta$ is the viscosity of the blood, and $\pi/8$ is the constant of proportionality. Examining the terms of Poiseuille law, a greater change in pressure will produce an increase in flow (provided the other components stay the same). If the viscosity of the blood increases, flow will decrease (remember the example of pouring honey vs. water). If the radius of a vessel changes, this will have a significant impact on flow because it is the radius to the fourth power, which is directly proportional to flow (Fig. 5-4). In the human body, vessel radius is the most important determinant of blood flow.

## RESISTANCE TO FLOW

Hemodynamic resistance is analogous to electrical resistance as described by Ohm law. Ohm law states that the current (flow) through two points is directly proportional to the potential difference or voltage across the two points and inversely proportional to the resistance between them.

$$I = \frac{V}{R}$$

where $I$ is the current, $V$ is the voltage, and $R$ is the resistance. If the terms are rearranged to solve for resistance, the expression becomes $R = V/I$. In the vascular system, this is represented as resistance being equal to the pressure drop divided by the flow:

$$R = \frac{\Delta P}{Q}$$

Looking back to the components of Poiseuille law, it can be determined that resistance can be expressed as:

$$R = \frac{8\eta l}{\pi r^4}$$

In the circulatory system, the length of a given vessel is virtually constant and the blood viscosity does not vary. Thus, changes in resistance are virtually all because of variations in radius. It is the smooth muscle cell layer within the media of the wall of a vessel that varies resistance by altering vessel radius.

In the vascular system, various types of vessels lie in series with one another, that is, one after another. For instance, blood flowing down to the leg goes through the aorta, then the iliac arteries, then common femoral artery, then superficial femoral artery, and so on. For resistances in series, the total resistance of the entire system equals the sum of the individual resistances (Fig. 5-5):

$$R_T = R_1 + R_2 + R_3$$

Thus, multiple stenoses along the same blood vessel will increase the total resistance.

Another arrangement in the vascular system has vessels that are arranged in parallel (or side by side) with each other. For resistances in parallel, the reciprocal of the total resistance of the system equals the sum of the reciprocals of the individual resistances (Fig. 5-6):

$$\frac{1}{R_T} = \frac{1}{R_1} + \frac{1}{R_2} + \frac{1}{R_3}$$

The more parallel elements in a network, the lower the overall resistance of the network will be. An example of a resistance in parallel is a collateral artery. A collateral artery dilates in response to ischemia produced by a flow-limiting stenosis in a main artery such as the superficial femoral artery. When adding a collateral pathway, around a stenosis, this will have the effect to lower the total resistance.

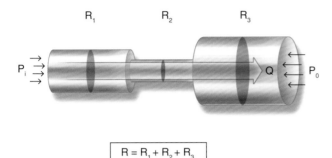

$$R = R_1 + R_2 + R_3$$

**FIGURE 5-5** A diagram illustrating multiple resistances in series.

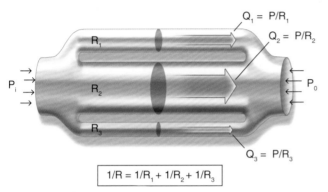

$$Q_1 = P/R_1$$
$$Q_2 = P/R_2$$
$$Q_3 = P/R_3$$

$$1/R = 1/R_1 + 1/R_2 + 1/R_3$$

**FIGURE 5-6** A diagram illustrating multiple resistances in parallel.

## PERIPHERAL RESISTANCE

Most flow can be described as either high or low resistance flow. A low resistance flow profile characteristically has antegrade flow throughout the cardiac cycle (Fig. 5-7). This is the result of dilation of the arteriolar bed. The internal carotid, vertebral, celiac, splenic, hepatic, and renal arteries will display low resistance flow. These vessels feed regions with constant high metabolic demand. The brain, liver, spleen, and kidneys are continually working at a rate that requires a great deal of oxygen and nutrients. Thus, the arterioles are open to allow for flow to meet the demand of these organs.

A high resistance flow profile displays both antegrade and retrograde flow (Fig. 5-8). In systole, flow is antegrade. In early diastole, flow reversal occurs. This is because of

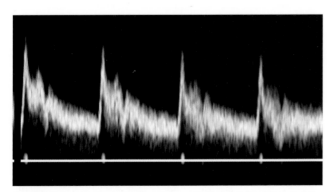

**FIGURE 5-7** A low resistance flow profile with antegrade flow throughout the cardiac cycle.

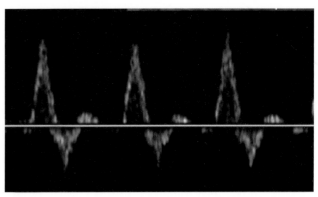

**FIGURE 5-8** A high resistance flow profile with both antegrade and retrograde flow.

slight vasoconstriction of the distal arterioles. The radius of these vessels is decreased, thus increasing the resistance to flow. As the flow traveling down the vessel encounters the high-resistance arteriolar bed, some flow is reflected back up the vessel. This produces a "reflected wave," which is apparent on ultrasound spectral analysis as well as on continuous-wave Doppler tracings and plethysmographic waveforms. Depending on the compliance of the more proximal vessels, a third antegrade flow component may be present. This feature of distensible vessels will be discussed later in this chapter. Vessels that normally display high resistance flow patterns include the external carotid, subclavian, distal aorta, iliac, fasting superior mesenteric, and resting peripheral arteries. Although these regions have a baseline demand for oxygen and nutrients, their demand is not continually elevated.

Some high-resistance tissue beds can change into low-resistance beds. This happens with extremity arteries after exercise. During exercise, the demand for oxygen and nutrients increases in the exercising muscle. Exercise produces vasodilation, which decreases the resistance to flow. This results in changing the flow profile into a low-resistance pattern with antegrade flow throughout the cardiac cycle. The same change can occur within the superior mesenteric artery. After eating, this tissue bed also vasodilates, changing the flow profile into a low-resistance pattern. In both these circumstances, the low-resistance pattern results in an increase in blood flow to meet the increased metabolic demand.

## LAMINAR AND TURBULENT FLOW

Under certain conditions, flow in a cylindrical tube (or blood vessel) will be laminar or streamlined. At the entrance to a vessel, all elements of the blood flow stream will have the same velocities (often referred to as plug flow). As the flow progresses in the vessel, a thin layer in contact with the wall will adhere to the wall and become motionless. The layer of fluid next to this layer must move against this motionless layer and therefore moves slowly because of friction between the layers. The adjacent more central layer travels a little more rapidly. The layers at the center of the tube move the fastest, and their velocity is equal to approximately twice the mean velocity across the entire cross-section of the tube. At a distance equal to several tube diameters away from the entrance, laminar flow becomes

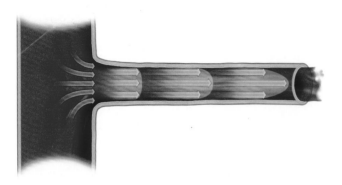

**FIGURE 5-9** Flow through a tube illustrating plug flow at the entrance of the tube and parabolic flow distal to the entrance.

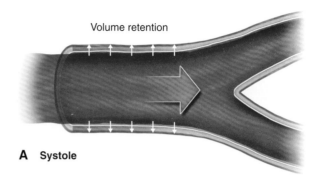

**A  Systole**

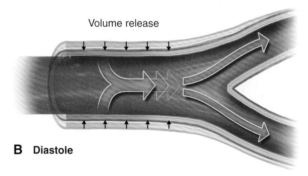

**B  Diastole**

**FIGURE 5-10** A diagram illustrating the distensibility of the arterial walls. Systole expanding the vessel walls (**A**), antegrade flow in diastole produced by the elastic recoil of the vessels (**B**).

fully developed. Thus, at the beginning of a vessel, the flow profile is rather blunted. The longitudinal velocity profile becomes parabolic at a point several diameters away from the entrance of a vessel (Fig. 5-9).

Turbulent flow is described as irregular motions of the fluid elements. Definite laminae are no longer present, but rapid radial mixing occurs. A greater pressure is required to move a given flow of fluid through a tube under turbulent conditions as compared to those for laminar flow.

Turbulence is best defined in terms of a dimensionless quantity, the Reynolds number (Re). The Reynolds number is proportional to the inertial forces and to the viscous forces acting on a fluid. In the vascular system, the Reynolds number is directly proportional to the velocity of the blood, the density of the blood, and the radius of the blood vessel. It is inversely proportional to the viscosity of the blood. Because blood density and viscosity are relatively constant, turbulence develops mainly because of changes in the velocity of blood and size of the blood vessel. For Re below 2,000, flow will be laminar. For Re above 2,000, turbulence will develop. As blood flows through a stenosis, the vessel radius is reduced by the presence of atherosclerotic disease and velocity increases. This results in turbulence, which is routinely documented as the flow exits the stenotic area.

## THE ARTERIAL SYSTEM: A HYDRAULIC FILTER

The principal function of the arterial system is to distribute blood to the capillary beds throughout the body. The arterial system consists of various sized vessels with varying volumes and distensibility. The arterial system, composed of elastic conduits and high-resistance terminals, constitutes a hydraulic filter analogous to resistance–capacitance filters of electrical circuits. Hydraulic filtering converts the intermittent (pulsatile) output of the heart to a steady flow through the capillaries. Steady flow in the capillaries ensures adequate exchange of nutrients and wastes.

The entire stroke volume is discharged from the heart during systole. Part of the energy of the cardiac contraction is dissipated as the kinetic energy of the forward blood flow. The remainder is stored as potential energy by the distensible arteries. During diastole, the elastic recoil of the arterial walls converts the potential energy into blood flow. This produces antegrade flow in late diastole (Fig. 5-10). If the arterial walls were rigid, no capillary flow would occur during diastole.

Arterial elasticity and capacitance are essential properties to allow for proper blood flow. The change in volume divided by the change in pressure represents capacitance or compliance. Normal capacitance of arteries is greatest over a median range of pressure variations. (Just like a balloon, it is hardest to inflate at the very beginning and again just before it is completely full, but it is easiest to inflate at intermediate volumes.) Capacitance decreases with age as the vessel walls become rigid. As a vessel wall becomes stiffer with age, this results in an increase in systolic pressure as well as pulse pressure. Pulse pressure is the difference between the systolic and diastolic pressures.

## CONTROL OF PERIPHERAL CIRCULATION

The peripheral circulation is controlled centrally by the nervous system and locally by conditions at the tissue bed. Vessels involved in regulating blood flow are the resistance vessels, namely the arterioles. The vessel diameter is varied by contracting or relaxing the smooth muscle cells in the medial layer of the vessel wall. The constant contraction of these muscle cells provides a degree of vasomotor tone.

The arterioles that control blood flow to a particular region or organ lie within the area or organ tissue itself. These arterioles are exposed to various chemicals in

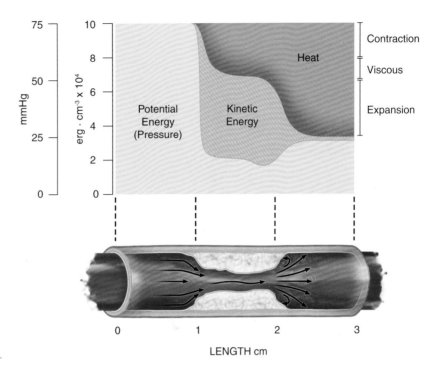

**FIGURE 5-11** Energy losses across a stenosis.

that region, and changes in concentrations of many substances can impact the arterioles. For instance, if interstitial oxygen levels fall because the cells are using more oxygen, this results in the arterioles dilating. When this vasodilation occurs, blood flow to the area will increase and bring more oxygen. This is an example of a local feedback mechanism that controls blood flow. Not only will oxygen levels alter the vasomotor tone, but carbon dioxide, hydrogen ions, and potassium ions will also have an effect. These are just a few of the substances that can locally impact blood flow.

There are nerve fibers of the sympathetic nervous system that innervate the arterioles. These nerve fibers release norepinephrine, which causes an increase in the tone of the arterioles. These vasoconstrictor nerves normally have a continual activity, resulting in a contractile tone of the arterioles.

At any given point in time, some arterioles are open and some are closed. If all arterioles were open at the same time, it would result in very low blood pressure values. Flow into many tissue beds is autoregulated. This means a constant level of blood flow is maintained over a wide range of perfusion pressures. Resistance vessels dilate in response to high blood pressure and constrict in response to low blood pressure. These actions help maintain a constant flow of oxygen and nutrients to vital organs. The heart, brain, and kidneys are all areas where autoregulation is clearly observed.

## HEMODYNAMICS OF ARTERIAL DISEASE

The development of atherosclerosis is a multifactorial process. Atherosclerotic changes begin with a lipid streak that consists of subintimal deposits of fat. Lesions that are of concern include fibrous and complicated plaques. Fibrous plaque has a smooth surface and is composed of smooth muscle and fibrous tissue and lacks calcification. Complicated plaque has an irregular surface, and loss of the normal endothelium and calcification is present. The exposure of the subendothelial collagen matrix is thrombogenic and may cause platelets to accumulate. Atherosclerosis typically develops in reproducible regions of the arterial tree including at branch points and at bifurcations. It is thought low or changing endothelial shear stress can bring about the start of atherosclerosis.

Most abnormal energy losses in the arterial system result from stenoses or obstruction of the vessel lumen (Fig. 5-11). According to Poiseuille law, viscous energy losses within a stenosis are inversely proportional to the fourth power of the radius and directly proportional to its length. Thus, the radius of a stenosis is more important than its length. Even a small change in radius will result in large changes in flow. A doubling in the length of a stenosis will yield a doubling in the associated energy losses. A decrease in the radius of a vessel by half will increase the energy losses by a factor of 16 (because it is the radius to the fourth power in Poiseuille law).

Inertial energy losses are encountered at the entrance and exit of a stenosis. More energy is lost at an abrupt change rather than a gradual tapering. A great deal more inertial energy is lost when blood exits a stenosis because the kinetic energy may be dissipated in the turbulent jet.

A critical stenosis is defined as a degree of narrowing at which pressure and flow begin to be affected. Experimentally, changes in pressure and flow do not occur until the cross-sectional area has been reduced by 75% (or 50% diameter reduction). Because energy losses also depend on the velocity of blood flow, in high-flow (low-resistance) systems, significant drops in pressures and flow occur with

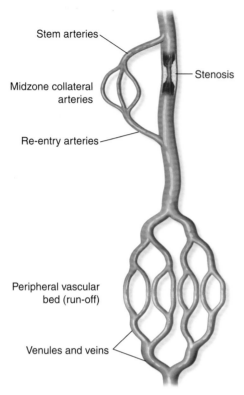

Stem arteries

Stenosis

Midzone collateral arteries

Re-entry arteries

Peripheral vascular bed (run-off)

Venules and veins

**FIGURE 5-12** Collateral arteries including stem arteries, midzone collaterals, and reentry arteries.

less severe narrowing than in low-flow systems. Therefore, a critical stenosis varies with the resistance of the run-off bed. In the carotid or coronary systems (low-resistance systems), a critical stenosis may be reached with less narrowing than in the resting lower extremity (high resistance). In the exercising leg, resistance drops, flow increases, and a stenosis may become critical or flow limiting.

Collateral vessels are preexisting pathways that enlarge with a stenosis or occlusion. They are one of the main mechanisms to compensate for a stenosis. Collateral arteries can be divided into (1) stem arteries, which are the large branches; (2) midzone collaterals, which are the small intramuscular branches; and (3) reentry arteries, which are the vessels that rejoin a major artery distal to the area of stenosis or occlusion (Fig. 5-12). The resistance of the collateral bed is almost fixed and will only slightly dilate gradually. Exercise, sympathectomy, and vasodilator drugs have little effect on collaterals unlike the peripheral run-off bed.

Blood flow increases with exercise to at least three to five times resting flow in normal limbs. In limbs with mild to moderate disease, blood flow is increased far less. In patients with multilevel disease, flow after exercise may change very little. At rest, blood pressure distal to an arterial lesion will be decreased with mild to moderate disease and even more with severe disease. Exercise will cause a further decrease in peripheral pressure.

## SUMMARY

- Energy within the vascular system is made up of potential energy stored as intravascular pressure and kinetic energy represented by the velocity of moving blood.
- The hemodynamics of the arterial system includes unique relationships between pressure, resistance, and flow.
- Blood flow will follow the same rules that govern the movement of other fluids.
- Blood flow is determined by changes in pressure and resistance.
- The greatest impact to blood flow is the radius of a blood vessel.
- Arterioles are the main source of resistance within the vascular system.
- There are high-resistance and low-resistance vascular beds, which are determined by their metabolic demands.
- Changes across a stenosis will result in changes in pressure and velocity distal to the stenosis.
- Understanding the factors that influence the movement of blood flow in the arterial system will make it easier to understand the velocities and waveforms encountered during ultrasound examinations.

## CRITICAL THINKING QUESTIONS

1. You are examining a patient with a lower extremity bypass graft from the common femoral artery to the popliteal artery. The flow is constant throughout the graft but at one point you detect a velocity increase on spectral analysis. What must be happening in this area?
2. Would increasing the viscosity of blood or increasing the length of a conduit have a greater effect on decreasing blood flow?
3. You examine a popliteal artery that displays continuous forward (antegrade) flow throughout the entire cardiac cycle. In the absence of any disease or pathology, what is the most likely explanation of these findings?

## MEDIA MENU

Student Resources available on thePoint® include:
- Audio glossary
- Interactive question bank
- Videos
- Internet resources

### SUGGESTED READINGS

Carter SA. Hemodynamic considerations in peripheral vascular and cerebrovascular disease. In: Zwiebel WJ, Pellerito JS, eds. *Introduction to Vascular Ultrasonography*. 5th ed. Philadelphia, PA: Elsevier Saunders; 2005:3–17.
Guyton AC, Hall JE. *Textbook of Medical Physiology*. 11th ed. Philadelphia, PA: Saunders; 2005.
Koeppen BM, Stanton BA. *Berne & Levy Physiology*. 6th ed. Philadelphia, PA: Mosby; 2009.

Mohrman DE, Heller LJ. *Cardiovascular Physiology*. New York, NY: McGraw-Hill; 1997.
Oates C, ed. *Cardiovascular Haemodynamics and Doppler Waveforms Explained*. Cambridge, England: Cambridge University Press; 2001.
Zierler RE. Hemodynamics of normal and abnormal arteries. *Strandness's Duplex Scanning in Vascular Disorders*. 4th ed. Philadelphia, PA: Lippincott Williams & Wilkins; 2010:47–55.

# Venous Physiology

ANN MARIE KUPINKSI

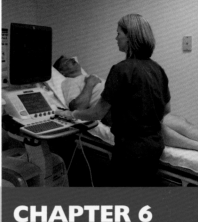

## CHAPTER 6

## OBJECTIVES

- List the hemodynamic factors that affect venous blood flow
- Describe the components of hydrostatic pressure
- Identify the forces that lead to edema formation
- Define the changes that occur at rest and with exercise in the venous system

## KEY TERMS

**calf muscle pump**

**edema**

**hydrostatics**

**resistance**

**transmural pressure**

**valvular incompetence**

## GLOSSARY

**edema** Excessive accumulation of fluid in cells, tissues, or cavities of the body

**hydrostatic pressure** The pressure within the vascular system because of the weight of a column of blood

**transmural pressure** The pressure on the walls of a vessel

**valvular insufficiency** Retrograde flow across a venous valve of an abnormal duration

The venous system is usually perceived to be rather passive. It is generally believed that the arterial system does all the work and the veins just simply return the blood back to the heart. However, veins act as an important reservoir for blood volume and are required to efficiently return blood to the heart. Changes in venous blood flow can cause various complications from varicose veins to pulmonary emboli, in addition to cardiac problems as a result of abnormal venous return. Venous disease affects a significant portion of the population. Several factors impact the movement of blood throughout the venous system. The following chapter will present the major features of venous physiology and pathophysiology.

## VENOUS CAPACITANCE

Veins are known as the capacitance vessels of the body. They serve an important role acting as a reservoir. The venous side of the circulatory system holds approximately two-thirds of the total blood volume of the body (Fig. 6-1). The arterial side of the circulatory system typically holds about 30% of the blood volume, with the remaining 3% to 4% within the capillaries. The cross-sectional area of a fully distended vein can be three to four times that of the

corresponding companion artery. Often, the veins are paired structures and this adds to their ability to hold blood.

## VENOUS RESISTANCE

By changing the cross-sectional area, veins can vary their resistance to blood flow. When partially empty, they assume an elliptical cross-sectional shape, which offers a great deal of resistance to blood flow. When distended, veins offer almost no resistance to blood flow as they take on a more circular shape. Remember the importance of the radius of a vessel to the resistance. Their ability to change shape permits veins to accommodate increases in blood flow without causing increases in the pressure gradient to the heart.

At several areas within the body, veins naturally offer resistance to flow. Veins tend to collapse as they enter the thorax. The subclavian veins are compressed by the first rib. The jugular veins collapse because of atmospheric pressure. Changes in resistance to flow within these upper extremity veins are usually minimal but can vary depending on the patient position and intravascular pressures. The inferior vena cava can be compressed by abdominal organs and intraabdominal pressure, both of which will impact the venous return through the vena cava. The impact of

| Arteries | Capillaries | Veins |
|----------|-------------|-------|
| 30% | 2% | 60% |

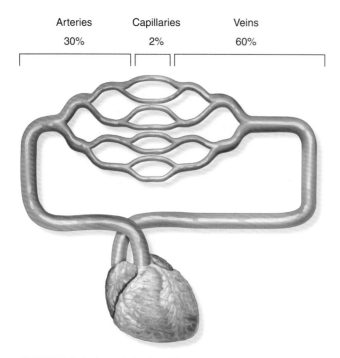

**FIGURE 6-1** A schematic drawing of the distribution of blood volume through the circulatory system.

**Arterial**

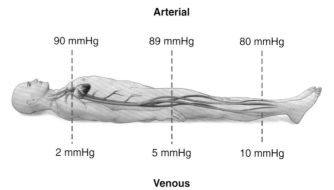

| 90 mmHg | 89 mmHg | 80 mmHg |
|---------|---------|---------|
| 2 mmHg | 5 mmHg | 10 mmHg |

**Venous**

**FIGURE 6-3** Pressures within the arteries and veins in a supine individual.

intraabdominal pressure on resistance to venous flow will be discussed in more detail when describing resting venous dynamics later in the chapter.

## HYDROSTATICS

A major force affecting the venous system is hydrostatic pressure. Hydrostatic pressure is caused by the weight of a fluid as measured compared to a reference point. As stated in the preceding chapter, the reference point of the human body is the right atrium. Hydrostatic pressure is equal to $\rho \times g \times h$, where $\rho$ is the density of blood, $g$ is the acceleration due to gravity, and $h$ is the height of the column of blood.

Pressure within a blood vessel is equal to the dynamic pressure supplied by the contraction of the heart plus the hydrostatic pressure (Fig. 6-2). Hydrostatic pressure affects both the arteries and the veins equally. Because the dynamic pressure is so low in the veins, the hydrostatic pressure plays a greater role in determining the overall venous pressure. When supine, all the arteries and veins are roughly at the same level as the right atrium; therefore, the hydrostatic pressure is negligible (Fig. 6-3). Pressure throughout the vascular system is roughly equal to the dynamic pressure. In this position, the pressure in the veins at the ankle level is about 10 to 15 mm Hg. The pressure decreases steadily as the blood is returned to the right side of the heart where right atrial pressure is 2 to 6 mm Hg.

When standing, an individual (who is approximately 6 ft tall) will add a hydrostatic pressure component of about 102 mm Hg at the ankle. This occurs in both the arteries and the veins so that the pressure gradient across the capillary bed is the same as it was in the supine position (about 80 mm Hg).

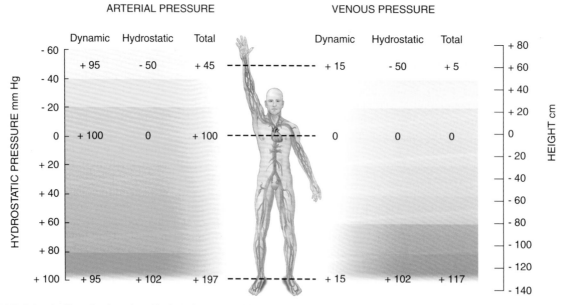

**FIGURE 6-2** A drawing illustrating dynamic and hydrostatic pressure within the vascular system.

During exercise, the pressure in the veins falls to below 20 mm Hg. This has the result of increasing the pressure gradient (to about 177 mm Hg) across the capillaries. This increased pressure gradient will increase blood flow needed during exercise. Remember from the preceding chapter that blood will move down an energy (pressure) gradient, and the bigger the gradient, the more the flow.

In an uplifted arm, the hydrostatic pressure is negative. The hydrostatic pressure at the wrist would be approximately −50 mm Hg. Combining the hydrostatic pressure with a dynamic pressure of 15 mm Hg would yield a total intravascular pressure of −35 mm Hg. However, pressure within the veins cannot fall to below the tissue pressure of 5 mm Hg or the veins would collapse and no blood flow would occur. The pressure gradient across the capillary in this uplifted arm does decrease to 40 mm Hg as compared to 80 mm Hg in the supine position. The decrease in the pressure gradient explains why it is more difficult to work with the arm raised above the head.

## PRESSURE–VOLUME RELATIONSHIPS

Because veins are collapsible tubes, their shape is determined by transmural pressure. Transmural pressure equals the difference between the pressure within the vein and the tissue pressure. At low transmural pressure, a vein will assume a dumbbell shape. As the pressure within a vein increases, the vein will become elliptical. At high transmural pressures, the vein will become circular (Fig. 6-4).

Changes in vein shape are associated with large increases in venous volume (Fig. 6-5). As such, veins can accommodate large changes in volume with very little changes in pressure. This occurs over a pressure range of 5 to 25 mm Hg. The walls of a vein are rather elastic, but a very large change in pressure is needed to change the volume of the vein when it is circular as compared to partially collapsed and elliptical. When supine, the transmural pressure is low. However, upon standing, the pressure increases and the walls stiffen such that the venous volume will change little even with large changes in pressure.

Elastic compression stockings are available in varying degrees of pressure, with some patients wearing stockings with 15 mm Hg pressure. This pressure is exerted on the limb, producing an increase in the tissue pressure. Thus, with 15 mm Hg stockings, the tissue pressure increases from about 5 to 15 mm Hg. This results in a net decrease in the transmural pressure of 10 mm Hg. When supine, this 10 mm Hg

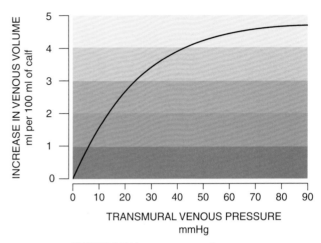

**FIGURE 6-5** Venous pressure–volume curve.

difference will greatly reduce venous volume. However, when standing, these low-pressure compression stockings will have little effect because of the increased pressure within the vein as a result of the hydrostatic pressure. This is one reason why higher pressure compression stockings are often employed to aid individuals while sitting or standing.

## EDEMA

Edema is a consistent sign of increased venous pressure. The Starling equilibrium describes the movement of fluid across the capillary (Fig. 6-6). Forces that act to move fluid out of the capillary are the intracapillary pressure and the interstitial osmotic pressure. Forces that tend to favor the reabsorption of fluid from the interstitium are the interstitial pressure and the capillary osmotic pressure. Osmotic pressure is the pressure exerted by the fluid when there is a difference in the concentrations of solutes across a semipermeable membrane, in this case the capillary endothelium. Normally, the forces are fairly balanced so that there is little overall fluid loss. What little fluid normally moves out into

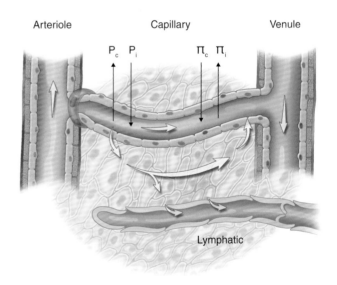

**FIGURE 6-6** The Starling forces governing the movement of fluid across the capillary bed.

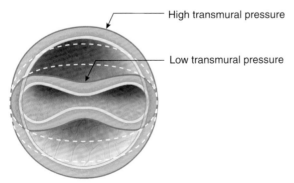

**FIGURE 6-4** The effects of transmural pressure on the shape of a vein.

**Inspiration**

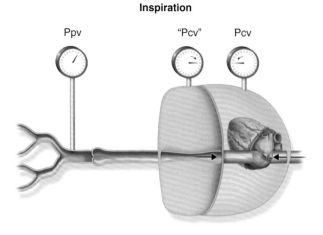

**Expiration**

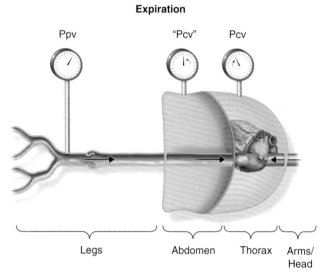

Legs　　Abdomen　Thorax　Arms/
　　　　　　　　　　　　　　　Head

**FIGURE 6-7** Resting venous flow and changes with respiration.

the interstitial space is picked up by the lymphatics. While standing, the increased capillary pressure is no longer balanced by the reabsorptive forces, and fluid loss occurs. Edema formation is limited by the action of the calf muscle pump. The contraction of the calf muscles acts to empty the veins and decrease the venous pressure. In the presence of venous thrombosis, the venous pressure is increased. The increased venous pressure will be transmitted back through the venous system, into the smaller veins, venules, and finally the capillaries. This increase in pressure at the capillary level will result in edema formation. As described earlier, the use of compression stockings will increase the interstitial pressure, which will favor an increase in fluid reabsorption, thus decreasing edema. Elevating the legs will reduce the intracapillary pressure (by lowering the hydrostatic pressure), which also limits edema formation.

## VENOUS DYNAMICS AT REST

Changes in intrathoracic and intraabdominal pressure have a profound effect on the venous return to the heart. During inspiration, the diaphragm descends, which decreases the pressure in the chest cavity. This causes blood to pool into the pulmonary vascular bed and also pulls air into the lungs. Also during inspiration, the descending movement of the diaphragm results in an increase in intraabdominal pressure. This partially collapses the inferior vena cava, which impedes venous return from the legs. Upon expiration, the diaphragm moves upward, which decreases intraabdominal pressure. This results in an increase in blood flow from the legs and a decrease in blood flow into the thorax (Fig. 6-7).

In the presence of a deep venous thrombosis, venous pressure is increased in the legs because of an increase in venous resistance caused by the occluded or partially occluded veins (Fig. 6-8). Variations in abdominal pressure

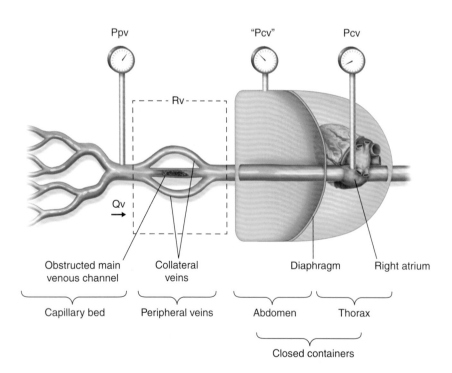

Obstructed main　　Collateral　　　Diaphragm　　Right atrium
venous channel　　　veins

Capillary bed　　Peripheral veins　　Abdomen　　　Thorax

Closed containers

**FIGURE 6-8** Venous pressure changes associated with deep venous thrombosis.

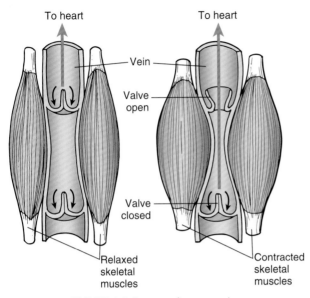

To heart        To heart

Vein

Valve
open

Valve
closed

Relaxed
skeletal
muscles

Contracted
skeletal
muscles

**FIGURE 6-9** Structure of a venous valve.

within the gastrocnemius and soleus muscles as well as the deep and superficial veins all play a part in this mechanism. The venous valves are necessary to ensure efficient action of the muscle pump (Fig. 6-9). Closure of the valves in the deep veins decreases the length of the column of blood, which helps reduce the venous pressure.

At rest, blood pools in the leg and is only propelled passively by the dynamic pressure gradient created by the contraction of the left ventricle. Contraction of the calf muscles can generate pressures greater than 200 mm Hg. This compresses the veins, forcing blood upward (back to the heart) in both the deep and superficial veins. The valves are closed in the perforating veins and in the veins of the distal calf to prevent reflux or retrograde flow of the blood. Upon relaxation, because the veins in the calf are empty, blood is drawn into the area from the superficial veins via perforators. More distal veins also help to fill the calf veins upon relaxation (Fig. 6-10). In the more proximal segments of the leg, the valves close to prevent reflux of blood from these segments.

with respiration have little effect on the pressure gradient from the legs. Normal phasic venous flow from the lower extremity may be reduced or absent. Venous flow from the legs may become continuous as the venous pressures in the legs exceed the normal changes in intraabdominal venous pressures.

## VENOUS DYNAMICS WITH EXERCISE

The calf muscle pump aids in the return of blood from the legs against the force of gravity (hydrostatic pressure). The muscles act as the power source. The intramuscular sinusoids

## DISORDERS

### Primary Varicose Veins

Varicose veins that develop in the absence of a deep venous thrombosis are referred to as primary varicose veins. In the presence of primary varicose veins, incompetent valves may be found in the common femoral and great saphenous veins. In some patients, valves may be congenitally absent from the common femoral and iliac veins. Only rarely are primary varicose veins associated with the small saphenous vein. With primary varicose veins, the calf muscle pump still works to propel blood upward during a contraction.

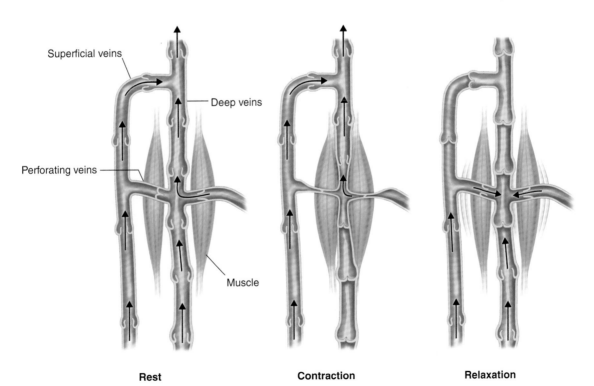

Superficial veins

Deep veins

Perforating veins

Muscle

**Rest**        **Contraction**        **Relaxation**

**FIGURE 6-10** Patterns of normal venous flow at rest and with calf contraction.

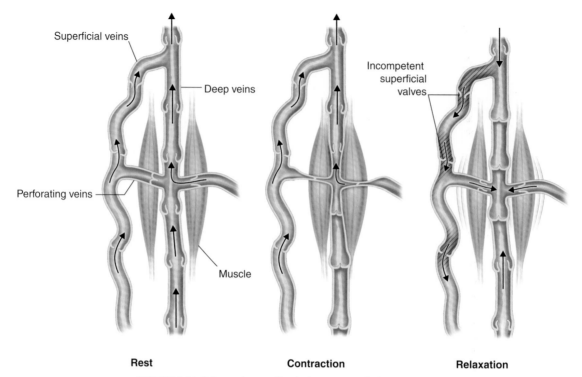

**FIGURE 6-11** Patterns of venous flow in the presence of primary varicose veins.

However, during relaxation, blood falls back down the superficial veins because of valvular incompetence (Fig. 6-11). This blood then reenters the deep system through the perforators. This creates an inefficient circular motion of blood. Venous pressure is increased because of the presence of a long column of blood caused by the incompetent valves.

## Secondary Varicose Veins

Secondary varicose veins are mainly the result of deep venous thrombosis. The valves in the deep, superficial, and perforating veins are incompetent, and there may be a degree of residual venous obstruction (Fig. 6-12). Because

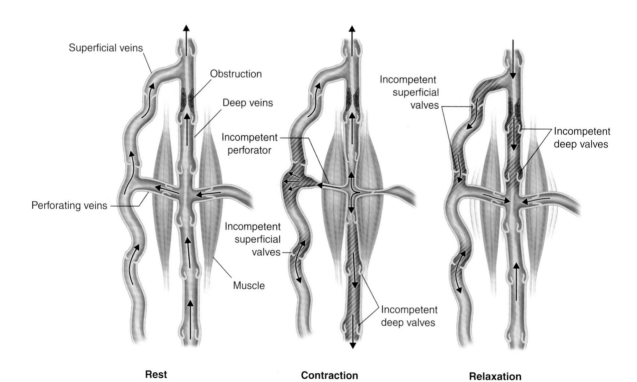

**FIGURE 6-12** Patterns of venous flow in the presence of secondary varicose veins.

of the obstruction, the superficial veins may function as collaterals, and blood may flow out from the deep to the superficial veins even at rest. Venous flow patterns are completely disrupted in these patients. The flow through the perforators can be bidirectional, thus increasing pressure within the superficial system. More blood is forced distally because of the incompetent valves in both the deep and superficial systems, resulting in increased venous pressure. If residual thrombus is present, the proximal obstruction to flow will also add to increased venous pressure in the leg.

## Venous Stasis Ulcers

The effect of persistent increased venous pressure or venous hypertension is distention of the capillaries and increased capillary pressure. This results in slightly opening the junctions between the endothelial cells. This will cause plasma proteins to move out of the vascular space and into the tissue. As a consequence of this protein movement, additional fluid will also enter the interstitial space. There are several theories as to how tissue damage occurs leading to ulceration. One theory involves fibrin accumulating around the capillaries in the interstitial space. This collection of fibrin, termed a fibrin cuff, leads to limited oxygen transfer across the capillaries. Another theory involves the migration and trapping of white blood cells in the capillaries and venules. The plugging of the capillaries and venules by these white blood cells also results in limited oxygen transfer into the tissue bed. The decreased oxygen transfer produces tissue ischemia. As the ischemia progresses, ulceration occurs. Venous stasis ulcers are a serious end result of this extreme form of venous disease.

## Pregnancy and Varicose Veins

During pregnancy, the inferior vena cava and the iliac veins can be compressed by the enlarged gravid uterus while lying supine, particularly in the third trimester. This can produce a continuous venous outflow signal from the legs that is no longer responsive to changes in pressure brought on by respiration. This change in lower extremity venous flow is a result of increased venous pressure because of compression of the pelvic veins. This can be alleviated somewhat by turning the patient on her side so that the weight of the gravid uterus no longer impinges on the venous structures.

Humoral factors circulating during pregnancy cause the veins to be more compliant. This increase in compliance plus the increased venous pressure that occurs later in pregnancy because of the size of the uterus can cause significant venous distention. The final result is a decrease in the velocity of venous flow out of the legs. This can contribute to the development of a deep venous thrombosis.

Pregnancy does not cause varicose veins. Increased venous pressure and venous distention can magnify predisposing factors. Thus, varicose veins often first appear during pregnancy. Typically, varicose veins become more severe with subsequent pregnancies.

### SUMMARY

- Veins are the capacitance vessels of the body.
- By changing shape, veins can offer resistance to flow.
- Pressure caused by the weight of a fluid as measured to a reference point is known as hydrostatic pressure.
- Venous capacitance, transmural pressure, hydrostatic pressure, as well as other anatomic and physiologic components help to govern venous flow.
- When transmural pressure is low, veins are elliptical. When transmural pressure is high, veins are circular.
- Edema is a sign of increased venous pressure.
- The calf muscle pump and venous valves help move blood from the legs back to the heart in an efficient manner.
- Primary varicose veins are associated with incompetent valves within the superficial veins.
- Secondary varicose veins are associated with prior deep venous thrombosis. Valves in the deep, superficial, and perforating veins may be incompetent.
- Venous physiology impacts what is observed on the ultrasound image as well as the venous Doppler signals obtained during a duplex ultrasound examination.

### CRITICAL THINKING QUESTIONS

1. You are examining a patient's calf veins with ultrasound and the veins appear small and difficult to visualize. The patient is lying supine with their head slightly elevated. What is one simple change not involving the ultrasound system that can be done to make the veins easier to image?
2. Is the venous pressure higher or lower than normal in a common femoral vein that demonstrates a continuous venous Doppler signal with no respiratory phasicity?
3. A patient presents for a venous examination with clinically evident varicose veins and no history of a deep vein thrombosis or venous ulceration. Would venous insufficiency be more likely in the deep or superficial system or both?

### MEDIA MENU

Student Resources available on thePoint® include:
- Audio glossary
- Interactive question bank
- Videos
- Internet resources

## SUGGESTED READINGS

1. Carter SA. Hemodynamic considerations in peripheral vascular and cerebrovascular disease. In: Zwiebel WJ, Pellerito JS, eds. *Introduction to Vascular Ultrasonography*. 5th ed. Philadelphia, PA: Elsevier Saunders; 2005:3–17.
2. Eberhardt RT, Raffetto JD. Chronic venous insufficiency. *Circulation*. 2005;111:2398–2409.
3. Guyton AC, Hall JE. *Textbook of Medical Physiology*. 11th ed. Philadelphia, PA: Saunders; 2005.
4. Koeppen BM, Stanton BA. *Berne & Levy Physiology*. 6th ed. Philadelphia, PA: Mosby; 2009.
5. Kupinski AM. Dynamics of venous disease. *Vascular US Today*. 2006;11:1–20.
6. Meissner MH. Venous anatomy and hemodynamics. In: Zierler RE, ed. *Strandness's Duplex Scanning in Vascular Disorders*. 4th ed. Philadelphia, PA: Lippincott Williams & Wilkins; 2010:56–60.
7. Mohrman DE, Heller LJ. *Cardiovascular Physiology*. New York, NY: McGraw-Hill; 1997.
8. Oates C, ed. *Cardiovascular Haemodynamics and Doppler Waveforms Explained*. Cambridge, England: Cambridge University Press; 2001.

# PART THREE

# CEREBROVASCULAR

# The Extracranial Duplex Ultrasound Examination

KARI A. CAMPBELL    |    R. EUGENE ZIERLER

## CHAPTER 7

## OBJECTIVES

- List the essential components of a carotid duplex ultrasound examination
- Describe the normal waveform characteristics of the extracranial carotid vessels
- Define the common diagnostic criteria used to evaluate the extracranial carotid vessels
- Describe common pathology observed during a carotid duplex ultrasound examination

## KEY TERMS

**carotid artery**

**carotid duplex**

**Doppler waveform**

**extracranial cerebrovascular disease**

**spectral analysis**

**stroke**

**vertebral artery**

**transient ischemic attack (TIA)**

## GLOSSARY

**bruit** An abnormal "blowing" or "swishing" sound heard with a stethoscope while auscultating over an artery such as the carotid. The sound results from vibrations that are transmitted through the tissues when blood flows through a stenotic artery. Although the presence of a bruit is a sign of arterial disease, the absence of a bruit is less diagnostic, because all stenoses are not associated with bruits

**carotid bulb** A slight dilation involving variable portions of the distal common and proximal internal carotid arteries, often including the origin of the external carotid artery. This is where the baroreceptors assisting in reflex blood pressure control are located. The carotid bulb tends to be most prominent in normal young individuals

**Doppler angle** Most commonly defined as the angle between the line of the Doppler ultrasound beam emitted by the transducer and the arterial wall (also referred to as the "angle of insonation"). This is a key variable in the Doppler equation used to calculate flow velocity

**spectral analysis** It is a signal processing technique that displays the complete frequency and amplitude content of the Doppler flow signal. The spectral information is usually presented as waveforms with frequency (converted to a velocity scale) on the vertical axis, time on the horizontal axis, and amplitude indicated by a gray scale

**spectral broadening** An increase in the "width" of the spectral waveform (frequency band) or "filling-in" of the normally clear area under the systolic peak. This represents turbulent blood flow associated with arterial lesions

**transient ischemic attack (TIA)** An episode of stroke-like neurologic symptoms that typically lasts for a few minutes to several hours and then resolves completely. This is caused by temporary interruption of the blood supply to the brain in the distribution of a cerebral artery

Evaluation of the extracranial cerebral vasculature was the first clinical application of the duplex ultrasound device that was developed at the University of Washington in the late 1970s.[1,2] Although B-mode imaging and Doppler flow detection had been used separately to characterize vascular disorders, the duplex concept combined real-time B-mode imaging and pulsed Doppler flow detection in a single instrument to obtain both anatomic and physiologic information on the status of blood vessels. In addition to the B-mode imaging and pulsed Doppler systems, the first duplex scanning instrument contained a spectrum analyzer for generating Doppler spectral waveforms. The position of the Doppler beam and the pulsed Doppler sample volume were indicated by a line and a cursor superimposed on the B-mode image. Ultrasound technology has advanced significantly since the introduction of the duplex scanner, with improved B-mode image resolution, a wider selection of transducers, and alternative approaches to displaying flow information such as color Doppler and power Doppler. Unlike contrast arteriography, which can be interpreted in terms of a specific percentage of diameter reduction, duplex scanning classifies arterial lesions into categories that include ranges of stenosis severity.

The primary goal of noninvasive testing for extracranial cerebrovascular disease is to identify patients who are at risk for stroke due to atherosclerotic plaque and facilitate treatment by either carotid endarterectomy (CEA), stenting, or aggressive medical management of modifiable risk factors. A secondary goal is to document progressive disease in patients already known to be at risk or recurrent stenosis after intervention. Duplex scanning can also detect a variety of nonatherosclerotic conditions that involve the extracranial carotid and vertebral arteries, such as dissection, fibromuscular dysplasia, trauma, arteritis, radiation effects, and aneurysms.

## SONOGRAPHIC EXAMINATION TECHNIQUES

The major indications for a duplex scan of the carotid and vertebral arteries include an asymptomatic neck bruit; hemispheric cerebral or ocular transient ischemic attacks (TIAs); a history of stroke; screening prior to major cardiac, peripheral vascular, or other surgery; and follow-up after CEA or stenting. Atherosclerotic lesions of the extracranial carotid arteries can be present without neurologic symptoms, and some may produce a neck bruit. Experience has shown that only about one-third of bruits are related to high-grade (≥50% diameter reducing) internal carotid stenoses.[3,4] Symptoms of cerebrovascular disease can be produced by emboli from atherosclerotic plaques, reduction of flow caused by high-grade stenoses, and arterial thrombosis. An important mechanism for both transient and permanent neurologic deficits appears to be small emboli consisting of platelet aggregates or atheromatous debris arising from ulcerated plaques in the extracranial carotid system. Hemorrhage or necrosis within a plaque may lead to ulceration and the appearance of symptoms. Although high-grade stenoses can reduce flow through the involved internal carotid artery (ICA), this is rarely a primary cause of symptoms because of the collateral circulation available through the circle of Willis.

Symptoms typically associated with extracranial carotid artery lesions include TIAs, amaurosis fugax, reversible ischemic neurologic deficits (RINDs), and strokes. A TIA is sometimes referred to as a "mini stroke" and is characterized by focal weakness (paralysis) or numbness (paresthesia) involving some combination of the face, arm, and leg on one side of the body. Difficulty in speaking (aphasia) may also occur. These symptoms occur on the side of the body opposite to the affected carotid artery and cerebral hemisphere. Symptoms of a TIA typically last from several minutes to a few hours, but not longer than 24 hours. Amaurosis fugax is a TIA of the eye that produces transient monocular blindness on the same side as the responsible carotid artery lesion. A RIND is similar to a TIA but with symptoms lasting between about 24 and 72 hours. A stroke, also known as a cerebrovascular accident (CVA), results in fixed or permanent neurologic deficits. The symptoms of vertebrobasilar arterial insufficiency are less specific than those related to the carotid circulation and include dizziness, diplopia, and ataxia. In general, patients with transient neurologic symptoms in the distribution of an ICA (TIAs, RINDs, and amaurosis fugax) are considered to be at risk for stroke.[5] For patients with TIAs, the overall stroke risk is about 6% per year, with a 12% risk of stroke during the first year after onset of symptoms. Patients who survive their initial stroke have a continuing stroke risk in the range of 6% to 11% per year.[6]

## Patient Preparation

In preparation for a carotid artery duplex evaluation, the patient should remove jewelry and tight clothing from the neck area, allowing unobstructed access to the cervical carotid artery segments. Interview the patient to obtain the pertinent past medical history and current signs or symptoms that prompted the request for a carotid duplex evaluation (Table 7-1). A brief physical examination can

---

**TABLE 7-1  Patient Interview for Pertinent Medical History**

- Are you being treated for high blood pressure (hypertension)?
- Are you being treated for high cholesterol (hypercholesterolemia)?
- Do you have diabetes? If so, for how long? Is it treated with diet control, oral medication, or insulin?
- Have you ever had a heart attack (myocardial infarction) or chest pains?
- Have you ever had surgery or other interventions on any of your blood vessels (coronary artery bypass graft or stent placement, carotid endarterectomy or stent placement, peripheral arterial revascularization)?
- Have you had a stroke or "mini stroke" (CVA, TIA) in the past?
- Have you recently experienced or are you currently experiencing stroke-like symptoms:
  - weakness or numbness down one side of your body
  - difficulty with balance or walking
  - slurred speech or difficulty forming words
  - dizziness, nausea, or vomiting
  - severe headache
  - vision disturbances such as "cloudiness" or perhaps like a "shade" coming down over one eye or the other

be performed that includes palpation of pulses for strength and symmetry (carotid, axillary, brachial, and radial) and auscultation with a stethoscope for bruits (high, mid, and low neck, and in the region of the clavicle).

## Patient Positioning

Place the patient in a supine position on the stretcher. The head of the bed may be elevated, and a pillow placed beneath the patient's knees for comfort. In rare instances when the patient cannot tolerate lying supine, the examination may be performed with the patient sitting in a chair, although this is not an ideal position because of potential patient movement and poor ergonomics for the sonographer or vascular technologist. Position a pillow beneath the patient's head and shoulders, and adjust it to have the patient's chin tilted up toward the ceiling, rather than down toward the chest. If this cannot be accomplished, forego the pillow and place a towel underneath the patient's neck for support. The patient's head should be turned away from the side examined, approximately 45 degrees from the midline (Fig. 7-1).

### Avoiding Repetitive Stress Injury

Sonographer/technologist comfort and career longevity depend greatly on avoiding repetitive stress injuries (RSI) by proper positioning during the examination. Being ambidextrous, practicing flexibility, and careful placement of equipment can help lessen the severity of RSI symptoms. Being ambidextrous can be particularly helpful. A sonographer or technologist should develop the ability to scan with either hand. Alternating scanning hands will extend the life of hands, arms, and shoulders by taking stress off one set of muscles at various times throughout the day. Practice flexibility by keeping muscles limber and stretched while keeping hydrated. Taking time to stretch the hands, arms, shoulders, and back before and after each examination is imperative to the prevention of RSI. There are many written, diagrammatic, and video resources available demonstrating these techniques. Maintaining proper hydration allows muscles to be less vulnerable to injury and promotes

healing. Position the equipment properly by taking time to arrange the stretcher or bed and the ultrasound machine, getting as close to the patient as possible. Particularly on an inpatient floor, this often involves moving equipment and furniture around the room to allow access close to the patient. Develop the ability to scan from the right and left sides as well as from the head of the bed. To decrease strain on the neck and shoulder muscles, the scanning arm should be maintained as close to the technologist's body as possible. Rolled towels or the bed can be used to support the scanning arm.

## Equipment

Proper transducer selection is essential to successfully completing the carotid artery duplex evaluation. The two key factors to consider when selecting a transducer are the transmit frequency for image quality and the transducer "footprint" for ultrasound access to the area of interest (Fig. 7-2). A linear array transducer with a 7 to 4 MHz frequency will generally provide the best image resolution and most options for Doppler angle correction; the midrange transmit frequencies provide high-resolution image at depths of 2.0 to 10.0 cm. The footprint of this transducer is rectangular (approximately 4.0 cm long) and narrow (approximately 1.0 cm wide).

An alternative transducer selection may be warranted in certain circumstances. A curvilinear array with a frequency range of 8 to 5 MHz is preferred when access to the neck is limited, as is the case with a short neck, internal jugular intravenous lines, or tracheotomy ties. This transducer provides similar image quality to a 7 to 4 MHz linear array because of similar midrange transmit frequency, but the face of the transducer is slightly curved, with a small rectangular footprint that is approximately 2.5 cm in length and narrow (approximately 0.5 cm wide). This is an excellent type of transducer to access areas around lines and bony structures. Use of a phased array, sector 4 to 1 MHz or curvilinear 5 to 2 MHz transducer may be necessary when vessels are located more deeply than usual in the neck.

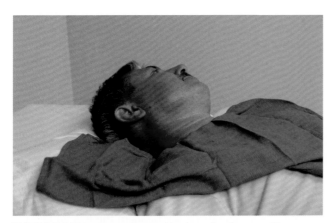

**FIGURE 7-1** The correct patient position for performing a carotid artery duplex evaluation. The patient's chin is elevated, and the head is turned 45 degrees away from the side being examined.

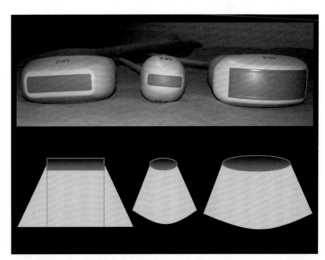

**FIGURE 7-2** Suitable transducers and image shapes for performing a carotid artery duplex evaluation: linear 9 to 3 MHz (for average size necks), curvilinear 8 to 5 MHz (for short necks and small spaces), and curvilinear 5 to 2 MHz (for deeper depths).

## Scanning Technique

The carotid artery duplex evaluation generally includes bilateral examination of the common carotid artery (CCA), ICA, and external carotid artery (ECA), as well as the vertebral artery at midneck and proximal subclavian artery. In special circumstances, a unilateral or limited evaluation may be performed. The carotid arteries are interrogated in both transverse- and long-axis orientations using grayscale B-mode imaging, color Doppler ultrasound and pulsed wave (PW) spectral Doppler.

Beginning with B-mode imaging, place the transducer on the anterolateral neck midway between the clavicle and the angle of the mandible to locate the vessels. Sweep along the carotid arteries in transverse orientation from the clavicle to the angle of the mandible. Move the transducer to the more anterior and posterior aspects of the neck to locate the clearest image path, and observe the location of the arteries and veins relative to one another. Turn the transducer into the long-axis plane, and image the length of the CCA, ICA, and ECA from the clavicle to above the angle of the mandible. Document intraluminal echoes representing plaque or other intimal defects, as well as any other areas of interest throughout the carotid arteries and surrounding tissues. Minimal B-mode image documentation should include long-axis views of the CCA, bifurcation region, and ICA.

Next, use the color Doppler modality to image the carotid segments in transverse orientation, and sweep once again from the clavicle to the angle of the mandible. The color Doppler scale is based on mean flow velocity, and this scale should generally be set in the range of 20 to 40 cm/s. Document the distal CCA and the proximal ICA and ECA at the bifurcation in both transverse and long-axis or longitudinal orientations. In addition, document any color Doppler disturbance, areas of aliasing, or mosaic flow patterns, and observe any color Doppler speckling in the tissues that may indicate a color Doppler bruit.

The PW spectral-Doppler modality is then selected, beginning low in the neck on the right, insonating the brachiocephalic (innominate) artery if possible. As previously stated, utilization of a smaller footprint transducer is often ideal for insonating behind the clavicle or sternum. Evaluations of the distal segment of the brachiocephalic artery and origins of the right and left CCA are considered optional for most examinations. However, when turbulent Doppler flow is found in the proximal and mid segments of either CCA, this step becomes imperative. With the left CCA originating directly off the aortic arch, this portion of the vessel cannot be imaged with a standard linear array transducer, and additional transducers and approaches are necessary. Sweep the Doppler sample volume throughout the proximal, mid, and distal segments of the CCA, documenting representative peak systolic Doppler flow velocities (PSV). It is not always necessary to document the end-diastolic Doppler flow velocities (EDV) throughout the CCA. However, measure the EDV when the flow appears more resistive, and compare to the contralateral segment.

Clearly differentiate the ICA from the ECA using one or both of the following methods. The ECA is typically located anterior and medial to the ICA and can be identified by finding the artery with multiple branches beyond

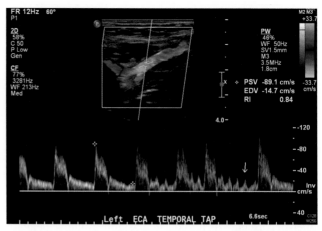

**FIGURE 7-3** Duplex image of the external carotid artery showing a "temporal tap." The Doppler waveform is affected by rapid oscillations on the ipsilateral temporal artery (*arrow*).

the carotid bifurcation. Of note, there are normal anatomic variants in which a branch may arise from the proximal ICA or the distal CCA (this is generally the superior thyroid artery). A second technique involves palpation of the pulse in the superficial temporal artery just anterior to the ear, then oscillating the flow by "tapping" on the artery (the "temporal tap" maneuver) while insonating flow in the proximal segment of the ECA (Fig. 7-3). An artifact from the tapping (oscillations) should be visible in the spectral waveform from the ECA but not from the ICA. The temporal tap technique is not always accurate, particularly in patients with an ICA occlusion and ECA collateralization. In some patients, the temporal tap may also produce oscillations within the ICA if the superficial temporal artery is tapped too vigorously. In addition, if the superficial temporal artery is tapped too softly, oscillations will not be generated within the ECA Doppler spectral waveform. Therefore, the temporal tap can be helpful in many patients, but it should be used with caution.

Sweep the Doppler sample volume from the distal CCA into the ECA, continuously insonating to document the highest PSV in the proximal ECA segment. Continue to move the Doppler sample volume through the proximal and mid segments to determine whether any waveform changes are present. When elevated flow velocities are obtained in the ECA, document the presence or absence of poststenotic turbulence to help determine hemodynamic significance.

Return to the distal CCA and sweep the Doppler sample volume into the proximal ICA to detect the presence of stenosis at the ICA origin. Document flow separation in the carotid bulb, if present, which appears as a small area of flow reversal. This typically is located along the outer wall of the bulb on the side opposite to the flow divider, as shown in Figure 7-4. As plaque formation progresses and fills in the carotid bulb, the area of flow separation disappears. It is not necessary to measure the flow velocity of this reversal component. Move the sample volume throughout the carotid bulb to detect the highest PSV and EDV present in that location. Continue to sweep through the origin, proximal, mid, and distal segments of the ICA. Often, the distal segment of the ICA is difficult to visualize or insonate beyond the angle of the mandible. It is particularly important

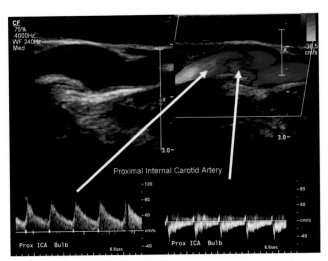

**FIGURE 7-4** Duplex image showing the normal area flow separation in the proximal internal carotid artery (carotid bulb).

to evaluate this segment of the ICA in patients who are at risk for fibromuscular dysplasia (young to middle-aged females). Curved or phased array transducers are ideal for evaluating the distal ICA.

The next vessel evaluated is the vertebral artery. Place the transducer at the anteriomedial aspect of the midneck in the long-axis position. Once the CCA has been identified, slowly slide or angle the transducer posteriorly, focusing deep to the CCA to view the vertebral artery between the transverse processes of the cervical vertebrae. Take care to properly identify the flow direction and document waveform contour at the midneck level. Abnormal waveform contour or flow direction indicates hemodynamically significant stenosis of the ipsilateral proximal subclavian artery and will be discussed later. When turbulent Doppler flow is detected in the vertebral artery at low-to-mid neck, evaluate the origin and proximal segments to identify a stenosis.

Finally, place the transducer in transverse orientation at the base of the neck to insonate the supraclavicular subclavian artery. Set the Doppler sample volume as far proximally in the vessel as possible, then sweep distally to obtain the highest PSV and most laminar Doppler spectral waveform. If elevated velocities are detected, determine hemodynamic significance by sampling distally in the infraclavicular segments of the subclavian artery, documenting the presence or absence of poststenotic turbulence.

## Pitfalls

The majority of patients' carotid arteries are difficult to visualize high in the neck (distal ICA) and very low in the neck (proximal CCA or brachiocephalic artery). Patients with short and thick necks will likely have the most difficult visualization because of vessel depths and difficult access. The low-range transmit frequencies allow for better ultrasound penetration and image capability at deeper depths. A 4 to 1 MHz phased array transducer has a flat, small footprint that is approximately 3.0 cm in square. A 5 to 2 MHz curvilinear transducer also has low- to midrange transmit frequencies and better image resolution than the

phased array transducer. The curvilinear transducer has a curved and rectangular footprint, approximately 6.0 cm in length and 1.5 cm wide, which is a larger footprint than the phased array. The primary challenge when using these alternative transducers is the limited options for angle correction and beam steering. The sector, wedge-shaped imaging format does not allow for Doppler beam steering as with a linear array transducer.

## DIAGNOSIS

The ultrasound image quality of modern duplex scanners is vastly improved compared to early ultrasound systems. In the early days of duplex scanning, the B-mode image was primarily used for locating the vessels of interest, and Doppler spectral waveforms provided nearly all the information on vessel patency. Today, Doppler continues to provide the most reliable data on the degree of stenosis. However, owing to the higher resolution of B-mode images generated by current instruments and the use of harmonic imaging techniques, great amounts of data are being gleaned by researchers on plaque composition, intimal–medial thickness, and overall vessel wall properties.[7,8] Common findings are summarized within Pathology Box 7-1.

### B-Mode Characteristics

A normal carotid artery has smooth vessel walls with no appreciable plaque extending into the vessel lumen. The intimal–medial layer is clearly visible as a thin gray-white line on the innermost part of the wall and is uniform throughout the length of the visualized vessel (Fig. 7-5). The adventitial layer is visible outside the intimal–medial layer, appearing as brighter white than the adjacent tissues. The lumen of the vessel is anechoic. It is not unusual for a mobile appearing echo to be present within the lumen of the carotid artery in both planes; this represents a normally occurring reverberation artifact of the wall of the adjacent internal jugular vein.

Most abnormalities of the carotid artery are detectible on B-mode imaging. These include plaque formation, intraluminal defects (such as intimal dissection or thrombus), and iatrogenic injuries (such as pseudoaneurysm or arteriovenous fistula involving the adjacent internal jugular vein).

### Plaque

Modern B-mode imaging can provide detailed information on both the surface features and internal composition of atherosclerotic plaque. Plaque formation can occur along any segment of the extracranial carotid system; however, plaque most commonly forms at the common carotid bifurcation in the distal common, proximal internal, and proximal external carotid arteries. In the early stages, plaque appears as a thickening of the intimal–medial layers, and a fibrous cap may form between the bulk of the plaque and the lumen (Fig. 7-6). The surface of the plaque can be described as smooth or irregular, but use of the term "ulcerated" is generally discouraged. Strictly speaking, an ulcer refers to an area where there is loss of the vascular endothelium, and although some irregular plaques may be ulcerated, this is not a finding that is reliably documented by ultrasound

**PATHOLOGY BOX 7-1**
*Carotid Artery Pathology*

| Pathology | Sonographic Appearance | | |
|---|---|---|---|
| | **B-Mode Image** | **Color-Flow Doppler** | **Doppler Spectral Waveform** |
| Normal internal carotid artery | No plaque or wall thickening | Complete filling of the lumen<br>Flow separation zone along the outer wall of the bulb | PSV < 125 cm/s<br>Narrow frequency band with a "window" under the systolic peak<br>Flow (or boundary layer) separation along the outer wall of the bulb |
| Severe (80%–99%) internal carotid stenosis | Extensive plaque, often with acoustic shadowing due to calcification | Narrowing of the lumen<br>Aliasing in the color-flow image | PSV ≥ 125 cm/s and EDV ≥ 140 cm/s<br>Spectral broadening throughout the cardiac cycle |
| Internal carotid string sign | Extensive plaque, often with acoustic shadowing due to calcification | Severely narrowed lumen<br>Power Doppler may show a small lumen | Variable velocity (high, low, or undetectable flow)<br>May be decreased diastolic flow in the ipsilateral common carotid artery |
| Internal carotid occlusion | Extensive plaque filling the lumen, often with acoustic shadowing due to calcification | No filling of the lumen beyond the bulb by color-flow or power Doppler | No flow in the internal carotid artery<br>Decreased diastolic flow in the ipsilateral common carotid artery |
| Subclavian steal (brachial systolic pressure gradient > 15 mm Hg) | May be plaque in the subclavian artery on the side of the decreased pressure | Retrograde flow in the ipsilateral vertebral artery | Increased PSV in the subclavian artery on the side of the decreased pressure<br>Retrograde or "hesitant" flow in the ipsilateral vertebral artery<br>May be increased PSV in the contralateral vertebral artery |

PSV, Peak systolic velocity; EDV, End-diastolic velocity.

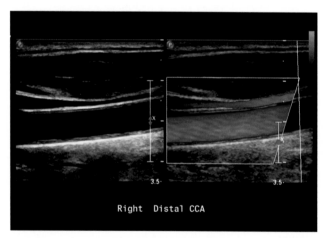

**FIGURE 7-5** B-mode image and color Doppler images of the common carotid artery, with the intimal–medial layer clearly visible.

(Fig. 7-7). Ulceration is best documented by a pathologic specimen at the time of surgery. The internal features of atherosclerotic plaque are often described qualitatively according to their echogenicity as either homogeneous or heterogeneous.

Homogeneous plaque is uniform in appearance and is often of relatively low echogenicity. In general, low echogenicity correlates with a high lipid content and the presence of fibrofatty tissue. A smooth appearing fibrous cap may also be present. Heterogeneous plaque, also described as mixed echogenicity plaque, may be comprised of fatty material and areas of calcium that tend to cause brighter

echoes and acoustic shadowing (Fig. 7-8). Acoustic shadowing occurs when calcium attenuates the transmission of ultrasound and creates a "shadow" deep to the calcified area. An echolucent region in a heterogeneous plaque may represent either lipid or hemorrhage (Fig. 7-9).

A plaque has the potential to rupture, exposing the plaque contents to the arterial lumen and flowing blood. Bleeding within the plaque beneath an intact fibrous cap is referred to as intraplaque hemorrhage and can cause the plaque to become "unstable." These unstable plaques can expand, increasing both the degree of stenosis and the potential to produce emboli to the brain. Ulceration or rupture of the fibrous cap is a feature of unstable plaque that also increases the risk of thrombus formation and subsequent embolization. The clinical value of characterizing plaque surface features and internal composition by B-mode imaging is controversial. Retrospective analyses suggest that plaques that are predominately echolucent or irregular are more likely to be associated with neurologic symptoms than predominately echo-dense or smooth plaques.[8-10]

### Intraluminal Defects

Intraluminal defects in the carotid arteries include disruption of the intima with blood from the true lumen flowing between the layers of the vessel wall. This separation of the layers is referred to as an arterial dissection, and it creates a second (false) flow lumen within the vessel. Dissections tend to progress in a spiral pattern along the vessel, narrowing the true lumen and creating a generally nonfunctional false lumen that may go on to thrombose. Intimal dissections

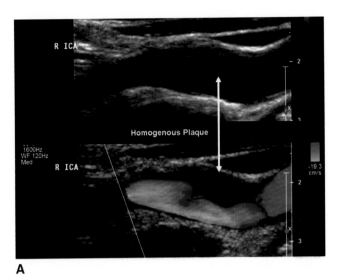
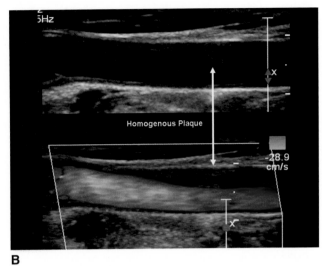

**A**　　　　**B**

**FIGURE 7-6** B-mode and color Doppler images demonstrating smooth homogeneous plaque in the carotid arteries. **A:** Homogeneous plaque in an internal carotid artery. **B:** Homogeneous plaque in a common carotid artery; the fibrous cap is visible as a brighter line along the intraluminal aspect of the plaque.

can occur either spontaneously or because of trauma. It is crucial to differentiate a carotid artery dissection from an internal jugular vein wall artifact. Multiple views should be used to confirm the presence of dissection. Interrogate with color Doppler for disturbed flow patterns which often indicate opposite directions of flow within the two lumens (Fig. 7-10). It is usually possible to identify distinctly different flow patterns within the separate true and false lumens with Doppler spectral waveforms. Flow patterns may reveal normal or stenotic characteristics in the first lumen and delayed backfilling into the second lumen.

Spontaneous dissections commonly begin at the aortic root and may be associated with thoracic aortic aneurysm formation. Once the dissection process has begun, the vessel walls continue to separate along the length of the artery with the force of blood through each cardiac cycle. Traumatic dissections can begin at any point along the vessel wall following blunt trauma or torsion. Examples include injury by the cross-chest component of a seat belt during a motor vehicle accident, blunt force from sports activities or equipment, and chiropractic manipulation of the neck. Smaller intimal defects can occur, presenting as short intimal flaps that do

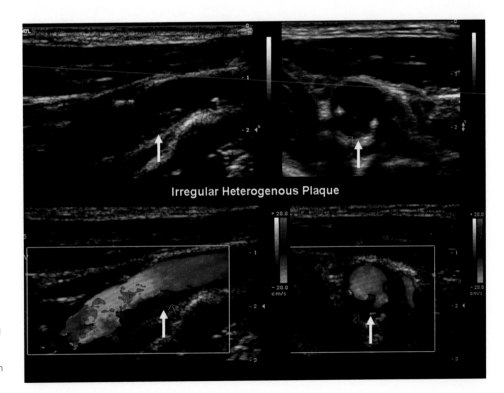

**FIGURE 7-7** B-mode and color Doppler images of heterogeneous irregular plaque in the proximal internal carotid artery. Note the color Doppler flow eddy at the area of apparent plaque compromise, possible ulceration (*arrows*).

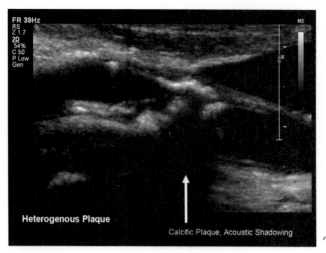

**FIGURE 7-8** B-mode image of the carotid bifurcation demonstrating heterogeneous plaque with mixed echogenicity, calcification, and acoustic shadowing.

not extend far along the length of the vessel. Although some of these defects resolve spontaneously, some may extend and be associated with thrombosis or embolization.

Carotid artery thrombosis is rare, and differentiation of thrombus from softly echogenic homogeneous plaque can be challenging. The soft uniform echoes are similar in both acute thrombus and some homogeneous plaques (Fig. 7-11). The etiology of carotid artery thrombosis is most often related to progressive atherosclerotic plaque with eventual obliteration of the remaining vessel lumen by thrombus.

Other possible contributing factors include cardiogenic embolus, trauma, and dissection.

### Iatrogenic Injury

Iatrogenic injury is defined as any adverse patient condition that is induced inadvertently by a health care provider in the course of a diagnostic procedure or therapeutic intervention. Iatrogenic injury to the carotid artery can occur during catheter interventions or venous line placement. Inadvertent puncture of the carotid artery has the potential to cause a pseudoaneurysm at the puncture site, an arteriovenous fistula between the CCA and the internal jugular or external jugular veins, or intimal dissection (Fig. 7-12). Intraluminal arterial injury can be caused by instrumentation with catheters and wires during procedures on the extracranial or intracranial carotid segments, including balloon angioplasty and stent deployment.

### Spectral Doppler Characteristics

In addition to what the B-mode image reveals about the carotid arteries, each segment must be insonated and flow velocity and waveform contour carefully evaluated with Doppler spectral waveform analysis. Duplex ultrasound is unique in that the information collected is both anatomic and physiologic, as compared to the purely anatomic information provided by standard intra-arterial contrast arteriography and computed tomography arteriography (CTA). The physiologic data provides hemodynamic information for interpretation of flow changes proximal and distal to any given insonated location. The spectral Doppler component provides the most

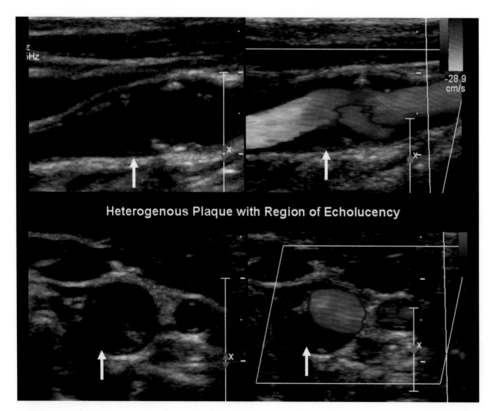

**FIGURE 7-9** B-mode and color Doppler image of the proximal internal carotid artery demonstrating plaque with echolucency (*arrow*); these findings may represent lipid core versus intraplaque hemorrhage.

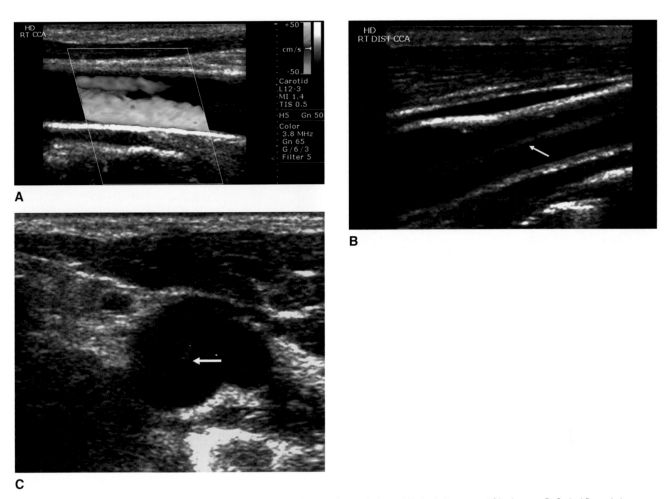

**FIGURE 7-10** **A:** A common carotid artery dissection illustrating color Doppler flow variations within both the true and false lumens. **B:** Sagittal B-mode image of the distal common carotid artery illustrating an intraluminal defect (*arrow*). **C:** Transverse B-mode image across the carotid bifurcation with the dissected lumen (*arrow*) visible within the internal carotid artery.

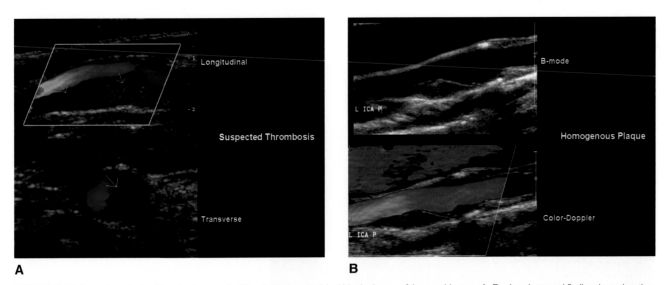

**FIGURE 7-11** B-mode and color Doppler images of softly echogenic material within the lumen of the carotid artery. **A:** Duplex ultrasound findings in conjunction with patient history indicate carotid artery partial (nonocclusive) thrombosis. **B:** Findings indicate soft homogeneous plaque.

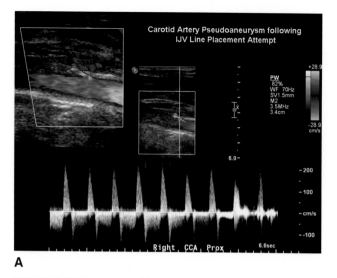

**A**

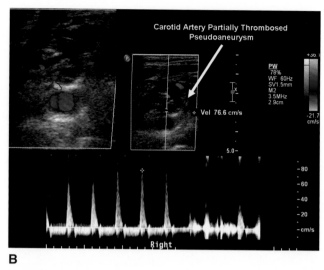

**B**

**FIGURE 7-12** Common carotid artery pseudoaneurysm following attempted internal jugular vein line placement. **A:** Duplex ultrasound demonstration of to-and-fro flow in the neck of the pseudoaneurysm, arising from the common carotid artery. **B:** Duplex image of the pseudoaneurysm which is mostly thrombosed.

reliable means for assessing vessel patency and classifying the degree of stenosis.

## Doppler Waveform Contour

Doppler waveform contour is directly related to cardiac output, vessel compliance, and the status of the distal vascular bed (peripheral resistance). The Doppler waveform contour in a normal CCA, ICA, or ECA has a rapid systolic upstroke (acceleration), sharp systolic peak, and a clear spectral "window" under the peak (Fig. 7-13). Because the ICA supplies the brain directly, it has the lowest peripheral resistance and shows the highest diastolic flow velocities with forward flow throughout the cardiac cycle. The ECA normally supplies a relatively high-resistance vascular bed that includes the muscles of the face and mouth. This produces lower diastolic flow velocities and often results in a multiphasic waveform similar to that of a peripheral artery. The Doppler

waveform from the CCA takes on the characteristics of both the internal and external carotid arteries, because it supplies both branches; however, about 70% of the normal CCA flow volume passes through the ICA, so the CCA usually has a low-resistance flow pattern with forward flow throughout the cardiac cycle (Fig. 7-14). The brachiocephalic artery has a higher resistance flow pattern that reflects the status of the multiple vascular beds that it supplies: arm (high resistance), face (high resistance), and brain (low resistance).

The carotid sinus or carotid bulb is a slight focal dilation in the artery where baroreceptors assisting in reflex blood pressure control are located. The carotid bodies, which are chemoreceptors involved in the control of respiratory rate, are also nearby. The carotid bulb typically involves the origin and proximal segments of the ICA, but the dilated segment may also include the distal CCA or the origin of the ECA. How to classify the severity of an ICA stenosis within the

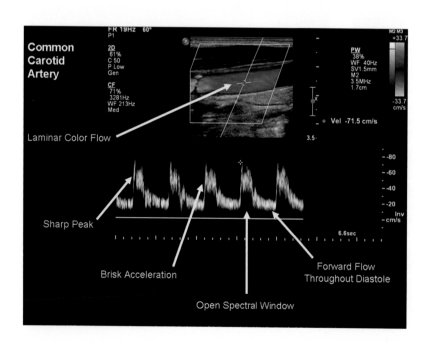

**FIGURE 7-13** Normal spectral waveform of Doppler flow through the common carotid artery.

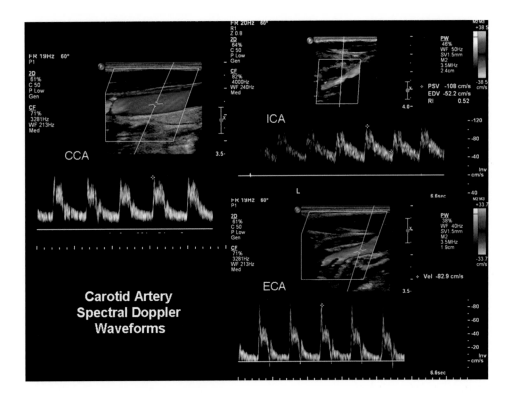

**FIGURE 7-14** Duplex images of normal Doppler flow through the common carotid, external carotid, and internal carotid arteries.

carotid bulb has been the subject of much research. The normal carotid bulb will have an area of flow separation along the outer wall on the side opposite to the flow divider, as discussed previously. This area of flow separation is created when flow from the CCA enters the widened bulb segment, and this change in vessel geometry creates a helical flow pattern that includes a zone of reversed, lower velocity flow (Fig. 7-15). The appearance of flow separation in this situation is considered to be normal and usually correlates with minimal or no plaque in the bulb. A more characteristic low-resistance ICA flow pattern is present in the bulb along the flow divider and in the mid and distal ICA

segments beyond the bulb. As plaque develops, it tends to fill in the bulb, leaving a residual segment of vessel that is more uniform in diameter, and the area of flow separation disappears. Therefore, even though the Doppler spectral waveform contour may be normal, the absence of flow reversal in the bulb can be considered "abnormal."

Changes in the contour of the Doppler spectral waveform associated with arterial disease depend greatly on the site of insonation relative to the stenosis or obstruction. In addition, collateral pathways can influence waveform contour, depending on the location of the stenosis relative to proximal and distal arterial branches. Hemodynamic principles

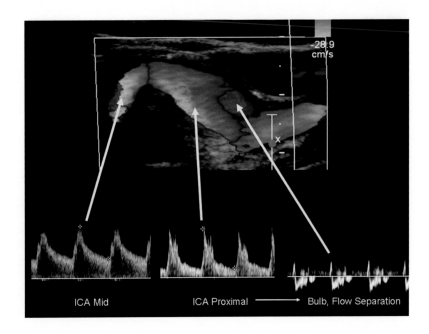

**FIGURE 7-15** Duplex image of normal Doppler flow characteristics through the carotid bulb and internal carotid artery.

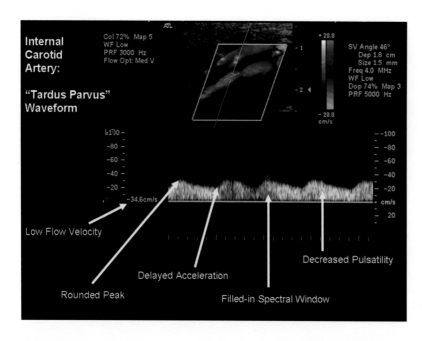

Internal Carotid Artery:

"Tardus Parvus" Waveform

Low Flow Velocity

Rounded Peak

Delayed Acceleration

Filled-in Spectral Window

Decreased Pulsatility

**FIGURE 7-16** Abnormal dampened Doppler spectral waveform contour in the internal carotid artery, described as "tardus and parvus."

dictate that the flow pattern within a significant stenosis will be characterized by a high-velocity jet. The waveform contour distal to a significant stenosis will be dampened, with decreased flow velocity, delayed acceleration, and a rounded peak. This is sometimes referred to as a "tardus–parvus" pattern (Fig. 7-16). When the site of insonation is immediately distal to the stenotic lesion, poststenotic turbulence will be present, resulting in a waveform with spectral broadening. The high-velocity jet and the maximal spectral broadening may be evident only for a few vessel diameters distal to the stenosis, so it is important to sample flow with

the PW Doppler relatively close to the lesion. Because the severity of stenosis increases, the downstream extent of the high-velocity jet and dampened poststenotic flow tend to increase. The features of Doppler spectral waveforms obtained proximal to a stenosis depend on the severity of the lesion and the intervening collateral vessels. If there are abundant collateral vessels, the waveform may appear essentially normal. If collateral flow is limited and the stenosis is severe, the waveform will have a "high-resistance" pattern with low-velocity or absent diastolic flow (Fig. 7-17). As will be discussed, the most severe stenoses that are nearly

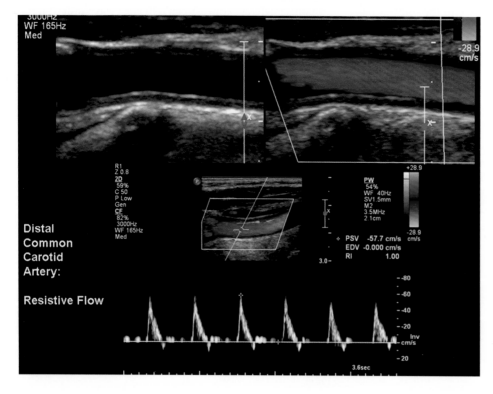

Distal Common Carotid Artery:

Resistive Flow

**FIGURE 7-17** Abnormal, resistive Doppler flow through the common carotid artery in the setting of ipsilateral internal carotid artery occlusion.

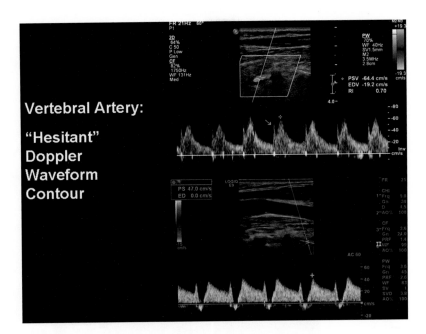

**FIGURE 7-18** Duplex images of abnormal "hesitant" Doppler vertebral artery flow, indicating a latent subclavian steal phenomenon.

occlusive will produce the most abnormal, preocclusive waveform contour, known as "string sign" flow.

### "Steal" Waveform Contours

Another spectral waveform abnormality is the "steal" phenomenon. This describes the situation where one vascular bed draws blood away or steals from another and tends to occur when two runoff beds with different resistances are supplied by a limited source of inflow. The degree of arterial steal depends on the severity of the stenosis and the resistance offered by the various downstream vascular beds.

A "latent" steal describes flow that is beginning to show signs of reversal, but is not yet completely retrograde. There are progressing stages of abnormal flow that indicate an impending steal. "Hesitant" waveforms possess a deep flow reversal notch when flow pauses before progressing cephalad (Fig. 7-18). When the deep notch in the Doppler waveform extends below the baseline, with a portion of the flow fully retrograde during part of the cardiac cycle, these waveforms are described as "alternating" or bidirectional. In the case of a progressive proximal subclavian artery stenosis, changing pressure gradients at the origin of the ipsilateral vertebral artery can alter the ratio of antegrade to retrograde flow in the vertebral artery to the point where flow is entirely in the retrograde direction—a "complete" steal. In this setting, it is important to determine the flow direction based on the color Doppler and spectral Doppler settings. Abnormal steal patterns can also develop in the presence of a severe stenosis or occlusion of the brachiocephalic artery. In either of these instances, blood flow will be affected in the carotid distribution (Fig. 7-19A) as well as within the subclavian and vertebral arteries (Fig. 7-19B).

### Vessel-Specific Abnormal Waveform Contours

"String sign" flow is characterized by blunted, low-velocity, somewhat resistive waveforms and is the pattern that precedes complete occlusion of the vessel (Fig. 7-20). This is most likely to be found in a severely diseased ICA in which only a small, string-like lumen remains. It is important to differentiate "string sign" flow from complete vessel occlusion. With a "string sign," the ICA is patent and the patient may still undergo an endarterectomy, whereas with a completely occluded ICA, the patient will not be a surgical candidate. To aid in this differentiation, the vessels should be imaged in both long-axis and transverse planes using color Doppler (with settings of low scale and high gain) and power Doppler to detect the presence of any flow. Careful interrogation of the most distal extracranial ICA segment is important to avoid overlooking a patent but small lumen in that location.

Markedly decreased diastolic flow or a highly resistive component and overall "blunted" appearing waveform in the extracranial ICA indicates a severe stenosis or occlusion in the more distal or intracranial segments (Fig. 7-21). This may be associated with severe distal extracranial ICA stenosis due to fibromuscular dysplasia or segmental dissection. These changes will be observed even when there is a stenosis in the proximal ICA. Resistive and blunted flow in the ICA will also be reflected in the CCA waveform. This is similar to the setting of extracranial ICA occlusion, where the flow pattern in the CCA takes on the features of the patent ECA. Careful comparison of the bilateral ICA EDVs is imperative to verify hemodynamic significance of a unilateral distal stenosis.

Recognition of a severe, hemodynamically significant ECA stenosis is generally straightforward. Atherosclerotic lesions of this vessel tend to involve the origin and proximal segments and are associated with a focal velocity increase, poststenotic turbulence (spectral broadening), and a dampened waveform distally. Diffuse increases in ECA velocity caused by intracranial collateralization and compensatory flow may be found when the ipsilateral ICA is occluded.

Aortic valve or root stenosis will generate symmetrically abnormal Doppler arterial waveform contour in the right

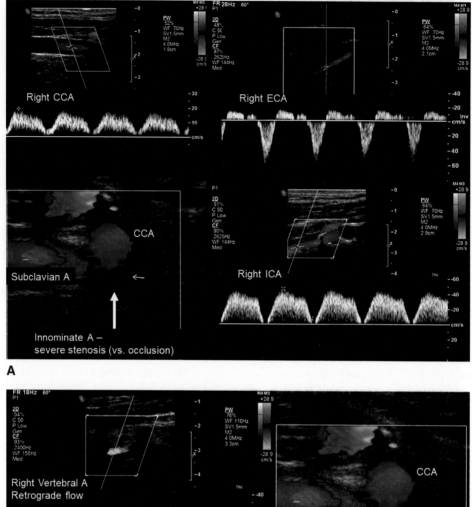

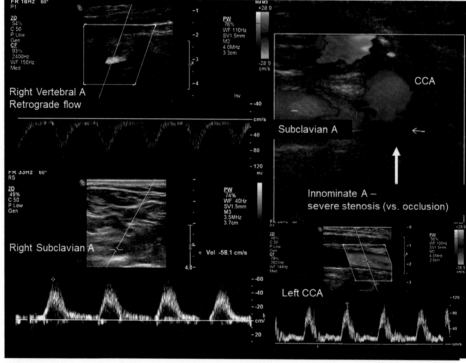

**FIGURE 7-19** Duplex images associated with a severe brachiocephalic artery stenosis. **A:** Abnormal Doppler arterial flow through the right carotid distribution. A low-velocity "hesitant" flow pattern is present in the right common carotid and internal carotid arteries, and there is alternating or to-and-fro flow in the external carotid artery. **B:** Abnormal Doppler arterial flow through the right subclavian and vertebral distribution. There is a dampened flow pattern in the right subclavian artery and retrograde flow in the right vertebral artery. The left common carotid flow waveform is shown for comparison.

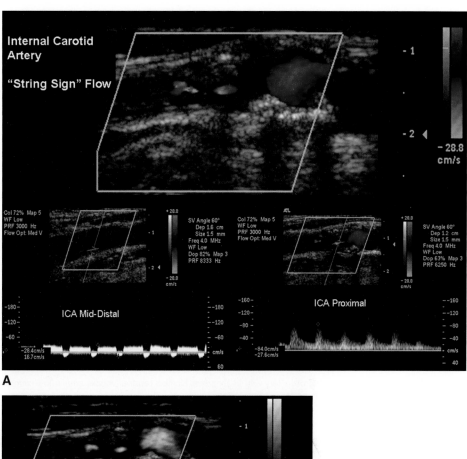

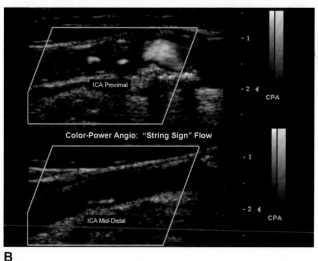

**FIGURE 7-20** Duplex images of a functionally occluded internal carotid artery with "string sign" Doppler flow. **A:** Utilization of color Doppler and Doppler spectral waveform modalities. **B:** Utilization of color power angio modality.

and left carotid systems (Fig. 7-22). Brachial systolic pressures may also be symmetrically low, depending on the severity of the stenosis. Severe stenosis or occlusion of the brachiocephalic artery creates decreased pressure and waveform changes in the right CCA and subclavian artery and their distal branches. Therefore, when the brachiocephalic artery bifurcation is patent, there is the potential for a steal from the subclavian and the vertebral arteries to supply the common carotid circulation.

Severe stenosis or occlusion of the proximal, mid, or distal CCA will affect the Doppler arterial waveforms in the remaining peripheral segments of the CCA, as well as the ICA and ECA. A severe distal CCA obstruction with continued patency of the carotid bifurcation is often referred to as a "choke lesion" (Fig. 7-23). Flow direction distal to a "choke lesion" depends on the local pressure gradients and can result in varying degrees of steal. In this situation, flow will typically reverse in the ECA to supply the ICA (Fig. 7-24). Rarely, flow will reverse in the ICA to supply the ECA in response to unusual intracranial collateral pathways. In these cases, it is important to make sure that the vessels have been correctly identified. When the ICA is

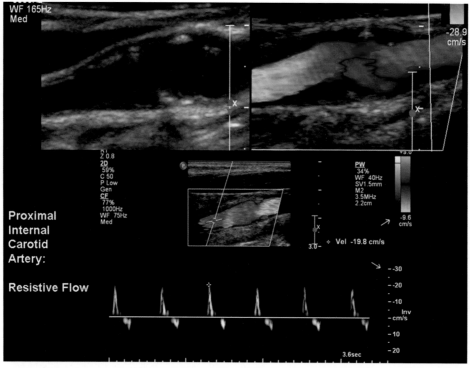

**FIGURE 7-21** Duplex images of a patent proximal internal carotid artery with an abnormal, blunted, resistive Doppler arterial flow pattern. Findings indicate distal extracranial versus intracranial severe stenosis or occlusion of the internal carotid artery.

occluded, Doppler arterial waveforms throughout the CCA will be more resistive and identical to the ECA (Fig. 7-25). Complete ECA occlusion is uncommon because of multiple branches and abundant collateral pathways.

### Special Considerations

Low cardiac output and poor ejection fraction can affect systemic arterial pressure and Doppler arterial waveform contour throughout the carotid system. Doppler waveforms will be dampened with delayed acceleration in every artery evaluated, yet no stenosis or poststenotic turbulence will be identified. Differentiating low cardiac output from aortic stenosis can be difficult with duplex ultrasound; however, an unusual waveform with two prominent systolic peaks separated by a midsystolic retraction called "pulsus bisferiens" has been described in the carotid arteries of a patient with aortic valvular disease and hypertrophic obstructive cardiomyopathy.[11] Cardiac arrhythmias (abnormal heart rhythms or rates) can also make interpretation of Doppler waveforms difficult, because standard velocity criteria may not apply and waveform contour is altered (Fig. 7-26).

Cardiac assist devices are used in patients with heart failure to support cardiac function, often while they are recovering from myocardial infarction or heart surgery. Some cardiac assist devices are intended for short-term use, whereas others may be in place for long periods as a bridge to cardiac transplantation. A left ventricular assist device (LVAD) and an intra-aortic balloon pump (IABP) are two examples of cardiac assist devices. The effect of cardiac assist devices on Doppler arterial waveform contour is profound, creating patterns that may be unrecognizable as arterial flow. An example of a carotid artery Doppler waveform in a patient with an IABP is shown in Figure 7-27. In these cases, the

vascular laboratory report should contain a "disclaimer" stating that waveform contour cannot be interpreted according to standard criteria. Hospital-based vascular laboratories are most likely to encounter these patients, because they are usually inpatients. However, some of these devices are portable, so occasionally an outpatient may present to the vascular laboratory with one of these devices in place.

### Measurement of Doppler Flow Velocity

Flow velocity obtained from Doppler spectral waveforms serves as the primary criterion for classification of stenosis severity with duplex ultrasound. Obtaining accurate Doppler information is highly dependent on proper examination technique, particularly using the correct angle of insonation. The Doppler angle of insonation is traditionally defined as the angle between the line of the ultrasound beam and the arterial wall at the site of the PW Doppler sample volume. This assumes that the direction of flow is parallel to the wall of the artery and requires that the angle cursor be aligned parallel to the vessel wall. However, "off-axis" flow (flow not parallel to the wall) is common in diseased arteries. When the direction of an off-axis flow jet can be determined on the basis of the color Doppler image, some laboratories set the angle cursor parallel to the flow jet, but it has not been established that this is more accurate than setting the angle cursor parallel to the vessel wall.

All arterial velocity measurements should be obtained using an angle of insonation of 60 degrees or less. This is accomplished by adjusting the steering of the Doppler beam or by a transducer maneuver called "toe–heel." This maneuver involves slight transducer pressure at either end of the transducer (the toe or the heel) to push the vessel into a slight angle. This moves the vessel enough to create an

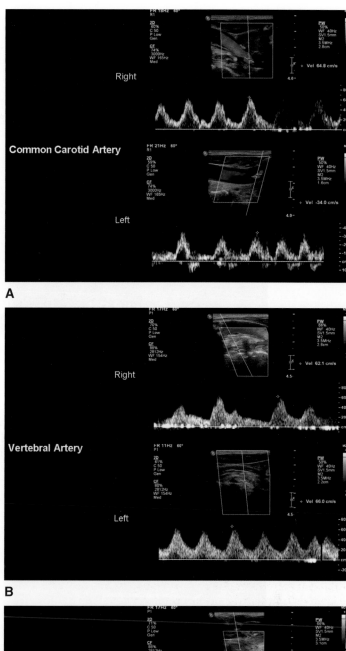

**A**

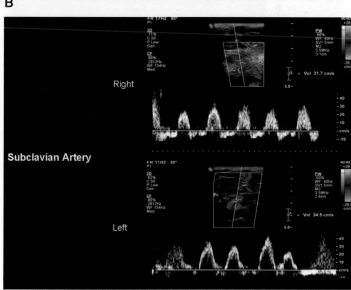

**C**

**FIGURE 7-22** Duplex images showing symmetrically abnormal Doppler arterial flow patterns in the presence of known aortic stenosis (demonstrated in the right and left)—**A:** common carotid arteries, **B:** vertebral arteries, and **C:** subclavian arteries.

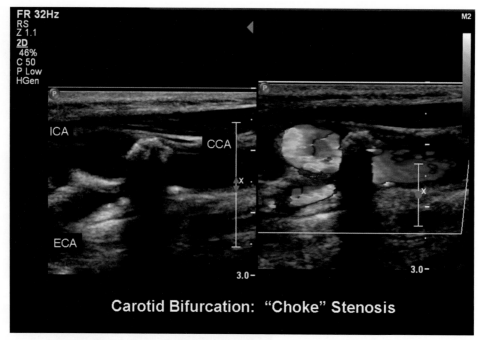

**FIGURE 7-23** B-mode and color Doppler images of a distal common carotid artery stenosis, or "choke lesion." The plaque is heavily calcified with prominent acoustic shadowing.

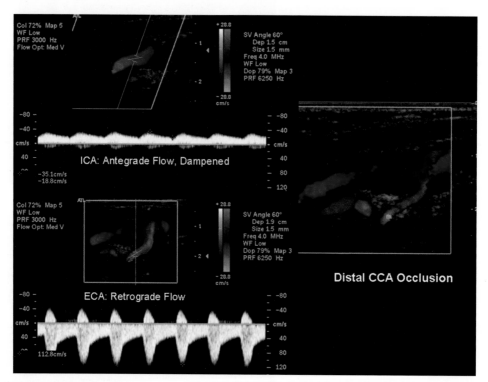

**FIGURE 7-24** Duplex images demonstrating distal common carotid artery occlusion with retrograde Doppler flow through the external carotid artery and dampened antegrade flow through the proximal internal carotid artery.

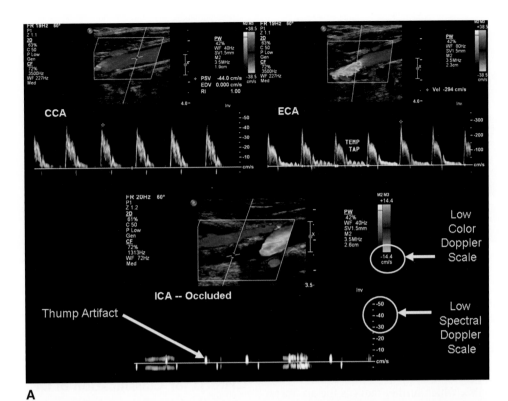

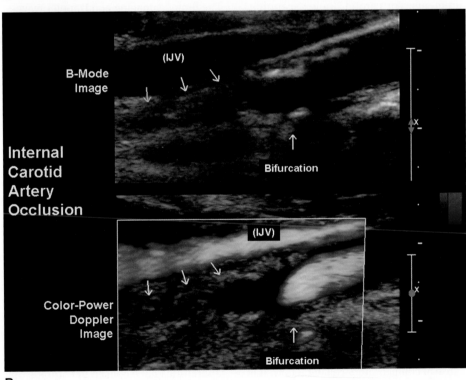

**FIGURE 7-25** Duplex images of an internal carotid artery occlusion with no obtainable Doppler flow. **A:** Utilization of color Doppler and Doppler spectral waveform modalities. **B:** Utilization of color power angio modality.

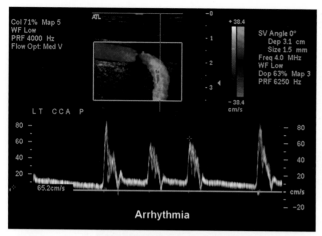

**FIGURE 7-26** Doppler spectral waveform obtained from the common carotid artery in a patient with an arrhythmia.

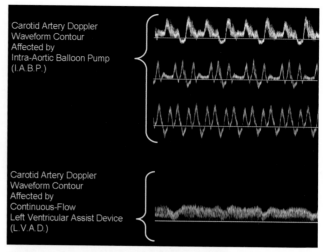

**FIGURE 7-27** Carotid artery Doppler flow patterns associated with cardiac assist devices: intra-aortic balloon pump (IABP) and left ventricular assist device (LVAD).

angle of 60 degrees or less. Although an in-depth discussion of Doppler physics is beyond the scope of this chapter, this recommendation is based on the concept that errors related to Doppler angle are more critical at large angles because the cosine changes more rapidly at angles approaching 90 degrees.[12] Doppler shift frequencies also become very small at larger angles, which further reduces the accuracy of velocity measurements. For carotid duplex scanning, experience has shown that a Doppler angle of 60 degrees or less results in clinically valid velocity information for classification of stenosis severity.

Obtaining the most complete and accurate representation of flow velocity changes throughout the carotid arteries requires that the PW Doppler sample volume be moved slowly and continuously ("swept") along the vessel. Simply "spot checking" the flow pattern may overlook very focal or localized flow disturbances. In a segment where stenosis is suspected, sweep the sample volume cursor through the area from proximal to distal, evaluating flow at closely spaced intervals and moving the sample volume across the lumen to identify the highest velocity flow jet. As this is being done, the Doppler angle must be continually evaluated and adjusted to maintain proper alignment through each segment.

The carotid and vertebral artery systems are connected by the circle of Willis at the base of the brain. The branches of the circle of Willis are variable and provide numerous collateral pathways to compensate for extracranial cerebrovascular disease. Potential collateral routes include posterior to anterior, side to side, and extracranial to intracranial. When there is a severe stenosis or complete occlusion of one ICA, velocities may be increased in the contralateral carotid system because of compensatory collateral flow. It is important to recognize this situation to avoid overestimating the extent of disease on the contralateral side. Compensatory flow is generally associated with a diffuse increase in flow velocity throughout the contralateral CCA and ICA, without a focal high-velocity jet or other localized flow disturbance. Even when a hemodynamically significant ICA stenosis is identified contralateral to a severe stenosis or occlusion, it is appropriate to comment that the Doppler flow velocity elevation may be caused in part by the contralateral disease. More detailed information on specific intracranial

collateral pathways can be obtained by a transcranial Doppler examination.

## Criteria for Classification of Disease

The B-mode imaging and Doppler waveform parameters for classification of carotid artery disease have been developed by comparing the results of duplex scanning with "gold standard" imaging modalities or surgical findings. These alternative standard imaging approaches include intra-arterial catheter contrast arteriography, CTA, and magnetic resonance arteriography (MRA). The majority of duplex ultrasound carotid criteria have been validated for the ICA. Therefore, it must be emphasized that such criteria developed for the ICA cannot be applied to the CCA or ECA.

### Internal Carotid Artery

One of the most widely applied duplex classification schemes for ICA stenosis was developed at the University of Washington under the direction of Dr. D. Eugene Strandness, Jr. These criteria classify ICA lesions into the following ranges of stenosis: Normal, 1% to 15%, 16% to 49%, 50% to 79%, 80% to 99%, and occlusion (Table 7-2). The primary threshold criterion for 50% ICA stenosis is a PSV at the stenotic site of 125 cm/s or greater. The stenosis categories below the 50% threshold (Normal, 1% to 15%, and 16% to 49%) are distinguished by the presence or absence of flow separation in the carotid bulb, the extent of spectral broadening, and the amount of plaque visualized. Evaluation of these features is often subjective, and some laboratories have chosen to combine one or more of these categories. Once the 50% stenosis threshold is exceeded, the secondary criterion is an EDV of 140 cm/s or greater, which indicates a stenosis in the 80% to 99% category. A 50% to 79% stenosis is indicated by a PSV 125 cm/s or greater and EDV < 140 cm/s. The identification of an ICA occlusion is based on multiple parameters, including absence of flow with plaque or thrombus in the ICA lumen, decreased or absent diastolic flow in the ipsilateral CCA, and evidence of compensatory collateral flow in the contralateral carotid system. Prospective validation of

**TABLE 7-2    University of Washington Criteria for Classification of Internal Carotid Artery Disease**

| Arteriographic Diameter Reduction[a] | Peak Systolic Velocity (PSV, cm/s) | End-Diastolic Velocity (EDV, cm/s) | Spectral Waveform Characteristics | B-Mode Image | Other Parameters |
|---|---|---|---|---|---|
| 0% (Normal) | <125 | – | Minimal or no spectral broadening; flow separation present in the carotid bulb | Normal arterial wall | |
| 1%-15% | <125 | – | Spectral broadening during deceleration phase of systole only | Wall thickening | |
| 16%-49% | <125 | – | Spectral broadening throughout systole | Plaque | |
| 50%-79% | ≥125 | <140 | Marked spectral broadening | Plaque | PSV ≥ 230 cm/s or ICA/CCA ratio ≥ 4.0 indicates a ≥70% NASCET stenosis |
| 80%-99% | ≥125 | ≥140 | Marked spectral broadening | Plaque | |
| 100% (occlusion) | – | – | No flow signal in the internal carotid artery; decreased or absent diastolic flow in the ipsilateral common carotid artery | Plaque or thrombus in the internal carotid artery lumen | There may be diffusely increased PSV in the contralateral carotid system or increased diastolic flow in the ipsilateral external carotid artery caused by compensatory collateral flow |

Velocity threshold criteria are based on the angle-adjusted velocity obtained with a Doppler angle of 60 degrees or less. ICA/CCA ratio is defined as maximal internal carotid PSV divided by the common carotid PSV.

NASCET, North American Symptomatic Carotid Endarterectomy Trial.

[a]Diameter reduction is based on arteriographic methods that compared the residual internal carotid artery lumen diameter to the estimated diameter of the carotid bulb.

these criteria has demonstrated a 99% sensitivity for the detection of carotid disease and an 84% specificity for the identification of normal arteries.[13]

The carotid duplex criteria have undergone period updating to remain relevant to current clinical practice. For example, the randomized trials that evaluated the efficacy of CEA in the 1990s prompted the development of some new interpretation criteria.[14-16] In the North American Symptomatic Carotid Endarterectomy Trial (NASCET), patients with symptomatic internal carotid stenosis of 70% to 99% had significant benefit from endarterectomy. Based on a detailed review of multiple Doppler waveform parameters, the best criteria for identifying a 70% or greater internal carotid stenosis, as defined in the NASCET, was a PSV of 230 cm/s or greater, or an internal carotid to common carotid PSV ratio (ICA/CCA ratio) of 4.0 or greater.[17] When calculating the ICA/CCA ratio, it is important to use the highest PSV from the stenotic site for the ICA value and the PSV in a normal mid to distal CCA segment (where the imaged arterial walls are parallel) for the CCA value (Fig. 7-28). The ICA/CCA ratio is not valid in the presence of significant CCA disease.

In the major North American CEA trials, the severity of internal carotid stenosis was calculated from arteriograms by comparing the diameter of the minimal residual lumen at the stenotic site to the diameter of the normal distal cervical ICA.[14] This approach to measuring the stenosis is now often referred to as the "NASCET method." The categories of internal carotid stenosis in the University of Washington criteria were also based on arteriograms but were developed long before the CEA trials by comparing the diameter at

the stenotic site to an estimate of the largest diameter of the normal carotid bulb that typically included the origin and proximal segments of the ICA. However, because the bulb often has a larger diameter than the distal ICA, the two methods of measuring stenosis do not give the same percentage of arteriographic stenosis for the same lesion. Calculations of arteriographic stenosis using the distal ICA as the reference vessel result in lower stenosis percentages than calculations using the bulb as the reference site. This effect is particularly striking for lesions in the middle of the stenosis range, and the differences decrease with increasing stenosis severity.

Recognizing the wide variability in the performance and interpretation of carotid duplex scans, a panel of authorities from a variety of medical specialties met in 2002 to develop a consensus regarding the key components of the carotid ultrasound examination and the most appropriate criteria for classification of disease.[18] The panelists recommended the consistent use of relatively broad categories to classify the degree of ICA stenosis. The panel also concluded that Doppler parameters are relatively inaccurate for subcategorizing stenoses of less than 50% diameter reduction and recommended that these lesions be reported under a single stenosis category. They noted that although PSV is a primary parameter for interpretation, its measurement is subject to significant variability. To minimize this variability, it was recommended that Doppler waveforms be obtained with an insonation angle of as close to 60 degrees as possible, but not exceeding 60 degrees, and that the sample volume be placed within the area of maximal stenosis. Additional parameters such as the ICA/CCA ratio and EDV were regarded

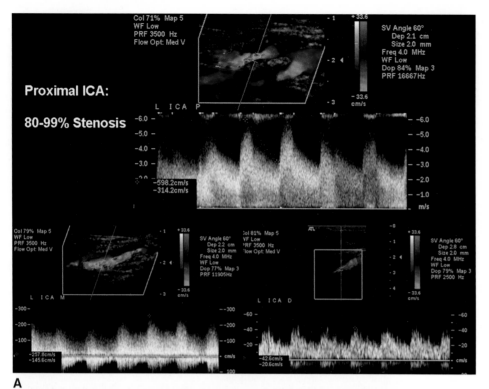

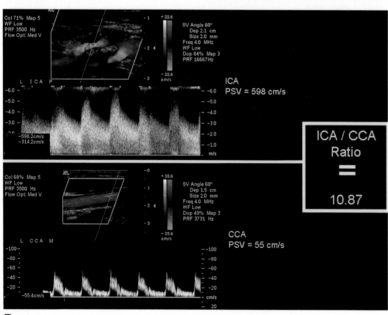

**FIGURE 7-28** Duplex images demonstrating high-grade stenosis of the internal carotid artery (ICA). **A:** 80% to 99% stenosis of the proximal ICA with poststenotic turbulence. **B:** Calculation of the ICA to common carotid artery (CCA) ratio.

as secondary parameters. A summary of the consensus panel recommendations is given in Table 7-3. It is important to emphasize that the specific thresholds listed in this table have not been subjected to rigorous prospective evaluation as a single set of duplex criteria, and they do not represent the results of any one laboratory or study. However, they can serve as a general reference for those laboratories that have not been able to internally validate their own criteria.

## Common Carotid and External Carotid Arteries

As previously stated, the criteria used for classifying ICA disease cannot be applied to lesions in the CCA or ECA.

However, sites of stenosis or occlusion in these vessels can still be identified by noting the presence of plaque on B-mode imaging and associated flow disturbances. As for stenotic lesions in the peripheral arteries, the duplex diagnosis of hemodynamically significant stenoses in the CCA and ECA can be based on the presence of a focally increased PSV followed by poststenotic turbulence. One general threshold criterion for greater than 50% arterial stenosis is a focal increase of twice the PSV or more compared to the PSV at a normal proximal site.[19,20] This parameter is commonly referred to as the "velocity ratio" and can be used for some lesions in the CCA; however, it is not suitable for most ECA

---

**TABLE 7-3    Consensus Panel Recommendations for Classification of Internal Carotid Artery Stenosis[18]**

**Normal:** The ICA PSV is less than 125 cm/s, and there is no visible plaque or intimal thickening. Normal arteries should also have an ICA/CCA ratio of less than 2.0 and ICA EDV of less than 40 cm/s.

**ICA stenosis <50%** is present when the ICA PSV is less than 125 cm/s and there is visible plaque or intimal thickening. Such arteries should also have an ICA/CCA ratio of less than 2.0 and an ICA EDV of less than 40 cm/s.

**ICA stenosis of 50%–69%** is present when the ICA PSV is 125–230 cm/s and there is visible plaque. Such arteries should also have an ICA/CCA ratio of 2.0 to 4.0 and an ICA EDV of 40–100 cm/s.

**ICA stenosis ≥70%–99%** but less than near occlusion is present when the ICA PSV is more than 230 cm/s and there is visible plaque with lumen narrowing on grayscale and color Doppler imaging. The higher the PSV, the more likely it is (higher positive predictive value) that there is severe disease. Such stenoses should also have an ICA/CCA ratio of more than 4.0 and an ICA EDV of more than 100 cm/s.

**Near occlusion of the ICA:** The velocity parameters may not apply. "Preocclusive" lesions may be associated with high, low, or undetectable velocity measurements. The diagnosis of near occlusion is therefore established primarily by demonstration of a markedly narrowed lumen with color Doppler. In some near occlusive lesions, color or power Doppler can distinguish between near occlusion and occlusion by demonstrating a thin channel of flow traversing the lesion.

**Occlusion:** There is no detectable patent lumen on grayscale imaging and no flow with pulsed Doppler, color Doppler, or power Doppler. Near occlusive lesions may be misdiagnosed as occlusions when only grayscale ultrasound and pulsed Doppler spectral waveforms are used.

ICA, Internal carotid artery; PSV, Peak systolic velocity; CCA, Common carotid artery; EDV, End diastolic velocity; ICA/CCA ratio, Maximal ICA PSV divided by the CCA PSV.

---

stenoses which typically involve the origin of that vessel where a normal proximal PSV cannot be obtained.

At the University of Washington vascular laboratory, stenotic lesions in the CCA and ECA are classified as Normal, less than 50%, and 50% to 99%, based on the presence or absence of plaque on B-mode imaging and a focal flow disturbance with a PSV of two or more times the expected normal PSV at that site. Classification schemes for the CCA and ECA with smaller ranges of stenosis and more categories have not been validated and are unlikely to be clinically useful. In general, focal increases in PSV of 200 cm/s or more should raise suspicion for a 50% to 99% stenosis in either the CCA or ECA. Increases in ECA PSV can also be because of compensatory collateral flow when the ipsilateral ICA is occluded. Increased PSV in spectral waveforms from the origin and proximal segments of the CCA can be associated with tortuosity. When there is a significant stenosis at the origin of the CCA, the more distal CCA waveforms will be dampened, with low PSV and a slow systolic acceleration. These CCA waveform changes are important diagnostically because the overall reduction in flow velocity may artificially lower velocities in an ipsilateral ICA stenosis, leading to underestimation of the severity of that lesion.

One relatively small study that compared duplex parameters to findings on contrast arteriography or CTA concluded that a CCA PSV ≥ 250 cm/s and EDV ≥ 60 cm/s were highly accurate threshold criteria for >60% CCA stenosis.[21] A similar study also evaluated duplex parameters from the CCA but compared them to the percent area stenosis determined by CTA and found that a PSV > 182 cm/s was the best criterion for a >50% stenosis.[22] Several studies have proposed threshold velocity criteria for ECA stenosis. One report compared B-mode image features and PSV measurements to the severity of stenosis determined by MRA and found that an ECA PSV < 150 cm/s predicted <50% stenosis, whereas a PSV > 250 cm/s was associated with >60% stenosis.[23] A study that focused on the status of the ECA following carotid interventions described the use of an ECA/CCA velocity ratio (similar to the previously described ICA/CCA ratio) for identifying 80% or greater ECA stenosis, with a threshold value of 4.0.[24]

## Color and Power Doppler Findings

The ability to display flow information using color Doppler and power Doppler has improved remarkably in recent generations of ultrasound machines. However, the diagnostic importance of these methods for the carotid duplex evaluation remains secondary to Doppler spectral waveforms and the associated velocity measurements. The main benefit from utilizing the color Doppler and power Doppler modalities is the rapid identification of flow disturbances and determining the location and direction of high-velocity jets. When set with appropriate sensitivity, the flow disturbances associated with poststenotic turbulence are readily demonstrated with color Doppler imaging (Fig. 7-29). Power Doppler is particularly helpful in detecting extremely low flow velocities, including "string sign" flow (Fig. 7-20).

There are several adjustments that can to be made to optimize the color Doppler image and maintain proper sensitivity. Whenever possible, the color Doppler scale should be set high enough so that no color aliasing is present during any phase of the cardiac cycle and low enough so that color fills the patent lumen with even the lowest velocities (Fig. 7-30). This may not be feasible when a wide range of velocities is present, and in this setting color aliasing can be used to identify the sites of high-velocity flow. The color Doppler transmit frequency can be adjusted to provide better resolution or penetration, depending on vessel depth.

A uniform, single color in the low- to medium tone range indicates laminar flow. When the flow velocity exceeds the color Doppler scale, aliasing occurs with brighter tones of color progressing to the opposite direction color (e.g., red to blue). Turbulent flow produces a typical mosaic color Doppler pattern (Fig. 7-31). Regardless of the color Doppler flow characteristics, Doppler spectral waveforms must always be used to classify the severity of disease.

The power Doppler modality displays flow based on the amplitude of the Doppler signal rather than the frequency shift and thus does not give any information on flow direction. This representation of blood flow is relatively independent of the angle of insonation. The main advantage of power Doppler is its ability to detect low-flow states.

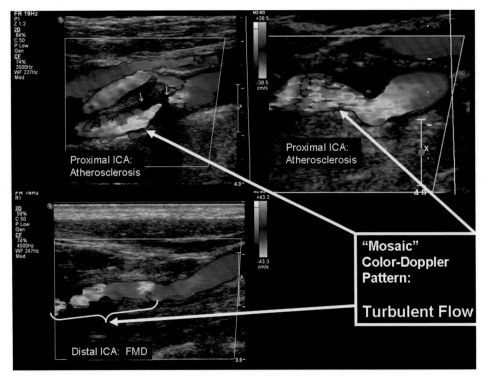

**FIGURE 7-29** Turbulent arterial flow demonstrated with a mosaic color Doppler pattern.

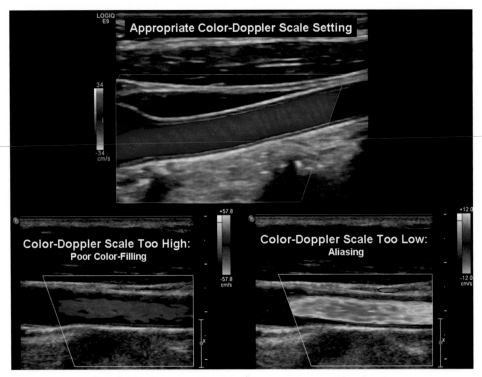

**FIGURE 7-30** Color Doppler scale settings: appropriate, too high and too low.

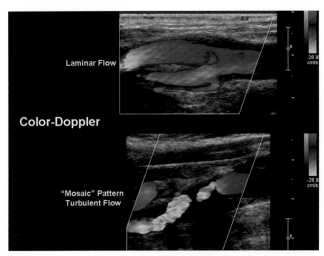

**FIGURE 7-31** Color Doppler images comparing laminar color Doppler flow and abnormal turbulent color Doppler flow (mosaic pattern).

## Vertebral Artery Stenosis

Although the vertebral artery cannot be visualized in its entirety owing to acoustic shadowing as the vessel courses through the transverse processes of the cervical vertebrae, the proximal vertebral artery should be evaluated during a routine carotid duplex scan. Normal vertebral artery flow has the same characteristics as the ICA, with a low-resistance pattern and antegrade (toward the brain) flow direction throughout the cardiac cycle. There will also be rapid systolic acceleration, a sharp peak, and relatively high diastolic flow (Fig. 7-32). Vertebral artery stenoses generally occur at the origin of the vessel from the subclavian artery. A proximal

vertebral artery stenosis will produce abnormal dampened waveforms distally, with delayed acceleration, a rounded peak, and possibly poststenotic turbulence.

Stenosis or occlusion in the more distal segments of the vertebral artery (extracranial or intracranial vertebral) will be apparent in spectral waveforms from the cervical segments. In this situation, waveforms will have rapid systolic acceleration and a sharp peak, but there will be a high-resistance pattern with minimal or no forward flow in diastole (Fig. 7-33). This waveform characteristic is referred to as resistive or blunted. When these findings are present, flow should be evaluated in the contralateral vertebral artery to help determine whether the distal lesion is in the ipsilateral vertebral or the basilar artery. When clinically indicated, transcranial Doppler may be utilized to assess the intracranial vertebral arteries and basilar artery directly.

Normal PSV in the vertebral artery is typically in the range of 30 to 50 cm/s; however, a PSV up to 80 to 90 cm/s is frequently found without any apparent abnormality. This variability may represent increased flow through a dominant vertebral artery or a small but otherwise normal vertebral artery. Detection of poststenotic turbulence distally can help to determine which increases in PSV are associated with a vertebral artery stenosis. Flow patterns are usually similar in the two vertebral arteries, but systolic and diastolic velocities may differ if vertebral artery diameters are asymmetrical. Therefore, recording of vertebral artery diameters is important if there is asymmetry in the vertebral artery flow patterns.

There are no well-established velocity criteria for vertebral artery stenosis, but the same general principles described for CCA and ECA stenosis can be applied. At the University of Washington vascular laboratory, the finding

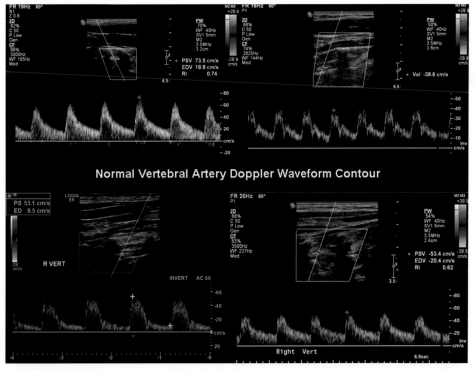

**FIGURE 7-32** Duplex images demonstrating various normal vertebral artery Doppler spectral waveform patterns.

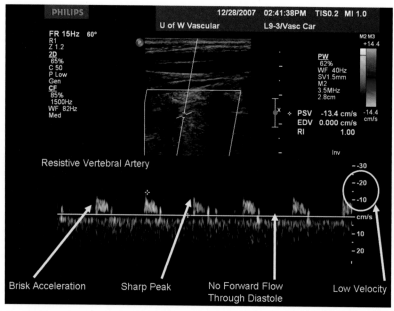

**FIGURE 7-33** Abnormal, resistive, and blunted vertebral artery Doppler spectral waveform patterns indicating distal (vs. intracranial) severe stenosis or occlusion.

of a focal vertebral artery PSV of around 150 cm/s or more is regarded as an indicator of a possible ≥50% stenosis; however, this velocity threshold has not been rigorously validated. One report evaluated various duplex parameters for identifying ≥50% vertebral artery stenosis, including a velocity ratio defined as the maximum PSV in the proximal vertebral artery (V1 segment) divided by the PSV from the normal distal vertebral artery (V2 segment).[25] In that study, a vertebral artery velocity ratio of >2.2 resulted in the highest sensitivity and specificity, but a PSV threshold of >108 cm/s also showed significant diagnostic value for vertebral artery stenosis.

## Subclavian Artery and Subclavian Steal

The general features of a vascular steal have been discussed previously. A hemodynamically significant stenosis in the proximal subclavian artery will result in a brachial systolic pressure gradient of more than 15 to 20 mm Hg. In addition to a significant pressure gradient, a velocity ratio of 2 or greater and a monophasic flow pattern in the distal subclavian artery are reliable indicators of a ≥50% subclavian artery stenosis.[26] Whenever such a brachial systolic pressure gradient is present, the vertebral arteries should be evaluated for a possible steal phenomenon. Subclavian steal occurs with severe stenosis or occlusion of the subclavian artery (or brachiocephalic artery on the right) proximal to the origin of the vertebral artery. This causes decreased pressure at the origin of the ipsilateral vertebral artery that can lead to reversed flow in that artery, because the abnormal pressure gradient "steals" blood from the vertebral circulation to supply the arm.

As upper extremity arterial inflow obstruction progresses, the vertebral artery flow pattern changes from normal antegrade to antegrade with a deep notch at mid-cardiac cycle (hesitant) and eventually to alternating (to-and-fro) flow and finally to fully retrograde flow, indicating a complete subclavian steal (Fig. 7-34).

### Reactive Hyperemia

Reactive hyperemia is a provocative noninvasive test that can be used to augment a subclavian steal from the latent or hesitant stages to the complete stage, making it easier to recognize. A blood pressure cuff is placed on the upper arm and inflated to a pressure that is more than systolic for 3 to 5 minutes, and duplex scanning is performed to continuously monitor the flow pattern in the vertebral artery. At the end of the inflation period, the cuff is rapidly deflated while the ipsilateral vertebral artery flow is observed. Tissue ischemia produced by the period of arterial occlusion results in vasodilation and an increase in the brachial systolic pressure gradient. The test is considered positive when flow in the vertebral artery completely reverses direction.

In cases where one vertebral artery is congenitally or pathologically small in caliber, the contralateral vertebral artery will often dilate and carry increased flow to compensate. In the case of severe subclavian steal, the contralateral vertebral artery flow velocity may be elevated. In complex cases where one or both common carotid or internal carotid arteries are obstructed, flow velocities will be elevated through the vertebral arteries to compensate through collateral pathways involving the circle of Willis.

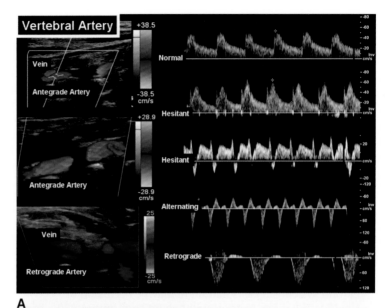

**A**

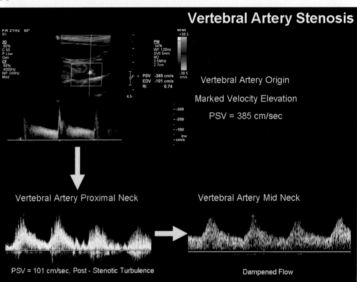

**B**

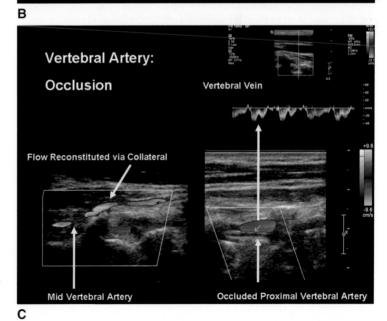

**C**

**FIGURE 7-34** Abnormal vertebral artery Doppler spectral waveform patterns. **A:** Progression from normal waveform contour through hesitant and alternating flow to retrograde vertebral artery flow. **B:** Vertebral artery stenosis. **C:** Proximal extracranial vertebral artery occlusion with collateral artery reconstitution.

## SUMMARY

- Duplex ultrasound for the diagnosis of extracranial carotid disease has become a standard tool utilized by clinicians.
- The combination of real-time B-mode imaging, Doppler spectral waveform analysis, and color Doppler imaging has proven to be accurate and clinically valuable in spite of variability in reported comparisons of velocity threshold criteria to the severity of arteriographic stenosis.[27]
- Multiple studies have established reliable criteria by which to classify carotid stenosis and occlusion.
- Atherosclerotic disease and other arterial abnormalities can be easily detected and monitored with ultrasound to prevent serious consequences such as stroke.

## CRITICAL THINKING QUESTIONS

1. Your initial B-mode and Doppler evaluation of the left carotid system suggests that there may be occlusion of the ICA. What key features will help to confirm occlusion of this vessel?

2. A carotid–vertebral artery duplex examination has been requested on a patient who is in the cardiac intensive care unit awaiting cardiac transplantation. The patient has an IABP. Doppler waveform contour is markedly altered, and there is an arrhythmia. What is the best way to approach this duplex examination in terms of interpreting the Doppler velocities and flow patterns and application of other diagnostic criteria?

3. During a carotid–vertebral artery duplex examination, you document high-grade, 80% to 99% stenosis of the left proximal ICA. There is minimal plaque visible in the right proximal ICA (and through the carotid bifurcation), yet the PSV is diffusely increased at 165 cm/s. Is this a 50% to 79% stenosis? What may account for the elevated Doppler flow velocities contralateral to the 80% to 99% stenosis? How would you describe this in the vascular laboratory report?

4. Brachial systolic pressures are asymmetrical: right = 86 mm Hg, left = 138 mm Hg. As you begin the carotid–vertebral artery duplex, you find abnormal, dampened, and hesitant Doppler waveform contour through the right proximal CCA. What do you expect the remainder of the carotid–vertebral artery duplex examination to reveal?

## MEDIA MENU

Student Resources available on the**Point**® include:
- Audio glossary
- Interactive question bank
- Videos
- Internet resources

## REFERENCES

1. Barber FE, Baker DW, Nation AWC, et al. Ultrasonic duplex echo-Doppler scanner. *IEEE Trans Biomed Eng*. 1974;21:109–113.
2. Beach KW. D. Eugene Strandness, Jr, MD, and the revolution in noninvasive vascular diagnosis. Part 1: foundations. *J Ultrasound Med*. 2005;24:259–272.
3. Fell G, Breslau P, Knox RA, et al. Importance of noninvasive ultrasonic Doppler testing in the evaluation of patients with asymptomatic carotid bruits. *Am Heart J*. 1981;102:221–226.
4. Fell G, Phillips DJ, Chikos PM, et al. Ultrasonic duplex scanning for disease of the carotid artery. *Circulation*. 1981;64:1191–1195.
5. Johnston SC, Gress DR, Browner WS, et al. Short-term prognosis after emergency department diagnosis of TIA. *JAMA*. 2000;284:2901–2906.
6. Whisnant JP. The role of the neurologist in the decline of stroke. *Ann Neurol*. 1983;14:1–7.
7. Santos RD, Nasir K. Insights into atherosclerosis from invasive and non-invasive imaging studies: should we treat subclinical atherosclerosis? *Atherosclerosis*. 2009;205:349–356.
8. Grogan JK, Shaalan WE, Cheng H, et al. B-mode ultrasonographic characterization of carotid atherosclerotic plaques in symptomatic and asymptomatic patients. *J Vasc Surg*. 2005;42:435–441.
9. El-Barghouty N, Geroulakos G, Nicolaides A, et al. Computer assisted carotid plaque characterization. *Eur J Vasc Endovasc Surg*. 1995;9:389–393.
10. Takiuchi S, Rakugi H, Honda K, et al. Quantitative ultrasonic tissue characterization can identify high-risk atherosclerotic alteration in human carotid arteries. *Circulation*. 2000;102:776–770.
11. Rohren EM, Kliewer MA, Carroll BA, et al. A spectrum of Doppler waveforms in the carotid and vertebral arteries. *AJR* 2001;181:1695–1704.
12. Kremkau FW. *Diagnostic Ultrasound Principles and Instruments*. St. Louis, MO: Saunders Elsevier; 2006.
13. Moneta GL, Mitchell EL, Esmonde N, et al. Extracranial carotid and vertebral arteries. In: Zierler RE, ed. *Strandness's Duplex Scanning in Vascular Disorders*. 4th ed. Philadelphia, PA: Lippincott Williams & Wilkens; 2010:87–100.
14. North American Symptomatic Carotid Endarterectomy Trial Collaborators. Beneficial effect of carotid endarterectomy in patients with high-grade carotid stenosis. *N Engl J Med*. 1991;325:445–453.
15. European Carotid Surgery Trialists' Collaborative Group (ECST). MRC European Carotid surgery Trial: interim results for symptomatic patients with severe (70-99%) or with mild (0-29%) carotid stenosis. *Lancet*. 1996;347:1591–1593.
16. Executive Committee for Asymptomatic Carotid Atherosclerosis Study. Endarterectomy for asymptomatic carotid artery stenosis. *JAMA*. 1995;273:1421–1428.
17. Moneta GL, Edwards JM, Papanicolaou G, et al. Screening for asymptomatic internal carotid artery stenosis: duplex criteria for discriminating 60% to 99% stenosis. *J Vasc Surg*. 1995;21:989–994.
18. Grant EG, Benson CB, Moneta GL, et al. Carotid artery stenosis: gray-scale and Doppler US diagnosis—Society of Radiologists in Ultrasound Consensus Conference. *Radiology*. 2003;229:340–346.
19. Whyman MR, Hoskins PR, Leng GC, et al. Accuracy and reproducibility of duplex ultrasound imaging in a phantom model of femoral artery stenosis. *J Vasc Surg*. 1993;17:524–530.
20. Leng GC, Whyman MR, Donnan PT, et al. Accuracy and reproducibility of duplex ultrasonography in grading femoropopliteal stenoses. *J Vasc Surg*. 1993;17:510–517.
21. Matos JM, Barshes NR, Mccoy S, et al. Validating common carotid stenosis by duplex ultrasound with carotid angiogram or computed tomography scan. *J Vasc Surg*. 2014;59:435–439.
22. Slovut DP, Romero JM, Hannon KM, et al. Detection of common carotid artery stenosis using duplex ultrasonography: a validation study with computed tomographic angiography. *J Vasc Surg*. 2010;51:65–70.
23. Ascer E, Gennaro M, Pollina RM, et al. The natural history of the external carotid artery after carotid endarterectomy: implications for management. *J Vasc Surg*. 1996;23:582–586.
24. Casey K, Zhou W, Tedesco MM, et al. Fate of the external carotid artery following carotid interventions. *Int J Angiol*. 2009;18:173–176.
25. Yurdakul M, Tola M. Proximal vertebral artery stenosis of 50% or more. *J Ultrasound Med*. 2011;30:163–168.
26. Yurdakul M, Tola M, Uslu OS. Color Doppler ultrasonography in occlusive diseases of the brachiocephalic and proximal subclavian arteries. *J Ultrasound Med*. 2008;27:1065–1070.
27. Beach KW, Leotta DF, Zierler RE. Carotid Doppler velocity measurements and anatomic stenosis: correlation is futile. *Vasc Endovascular Surg*. 2012;46:466–474.

# Uncommon Pathology of the Carotid System

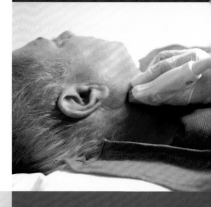

EILEEN FRENCH-SHERRY

## CHAPTER 8

## OBJECTIVES

- Recognize patient signs and symptoms of carotid artery pathology beyond atherosclerosis
- Identify uncommon pathology in the carotid arteries
- Plan an appropriate duplex examination to assist in the diagnosis of unusual pathology in the carotid arteries
- Create interpretable images of unusual carotid pathology using B-mode, Doppler, and color duplex ultrasound techniques
- Avoid pitfalls in scanning and documenting unusual pathology in the carotid arteries

## GLOSSARY

**aneurysm** A localized dilatation of the wall of an artery that involves all layers of the arterial wall

**arteritis** Inflammation of an artery

**carotid body tumor** A benign mass (also called paraganglioma or chemodectoma) of the carotid body that is a small round mass at the carotid bifurcation

**dissection** A tear along the inner layer of an artery that results in the splitting or separation of the walls of a blood vessel

**fibromuscular dysplasia** Abnormal growth and development of the muscular layer of an artery wall with fibrosis and collagen deposition causing a localized series of stenoses

**intimal flap** A small tear in the wall of a blood vessel resulting in a portion of the intima and part of the media protruding into the lumen of the vessel; this free portion of the blood vessel wall may appear to move with pulsations in flow

**pseudoaneurysm** The disruption of an arterial wall or anastomosis that results in a pulsating or expanding hematoma outside the artery, also called false aneurysm

**tortuosity** The quality of being tortuous, winding, turning, twisting

## KEY TERMS

**aneurysm**

**arteritis**

**carotid body tumor**

**dissection**

**fibromuscular dysplasia**

**intimal flap**

**pseudoaneurysm**

**radiation injury**

**tortuosity**

Atherosclerosis is clearly the most common pathology that is encountered during a carotid ultrasound examination. However, the vascular sonographer will be faced with other forms of disease and abnormalities while scanning the carotid arteries. Some of these abnormalities will be observed more frequently, such as tortuosity, whereas others are fairly rare, such as carotid artery aneurysms. It is important to know the ultrasound presentation and scanning requirements when presented with nonatherosclerotic carotid disease. This chapter will review several of these less common findings observed during carotid duplex scans.

## TORTUOSITY AND KINKING

Sonographers frequently encounter tortuous carotid arteries with varying degrees of winding and bending. Some of these vessels will be kinked with a very sharp angulation of the artery. As many as one-quarter of adults will have some degree of angulation within their internal carotid artery (ICA). Often, this is a bilateral finding.

## Signs and Symptoms

Tortuous carotid arteries are usually asymptomatic, but a kinked artery may cause symptoms of stroke or transient ischemic attack (TIA), particularly upon turning the head. Tortuous carotid arteries may be congenital, affecting more women than men, but most patients with symptoms are in the older adult population.[1] Frequently, a referring physician will mistake a very tortuous proximal common carotid artery (CCA) or brachiocephalic (innominate) artery for a carotid aneurysm, because a large tortuous vessel that courses superficially may appear to be a very pulsatile mass upon palpation and/or seen pulsing in the proximal neck. A duplex ultrasound scan can easily differentiate the two.

## Sonographic Examination Techniques

Although tortuosity is not uncommon in the CCA, the ICA is actually more likely to be redundant. It is a challenge to follow these vessels in long and transverse views, and takes considerable skill and experience to identify the course of the vessel as it changes planes while it curves, loops, and sometimes kinks (Fig. 8-1). Color is nearly essential to follow tortuous arteries, and care must be taken not to accidentally move on to a branch that the tortuous artery may be crossing. Moving slowly up the neck while concentrating only on the next half centimeter at a time will enable the sonographer to move the transducer along the plane needed to follow the vessel. The sonographer will be forced to move the transducer along unusual oblique angles and planes and, in transverse view, even move it proximally at times while the vessel turns upon itself. It is often not possible to obtain a picture of the entire tortuous segment in one image, but if it can be done, it creates a beautifully complex color picture (Fig. 8-2). Although Doppler angles close to

zero degrees may occur causing color aliasing in the vertical segments of the artery, flow also naturally increases along the outer edges of a curve and may also cause aliasing in the color display. Although a traditional velocity color image is important to demonstrate direction of flow, power color may also be used to demonstrate the course of the vessel without the potentially distracting color changes seen with velocity color in a tortuous vessel. It is very important to avoid moving on to a nearby vein or artery using power color while following a twisting vessel.

The next challenge is to obtain interpretable Doppler waveforms and velocities on a tortuous carotid artery. If there is no atherosclerotic disease or tight kink, Doppler waveforms should preferentially be taken on a straighter portion of the vessel, just before and after a curve, rather than directly at the point of the tightest curve. If a velocity measurement must be made on a curved segment of artery, the angle cursor is set so that the very middle of the angle correct cursor is parallel to the walls of the artery, even though one or both ends of the cursor may not appear to be aligned correctly (Fig. 8-3). Only the Doppler frequencies at the point of the sample volume are used to calculate the velocity, so the only angle needed is exactly at the point of the sample volume, not before or after it.

As in any carotid duplex examination, the sample volume should be kept center stream and small, despite the fact that velocities are higher along the outside of the curve. The inside of a curve may have lower velocities and demonstrate flow separation at or just distal to the curve. Some laboratories may choose to place the sample volume at the highest point of velocity, no matter whether it is along the wall or not. Although this process will ensure that no high velocities will be missed, in the case of the curved vessel a sample volume placed along the outer wall will possibly make the interpretation even more difficult because the velocities measured here will be more likely to enter the abnormal range even in a normal artery. It remains challenging to interpret the velocities around a curved vessel, and it

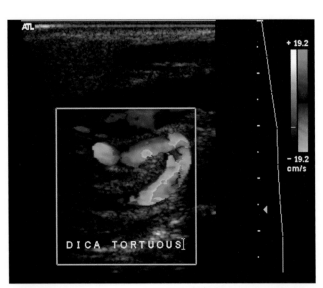

**FIGURE 8-1** Color is a useful tool to appreciate the tortuous course of the distal ICA. (Image courtesy of Kimberly Gaydula, BS, RVT, University of Chicago, Vascular Laboratory.)

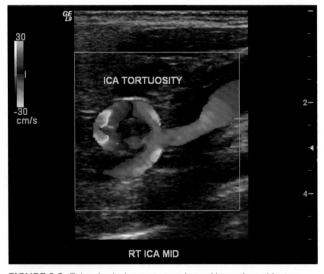

**FIGURE 8-2** Color clearly demonstrates a looped internal carotid artery with higher velocities (aliasing) along the outer walls of the vessel as the flow courses upward on the left side of the image and as it moves downward in the red segment in the middle of the image. (Image courtesy of Damaris Gonzalez, RVT, RDMS, Rush University, Vascular Laboratory.)

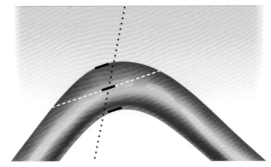

**FIGURE 8-3** Appropriate angle correction techniques when sampling along a curved portion of the vessel. The center part of the angle correct cursor needs to be parallel to the walls of a curved vessel.

is recommended that a combination of B-mode in multiple views together with Doppler velocities will demonstrate a suspected area best.

### Technical Considerations

A standard carotid duplex examination, as described in the preceding chapter, should be completed first. Additional transverse and longitudinal color images of the tortuous carotid segments should be obtained. Scroll the sample volume through the tortuous segment or kink and document Doppler velocities pre- and postcurve or kink, setting the middle of the angle correct cursor parallel to the walls of the vessel, as described above. Transverse and longitudinal B-mode images should be used to identify any plaque along the curved segment. A transverse B-mode image may be helpful in identifying the diameter of the artery at a tight kink. Some laboratories may document flow changes past a kink and/or symptoms while the patient turns the head.

### Diagnosis

High velocities naturally occur past a curve, making it difficult to apply strict velocity criteria on tortuous vessels. However, recognizing this normal flow phenomenon should be helpful to identify false positive velocity increases when the arterial lumen appears normal. Unfortunately, there is no specific velocity criterion to apply to tortuous vessels owing to the variety of angulations that may occur. Careful analysis of B-mode images with and without color in multiple planes can be helpful as adjunct data to confirm that velocity changes around the curve are caused by plaque formation or a significant kink rather than just a normal flow response to a curve in the vessel. In the case of a significant stenosis, poststenotic turbulence will be present and persist beyond the area in question.

## DISSECTIONS/INTIMAL FLAPS

An arterial dissection is simply a separation of the layers of an artery, typically the intima from the media, caused by a tear in the intima or a separation within the layers possibly from a rupture of the vasa vasorum.[2] The dissected intima, which may include some of the media, typically flaps or flutters freely in the arterial lumen, although some may appear stable. As the dissected intima flutters in the lumen with each pulse, it may temporarily cover a branch of the artery (i.e., renal artery off the aorta), stopping flow into the

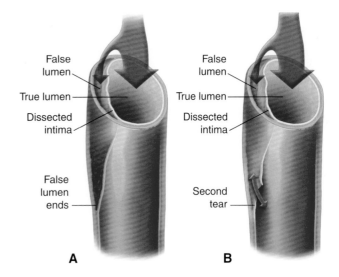

**FIGURE 8-4 A:** Diagram of a blind-ended dissection. **B:** Diagram of a dissection with a secondary tear.

branch for a segment of each pulse. Some dissections may result in a pseudoaneurysm (PA) because of the weakening in the arterial wall caused by the splitting of the layers.

The intimal tear creates a false lumen, where blood can enter through the tear and either flow or form a thrombus. Blood can exit the false lumen in either of two ways. It can enter and exit the false lumen through the same tear, or exit via a secondary tear either distal or proximal to the original tear (Fig. 8-4A and B). Either configuration will result in differing flow patterns in the false lumen compared to the true lumen. Flow in a false lumen may (1) demonstrate antegrade flow caused by the blood continuing through a distal secondary tear into the true lumen, (2) move in and out of the false lumen in a to-and-fro pattern, (3) thrombose to form a stenosis or occlusion by stretching into the true lumen, or (4) demonstrate reversed flow direction, with flow exiting the false lumen through a secondary proximal tear.

### Signs and Symptoms

A carotid artery dissection may originate in the aortic arch and extend into the CCA. Some of the dissections may be associated with diseases such as Marfan's syndrome or Ehler-Danlos syndrome. However, dissections may also originate in the mid/distal ICA 2 to 3 cm distal to the bulb and extend proximally or appear at the distal end of the carotid bifurcation. These dissections can be either spontaneous or traumatic. Following carotid endarterectomy, an intimal flap may occasionally form in the area of the endarterectomized segment.

A carotid dissection may be an unexpected finding in those patients where the dissection extends from the aorta because these dissections may cause no cerebral symptoms or pain. However, other patients with a dissection, particularly one that begins in the ICA, may present with pain in the head, face, or neck or with or without hemispheric symptoms. Dissection is usually suspected when a young patient (typically 35 to 50 years old) presents with symptoms of stroke despite having no risk factors for atherosclerosis, and particularly with a history of trauma. The trauma that

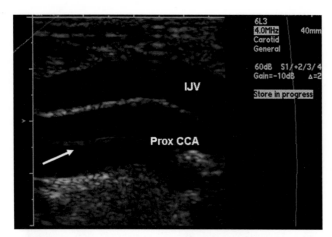

**FIGURE 8-5** A longitudinal view of the thin, bright structure (*arrow*) in the lumen of the proximal common carotid artery (prox CCA) clearly documents a dissection. The internal jugular vein (IJV) is shown anterior to the CCA. (Image courtesy of Damaris Gonzalez, RVT, RDMS, Rush University, Vascular Laboratory.)

may cause a dissection may not be evident at first, because it could be as subtle as a cough or turning the head or be a more obvious blunt trauma to the head or neck. A stretching of the artery may have occurred during these events, causing a tear in the arterial wall, or there may be an intimal weakness predisposing the individual to this consequence. With dissections that appear to be spontaneous, the primary risk factor is often hypertension.[3-6]

## Sonographic Examination Techniques

The first duplex ultrasound finding indicating that a dissection may be present is either an unusual color pattern in a section of an artery that otherwise shows no signs of atherosclerosis or the presence of a thin white line in the lumen that appears to flutter with each pulse. In B-mode, it is important to investigate the continued presence of the white line in both longitudinal and transverse views, and to be sure that it is not a refraction artifact from a nearby venous valve (Figs. 8-5 and 8-6). If the white structure can be visualized in multiple views, including anterior–posterior

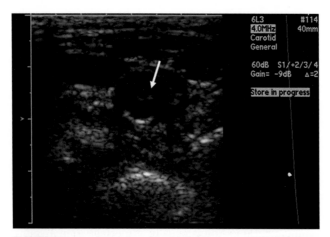

**FIGURE 8-6** A transverse view of the thin, bright structure in the lumen of a common carotid artery clearly documents the dissection (*arrow*). (Image courtesy of Damaris Gonzalez, RVT, RDMS, Rush University, Vascular Laboratory.)

(AP) and lateral planes, it is much more likely to be a dissection rather than an artifact. If the media is also involved, the white structure may appear thicker and move less.

The flow patterns on each side of the dissected intima (true and false lumens) need to be investigated with Doppler, and will be quite different from each other (Fig. 8-7A–C). In the case where there is only one tear in the intima, blood flow in the true lumen may continue to show a low-resistance Doppler signal, but the false lumen will have a different flow pattern, probably high resistance in nature. If the false lumen has enough thrombus or blood within it to block a significant portion of the artery, it will form a stenosis of the true lumen and demonstrate a stenotic velocity pattern. The stenosis formed by a thrombosed false lumen is typically very smooth and tapered, and may be longer than the stenosis formed by atherosclerotic plaque. If the thrombosed false lumen causes a tight stenosis or occlusion of the distal ICA, the proximal and mid-ICA may have a high-resistance flow pattern typical of a distal ICA occlusion with little or no diastolic flow.

If there is still flow in the false lumen with a blind end, the flow pattern will be highly resistant. There may be portions of the false lumen with reversed flow direction because the blood has nowhere else to go but back into the true lumen through the original tear in the intima.

In the case where there is both an inflow and outflow tear in the intima, the flow patterns within the true and false lumens can demonstrate forward flow, but each will be different, and one may demonstrate a reversed flow direction.

Do not confuse an apparent change in direction of flow from the helical or corkscrew flow pattern (sometimes seen in the CCA) with a true dissection. The true dissection will typically reveal a white line between the differing flow patterns that will be absent in a corkscrew pattern of flow in the normal CCA seen in transverse view.

### Technical Considerations

Following the completion of a standard carotid duplex examination, additional images are required. B-mode images of the dissection should be documented using longitudinal, transverse, and multiple planes if possible. Obtain Doppler waveforms and velocities in both the false and true lumen for a dissection, and pre-, at, and postflap for a short intimal flap. Color images can be used to demonstrate location, proximal and distal ends of dissection, open or thrombosed lumen, tapering of stenosis, length of stenosis, and dissection.

## Diagnosis

In the presence of a carotid dissection, the carotid duplex examination may not show any evidence of atherosclerotic disease, particularly in a young patient. Careful evaluation of the B-mode image will reveal a thin white structure in the arterial lumen. This represents the dissected intimal layer as well as some connective tissue and may be fluttering or still, depending on whether the medial layer is included in the dissected segment, making it thicker, or on whether the false lumen is completely or partially thrombosed. The stenosis in this case is typically smooth and tapered in nature, in the proximal/mid-CCA or mid-/distal ICA beyond the bifurcation. It is difficult to completely differentiate between this situation and a long smooth atherosclerotic plaque; however, there will likely be more evidence of

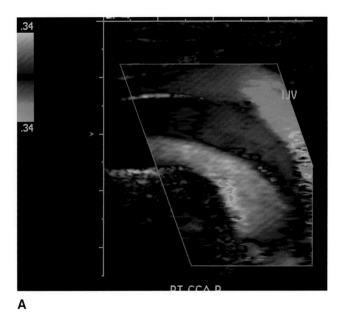

A

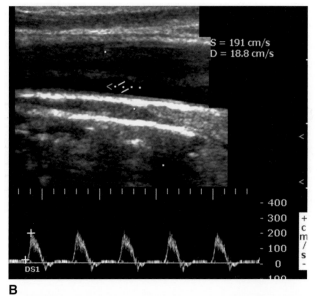

B

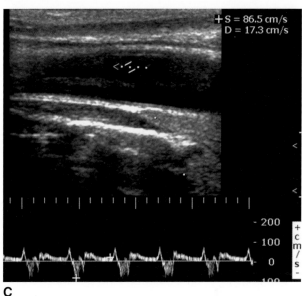

C

**FIGURE 8-7 A:** Color filling of the true and false lumens of the dissected artery documents different directions of flow in each. The uppermost blue lumen is the IJV. The two lower flow channels are the true and false lumens of the CCA. (Image courtesy of Damaris Gonzalez, RVT, RDMS, Rush University, Vascular Laboratory.) **B:** Spectral Doppler waveforms taken from the true lumen of a CCA dissection. Note the increased resistance to flow. **C:** Spectral Doppler waveforms taken from the false lumen of a CCA dissection. Note the to-and-fro (pendulum) flow pattern.

atherosclerosis in adjacent arteries in the latter case. Color changes are likely to be noticed either in the proximal and mid-CCA or in the mid-/distal ICA beyond the bifurcation. An important characteristic to identify the dissected artery is to demonstrate distinctly different flow patterns in the true and false lumens by analysis of the Doppler waveforms.

## FIBROMUSCULAR DYSPLASIA

Fibromuscular dysplasia (FMD) is a disease involving abnormal growth of the arterial wall and may involve the intima, media, and/or adventitia. The media is the most common location for the abnormal growth of smooth muscle cells and fibrous tissue. The abnormal growth will sometimes cause narrowing of the arterial lumen in multiple sections with normal walls or slight aneurysmal dilatation in between the stenotic segments. This essentially causes a "string of beads" appearance of the artery on arteriography with larger and smaller diameters in sequence.

## Signs and Symptoms

FMD is primarily seen in young (25 to 50 years old) Caucasians, occurring in females three times more commonly than men.[4-7] The most common location of disease is the renal arteries, and hypertension is frequently seen with renal involvement. The second most common vessel impacted is the ICA. Patients with carotid FMD often have no symptoms and can present with a cervical bruit. Embolization may occur and cause TIA's. In addition, approximately 30% of patients with carotid FMD may also have cerebral aneurysms.

## Sonographic Examination Techniques

A young person who is referred to the vascular laboratory for a carotid duplex examination should be evaluated for evidence of FMD. Bilateral disease is typical. The typical "string of beads" appearance of the artery may not be clearly appreciated at first because this disease primarily involves

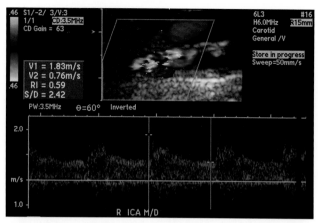

**FIGURE 8-8** An ICA with fibromuscular dysplasia. In the area of FMD in the mid-/distal ICA, the Doppler spectral waveform demonstrates marked turbulence with spectral broadening that is clearly different than the normal waveform seen in the proximal ICA. (Image courtesy of Besnike Ramadani, BS, RVT, University of Chicago, Vascular Laboratory.)

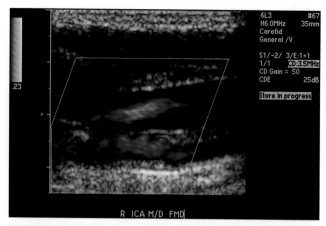

**FIGURE 8-10** Power color is helpful in documenting the dilatations and narrowing that are characteristic of FMD. (Image courtesy of Besnike Ramadani, BS, RVT, University of Chicago, Vascular Laboratory.)

the distal ICA, where the vessel often courses deeply into the tissue making detailed images difficult. The first sign of FMD during a duplex examination is most likely to be a sudden turbulence with high velocities in the distal ICA after the proximal arteries have shown no sign of atherosclerosis (Fig. 8-8). The sonographer may need to change to a lower frequency probe to visualize more distally in the ICA (Fig. 8-9). Power Doppler may be helpful in visualizing the characteristic beading in the artery, avoiding the distraction of aliasing from the marked turbulence (Fig. 8-10).

### Technical Considerations

The distal ICA should be carefully examined with color Doppler and B-mode looking for sudden turbulence distally after a normal appearing CCA and proximal ICA. A lower frequency probe may be needed to visualize the very distal ICA behind the ear.

Additional images are required when faced with the FMD patient. A color image of the distal ICA in longitudinal view

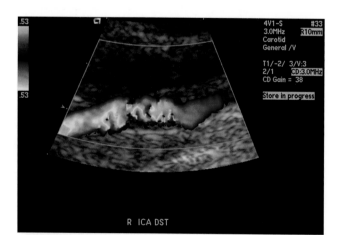

**FIGURE 8-9** FMD. This is an image obtained from the same patient illustrated in Figure 8-8. A 3 MHz transducer positioned posterior to the ear to obtain this view of FMD in the distal ICA. The image clearly depicts the turbulence and suggests a beading appearance of the artery. (Image courtesy of Besnike Ramadani, BS, RVT, University of Chicago, Vascular Laboratory.)

will demonstrate a change from normal color proximally to the turbulent area if FMD is present. A velocity waveform must be taken in the distal ICA at the point of highest velocity, confirming stenosis if present, and demonstrate a turbulent waveform configuration, whether a significant stenosis is present or not, in the presence of FMD. Power Doppler imaging can be used to attempt to demonstrate changes in diameter or "string of beads" appearance. In this same area, a B-mode image should be used to further demonstrate changes in diameter, especially if color bleeding is difficult to control.

If evidence of FMD is noted in the carotids, the referring physician may order a renal artery exam because FMD is often found in multiple vessels.

### Diagnosis

A young patient with no evidence of carotid atherosclerotic disease in the bifurcation who demonstrates marked turbulence in the distal ICA with increased velocities should be considered as having ultrasound characteristics consistent with FMD. A "string of beads" appearance of the distal ICA on B-mode, color Doppler, or power Doppler imaging aids in the confirmation of FMD. However, the gold standard for the diagnosis of FMD is angiography.

## CAROTID BODY TUMOR

The carotid body is a 1 to 1.5 mm structure located in the adventitia of the carotid bifurcation. It has a role in control of blood pressure, arterial pH, and blood gases. A carotid body tumor (CBT) may form that is easily seen with duplex ultrasound. These tumors are classified as paragangliomas and are usually not malignant.

### Signs and Symptoms

CBT are usually asymptomatic. Typically, patients notice a small lump in the anterior neck that has been growing slowly over a period of years. There may be a slight discomfort in the area, and some patients may notice dysphagia, headaches, or a change in their voice.[4,8]

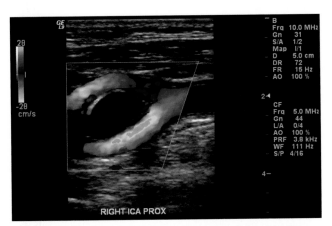

**FIGURE 8-11** Color image clearly demonstrates the splaying of the ECA (near field) and ICA (far field) by the mass of a CBT. (Image courtesy of Damaris Gonzalez, RVT, RDMS, Rush University, Vascular Laboratory.)

## Sonographic Examination Techniques

CBTs are easily seen on duplex ultrasound as a well-defined mass located between the ICA and external carotid artery (ECA) at the bifurcation, splaying the two vessels apart (Fig. 8-11). These tumors are highly vascular in nature, being fed by the ECA and its branches that can often be seen entering the mass with color flow. The color scale may need to be decreased to identify these small vessels (Fig. 8-12). Doppler will typically demonstrate low-resistance waveforms within the tumor.

### Technical Considerations

When scanning a patient with a CBT, a color image of the mass is recorded to document its vascularity. Color imaging should also be used to determine the proximity of the ICA and ECA to the mass.[4] Multiple B-mode images in various planes are used to determine the overall dimensions of the tumor with measurements in longitudinal and transverse planes.

## Diagnosis

Location of a highly vascularized mass most clearly identifies a CBT on duplex ultrasound. The CBT is clearly located

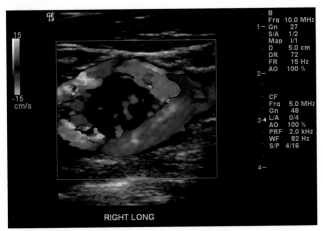

**FIGURE 8-12** The color scale was decreased in order to appreciate color within the mass of a CBT. (Image courtesy of Damaris Gonzalez, RVT, RDMS, Rush University, Vascular Laboratory.)

at the carotid bifurcation, splaying the ICA and ECA. It is typically highly vascular and fed by ECA branches. Doppler waveforms within the tumor are typically low resistance. It is important to the surgeon to document the length of the tumor and whether the tumor just touches the carotid vessels, partially surrounds them, or completely encases the ICA, ECA, and/or CCA.

## CAROTID ANEURYSM

An aneurysm is a dilatation of the artery that involves all three layers of the arterial wall. True carotid aneurysms are extremely uncommon. Carotid artery aneurysms are most commonly located within the CCA and often at the bifurcation, although the ECA may also develop aneurysms.[9] Atherosclerosis appears to be the cause in the majority of cases. Some carotid aneurysms are the result of infection and are termed mycotic aneurysms.[10]

### Signs and Symptoms

Usually, the patient with suspicion of a carotid aneurysm presents with a nontender, pulsatile mass in the neck. The patient may be asymptomatic or have symptoms of a TIA or stroke. Rupture is also rare, but there may be cranial nerve dysfunction such as a hoarseness of the patient's voice.[11]

### Sonographic Examination Techniques

Multiple B-mode images in longitudinal and transverse planes with diameter measurements are required to give a complete picture of the suspected aneurysm. Also compare the diameters of the CCA, ICA, and ECA to the contralateral carotid system.

### Technical Considerations

Longitudinal and transverse B-mode and color images of the widest area of the vessels should be documented and compared to the normal segments. Measure the widest diameter in the transverse view in both AP and lateral planes. To avoid overestimating the diameter, measure the widest diameter in longitudinal view *along the axis of flow* (90 degrees to flow or walls). This is a helpful confirmation of vessel diameter, particularly in a slightly tortuous vessel. Lastly, the diameter of the normal segments of the CCA and ICA should be measured bilaterally in longitudinal and transverse views for comparison to the dilated area.

### Diagnosis

True carotid aneurysms are extremely rare. It is difficult to differentiate a large carotid bulb from a medium or small aneurysm. Some authors have described the true aneurysm at the bulbous portion of the ICA or CCA as having a diameter >200% of the ICA or >150% of the CCA[10] (Fig. 8-13).

## PSEUDOANEURYSM

A PA, also known as a false aneurysm, is also very uncommon in the carotid arteries. PAs are typically caused by penetrating trauma or iatrogenic injury creating a perforation in the artery wall, whereby blood can extravasate out the

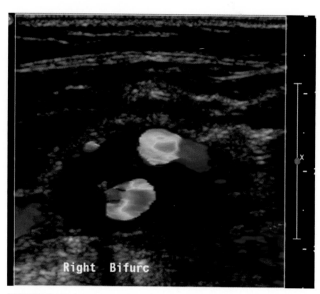

**FIGURE 8-13** A transverse view of a mycotic aneurysm at the carotid bifurcation. (Reprinted with permission from *Journal for Vascular Ultrasound* 2010;34:81.)

arterial wall into the surrounding tissue.[4] PAs may also form at an endarterectomy site or the anastomosis of a carotid bypass graft. The blood flow outside the artery wall forms a spherical or ovoid mass bordered by the surrounding tissues. There may or may not be thrombus formed within the external mass or sac. The channel connecting the PA mass to the artery is called the PA "neck" and may be short or long, wide or thin. Characteristically, blood flow within the neck has a to-and-fro appearance as blood flows out of the artery, to the mass, and back into the artery again.

## Signs and Symptoms

Patients will usually present with a palpable, pulsatile mass in the neck associated with a history of trauma, whether iatrogenic or otherwise. The presence of a carotid bypass graft with a pulsatile mass is also an appropriate indication for a duplex ultrasound examination. TIA or stroke is also possible, but rupture rarely occurs.

## Sonographic Examination Techniques

A transverse overview of the carotid arteries in color will typically be the easiest and fastest way to determine the area of interest for further examination. A mass, either partially or completely filled with a pulsatile color pattern, will be noted adjacent to the artery. Typically, the color flow within the PA in transverse view will demonstrate a "yin-yang" appearance, with red color on half the mass and blue color on the other half demonstrating flow into and out of the mass. Upon further investigation with careful color control of gain and scale, a point will be noted in the artery wall as the defect that allows blood flow to extend beyond the arterial wall into the color-filled "neck" of the PA. The neck may be short, with flow going directly into the mass, or long and winding. The diameter of the disruption in the wall and the neck of the PA is variable. However, the key feature of the neck is a to-and-fro Doppler flow pattern, usually with

high velocities. Velocities in the PA mass itself are typically much lower than in the neck because of the larger diameter. PAs may thrombose spontaneously, so a variable amount of thrombus may be present. The color scale may need to be decreased to obtain adequate color filling of the mass. Steering angles and planes of view may need to be varied to estimate the percentage of mass that is thrombosed.

A sonographer must be careful not to confuse a PA with an enlarged lymph node or a tumor. A lymph node or tumor may also appear to be a mass with color flow within it, but the flow patterns in a lymph node vessel or a branch feeding the node will have not the characteristic to-and-fro Doppler waveform but either a typical arterial waveform or a venous waveform pattern. A tumor vessel may demonstrate a low-resistance arterial waveform but will also be missing the pendulum flow pattern in the branches feeding it that are characteristic of a true PA.

## Technical Considerations

A transverse overview of the carotid arteries from clavicle to mandible is performed first to identify a mass adjacent to the artery. Color is very helpful in identifying a PA, especially if it is not completely filled with thrombus. Document the PA in color, demonstrating the red and blue color pattern associated with these structures. The largest diameter of the PA should be measured in both longitudinal and transverse views. Some laboratories choose to estimate the amount of thrombus in the PA, i.e., 30%, 50%, nearly completely thrombosed, because this will help the clinician to decide on a treatment. Many PAs thrombose spontaneously, and those with long necks that are nearly thrombosed are most likely to completely thrombose without intervention. B-mode images may document this estimate in multiple planes of view.

To identify the location of the source of the PA, color is used to follow the neck from the PA to the artery. In addition, there will be a color change along the wall of the native artery at the perforation (i.e., color aliasing) and possibly a color bruit. Spectral Doppler is used to identify and document the to-and-fro flow pattern associated with the neck of a true PA. If possible, try to measure the perforation in the artery wall using B-mode. This is not always possible, and the measurement should be taken very carefully. It can be used as an estimate of the size of the wall injury. Lastly, demonstrate Doppler flow patterns in the native artery pre- and post-PA.

## Diagnosis

Pulsatile color flow in the mass with a yin-yang (red and blue) appearance is the classic presentation of a PA. However, the most important characteristic to demonstrate for the diagnosis of a PA is the to-and-fro Doppler flow pattern in the neck of the PA. As mentioned in the preceding section, thrombus may or may not be noted in the mass, and an estimate of the percentage of the thrombus filling the mass may be helpful to the physician.

## RADIATION-INDUCED ARTERIAL INJURY

Radiation-induced arterial injury (RIAI) is caused by the use of therapeutic irradiation during treatment for various tumors. The treatment with radiation preferentially injures cancer cells, causing less injury to other tissues. However, there is a potential effect on blood vessels because of the presence of endothelial cells, which are sensitive to the radiation. Capillaries, arterioles, and venules are primarily involved, but it may also affect the carotid arteries in some patients. Injury to the vaso vasorum in the medial layer of the artery causes fibrosis. This injury and the repopulation of the endothelium may result in a narrowing of the lumen. Other risk factors such as hypercholesterolemia and hypertension may add to the effect of the radiation, but not all patients develop these lesions.[12]

## Signs and Symptoms

Patients will present with a history of radiation often several years prior to their examination. Often, these patients lack the typical risk factors for atherosclerosis. An atypical location of an atherosclerotic stenosis may tip the examiner to RIAI. In many patients, there is an absence of other atherosclerotic plaque in the carotids which makes a single unusually located stenosis suspicious. TIA or CVA may be effects of these lesions.

## Sonographic Scanning Techniques

The distribution, extent of stenosis, and sonographic characteristics of radiation-induced disease are different from the commonly encountered atherosclerotic disease. The ultrasound examination must include thorough B-mode imaging of the CCAs because there is a higher incidence of CCA radiation-induced stenosis as compared to bifurcation and ICA disease. Transverse and longitudinal B-mode images should be taken to document the echogenicity of these lesions. As with all carotid examinations, spectral Doppler and color-flow imaging are used to assess the areas of stenosis.

### Technical Considerations

A standard carotid duplex ultrasound examination is performed, although imaging may be difficult in some patients because of the changes in the tissue from the radiation. Poor echogenicity and hard, rather than supple, neck tissue is common in postradiated patients. Any surgery that may have altered the neck anatomy may also make the scan difficult, but rarely impossible, to obtain pertinent information. The patient's past medical history should be carefully reviewed for any earlier radiation treatment, and the exact location of the treatment can alert the interpreting physician to this phenomenon.

## Diagnosis

An atypical location of the carotid lesion with a history of radiation treatment in the past makes RIAI suggestive of the cause of the lesion. Radiation-induced stenotic lesions are significantly longer than the non–radiation-induced lesions. The area of maximum stenosis in the radiation-induced lesions also tends to be located at the distal end of the stenotic area. The stenotic lesions do not typically contain calcifications and may have hypoechoic foci (Figs. 8-14 and 8-15).

## ARTERITIS

Arteritis is an inflammation of the artery wall that results in breakdown of parts of the wall structure and may conclude

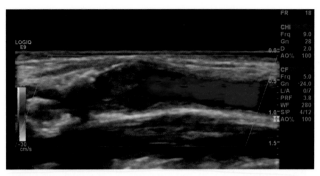

**FIGURE 8-14** RIAI. This image depicts an occlusion of the ICA in a 51-year-old man following radiation. There is no color filling of the ICA, only filling of the CCA. Note the several hypoechoic areas within the lesion. (Image courtesy of Kathleen Hannon, RN, MS, RVT, RDMS, Massachusetts General Hospital, Vascular Laboratory.)

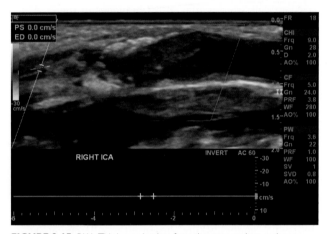

**FIGURE 8-15** RIAI. This image is taken from the same patient as shown in Figure 8-14. Spectral Doppler confirms the occlusion in the ICA. (Image courtesy of Kathleen Hannon, RN, MS, RVT, RDMS, Massachusetts General Hospital, Vascular Laboratory.)

in occlusion and sometimes distal ischemia. In the vascular laboratory, two forms of arteritis may be seen in a carotid artery examination, Takayasu's disease and temporal arteritis, a form of giant cell arteritis.

Takayasu's arteritis affects the aortic arch and great vessels, including the brachiocephalic, carotid, and subclavian arteries. Giant cell arteritis affects medium- and larger-sized arteries, so it may also affect the aortic arch and carotid arteries, but the vascular laboratory is usually asked to look specifically at the superficial temporal artery (STA) to assist in the diagnosis. There are no definitive ultrasound criteria for arteritis, and it is diagnosed through a series of blood tests and clinical presentations.

## Signs and Symptoms

There are a wide variety of clinical presentations for arteritis and no known etiology. However, autoimmune deficiencies are thought to be the suspect in these diseases, and women outnumber men 2:1. Although both young and old can be afflicted with arteritis, young people generally present with Takayasu's disease, and temporal arteritis generally affects the elderly. In Takayasu's disease, there may be claudication of the arms with no radial pulses if the subclavian arteries are affected. TIA, visual changes, stroke, and multiple bruits may also be encountered.[13] Temporal arteritis is likely to cause headache, low-grade fever, jaw claudication, tenderness in the temporal region, and visual problems, including blindness.

## Sonographic Examination Techniques

Takayasu's arteritis will generally be suspected in young people, especially young women. It may result in a vascular laboratory request for a carotid and renal examination because the obstruction of the arch and great vessels are most commonly seen in this order: subclavian, CCA, aorta, and, renal arteries. If lesions are seen in the carotid arteries, they are likely to appear as long, smooth, homogeneous narrowings in the artery, and appear to be more of a general wall thickening as opposed to typical atherosclerotic plaque within the lumen.

Giant cell arteritis may affect branches of the ECA, including the facial, occipital, and internal maxillary, but the most accessible branch is the STA. The STA can be scanned as it progresses up the temporal side of the head above the ear and across the forehead. If an echolucent or lightly echogenic "halo" surrounds the artery at any point, it is a positive sign of arteritis. The inflammation in this disease may be spotty, affecting segments of the artery and may include stenosis or occlusion. It is best to use the highest frequency transducer, such as a 12 or 15 MHz transducer. The STA is best located anterior to the ear, and if normal in that area, a pulse can be palpated. The course of the artery should be followed transversely along the side of the head and across the forehead where there are branches. Look for the characteristic "halo" to identify areas of inflammation, and avoid "spot checking" because the inflamed areas are intermittent and may be missed without a complete scan of the temporal artery. Look for areas of stenosis or occlusion if possible with color. It is best to obtain a Doppler waveform if any areas of aliasing are found in color. Otherwise,

a sample Doppler signal with a high-resistance waveform can be documented and is considered normal.

### Technical Considerations

When performing an ultrasound exam on a patient with Takayasu's arteritis, pay special attention to obtain Doppler waveforms in the most proximal areas possible, i.e., the brachiocephalic artery on the right and as proximal as possible on the left. Be sure to obtain bilateral brachial pressures and subclavian artery waveforms to assess the involvement of the subclavian arteries in the disease and/or the proximal or distal aorta. Take multiple B-mode images in longitudinal and transverse views and closely examine these for any arterial thickening or stenoses, especially in the CCAs.

With temporal arteritis, the entire course of the STA should be examined with transverse B-mode imaging. This approach is used to identify any areas with a halo or document no evidence of a halo with at least three representative images in transverse view. Use color-flow imaging to get an overview representation of flow within the temporal artery. Obtain a Doppler sample of a normal segment and any areas suspected of stenosis or occlusion.

## Diagnosis

Although there is no definitive test for these inflammatory diseases, duplex ultrasound can assist with information used to affirm the diagnosis. Takayasu's patients will typically have an unusual appearance of thickened artery walls, with some patients demonstrating long, narrowed stenoses of the CCAs. The echo texture will appear homogeneous. Often, the disease appears to be concentric and evenly distributed when imaged in transverse view (Fig. 8-16). This is in contrast to atherosclerotic disease, which is often eccentric and irregular. These patients will have abnormalities primarily related to the proximal CCAs and subclavian arteries, sometimes with abnormal waveforms indicating proximal

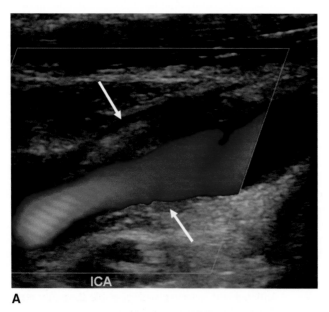

**A**

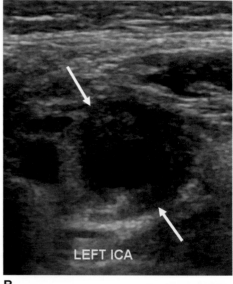

**B**

**FIGURE 8-16 A:** Sagittal view of arteritis impacting the carotid bifurcation extending into the proximal ICA. **B:** Transverse view of the same vessel demonstrating concentric wall thickening. Arrows in both images highlight the homogeneous wall thickening consistent with a vascular arteritis. (Images courtesy of Aria Levitas, BS and Richard Jackson, MD, Neurodiagnostics Laboratory, Glens Falls Hospital, Glens Falls, NY)

**PATHOLOGY BOX 8-1**
*Uncommon Carotid System Pathology*

| Pathology | B-Mode | Color | Doppler |
|---|---|---|---|
| Dissection or intimal flap | White line within lumen may be moving. Seen in transverse and longitudinal views. An occluded or thrombosed segment may cause smooth and tapered stenosis. | May be two colors on each side, aliasing if high velocities present. | Two clearly different flow patterns on each side of white line. May be occluded, high resistance, or reversed flow direction in one lumen. |
| Aneurysm | Section of artery at least 200% of normal ICA or 150% of normal CCA by some authors. Very rare. | Widened area of artery with flow separation and/or partial thrombosis. | Low velocities due to large diameter. |
| Pseudoaneurysm | Mass adjacent to artery post injury whether penetrating or iatrogenic. May have various levels of thrombosis or no evidence of thrombosis. | Color within mass has yin-yang (red/blue) pattern of color flow. | Distinct to-and-fro flow pattern in neck of pseudoaneurysm. |
| FMD | Difficult to see "string of beads" widening and narrowing in distal ICA. | Velocity and/or power color may demonstrate "string of beads." | Doppler waveforms typically show a sudden change from normal bulb and mid-ICA to markedly turbulent flow pattern with high velocities in distal ICA. |
| Temporal arteritis | Echolucent "halo" around sections of STA. | Color may show aliasing if stenoses occur. | Doppler pattern demonstrates high velocities if stenosis is present but not likely. |
| CBT | Mass between ICA and ECA splays arteries apart. | Color demonstrates highly vascular mass. ECA feeds mass. | Doppler demonstrates low-resistance waveforms within mass. |
| Tortuosity | Difficult to follow tortuous vessels with B-mode alone. | Color highly useful to follow tortuous vessels. Color aliasing seen frequently owing to sharp angulation (closer to zero degrees) and/or higher velocities past curve. Flow separation inside curve. | Velocities naturally increase as blood flows around a curve. Center of angle cursor (angle correct) set parallel to walls for velocity measurements. Edges of angle cursor may be off-parallel as long as center is parallel to walls. |

disease in the aorta or the origins of the great vessels. If the aortic arch is affected proximally, bilateral changes in the CCA waveforms will be noted, such as slow upstroke and lower than typical velocities bilaterally. If the aorta is stenosed in the area between the brachiocephalic and the left CCA, the left CCA and left subclavian artery waveforms may be turbulent, dampened, and display lower velocities than the right CCA and subclavian arteries.

An echolucent halo around the temporal artery is a strong indicator of temporal arteritis. Recent studies on the diagnostic value of the halo report sensitivity of 75% to 86% and specificity of 83% to 92% in patients with temporal arteritis.[14,15] Again, intermittent areas of focal velocity increases will be observed. Pathology Box 8-1 summarizes the various types of carotid pathology described in this chapter.

## SUMMARY

■ Sonographers expect to observe atherosclerotic plaque during carotid ultrasound examinations, but there are numerous other pathologies that can be encountered.
■ These additional carotid abnormalities include tortuosity, dissection, fibromuscular dysplagia, carotid body tumors, arteritis, pseudoaneurysms and rarely aneurysms.
■ Understanding the various pathologies and the associated ultrasound findings will aid in the proper diagnosis of these less commonly encountered carotid abnormalities.

## CRITICAL THINKING QUESTIONS

1. While examining a tortuous ICA, you observe an area of color aliasing. What can you do to determine if there is a stenosis?
2. When obtaining a Doppler waveform from the false lumen of a dissection, what direction would you expect the flow to be going?
3. A patient presents with a pulsatile neck mass. What would be helpful to differentiate the mass?

## REFERENCES

1. Lin PH, Lumsden AB. Carotid kinks and coils. In: Ernst CB, Stanley JC, eds. *Current Therapy in Vascular Surgery*. 4th ed. St. Louis, MO: Mosby; 2001:114–117.

2. Patel RR, Adam R, Maldjian C, et al. Cervical carotid dissection: current review of diagnosis and treatment. *Cardiovasc Rev*. 2012;20:145–152.

3. Treiman RL, Treiman GS. Carotid artery dissection. In: Ernst CB, Stanley JC, eds. *Current Therapy in Vascular Surgery*. 4th ed. St. Louis, MO: Mosby; 2001:108–111.

4. Zweibel WJ, Pellerito JS. Carotid occlusion, uncommon carotid pathology and tricky carotid cases. In: Zweibel WJ, Pellerito JS, eds. *Introduction to Vascular Ultrasonography*. 5th ed. Philadelphia, PA: Elsevier; 2005:191–210.

5. Morasch R, Pearce WH. Extracranial cerebrovascular disease. In: Fahey VA, ed. *Vascular Nursing*. 4th ed. Philadelphia, PA: Elsevier (USA); 2004:290–291.

6. Daigle R. Carotid color duplex imaging. In: Daigle RJ, ed. *Techniques in Noninvasive Vascular Diagnosis*. 2nd ed. Littleton, CO: Summer Publishing; 2002:23–48.

7. Kulbaski MJ, Smith RB. Surgical treatment of fibromuscular dysplasia of the carotid artery. In: Ernst CB, Stanley JC, eds. *Current Therapy in Vascular Surgery*. 4th ed. St. Louis, MO: Mosby; 2001:112–114.

8. Hallett JW. Carotid body tumors. In: Ernst CB, Stanley JC, eds. *Current Therapy in Vascular Surgery*. 4th ed. St. Louis, MO: Mosby; 2001:118–122.

9. El-Sabrout R, Cooley DA. Extracranial carotid artery aneurysms: Texas Heart Institute experience. *J Vasc Surg*. 2000;31:701–712.

10. Bekker D, Hannon K, Jaff MR, et al. Carotid artery mycotic aneurysm identified by duplex imaging. *J Vasc Ultrasound*. 2010;34:80–81.

11. Stanley JC. Extracranial carotid artery aneurysms. In: Ernst CB, Stanley JC, eds. *Current Therapy in Vascular Surgery*. 4th ed. St. Louis, MO: Mosby; 2001:104–107.

12. Modrall JG, Rosen SF, McIntyre KE. Radiation-induced arterial injury. In: Ernst CB, Stanley JC, eds. *Current Therapy in Vascular Surgery*. 4th ed. St. Louis, MO: Mosby; 2001:131–134.

13. Webb TH, Perler BA. Takayasu arteritis. In: Ernst CB, Stanley JC, eds. *Current Therapy in Vascular Surgery*. 4th ed. St. Louis, MO: Mosby; 2001:122–127.

14. LeSar CJ, Meier GH, DeMasi RJ, et al. The utility of color duplex ultrasonography in the diagnosis of temporal arteritis. *J Vasc Surg*. 2002;36:1154–1160.

15. Ball EL, Walsh SR, Yang TY, et al. Role of ultrasonography in the diagnosis of temporal arteritis. *Brit J Surg*. 2010;97:1765–1771.

# Carotid Intervention

ALI F. ABURAHMA

## CHAPTER 9

## OBJECTIVES

- Describe the ultrasound protocols unique for carotid scanning in postendarterectomy and poststent patients
- Define normal and abnormal diagnostic criteria associated with carotid stents
- List the pathology encountered in a postoperative or postinterventional carotid ultrasound

## KEY TERMS

**arteriotomy**

**carotid artery stenting**

**carotid endarterectomy**

**eversion carotid endarterectomy**

**in-stent restenosis**

## GLOSSARY

**arteriotomy** A surgical incision through the wall of an artery into the lumen

**carotid artery stenting** A catheter-based procedure in which a metal mesh tube is deployed into an artery to keep it open following balloon angioplasty to dilate a stenosis

**carotid endarterectomy** A surgical procedure during which the carotid artery is opened and plaque is removed in order to restore normal luminal diameter

**in-stent restenosis** A narrowing of the lumen of a stent which causes a stenosis

**polytetrafluoroethylene** Abbreviated PTFE, is a synthetic graft material used to create grafts and blood vessel patches; a common brand name is Gore-Tex

It is important for sonographers and clinicians to recognize that the duplex ultrasound data collected post-carotid artery stenting (CAS) will not be interpreted in the same way as for carotid endarterectomy (CEA). It is also important to recognize that although conventional duplex ultrasound velocity criteria may be applied in patients with CEA with primary closure, these criteria may not be applicable in CEA with patch closure. This chapter will review the techniques and criteria used with carotid artery ultrasound following surgery or stenting.

## CAROTID ENDARTERECTOMY

Carotid duplex ultrasound is usually used to evaluate the CEA patient either immediately postoperatively, within the first 30 days of surgery, or in long-term post-CEA duplex surveillance. The sonographer needs to be familiar with the operation and the complications that can arise during and subsequent to the procedure.

The traditional CEA is an open operation that is performed through an arteriotomy made longitudinally from the normalized internal carotid artery (ICA), through the bulb, and into the common carotid artery (CCA). Exposure is made sufficient to allow complete removal of the atheromatous plaque, which may extend from the distal CCA into the distal taper of the proximal ICA. Once the plaque is removed, the arteriotomy may be closed primarily by suturing together the cut edges of the arterial wall. In many patients, particularly women and patients with smaller diameter vessels, primary closure may narrow the lumen to the point of stenosis. This is more common at the distal end of the arteriotomy, where the ICA normalizes. At that point, common potential problems that may lead to a stenosis include: (1) narrowing as a result of closure, (2) plaque retained from an incomplete excision, and (3) a neointimal hyperplastic response to the operation which occurs within subsequent months (few to 18 months) of follow-up. Of these three potential problems, only the latter can truly be characterized as a restenosis. Other forms of stenosis are technical errors of the operation.

### CEA and Patch Closure

Because stenotic narrowing can result from closing the arteriotomy primarily, surgeons will often reduce the potential for stenosis by suturing in a patch to widen the lumen. The patch also reduces the potential intrusion of a hyperplastic response that may develop a restenosis.[1] Overall, patching will decrease perioperative carotid thrombosis, perioperative stroke, and late restenosis.[1,2]

The sonographer evaluating patients in follow-up to a CEA should expect to see most CEA patients with patches particularly in female patients, whose arteries tend to be narrower than that of males. Patches for CEA may be either autogenous vein or synthetic. The latter is constructed of either Dacron, polytetrafluoroethylene (PTFE), or bovine pericardial patches. The vein used for the patch may be a cervical vein exposed and harvested from the incision site or a segment taken from the great saphenous vein at the ankle or upper thigh. When a vein is used, the vein intima will face the lumen of the artery.[1]

## Eversion versus Traditional CEA

In recent years, some vascular surgeons are performing the operation using a technique called eversion CEA, which is more popular in Europe than the United States. Instead of using a long-axis arteriotomy and patch, the eversion CEA is performed with a complete transection of the ICA at the carotid bifurcation. The endarterectomy is performed by everting the cut ends of the arteries away from the incision and peeling the arterial wall away from the plaque as it is everted. The ends of the arteries are reverted to their normal position for subsequent reattachment. The procedure does not require a patch because the sutures are placed on the widened bulb of the ICA (Fig. 9-1).[2]

To the vascular sonographer, the eversion CEA will be less obvious in its presentation than the traditional CEA with patch. It will appear more like the traditional revascularization that was closed primarily (without a patch). Sutures if visible will surround the ICA circumferentially. In the standard CEA, the suture line will have an orientation along the long axis of the ICA, on its superficial wall. The eversion technique has the advantage of not requiring a patch because the full diameter of distal taper of the ICA is retained and possibly enlarged in the process of feathering the plaque beyond the bulb. The sonographer should expect to see less restenosis in the eversion CEA than in the CEA with primary closure, but eversion appears to have equivalent restenosis to the traditional CEA with patch.[2]

## Sonographic Examination Techniques

Most follow-up evaluations arise as scheduled outpatient appointments. Emergent testing is infrequently requested in an immediate postoperative patient, whether in the operating room or recovery room.

### Patient Preparation

The CEA duplex evaluation may be difficult in the immediate postoperative period. Sutures, staples, and dressings all compromise access for the sonographer. Sterile techniques, including sterile imaging pads, gel, transducer covers, or bio-occlusive dressings, should be used to minimize the risk of infection when scanning a patient in the first 48 hours

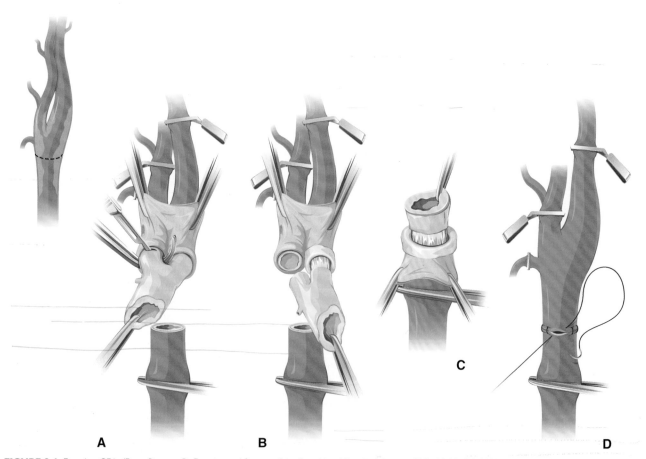

**A**          **B**          **C**          **D**

**FIGURE 9-1** Eversion CEA. (From Berguer R. *Function and Surgery of the Carotid and Vertebral Arteries.* Philadelphia, PA: Wolters Kluwer; 2013; Figure 5-17.)

following surgery. Once the skin has healed, there is little impedance to the ultrasound examination. No specific preparation is typically required other than to remove jewelry or clothing that may limit access to the neck.

In the long term, patients with CEA should be followed with duplex ultrasound testing. For any follow-up protocol, it is important that the first duplex examination be performed immediately postoperatively or within 1 month of CEA. This serves as the baseline study that will provide the velocity data to which all subsequent follow-ups should be compared.

## Patient Positioning

Patient positioning is the same used for a standard carotid ultrasound examination. The patient should be placed in a supine position with the head turned away from the side being examined. The chin should be tilted up slightly.

## Scanning Techniques

Ultrasound scanning techniques are similar to the standard preoperative scan. The CCA, ICA, and external carotid artery (ECA) are examined using B-mode and color-flow imaging techniques. Spectral Doppler is taken throughout the vessels at the typical levels specified in Chapter 7. There are particular areas to be closely examined, and these are described in the following section.

## Sonographic Technical Considerations

Primary concerns for the evaluation of the CEA patient include stenosis from residual plaque or intimal flap, suture narrowing, or thrombotic narrowing/occlusion. The ultrasound findings along the endarterectomy site as well as at the ends of the endarterectomy site must be carefully examined for any of these primary concerns. In the immediate postoperative period, specifically in patients whose CEA was closed using certain patches (e.g., PTFE), the information obtainable may be restricted to examining the CCA proximal to the patch and knowing whether there is flow or no flow in the distal cervical ICA. The quality of flow then also becomes important to determine whether poststenotic turbulence exists. These patches are not well visualized by ultrasound, in part, secondary to air trapped in the patch material.

The sonographer will, in all likelihood, not have any information on how the CEA was performed. It could be best to assume that a traditional CEA was performed and a patch was used. If a patch is identified, it should be determined whether the patch is synthetic or autogenous. A synthetic patch may appear to have a woven appearance to the walls (in the case of a Dacron patch, Fig. 9-2) or demonstrate two brightly echogenic lines (in the case of a double–layered PTTE). Vein patches will more closely resemble the native vessel. Eversion CEA will behave ultrasonographically similar to standard CEA with primary closure.

Any patient with neck swelling on the side of a CEA should be evaluated for the possibility of hematoma, infection, or pseudoaneurysm. All are associated with a synthetic patch. A vein patch may be associated with patch rupture. The intentions for a duplex evaluation should be to identify the presence of a fluid collection or encapsulated mass in the soft tissue that surrounds the patch, remembering that the patch and swelling associated with the CEA will typically lie superficial to the endarterectomy. An encapsulated mass is associated with hematoma or pseudoaneurysm but may also suggest the presence of inflammatory tissue associated with infection. The appearance of a perivascular fluid collection above an irregular buckling of the Dacron patch has also been described as indication of a pending or active infection (Fig. 9-2).[3]

An extravascular leak or pseudoaneurysm is not common but if detected in a synthetic patch, its most likely source is a suture disruption. Extravasation in a vein patch is associated with patch rupture. A hematoma can also occur as synthetic patches can have problems with suture hole bleeding that tends not to be seen in vein patches. A hematoma may also be the result of blood extravasated from surrounding tissue or loose ligatures. Early infection may present as a wound complication and hematoma. Late infection may be evident as neck swelling. According to Knight,[3] most cases of synthetic patch infections are painless, with no local or systemic signs of infection. Infection is typically not associated with vein patches and is rare with synthetic patches with an occurrence rate of 0.18% in the latter.[1] Given the low occurrence rate, sonographers may not consider this a problem of concern. Still, a duplex ultrasound evaluation is often the first diagnostic step, and the sonographer must know of these abnormalities in order to perform an adequate assessment when evaluating a swollen neck.

## Pitfalls

In the early postoperative period within the first few days after surgery, ultrasound visualization should be expected to be complicated by air entrapped in the matrix of a synthetic patch or introduced in hemostatic agents applied prior to closure, or by wound hematomas. Because entrapped air

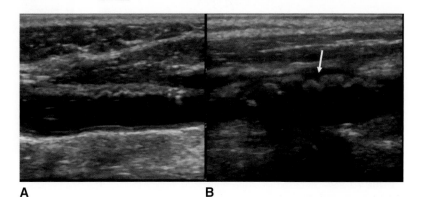

**FIGURE 9-2** Endarterectomy Dacron patch: **(A)** normal Dacron patch along the superficial wall of endarterectomy site and **(B)** abnormal Dacron patch with buckling of the patch and hypoechoic mass (*arrow*) suggestive of extraluminal fluid collection providing evidence of infection.

A                    B

often obliterates the ultrasound image directly above the CEA site, the sonographer is often required to visualize the carotid bifurcation from the most posterior approach possible. By the time of a first postoperative follow-up (usually at 30 days), the image is no longer compromised by entrapped air. Wound hematomas should also have been substantially reduced.

## Post-CEA Diagnostic Features

Vascular problems associated with the CEA may include both stenotic and nonstenotic pathology. One type of nonstenotic issue associated with the CEA includes an oversized or irregular patch that gives the vessel an aneurysmal appearance. Diameters are important measurements in these cases. It should be remembered that a patch identified as synthetic is more thrombogenic than an autogenous patch. Slower flows in an aneurysmal patch are more likely to laminate thrombus in a synthetic patch. Evaluating an oversized patch for mural thrombi can be significant. Another nonstenotic problem is loosely mobilized material may be detected within the lumen at the site of CEA. The material may be an intimal flap or loose strands of suture material. The intimal flap can be minimal or limited with no clinical significance, or it may be a significant flap, which may lead to carotid thrombosis or a source of thromboembolic material causing TIA or stroke. Intimal flaps will appear on the B-mode image as a small disruption along the wall with a short piece of material (the intimal and some additional wall material) protruding into the vessel lumen. Intimal flaps will produce disturbed color-flow patterns and depending on the extent, cause elevated velocities (Fig. 9-3).

Stenotic problems can be differentiated as technical problems of surgery or restenosis. Stenoses identified within the first postoperative month should be considered because of technical problems of surgery. They could be the result of narrowing in the primary closure or residual plaque that was not resected during the procedure. The latter is often called a "shelf lesion." The cut edge of the plaque is left and creates an abrupt, stepped edge in the arterial wall. A shelf lesion may be located at the proximal or distal edges of the CEA. It is more commonly associated with the distal edge, particularly when a "high bifurcation" limits surgical access and prevents an adequate feathering or tapering of the plaque. On B-mode image, the edge of the residual plaque will be easy to visualize adjacent to the endarterectomized segment of the vessel wall. A stenosis may also be caused by nonocclusive thrombus adherent to the wall that developed from the manipulations of surgery. This thrombus can be associated with the CEA site and patch.[4] Lastly, although the post-CEA examination is targeted at the operative site, there is still the possibility of missed lesions in the proximal CCA or the innominate artery (on the right) that had been overlooked in presurgical workup.

### Post-CEA Restenosis

Although a stenosis seen within 1 month of surgery is typically associated with the surgery in the form of retained plaque or thrombus, narrowing over the first 24 months of CEA is considered a result of neointimal hyperplasia. The hyperplastic lesion is considered relatively benign with the low thromboembolic potential of a fibrotic plaque. After 2 years, restenosis is considered progressive atherosclerotic and potentially more problematic with risks approaching that of the asymptomatic lesion. Restenosis rates vary widely in the literature, but Rosenborough estimates the incidence of restenosis as 6% to 14% after CEA[5] (Pathology Box 9-1).

When evaluating patients in follow-up, some laboratories may adjust velocity criteria post-CEA. Most will use the preprocedural velocity criteria established by the lab to identify the presence of stenosis. This is specifically applicable to CEA with primary closure or eversion CEA.

Because carotid duplex velocities have been tested on native (nonoperated) carotid arteries, these standard velocities may not be applicable to carotid restenosis after CEA with patch angioplasty. Elevated velocities have been noted in the ICA distal to patching because of the relative narrowing of the normal ICA distal to the patch.[6]

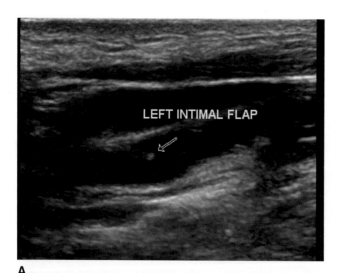

**A**

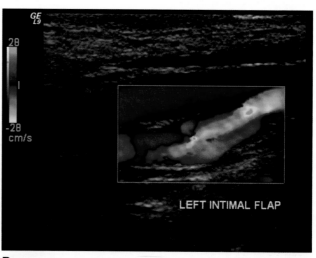

**B**

**FIGURE 9-3** Post-CEA carotid intimal flap. **A:** Grayscale image with defect projecting into lumen along anterior wall of the ICA. **B:** Color-flow imaging noting turbulence along the area of the flap.

**PATHOLOGY BOX 9-1**
*Common Pathology Associated with CEA*

| Pathology | Ultrasound Characteristics |
|---|---|
| Residual plaque | Plaque observed at end of CEA site, may have abrupt stepped edge (shelf lesion); color and spectral Doppler may display turbulence or elevated PSV depending on severity |
| Intimal flap | Disruption along vessel wall with moving material observed within lumen; disturbed color-flow patterns and elevated PSV often present |
| Occlusion | No color filling, no lumen detected, no spectral Doppler signal |
| Infected patch | Irregular buckling of patch material along vessel wall; perivascular fluid accumulation |
| Hematoma | Nonvascular mass adjacent to vessel; may appear cystic or contain various levels of echogenicity |
| Pseudoaneurysm | Dilated area attached to vessel with flow demonstrated on color and spectral Doppler; to-and-fro pattern flow may be detected in connection between dilated sac and native vessel; color swirling (yin-yang appearance) present within dilated sac |
| Restenosis | Focal area of elevated velocities with poststenotic turbulence; homogeneous material present along the wall in cases of restenosis due to hyperplasia |

CEA, carotid endarterectomy; PSV, peak systolic velocity.

A study was conducted in 200 patients to determine if patch angioplasty closure alters velocities just distal to CEA and to define the optimal velocities for detecting ≥30%, ≥50%, and ≥70% restenosis.[7] Ultrasound findings were compared with computed tomography angiogram (CTA). When the standard velocity criteria for nonoperated arteries were applied, 37% and 10% of patients were believed to have ≥50% to <70% and ≥70% to 99% restenosis versus 11.3% and 11.3% on CTA/angiography, respectively. The mean PSV for ≥30%, ≥50%, and ≥70% restenosis were 172, 249, and 389 cm/s, respectively ($p < 0.001$; Table 9-1). An ICA PSV of ≥155 cm/s was optimal for ≥30% restenosis with sensitivity and specificity of 98%. A PSV of ≥213 cm/s was optimal for ≥50% restenosis with sensitivity of 99% and specificity of 100%. An ICA PSV of 274 cm/s was optimal for ≥70% restenosis with sensitivity of 99% and specificity of 91% (Table 9-2). Receiver operating characteristic (ROC) curve analysis showed that the PSVs were significantly better than EDVs and ICA/CCA ratios in detecting ≥30% and ≥50% restenosis. The conclusion of this study was that the mean PSVs of a normal ICA distal to CEA patching were higher than normal nonoperated ICAs; therefore, standard duplex velocities criteria should be revised after CEA with patch closure.

Sonographers may question ... surveillance if the restenosis ra... with patching and the lesion ... respects, it matches the sur... lesion. Unlike the primary ... the hyperplastic response ... becoming virulent with a rapid ... particularly in patients with primary ... aims of the surgeon are to identify the ... and, when the disease is found to progress in ... to intervene before it reaches occlusion. Follow-up is ... important for the contralateral bifurcation. Atherogenesis has a degree of symmetry. Patients treated for disease in one carotid bifurcation are at risk of aggressive disease in the contralateral bifurcation. Postoperative surveillance should always be performed bilaterally.

An additional study was conducted on 489 patients (501 CEA) with patch closure examining the role of routine postoperative ultrasound.[8] All patients had immediate postoperative duplex ultrasounds and at regular intervals of 1, 6, 12 months, and every 12 months thereafter. The mean follow-up was 20.4 months. Overall, 15 patients (3.1%) had ≥50% restenosis: nine with 50% to <80% and four with 80% to 99%, and two had late carotid occlusion. All of these were asymptomatic, except for one who had a transient ischemic attack. The mean time to ≥50% to <80% restenosis was 14.7 months versus 19.8 months for ≥80% restenosis after the CEA. The results showed that the freedom from ≥50% and ≥80% restenosis rates were 98%, 96%, 94%, 94%, 94%, and 99%, 98%, 97%, 97%, 97% at 1, 2, 3, 4, and 5 years, respectively. The estimated charge of this surveillance was 3.6 (average number of ultrasounds per patient) × 489 (number of patients) × $800 (charge for carotid duplex ultrasound), which equals $1,408,320 to detect only four patients with ≥80% to 99% restenosis who may have been potential candidates for reintervention. Therefore, this study concluded that the value of routine postoperative duplex ultrasound surveillance after CEA with patch closure may be limited, particularly if the immediate postoperative ultrasound or the ultrasound performed at the 6-month follow-up was normal or had minimal disease.

## CAROTID ARTERY STENTING

CAS has been proposed as an alternative treatment to CEA for severe carotid artery stenosis, particularly in high-risk surgical patients.[9-11] In 2005, CAS accounted for approximately 10% of patients treated for extracranial cerebrovascular disease; because of concerns of high complication rates and low reimbursements, CAS has not benefitted from wide utilization.[12] However, complication rates for CAS continue to decrease with the increased use of cerebral embolic protective devices and retrograde flow flushing of the ICA during stenting. In spite of the controversial debate regarding the exact role of CAS as compared to CEA, its use in clinical practice has expanded all over the world. However, the favorable results of CAS in some of the carotid stenting trials have not been reflected in the real-world experience.

Between 2005 and 2009, over 22,000 patients were analyzed in a large retrospective cohort study of the Centers for Medicare and Medicaid Services CAS Database: 60% were men, one-half were symptomatic, 91% were at high surgical

## TABLE 9-1 Mean Velocities and Ratio and Degree of Restenosis[7]

| Variable | <30 (n = 112) | | | ≥30–50 (n = 39) | | | ≥50–70 (n = 22) | | | ≥70–99 (n = 22) | | | p Value |
| | Mean | Standard Deviation | Range | Mean | Standard Deviation | Range | Mean | Standard Deviation | Range | Mean | Standard Deviation | Range | |
|---|---|---|---|---|---|---|---|---|---|---|---|---|---|
| PSV | 107.13 | 30.75 | 44–162 | 172 | 14.35 | 150–213 | 248.5 | 61 | 201–327 | 389 | 84.22 | 221–525 | <0.0001 |
| EDV | 29.46 | 11.37 | 10–57 | 44 | 10.71 | 22–62 | 63.4 | 16.6 | 33–94 | 129 | 52.1 | 43–237 | <0.0001 |
| Velocity ratio | 1.28 | 0.52 | 0.49–3.1 | 1.93 | 0.77 | 0.62–4.35 | 2.35 | 1.02 | 0.88–4.61 | 3.68 | 1.58 | 1.14–6.51 | <0.0001 |

**TABLE 9-2   Cutoff of PSVs, EDVs, and ICA/CCA Ratios[7]**

| Percent Stenosis | PSV | | EDV | | Velocity Ratio | |
|---|---|---|---|---|---|---|
| | Cutoff | AUC (95% CI) | Cutoff | AUC (95% CI) | Cutoff | AUC (95% CI) |
| >30 | 155 | 99.8 (99.5–100) | 41 | 90.3 (86.1–94.4) | 1.64 | 84.0 (78.3–89.6) |
| >50 | 213 | 100 (99.5–100) | 60 | 95.3 (92.1–98.6) | 2.25 | 84.3 (77.1–91.5) |
| >70 | 274 | 99.2 (98.1–100) | 80 | 97.3 (93.9–100) | 3.35 | 88.6 (80.3–96.8) |

AUC, area under curve; CI, confidence interval.

risk and showed a periprocedural mortality of more than twice the rate in this patient population than those reported earlier in the CREST and SAPPHIRE trials.[9,13,14] Eighty percent of patients met the SAPPHIRE trial indications, and about one-half of them met at least one of the SAPPHIRE criteria for high surgical risk. The unadjusted 30-day risks were 1.7% for mortality, 3.3% for stroke, and 2.5% for myocardial infarction (MI). The mean follow-up was 2 years. Overall, the mortality rate was 42% for patients ≥80 years old and 37% in patients who were at high surgical risk. In high surgical risk symptomatic patients, the overall mortality rate was 37%. In asymptomatic patients, the mortality rate after CAS exceeded one-third of those patients who were at least 50 years old. Over 80% of physicians did not meet the minimum criteria of CAS volume requirements and/or minimal complication rates of the SAPPHIRE trial, and more than 90% of physicians did not meet the requirements for the CREST trial. The study concluded that a major concern must be raised regarding generalizing the results of randomized clinical trials in the real world.[13]

Still, the demonstration of equivalence between CEA and CAS in rigorously controlled usage speaks to increased utilization. Should indications and reimbursement for CAS relax, the vascular laboratory will see greater numbers of patients treated with CAS, and sonographers must become familiar with duplex ultrasound-related issues associated with CAS.

Pre- and postprocedure ultrasound testing for CAS is performed because it is related to technical issues associated with the CAS procedure and the stent that is implanted "for life." There are aspects of the procedure that are important for the sonographer and should be described. These not only relate to the carotid bifurcation but also to the path that the catheter follows toward the stenosis. The latter is important because the vascular sonographer may be involved in defining the status of that path before or after CAS is performed.

The reported incidence of carotid in-stent stenosis varies between 1% and 50%.[15–19] This variation has been attributed to multiple factors, for example, the method of stenosis calculation, the duration of follow-up, and the definition of severity of stenosis. In spite of the fact that carotid duplex ultrasound has been the procedure of choice to evaluate the incidence of post-CEA stenosis, its role in determining the incidence of carotid in-stent stenosis has been debated.[18–29]

## CAS Techniques

Catheter manipulations for CAS are typically performed after accessing the common femoral artery at the groin. This can also be done via the brachial artery approach. Postprocedure complications are not limited to the carotid bifurcation but may include dissection, thrombosis, or perforations within the path where devices encounter difficulty. This catheter is positioned first at the mid-CCA, proximal to the carotid bifurcation, then a fine filter wire is passed across the lesion. This is used to position a cerebral embolic protection device (EPD), then to position the balloon and stent catheters used subsequently. The EPDs must gain access to the ICA segment that lies distal to the lesion. Once the EPD is placed, a balloon catheter is typically used to predilate the lesion. Following this, a stent catheter is then positioned over the lesion, and deployment starts from beyond the distal border of the stenosis. The stent is unsheathed by retracting the stent catheter over the lesion. This deploys a self-expanding stent that should cover the entire lesion from its distal through proximal borders. A second balloon catheter may be used and inflated to ensure full expansion of the stent. For full coverage, a stent length should be selected that will extend a few millimeters beyond the lesion proximally and distally once it is deployed. The stent may extend from the CCA into the bulb, and coverage of the ECA is not considered a contraindication for the procedure.

## Sonographic Examination Techniques

Carotid duplex ultrasound has been used for detection of carotid stenosis for more than three decades. It can also be used to examine stented carotid arteries. Although the stent material is highly reflective, it does not produce significant artifacts to limit ultrasonic visualization of the stent. It can also provide image details of the stent, vessel wall characteristics, as well as any abnormalities.

The technique used for ultrasound after CAS is similar to that used for native carotid artery disease, with emphasis on B-mode imaging. A bilateral examination using a high-resolution linear array transducer should be done in longitudinal and cross-sectional scan planes beginning at the CCA, through the stented CCA/ICA and bifurcation, and into the distal ICA. The stent should be fully visible along its length by ultrasound.

All Doppler spectra are obtained using a Doppler sample volume of 1 to 1.5 mm and a Doppler angle of 60 degrees or less. The examination also includes grayscale B-mode imaging and color images of the CCA, carotid bifurcation, proximal, middle, and distal portions of the stent, the distal unstented portion of the ICA, and the ECA. Both color and/or power Doppler can be used to aid in confirming flow dynamics and potential luminal narrowing. The PSV and EDV of the

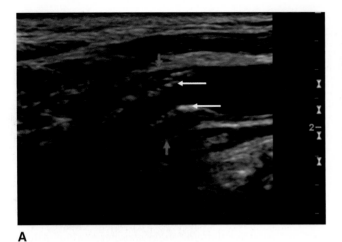
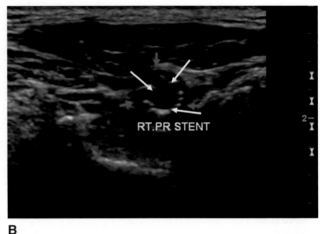

**A**    **B**

**FIGURE 9-4** B-mode images of a deformed stent. Stent walls (*white arrows*) are not apposed to vessel walls (*red arrows*). Extensive plaque is observed between vessels walls and stent. **A:** Longitudinal view. **B:** Transverse view.

ICA, CCA, and the ICA/CCA PSV ratios are recorded. The PSV velocities are taken as close as possible to the lesion. The highest velocities in the stented segment are used for analysis and comparison to other imaging modalities. The stent may traverse the orifice of the ECA, but flow through the stent interstices into the ECA is usually maintained. The stent is usually placed from the CCA into the proximal ICA.

A carotid stent should be imaged in multiple planes. The apposition of the stent to the surrounding plaque, luminal encroachment of neointimal hyperplasia, and expansion of the lumen should be noted. In addition, the B-mode image should be examined for any evidence of stent compression, incomplete deployment, or other deformation (Fig. 9-4). The luminal diameter and velocities should be measured at multiple locations (Fig. 9-5 and Fig. 9-6).

### Pitfalls

Dense calcification that produced shadows in a preprocedural ultrasound will be present in the follow-up CAS evaluation and will compromise the B-mode image and Doppler interrogation of the stented vessel. Multiple views should be used to avoid areas of acoustic shadowing. In some vessels, this is not possible; therefore, signals distal to the calcific areas will be important in determining the presence of disease. Turbulence distal to these areas likely indicates that a significant stenosis is present.

Dense circumferential calcification is problematic during the stent placement as well. It restricts balloon expansion of the lesion during stenting, which in turn increases procedural manipulation, and adds the risk of an inadequate stent expansion. Both are reasons for sonographers to pay particular attention to velocity changes with the area of calcification. Added manipulation may increase the hyperplastic response, and inadequate expansion may lead to residual stenosis.

## Post-CAS Diagnostic Features

The normal ultrasound appearance of a carotid stent should reveal the walls of the stent apposed to the walls of the vessel. These walls should be relatively uniform, and color filling should be observed out to the edges of the stent. The velocity spectra through the stent should not demonstrate any focal increases (Fig. 9-5). The CAS patient can present with some unique pathology. For the vascular sonographer, the forms of concern include stent fracture, stent migration, thrombus formation, dissection, intimal flap, intimal hyperplasia, and in-stent restenosis (Pathology Box 9-2).

### Duplex Ultrasound Velocity Criteria for In-Stent Restenosis

It has been speculated that stenting may diminish the compliance of the carotid artery, which may lead to elevated PSVs, even in stenting with normal lumen.[19–22] The enhanced stiffness of the stent–arterial wall complex renders the flow–pressure relationship of the carotid artery similar to that observed in a rigid tube, so that the energy normally applied to dilate the artery results in an increased velocity. In addition, because the plaque is not removed with CAS, this may also add to decreased compliance and elevated velocities. Although B-mode imaging data is useful, the primary ultrasound parameters utilized in most vascular laboratories to diagnose the severity of carotid artery stenosis have been the hemodynamic parameters, that is, PSV, EDV, and ICA/CCA PSV ratio, alone or in combination.

At the present time, ultrasound velocity criteria have not been standardized for patients undergoing CAS. An earlier study by Robbin et al.[20] concluded that the use of ultrasound in the follow-up of stented carotid arteries was unreliable in detecting in-stent stenosis based on variable velocity measurements. Similarly, Ringer et al.[21] reviewed their experience after CAS and concluded that strict velocity criteria for stenosis were unreliable.

A prospective study was conducted to define the optimal velocities in detecting various severities of in-stent stenosis: ≥30%, ≥50%, and ≥80% to 99%.[23] This study included 144 patients who underwent CAS as a part of clinical trials. All patients had completion arteriograms and underwent postoperative carotid ultrasound, which was repeated at 1 month and every 6 months thereafter. Patients with a PSV of the ICA of ≥130 cm/s underwent carotid CTA. PSVs and EDVs of the ICA and CCA and ICA/CCA PSV ratios were recorded. An ROC curve analysis

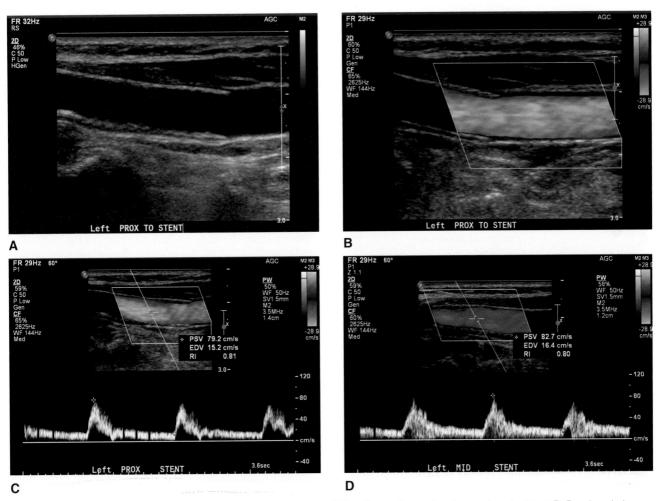

**FIGURE 9-5** **A**: B-mode image of normal stent. **B**: Color flow in normal stent. **C**: Doppler velocity waveform in normal proximal stent. **D**: Doppler velocity waveform in normal mid stent.

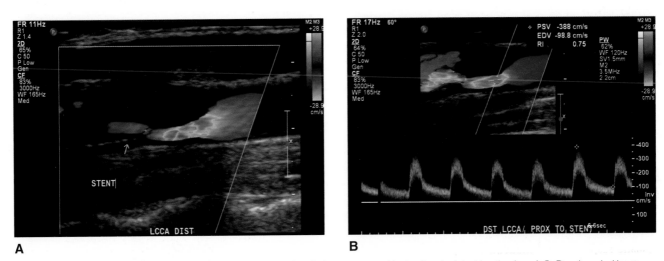

**FIGURE 9-6** **A**: B-mode with color flow showing severe stenosis at the distal common carotid artery/proximal stent location (*arrow*). **B**: Doppler velocities at same location of severe in-stent restenosis.

**PATHOLOGY BOX 9-2**
*Common Pathology Associated with CAS*

| Pathology | Ultrasound Characteristics |
|---|---|
| Restenosis | Focal area of elevated velocities with poststenotic turbulence; homogeneous material present along stent wall |
| Stent fracture | Irregular border of stent with abrupt edge apparent; color and spectral Doppler turbulence noted |
| Stent deformation | Border of stent appears to protrude into vessel lumen; color-flow channel is reduced; elevated PSV may be present depending on degree of deformation |
| Thrombus | Homogeneous, smooth-bordered material present within stent or native vessel; reduced color-flow lumen; elevated PSV |
| Dissection | White line seen within vessel lumen using multiple views, may be seen moving; disturbed color-flow and spectral Doppler will be present on both sides of dissection |
| Occlusion | No color filling, no lumen detected, no spectral Doppler signal |

CAS, carotid artery stenting; PSV, peak systolic velocity.

was used to determine the optimal velocity criteria for detection of ≥30%, ≥50%, and ≥80% in-stent stenosis. The mean velocities of various in-stent restenosis is summarized in Table 9-3.

The ROC curve analysis from this study demonstrated that an ICA PSV of ≥154 cm/s was optimal for ≥30% stenosis with a sensitivity of 99% and specificity of 89%. An ICA EDV of 42 cm/s had sensitivity of 86% and specificity of 62% in detecting ≥30% stenosis. An ICA PSV of ≥224 cm/s was optimal for ≥50% stenosis with a sensitivity of 99% and specificity of 90%. An ICA EDV of 88 cm/s had sensitivity of 96% and specificity of 100% in detecting ≥50% stenosis. An ICA/CCA ratio of 3.4 had sensitivity of 96% and specificity of 100% in detecting ≥50% stenosis. An ICA PSV of ≥325 cm/s was optimal for ≥80% stenosis with a sensitivity of 100% and specificity of 99%. An ICA EDV of 119 cm/s had sensitivity of 99% and specificity of 100% in detecting ≥80% stenosis (Table 9-4). The PSV of the stented artery was a better predictor for ≥50% in-stent stenosis than the EDV or ICA/CCA ratio (Fig. 9-7). The study concluded that the optimal duplex velocity criteria for in-stent stenosis of ≥30%, ≥50%, and ≥80% were the PSVs of 154, 224, and 325 cm/s, respectively. Using the ROC curve analysis data, clinicians can select thresholds with high-negative predictive values and sensitivity, which will ensure that fewer patients with in-stent stenosis will be missed using carotid ultrasound, which is usually used as a screening modality before further imaging is done prior to any intervention.

Recently, additional studies have reported on the optimal duplex velocity criteria in detecting ≥50% in-stent stenosis. Kwon et al.[30] reported that a PSV of 200 cm/s and an ICA/CCA ratio of 2.5 were optimal in the diagnosis of ≥50% in-stent stenosis with a sensitivity of 90% and specificity of 97%. Stanziale et al.[31] reported that a PSV of ≥350 cm/s and an ICA/CCA ratio of ≥4.75% were optimal in detecting ≥70% in-stent stenosis. They also concluded that a PSV of ≥225 cm/s and ICA/CCA ratio of ≥2.5 were compatible with carotid in-stent stenosis of ≥50%.

| TABLE 9-3 | Mean PSVs, EDVs, and Ratios for Severity of In-Stent Stenosis[23] | | | | | | | | | |
|---|---|---|---|---|---|---|---|---|---|---|
| | >30–50 (n = 38) | | | >50–80 (n = 11) | | | >80–99 (n = 8) | | | p Value |
| Variable | Mean | Standard Error | Range | Mean | Standard Error | Range | Mean | Standard Error | Range | |
| PSV | 178 | 4.02 | 142–265 | 278 | 17.32 | 201–408 | 403 | 59.58 | 58–613 | <0.0001 |
| EDV | 43 | 2.54 | 20–80 | 65 | 11.09 | 20–119 | 130 | 17.5 | 26–181 | <0.0001 |
| Velocity ratio[a] | 1.99 | 0.11 | 0.97–3.38 | 2.93 | 0.31 | 1.51–4.53 | 5.26 | 0.97 | 0.16–8.88 | <0.0001 |

[a]ICA/CCA ratio.

| TABLE 9-4 | Optimal Cutoff Values for PSV, EDV, and ICA/CCA Ratios in Carotid Stents[23] | | | | | | | | |
|---|---|---|---|---|---|---|---|---|---|
| Stenosis | PSV Cutoff | PSV AUC (95% CI) | SE | EDV Cutoff | EDV AUC (95% CI) | SE | ICA/CCA Ratio Cutoff | ICA/CCA Ratio AUC (95% CI) | SE |
| ≥30% | >154 | 0.97 (0.93–1) | 0.02 | >42 | 0.76 (0.68–0.84) | 0.04 | >1.533 | 0.83 (0.77–0.90) | 0.03 |
| ≥50% | >224 | 0.95 (0.84–1) | 0.05 | >88 | 0.82 (0.69–0.96) | 0.07 | >3.439 | 0.88 (0.77–0.99) | 0.06 |
| ≥80% | >325 | 0.88 (0.63–1) | 0.12 | >119 | 0.90 (0.72–1) | 0.09 | >4.533 | 0.86 (0.62–1) | 0.12 |

SE, standard error; AUC, area under curve.

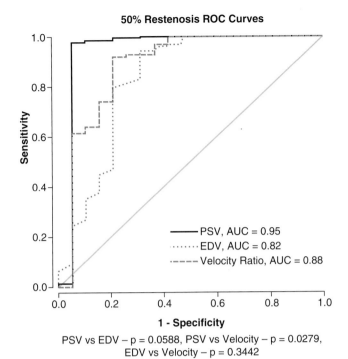

**50% Restenosis ROC Curves**

PSV vs EDV – p = 0.0588, PSV vs Velocity – p = 0.0279,
EDV vs Velocity – p = 0.3442

**FIGURE 9-7** ROC curve for ≥50% in-stent stenosis.

The report by Lal et al. on ultrasound criteria for stented carotid arteries was somewhat similar to the 2008 study by AbuRahma.[23,25] An ROC curve analysis demonstrated the following optimal threshold criteria: ≥20% stenosis (PSV ≥ 150 cm/s and ICA/CCA ratio ≥2.15), in-stent stenosis ≥50% (PSV ≥220 cm/s and ICA/CCA ratio ≥2.7), and in-stent stenosis ≥80% (PSV 340 cm/s and ICA/CCA ratio ≥4.15).

Peterson et al.[32] in analyzing ultrasound velocity criteria obtained in 158 patients who were treated with CAS, demonstrated the importance of obtaining a carotid ultrasound in the immediate postoperative period to serve as a reference for future follow-up, thus insuring early detection of in-stent stenosis. Similar observations were made by other studies.[21,23] Table 9-5 summarizes various velocity criteria for in-stent restenosis.

## Post-CAS Surveillance Frequency

Early poststenting surveillance is as important for the CAS patient as it is for CEA patients. The first ultrasound generally occurs within 1 month of the procedure to detect any technical problems associated with retained stenosis, thrombus, or stent deployment and to set baseline velocity data. Velocity elevations associated with changes in arterial compliance should be evident at this stage. Any subsequent velocity elevations should be considered potential evidence of restenosis.

After the 1 month evaluation, follow-up surveillance will typically address the development of restenosis in the hyperplastic lesion. As with CEA, restenosis develops asymptomatically, and duplex surveillance is intended to detect the aggressive disease. The goal of surveillance is to identify the restenosis that could advance to occlusion and the rate of progression is as important as the identification of the high-grade lesion. More frequent follow-up is indicated if significant changes in velocity are detected between surveillance scans.

All patients undergoing CAS should be placed in a routine follow-up protocol. The majority of stenosis ≥50% is seen to occur within 18 months.[23] Generally, CAS patients are evaluated every 6 months for the first 2 years and annually thereafter. These velocity measurements should be compared with the immediate post-CAS velocities (preferably during the same admission), and future results can be compared to these.

As noted earlier, duplex may not reliably detect the moderate stenosis following CAS. This softening of the velocity criteria post-CAS should not significantly compromise surveillance. An individual patient can still be followed serially over multiple scans through the development of a moderate stenosis if the angle correction is appropriately maintained. A PSV of 175 cm/s found in a stent at baseline should not raise concerns if it remained unchanged in serial testing. If on subsequent testing, PSV rose to 200 cm/s then 250 cm/s, these data are consistent with the rapid progression of a moderate stenosis. Intervention may be indicated with further workup before velocities reach the PSV threshold for a high-grade stenosis.

## Stent Fracture and Migration

Migration and fracture have to date not been seen as significant problems. Stent fractures are generally considered rare (1.9% in 78 patients).[34,35] Still, biomechanical forces associated with head tilting, neck rotations, and swallowing have been found to distort stents in carotid bifurcation. Temporary lengthening, twisting, and crushing deformations were demonstrated in cine fluoroscopy.[36] Long-term effects were evident in plain radiographic evaluations of patients followed an average of 18 months. Stent fractures, most benign, were found in 29% of 48 stents.[37] Only 3 of 14 were associated with flow velocity changes. Fracture was strongly associated with calcification, and it was suggested that torsional motions of a stent that repeatedly rubbed against a hard calcified surface during rotations of the neck may be at fault. Compromises to the architectural integrity of the stent should be considered as time dependent. Sonographers may need to be alert to the possibility that biomechanical distortion with repeated neck flexion could create a fracture and stimulate a late hyperplastic response. The natural history of a stent is still unknown, and the wearing of the device over the long-term may lead to late occurrences. In the case of a stent deformation, the border of the stent may appear to protrude into the vessel lumen (Fig. 9-4). A stent fracture will produce an abrupt edge within the stented portion with associated changes in the color-flow signals.

**TABLE 9-5   Post-CAS Duplex Ultrasound Criteria**

| Author/Series | Stenosis Threshold 20% | | | Stenosis Threshold 30% | | | Stenosis Threshold 50% | | | Stenosis Threshold 70% | | | Stenosis Threshold 75% | | | Stenosis Threshold 80% | | |
|---|---|---|---|---|---|---|---|---|---|---|---|---|---|---|---|---|---|---|
| | PSV | EDV | ICA/CCA | PSV | EDV | ICA/CCA | PSV | EDV | ICA/CCA | PSV | EDV | ICA/CCA | PSV | EDV | ICA/CCA | PSV | EDV | ICA/CCA |
| AbuRahma[19] | | | | 154 | 42 | | 224 | 88 | | | | | | | | 325 | 119 | |
| Setacci[33] | | | | 105 | | | 175 | | | 300 | 140 | 3.8 | | | | | | |
| Chi[27] | | | | | | | 240 | | 2.45 | 450 | | 4.3 | | | | | | |
| Chahwan[28] | 137 | 20 | | | | | 195 | 62 | | | | | | | | 300 | 96 | |
| Lal[22] | | | 2.15 | | | | 220 | | 2.7 | | | | | | | 340 | | 4.15 |
| Zhou[29] | | | | | | | | | | 300 | 90 | 4.0 | | | | | | |
| Armstrong[26] | | | | | | | | | | | | | 300 | 125 | | | | |
| Kwon[30] | | | | | | | 200 | | 2.5 | | | | | | | | | |
| Stanziale[31] | | | | | | | 225 | | 2.5 | 350 | | 4.75 | | | | | | |

## SUMMARY

- CEA remains the traditional approach toward treating carotid bifurcation lesions, and while new techniques are evolving, its issues are relatively stable.
- Issues in CAS are poorly defined but given recent findings in CAS, the vascular sonographer should anticipate that with the increased experience in CAS the volume of CAS is expected to increase.
- It is important for vascular sonographers to recognize that significant differences exist in the duplex evaluation of CEA and CAS patients seen in follow-up.
- Duplex velocity of native carotids cannot be applied to CAS patients or CEA patients with patch closure.
- Duplex ultrasound will be the most important way of characterizing the behavior of this implanted device over time.

## CRITICAL THINKING QUESTIONS

1. You are asked to do carotid ultrasound in the recovery room on a patient who just underwent a CEA. What approach would you use to image the CEA site and why?

2. You perform an ultrasound examination on a patient who is 2 weeks post-CEA. You observe echogenic material along the wall of the vessel with color aliasing and elevated velocities. What is the most likely cause of the stenosis?

3. When scanning patients who have had a CAS or CEA, will either patient group present a problem with acoustic shadowing and why?

## MEDIA MENU

Student Resources available on thePoint® include:
- Audio glossary
- Interactive question bank
- Videos
- Internet resources

## REFERENCES

1. Muto A, Nishibe T, Dardik H, et al. Patches for carotid artery endarterectomy: current materials and prospects. *J Vasc Surg.* 2009;50:206–213.
2. AbuRahma AF. Processes of care for carotid endarterectomy: surgical and anesthesia considerations. *J Vasc Surg.* 2009;50:921–933.
3. Knight BC, Tait WF. Dacron patch infection following carotid endarterectomy: a systematic review of the literature. *Eur J Vasc Endovasc Surg.* 2009;37:140–148.
4. Flanigan DP, Flanigan ME, Dorne AL, et al. Long-term results of 442 consecutive, standardized carotid endarterectomy procedures in standard-risk and high-risk patients. *J Vasc Surg.* 2007;46:876–882.
5. Roseborough GS, Perler BA. Carotid artery disease: endarterectomy. In: Cronenwett JL, Johnston KW, eds. *Rutherford's Vascular Surgery.* 7th ed. Philadelphia, PA: Saunders/Elsevier; 2010:1443–1468.
6. Hirsch M, Bernt RA, Hirschl MM. Carotid endarterectomy of the internal carotid artery with and without patch angioplasty: comparison of hemodynamic and morphological parameters. *Int Angiol.* 1989;8:10–15.
7. AbuRahma AF, Stone PA, Deem S, et al. Proposed duplex velocity criteria for carotid restenosis following carotid endarterectomy with patch closure. *J Vasc Surg.* 2009;50:286–291.
8. AbuRahma AF, Srivastava M, AbuRahma Z, et al. The value and economic analysis of routine postoperative carotid duplex ultrasound surveillance after carotid endarterectomy. *J Vasc Surg.* 2015;62:378–384.
9. Brott TG, Hobson RW, Howard G, et al. Stenting versus endarterectomy for treatment of carotid-artery stenosis. *N Engl J Med.* 2010;363:11–23.
10. Mas JL, Arquizan C, Calvet D, et al. Long-term follow-up study of endarterectomy versus angioplasty in patients with symptomatic severe carotid stenosis trial. *Stroke.* 2014;45:2750–2756.
11. Ricotta JJ, AbuRahma A, Ascher E, et al; Society for Vascular Surgery. Updated society for vascular surgery guidelines for management of extracranial carotid disease. *J Vasc Surg.* 2011;54:e1–e31.
12. Timaran CH, Veith FJ, Rosero EB, et al. Intracranial hemorrhage after carotid endarterectomy and carotid stenting in the United States in 2005. *J Vasc Surg.* 2009;49:623–628.
13. Jalbert JJ, Nguyen LL, Gerhard-Herman MD, et al. Outcomes after carotid artery stenting in medicare beneficiaries, 2005 to 2009. *JAMA Neurol.* 2015;72:276–286.
14. Yadav J; SAPPHIRE Investigators. Stenting and angioplasty with protection in patients at high risk for endarterectomy: the SAPPHIRE study. *Circulation.* 2002;106:2986–2989.
15. Ferguson RD, Ferguson JG. Carotid angioplasty. In search of a worthy alternative to endarterectomy. *Arch Neurol.* 1996;53(7):696–698.
16. New G, Roubin GS, Iyer SS, et al. Safety, efficacy and durability of carotid artery stenting for stenosis following carotid endarterectomy: a multicenter study. *J Endovasc Ther.* 2000;7:345–352.
17. Hobson RW, Lal BK, Chakhtoura E, et al. Carotid artery stenting: analysis of data for 105 patients at high risk. *J Vasc Surg.* 2003;37(6):1234–1239.
18. Lal BK, Hobson RW, Goldstein J, et al. In-stent recurrent stenosis after carotid artery stenting: life table analysis and clinical relevance. *J Vasc Surg.* 2003;38(6):1162–1168; discussion 9.
19. AbuRahma AF, Maxwell D, Eads K, et al. Carotid duplex velocity criteria revisited for the diagnosis of carotid in-stent stenosis. *Vascular.* 2007;15:119–125.
20. Robbin ML, Lockhart ME, Weber TM, et al. Carotid artery stents: early and intermediate follow-up with Doppler US. *Radiology.* 1997;205:749–756.
21. Ringer AJ, German JW, Guterman LR, et al. Follow-up of stented carotid arteries by Doppler ultrasound. *Neurosurgery.* 2002;51:639–643.
22. Lal BK, Hobson RW, Goldstein J, et al. Carotid artery stenting: Is there a need to revise ultrasound velocity criteria? *J Vasc Surg.* 2004;39:58–66.
23. AbuRahma AF, Abu-Halimah S, Bensenhaver J, et al. Optimal carotid duplex velocity criteria for defining the severity of carotid in-stent restenosis. *J Vasc Surg.* 2008;48:589–594.
24. Lal BK, Kaperonis EA, Cuadra S, et al. Patterns of in-stent restenosis after carotid artery stenting: classification and implications for long-term outcome. *J Vasc Surg.* 2007;46:833–840.
25. Lal BK, Hobson RW II, Tofighi B, et al. Duplex ultrasound velocity criteria for the stented carotid artery. *J Vasc Surg.* 2008;47:63–73.
26. Armstrong PA, Bandyk DF, Johnson BL, et al. Duplex scan surveillance after carotid angioplasty and stenting: a rational definition of stent stenosis. *J Vasc Surg.* 2007;46:460–465.
27. Chi YW, White CJ, Woods TC, et al. Ultrasound velocity criteria for carotid in-stent restenosis. *Catheter Cardiovasc Interv.* 2007;69:349–354.
28. Chahwan S, Miller MT, Pigott JP, et al. Carotid artery velocity characteristics after carotid artery angioplasty and stenting. *J Vasc Surg.* 2007;45:523–526.

29. Zhou W, Felkai DD, Evans M, et al. Ultrasound criteria for severe in-stent restenosis following carotid artery stenting. *J Vasc Surg.* 2008;47:74–80.

30. Kwon BJ, Jung C, Sheen SH, et al. CT angiography of stented carotid arteries: comparison with Doppler ultrasonography. *J Endovasc Ther.* 2007;14:489–497.

31. Stanziale SF, Wholey MH, Boules TN, et al. Determining in-stent stenosis of carotid arteries by duplex ultrasound criteria. *J Endovasc Ther.* 2005;12:346–353.

32. Peterson BG, Longo GM, Kibbe MR, et al. Duplex ultrasound remains a reliable test even after carotid stenting. *Ann Vasc Surg.* 2005;19:793–797.

33. Setacci C, Chisci E, Setacci F, et al. Grading carotid intrastent restenosis: a 6-year follow-up study. *Stroke.* 2008;39:1189–1196.

34. Varcoe RL, Mah J, Young N, et al. Relevance of carotid stent fractures in a single-center experience. *J Endovasc Ther.* 2008;15:485–489.

35. Surdell D, Shaibani A, Bendok B, et al. Fracture of a nitinol carotid artery stent that caused restenosis. *J Vasc Interv Radiol.* 2007;18:1297–1299.

36. Robertson SW, Cheng CP, Razavi MK. Biomechanical response of stented carotid arteries to swallowing and neck motion. *J Endovasc Ther.* 2008;15:663–671.

37. Ling AJ, Mwipatayi P, Gandhi T, et al. Stenting for carotid artery stenosis: fractures, proposed etiology and the need for surveillance. *J Vasc Surg.* 2008;47:1220–1226.

# Intracranial Cerebrovascular Examination

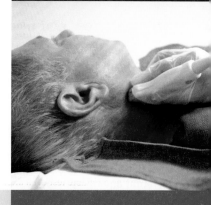

COLLEEN DOUVILLE

## CHAPTER 10

## OBJECTIVES

- Describe the arterial segments of the intracranial cerebral circulation that are standard to examine with transcranial Doppler (TCD) and transcranial duplex imaging (TCDI) techniques
- Describe the anatomic approaches used to insonate the intracranial vessels in adults
- List the current clinical applications for TCD examinations
- Describe normal velocities for each intracranial arterial segment examined with TCD and TCDI
- Define the diagnostic criteria used to make the interpretation of collateral flow
- List the values used for interpretation of >50% stenosis of the middle cerebral and intracranial internal carotid arteries
- List the criteria for vasospasm of the middle cerebral artery
- Define the use of extracranial to intracranial ratios in vasospasm

## GLOSSARY

**circle of Willis** A roughly circular anastomosis of arteries located at the base of the brain

**collateral** A vessel that is parallel to another vessel; a vessel that maintains blood flow around another stenotic or occluded vessel

**Lindegaard ratio** Middle cerebral artery (MCA) mean velocity divided by the sub-mandibular internal carotid artery (ICA) mean velocity. This ratio is useful in differentiating increased volume flow from decreased diameter when high velocities are encountered in the MCA or intracranial ICA

**pulsatility** Expressed as Gosling's pulsatility index (peak systolic velocity minus end-diastolic velocity divided by the time-averaged peak velocity)

**Sviri ratio** Ratio calculation used to determine vasospasm from hyperdynamic flow in the posterior circulation. The bilateral vertebral artery velocities taken at the atlas loop are added together and averaged. This averaged velocity is then divided into the highest basilar mean velocity

**transcranial Doppler (TCD)** A noninvasive test that uses ultrasound to measure the velocity of blood flow through the intracranial cerebral vessels

**transcranial duplex imaging (TCDI)** A noninvasive test on the intracranial cerebral blood vessels that uses ultrasound and provides both an image of the blood vessels and a graphical display of the velocities within the vessels

**vasospasm** A sudden constriction in a blood vessel causing a restriction in blood flow

## KEY TERMS

**anterior cerebral artery**

**anterior communicating artery**

**basilar artery**

**collateral flow**

**intracranial stenosis**

**middle cerebral artery**

**posterior cerebral artery**

**posterior communicating artery**

**transcranial duplex imaging**

**transcranial Doppler**

**vasospasm**

**vertebral artery**

Originally introduced by Rune Aaslid in 1982 and applied to patients with vasospasm secondary to subarachnoid hemorrhage (SAH), transcranial Doppler (TCD) and transcranial duplex imaging (TCDI) provide diagnostic information in patients with a variety of cerebrovascular diseases.[1] This ultrasound technology complements the neuroimaging techniques of computed tomography with contrast (CTA), magnetic resonance imaging with contrast (MRA), and cerebral angiography by providing physiologic data in real time that can be repeated, a valuable tool when considering the complex dynamics of cerebral blood flow (CBF).

## ANATOMY

TCD examinations directly study the intracranial conducting arteries that lie at the base of the brain, including the arterial anastomosis called the circle of Willis and the major anterior and posterior arteries that supply the circle. To put things in perspective, it is useful to understand that these are small targets; the center of the circle of Willis is about the size of a thumbnail, and on average, the diameter of the basal cerebral arteries range from approximately 2 to 4 mm.[2,3]

Most cerebral arteries have a numerical classification system that describes each arterial segment by name and number, with the number referring to either the anatomic course or a branch point. Variations in the circle of Willis are frequent in 18% to 54% of individuals and result from anomalies in vessel caliber, course, and origin of branches.[4-6]

The anterior circulation is formed by the intracranial continuation of the internal carotid artery (ICA), which first becomes accessible by TCD examination in the cavernous portion usually referred to as the carotid "siphon" because of its tortuous course (Fig. 10-1). The siphon is broken down into three segments: the parasellar ($C_4$), genu ($C_3$), and supraclinoid ($C_2$). The ICA pierces the dura, then enters the subarachnoid space, and terminates ($C_1$) by dividing into

the middle cerebral artery (MCA) and anterior cerebral artery (ACA). Significant branches to a TCD study that arise from the distal ICA are the ophthalmic artery (OA) and posterior communicating arteries (PCOAs).

The MCA branches and courses laterally from the ICA as the main trunk or $M_1$ segment and bifurcates or trifurcates into $M_2$ branches that quickly angle upward into the insular area. There is very little asymmetry between the left and right MCA. The ACA ($A_1$ or precommunicating segment) begins and courses medially from the ICA for a short distance before passing forward as the $A_2$ or postcommunicating segment. The two ACAs are connected above the optic chiasm by the anterior communicating artery (ACOA). There are frequent variations between the two ACAs mainly consisting of differences in diameter or curvature.[4-6]

The intracranial posterior circulation is a continuation of the vertebral arteries (VAs) once these vessels pass through the foramen magnum and enter the subarachnoid space ($V_4$ segment) and course beneath the brain stem. Major branches, the posterior inferior cerebellar arteries (PICAs), usually arise from the distal part of the vertebral ($V_4$) and supply the brainstem and cerebellum. The VAs may have a tortuous course and often are of unequal size.[7] The basilar artery (BA) is created by the joining together of the two VAs and ends by terminating into the right and left posterior cerebral arteries (PCAs). It gives rise to two paired sets of branches, the anterior inferior cerebellar and superior cerebellar arteries along with numerous, small penetrating branches.[7]

The initial short segment of the PCA arising from the BA and prior to the PCOA is called the $P_1$ or precommunicating segment. Beyond this point, it becomes the $P_2$, postcommunicating segment, which winds around the cerebral peduncle. The PCOA anatomically connects the anterior and posterior circulations but may be hypoplastic. The PCA normally arises from the BA but can have a "fetal origin" in 18% to 27% of the population, meaning it is dependent on the ICA for flow, either exclusively or in combination with the BA.[7]

## SONOGRAPHIC EXAMINATION TECHNIQUES

### Patient Preparation

There are numerous established clinical indications for TCD testing spanning multiple medical specialties. For example, a patient with a transient ischemic attack (TIA) and carotid stenosis may be seen at a traditional cardiac or vascular laboratory, but patients with SAH will be studied in the neurointensive care unit, and children with sickle cell disease (SCD) are managed by Hematology. Periprocedural monitoring during carotid stenting and endarterectomy requires knowledge of the interventions and environment. Because the clinical indications and venue vary widely, so does the information sought from a history and physical.

In 2010 the American Society of Neuroimaging published practice standards for TCD. A multidisciplinary panel of experts established appropriate clinical indications including SCD, cerebral ischemia, detection of right to left shunt, SAH, brain death, and periprocedural or surgical monitoring.[8]

Using simple language, explain the test to the patient, instruct them to be quiet and unless necessary, not to speak

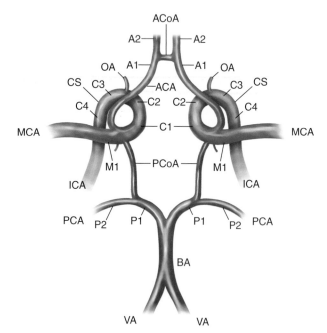

**FIGURE 10-1** Circle of Willis and branches with abbreviations used for each arterial segment.

during the examination. Take a relevant history from the patient or refer to their medical records and make note of relevant indications for the test (Table 10-1). When working in the intensive care unit (ICU) setting, check with the nurse before changing the level of the head. Take or record the blood pressure if the patient has an arterial line in place.

## Patient Position

The patient is examined supine with their head slightly elevated during examination of the anterior circulation when using the transtemporal, transorbital, and submandibular approaches. It is advisable to use a rolled hand towel or very small pillow to allow maximum access to the head and neck. The patient should be made as comfortable as possible because their co-operation and stillness is important to obtaining a good study. A semi-dark room facilitates relaxation as well as better image visualization on the ultrasound screen. To minimize variations in the spectral waveforms caused by fluctuating physiologic variables, allow time for the heart rate, respiratory rate, and blood pressure to reach a steady state before beginning the study.

The VAs and BA require insonation through the foramen magnum. Place the patient in the lateral decubitus position supporting the face and head with a small pillow or towel with the neck aligned centrally. Palpate at midline about 1.25 inches down from the skull base, flex the neck slightly. If the patient cannot be turned onto their side, the examination can be performed with the patient supine with the head rotated to the opposite side of insonation and the transducer placed just to the left or right side of the foramen magnum. For ambulatory patients, the upright sitting position is a feasible alternative with the neck flexed slightly and the head supported by the patient's arms and hands for stabilization. For ICU or other hospital inpatients that cannot be turned or optimally positioned the head can be propped up using a rolled towel and turned away from the side of insonation. This will create a space large enough for the transducer to be placed at either midline or just lateral to the foramen magnum and will usually provide adequate access to the VAs and BA.

## Technologist Position

The position of the sonographer may vary according to the setting. Outpatients are studied from the head or the side of the examination table, but for inpatients, the equipment and the sonographer are usually placed at the side of the bed. Dedicated TCD instruments often have remote controls allowing manipulation of the instrument at a distance from the machine. Duplex ultrasound systems are more limited and require closer proximity of the ultrasound system and the sonographer.

A nonimaging TCD transducer is smaller than most imaging probes, and unique ergonomic injuries can result from gripping the transducer too tightly and bending the thumbs and wrists backward. To avoid tendonitis and other injuries of the hands, grip the transducer with minimal pressure, rest when the hand becomes tired, and seek out preventative exercises from an ergonomics specialist.

## Equipment

A dedicated nonimaging TCD instrument uses a 1 to 2 MHz pulsed wave transducer, spectral analysis, and additionally may have M-mode capabilities. Software allows for the computation of peak systolic velocity (PSV), end-diastolic velocity (EDV), time-averaged peak velocity (TAP-V), and Goslings pulsatility index (PI) at a minimum. Cursors and spectral outline tracers are available to compute values when automatic computations are erroneous. Additional software will function for specific applications such as monitoring for emboli, trending velocities, and displaying temporal changes in velocity.

Power M-mode, introduced in 2002, uses simultaneous signal acquisition from 32 gates to create a display that demonstrates flow intensity and direction in bands of color (red is flow directed toward the transducer and blue away from the transducer). The display ranges from 25 to 85 mm and corresponds to the course and depth of the arteries. Information in the power M-mode display helps the user find signals by creating a kind of visual road map much in the way color flow facilitates duplex imaging.

## TABLE 10-1  Patient Interview

| Relevant Medical History | Risk Factors | Physical |
|---|---|---|
| Have you recently experienced any of these symptoms:<br>• Unilateral or bilateral face, leg and/or arm numbness, tingling, weakness<br>• Dysarthria, slurred, garbled, hesitant speech, inability to speak or understand speech<br>• Amaurosis fugax: transient monocular blindness; hemianopsia: loss of field of vision, unilateral, or bilateral; double vision<br>• Ataxia, gait disturbance, or drop attack: abrupt leg weakness and fall without loss of consciousness<br>• Vertigo, loss of consciousness<br>• Severe headache | • Diabetes<br>• Hypertension<br>• High cholesterol<br>• Tobacco abuse<br>• Cardiac disease, heart attack<br>• Claudication—leg muscle pain when walking<br>• Stroke or TIA<br>• Procedures to treat vascular disease (carotid endarterectomy/stent, coronary artery bypass graft/stent, peripheral arterial bypass graft/stent) | • Palpation of radial, carotid, and superficial temporal pulses<br>• Assess bilateral hand grip strength, ask patient to squeeze your hands as hard as possible; compare side to side strength<br>• Upper leg weakness assessed by having patient flex hip and knee about 8 inches off bed, instruct to maintain position and attempt to push down against thigh. Lower leg: stand at foot of bed and have patient push foot against your hand, then have them pull it up against your hand<br>• Bilateral brachial blood pressures<br>• Have patient smile, assess for symmetry |

Intracranial studies may or may not be conducted following a carotid duplex. Interview questions are similar for both study types when assessing for stroke or stroke risk.

Standard duplex ultrasound technology allows TCDI examinations through the use of a broadband phased array sector transducer with a 1 to 5 MHz frequency range. Software provides computational packages similar to those found on dedicated TCD systems; however, TCDI is not routinely used for monitoring applications because the transducer size is too large to attach to the headband, and most companies have not developed instruments hardware or software for these uses. With either TCD or TCDI examinations, the equipment settings should be optimized for each patient.

## Required Documentation

In general, documentation for both techniques (TCD and TCDI) will be based on spectral waveforms. The B-mode and color Doppler information yielded in TCDI studies primarily facilitates acquisition of spectral Doppler signals by providing a kind of color road map. Exceptions to this are color or power Doppler signals supporting identification of anomalous vessels and B-mode providing evidence of brain midline shifts and the visualization of masses. M-mode captures high-intensity transient signals (HITS), representing emboli. Documentation will vary according the type of study being performed and will be discussed for each application later in the chapter.

The intracranial arteries are a continuation of the cervical internal and VAs, and as such, examining them in a proximal to distal order will facilitate interpretation. Spectral Doppler waveforms from each of the listed arterial segments from the right and left cerebral hemispheres and posterior circulation constitute a complete study.[8] When pathology is present, additional waveforms may be required to demonstrate abnormal flow characteristics.

Limited TCDs may be done for a number of reasons, such as repeat examinations of affected vessels only, in acute stroke when using a fast protocol to determine single vessel patency,[9] when monitoring for microemboli or when monitoring during an intervention. Required documentation will depend on the specifics of the study, why it was

ordered, and which arteries are of interest. At a minimum, one spectral waveform from each artery or arterial segment studied is documented in normal examinations or multiple waveforms to demonstrate the pathology is required for an adequate interpretation to be made.

### Spectral Doppler Characteristics

Acquisition of a good spectral Doppler waveform from each required segment is essential because interpretation depends almost entirely upon these signals. In TCD studies, the sample volume size is relatively large in comparison to the size of the arteries, which are on average only 2 to 4 mm in diameter, and therefore, even normal waveforms have the appearance of spectral broadening. The biggest difference between TCD and extracranial velocity calculations is the common use of a TAP-V obtained from the entire cardiac cycle, which is used for interpretation rather than the single point PSV and EDV used in extracranial carotid studies. This value is described differently by various manufacturers, and for simplification is often referred to as the *mean* velocity as will be the case in this chapter. Quantitative values of mean velocity and pulsatility (PI) are used along with waveform morphology and specific signatures seen in the amplitude of the waveform to make the formal interpretation in adults. Very high velocities and turbulent flow can be simultaneously displayed in signals detected in severe stenosis, vasospasm, collateral and hyperdynamic flow creating complex waveforms. Instruments, generally, use an envelope trace that allows for real-time calculations of appropriate values; however, when the velocities become too complicated, these envelope tracers frequently fail to follow the true waveform outline, and manual calculations become necessary. Depending on the equipment different calculation methods are employed, one requires setting two cursors at the PSV and EDV and the second allows the user to trace the waveform contour with a cursor (Fig. 10-2).

With the exception of the OA, all of the arteries examined during a TCD examination supply the brain, a low resistance organ with relatively high flow during diastole, similar to the extracranial ICA. There are a wide range of normal values

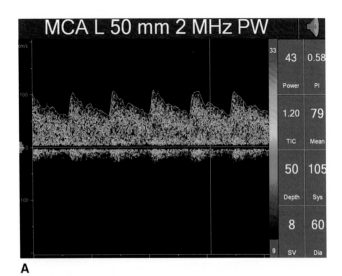

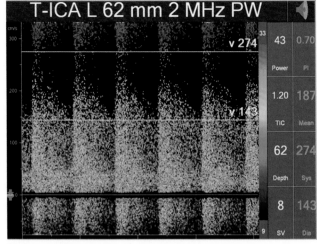

**A**                                    **B**

**FIGURE 10-2 A:** Spectral waveform from the MCA; envelope tracer calculates the time-averaged peak velocity (mean). **B:** Nonoptimal spectral waveform from the MCA with the envelope tracer turned off and manual cursors set to peak systole and end diastole resulting in a rough calculation of the mean velocity.

which vary primarily owing to age, gender, cardiac effects, and by other intrinsic and extrinsic physiologic factors. Waveforms are evaluated for both quantitative and qualitative characteristics and with knowledge of physiologic variables that can significantly influence flow findings.

### Audio Signals

Doppler signals are audible as well as visible in the spectral waveform. With the increased sophistication of ultrasound instrumentation, there has been a trend toward diminishing the importance of hearing Doppler sounds. The human ear and brain are exquisitely designed to perceive subtle audio nuances, and when used for vascular studies provide a feedback loop of information which aids in signal optimization. Developing good listening skills is especially important during nonimaging TCD and drives the acquisition of good signals, but should not be minimized during TCDI examinations.

## Anatomic Approaches

Both TCD and TCDI utilize the same regions of the cranium to access the basal cerebral arteries. Four approaches, also referred to as acoustic windows, are used: transtemporal,[1] transorbital,[10] suboccipital,[11,12] and submandibular (Fig. 10-3).[13,14] A fifth approach involves obtaining the VA signals at the atlas loop and is used to facilitate calculation of a ratio specific to BA vasospasm.[15,16]

### Transtemporal Approach

The transtemporal approach is located over the temporal bone, superior to the zygomatic arch, and anterior and slightly superior to the tragus of the ear conch. Despite the relative thinness of the temporal bone, there is significant attenuation of the ultrasound at this interface. Early experiments measuring ultrasound energy transmission through the temporal bone showed that a large range of energy losses occurred between different skull samples and depended on

the thickness of the bone.[17] There are individual variations in location of the temporal window, which is subdivided into posterior, middle, anterior, and frontal sites (Fig. 10-4). To find the site of optimal ultrasound penetration, all areas should be thoroughly explored. Window location determines the orientation of the transducer to the initial target, the MCA. Each area will require a somewhat different transducer angulation in order to be on axis with the arterial flow. From the posterior window, the beam is aimed slightly anterior, and from an anterior or frontal window, it is aimed more posterior. Generally, the middle window requires a direct, neutral orientation (Fig. 10-5A).

### Transorbital Approach

The orbital approach relies on the transmission of the ultrasound beam through the thin orbital plate of the frontal bone, optic canal, and superior orbital fissure, and signal attenuation is lower than for the temporal bone[10] (Fig. 10-5B). The power intensity is reduced to limit direct exposure to the eye and is guided by the manufacturers' recommendations and the ALARA (as low as reasonably achievable) principle.

### Foramen Magnum Approach

The foramen magnum approach takes advantage of the natural opening in the skull through which the spinal cord passes. The transducer is placed approximately 1¼ inches below the base of the skull, and the sound beam is aimed toward the nasion. The amount of soft tissue in this area varies considerably between individuals and will influence the depths at which the VA and BA are identified (Fig. 10-5C).

### Submandibular Approach

This approach to the extracranial ICA is notably different from the standard technique used to study the carotid arteries with a linear probe and a 60° angle. The power should be reduced because the sound is not penetrating bone.

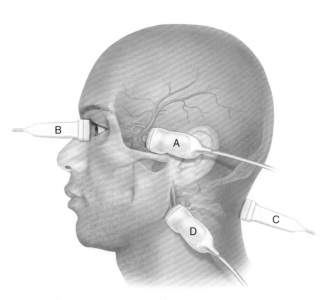

**FIGURE 10-3** Four approaches used for intracranial examinations: (**A**) transtemporal, (**B**) transorbital, (**C**) transoccipital, and (**D**) submandibular.

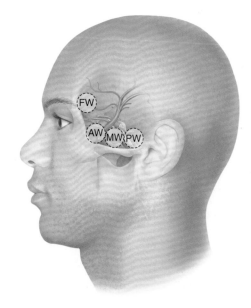

**FIGURE 10-4** The transtemporal window located above the zygomatic arch with four possibilities for obtaining access through the temporal bone.

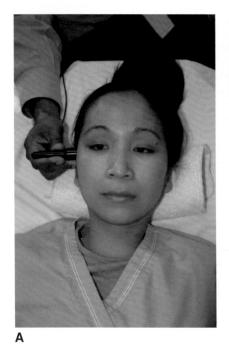
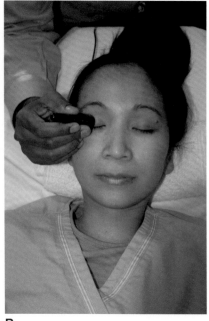
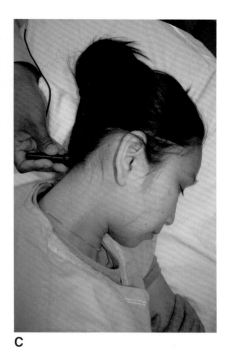

**A**  **B**  **C**

**FIGURE 10-5 A:** The most common position used for transtemporal access is the posterior window with the ultrasound beam oriented anteriorly. **B:** Transducer position for the orbit showing placement over the center of the eyelid with the beam aimed 15° to 20° medially. **C:** Midline transducer placement for the foramen magnum approach below the skull base and aimed toward the nasion.

The retromandibular ICA signal is obtained by using the TCD transducer and a zero degree angle of insonation. The transducer is placed at the angle of the jaw with the beam-directed cephalad. Signals obtained are usually used to calculate a Lindegaard ratio in patients with vasospasm secondary to SAH or for documenting distal ICA stenosis arising from fibromuscular dysplasia and dissections[11] (Fig. 10-6A).

### Atlas Loop Approach

Originally described by von Reutern to study the extracranial VA using continuous wave Doppler,[2] obtaining VA signals at this location is used to calculate the BA/VA ratio which, similar to the Lindegaard ratio, is useful to categorize BA vasospasm.[16] The transducer is placed approximately 1.25 inches below the mastoid process and behind the

sternocleidomastoid muscle. Again, the power can be lowered because this is an extracranial signal and does not require penetration of bone (Fig. 10-6B).

### Standard TCD Examination Technique

TCD studies are a diagnostic tool in the clinical management of patients with a variety of intracranial vascular abnormalities. The study provides physiologic information that complements anatomic imaging studies. The results may provide rationales for the treatment of brain ischemia and stroke.

Standard TCD examinations are performed on both inpatients and outpatients when ordered. A complete standard TCD examination consists of pulsed wave Doppler

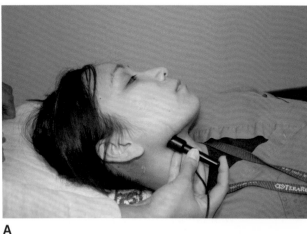
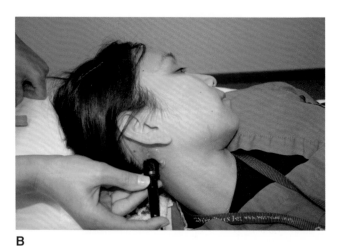

**A**  **B**

**FIGURE 10-6 A:** Obtaining the submandibular ICA at the angle of the jaw. **B:** Insonation of the vertebral artery in the region of the atlas loop.

insonation of the basal cerebral arteries, including the bilateral cavernous and terminal segments of the ICAs, OAs, MCAs, ACAs, PCAs, VAs, and the BA.[8] Additionally, in some populations, the extracranial retromandibular ICAs and VAs at the atlas loop will be examined to calculate vasospasm ratios (Table 10-2).

Doppler spectral waveforms are acquired in a blind fashion without the aid of B-mode or color Doppler requiring a good understanding of the anatomy and physiology of the intracranial vessels and a precise, systematic approach to the examination performance.

There are five primary criteria used for identification of each vessel segment:

1. Approach: each cranial window provides access to specific arteries only
2. Sample volume depth: each artery has a specific range of depths over which it courses
3. Direction of blood flow relative to the ultrasound transducer
4. The spatial relationship of one artery to another. For the anterior circulation, the reference vessel used to identify other arteries is the bifurcation of the terminal ICA.
5. Flow velocity: In general, the MCA > ACA > PCA = BA = VA. These relationships assist vessel identification and when reversed can be helpful in identifying pathologic flow states (Table 10-3).[18,19]

### Orbital Approach

Arteries identified through the orbital window include the OA and cavernous carotid (siphon). The acoustic intensity is lowered to the manufacturer's recommendations, and close observation of the ALARA principle is used. The patient is asked to close their eyes gently and keep them shut until the end of the orbital examination to avoid getting ultrasound gel into the eye. A small amount of ultrasound gel is placed on the transducer and or closed eyelid, and the transducer is placed gently over the center of the closed eyelid and aimed 15° to 20°, toward midline, without applying any pressure to the eye.

At sample volume depths ranging from 40 to 60 mm, the OA can be identified isolated away from the carotid siphon (CS). The unique waveform of the OA has low velocities, and because of the higher resistance bed of the eye compared with the brain typically has low diastolic flow. The OA is studied to determine whether flow is antegrade or retrograde, the latter indicative of external carotid artery (ECA) to ICA collateral flow.[10,11]

By increasing the sample volume to 60 to 70 mm, flow can be detected in the CS so named because of its tortuous course at this location, resulting in flow directionality that may be toward, away, or bidirectional, depending on the orientation of the vessel segment to the transducer, although normally the physiologic direction of flow is antegrade (Fig. 10-7).[10,11]

### Temporal Approach

The arteries identified through the transtemporal approach include the MCA ($M_1$ and proximal $M_2$ segments), ACA ($A_1$ segment), terminal internal carotid (TICA), and PCA ($P_1$ and proximal $P_2$ segments). The ACOA and PCOA are usually only identified when they are carrying an increased volume flow, because they are functioning as collaterals. Ample gel is applied to the transducer and to the patient's

### TABLE 10-2　Basal Cerebral Arteries Insonated during Intracranial Exam, Their Abbreviations, and the Minimum Documentation for a Complete, Normal TCD, or TCDI Study

| Artery | Abbreviations | Number of Waveforms | Comments |
|---|---|---|---|
| Ophthalmic | OA | 1 | |
| Carotid Siphon | CS | 1–3 | $C_2$ (supraclinoid), $C_3$ (genu), $C_4$ (parasellar) if accessible |
| Terminal internal carotid | TICA | 1 | $C_1$ |
| Middle cerebral | MCA and MCA2 | 3 | Proximal, mid, and distal, including MCA2 branches |
| Anterior cerebral (precommunicating segment) | ACA | 1 | |
| Anterior cerebral (postcommunicating segment) | ACA2 | 1 | Only applies to TCDI |
| Anterior communicating artery | ACOA | 1 | When functioning as collateral |
| Posterior cerebral (precommunicating segment) | $PCA_1$ | 1 | |
| Posterior cerebral (postcommunicating segment) | $PCA_2$ | 1 | |
| Posterior communicating | PCOA | 1 | When functioning as collateral |
| Submandibular internal carotid | SM-ICA | 1 | When calculating Lindegaard index or documenting distal narrowing |
| Vertebral | VA4 | 3 | Proximal, mid, and distal |
| Vertebral at the atlas loop ($V_3$) | VA3 | 1 | When calculating Sviri ratio for vasospasm |
| Basilar | BA | 3 | Proximal, mid, and distal |

**TABLE 10-3   Criteria Used to Identify Each Arterial Segment for a Full Diagnostic TCD Examination[18,19]**

| Cranial Approach | Arterial Segment | Flow Direction Relative to Transducer | Sample Volume Depth Ranges (mm) | Spatial Relationship to Landmark MCA/ACA Bifurcation | TCD Normal Mean Velocity Range and S/D (cm/s) | TCDI (Angle corrected) Normal Mean Velocity Range Age 20–39 (cm/s) | TCDI (Angle Corrected) Normal Mean Velocity Range Age 40–59 (cm/s) | TCDI (Angle Corrected) Normal Mean Velocity Range Age >60 (cm/s) |
|---|---|---|---|---|---|---|---|---|
| Temporal | MCA ($M_1$ and proximal $M_2$) | $M_1$—toward $M_2$—away | 30–60 | Identical | 55 ± 12 | 71–76 | 69–76 | 55–61 |
| Temporal | TICA ($C_1$) | Toward and/or away | 60–70 | Inferior | 39 ± 9 | | | |
| Temporal | ACA ($A_1$) | Away | 60–75 | Anterior and superior | 50 ± 11 | 57–62 | 57–64 | 48–54 |
| Temporal | PCA ($P_1$) | Toward | 60–75 | Posterior and inferior | 39 ± 10 | 51–55 | 48–51 | 40–45 |
| Temporal | PCA ($P_2$) | Away | 60–65 | Posterior and inferior | 40 ± 10 | 45–49 | 46–51 | 39–45 |
| Orbital | OA | Toward | 35–55 | | 21 ± 5 | | | |
| Orbital | Carotid siphon ($C_4$, $C_3$, $C_2$) | Toward, bidirectional, away | 65–80 | | $C_2$ 41 ± 11 $C_4$ 47 ± 14 | | | |
| Submandibular | ICA | Away | 35–80 | | 30 ± 9 | | | |
| Atlas loop | VA ($V_3$) | Away | 40–50 | | | | | |
| Foramen magnum | VA | Away | 60–90 | | 38 ± 10 | 42–47 | 38–43 | 30–36 |
| Foramen magnum | BA | Away | 70–120 | | 41 ± 10 | 47–53 | 39–48 | 31–40 |

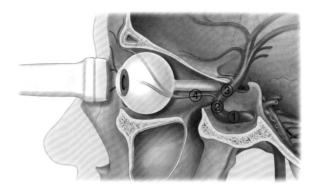

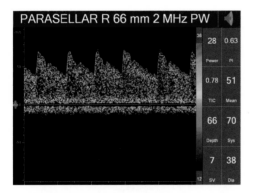

1 Parasellar

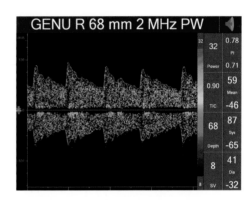

2 Genu

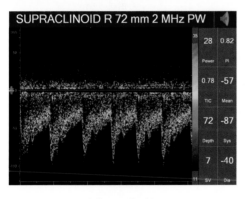

3 Supraclinoid

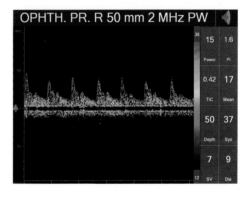

4 Ophthalmic

**FIGURE 10-7** Orbital approach showing a lateral view of the CS and ophthalmic arteries. **1:** Low-resistance waveform in parasellar segment of the intracranial ICA. **2:** Bidirectional signal seen at the genu. **3:** ICA siphon flow directed away from the transducer. **4:** Ophthalmic artery with high-resistant, low-velocity waveform.

skin to create a good interface for the transmission of the ultrasound.[11]

Finding the exact location on the temporal bone that allows the best ultrasound penetration can be challenging and will be facilitated by being systematic in the exploration of this area and using very fine hand movements. To facilitate finding, the temporal window power is set at maximum, and the sample volume is placed at a depth of 50 mm with the intention of finding the MCA.

The examination is begun by placing the transducer in the posterior window aiming the beam slightly anterior and superior and using a circular motion scanning for an audible Doppler signal and visual spectral display. If using, M-mode employs the same manual technique while also observing the M-mode display for a red color band at depths ranging from 30 to 65 mm.[20] If no or weak signals are obtained, the transducer is systematically moved to the middle and anterior or frontal locations, and scanning is repeated until signal acquisition is accomplished.

Once a suitable acoustic window is identified, emphasis changes to identifying each arterial segment. Initial signals directed toward the transducer at a depth of 50 mm most often arise from the MCA. The sample volume depth is then reduced in a stepwise manner, tracing the MCA distally in 2 to 5 mm increments. Distally, the main trunk of the MCA divides into the $M_2$ segment, and the branches course superior over the insula, have lower velocities, and flow direction may change to away from the transducer. Following the MCA2 branches will require aiming the beam slightly superior (Fig. 10-8).

The sample volume depth is then increased to trace the MCA proximally to its origin at 55 to 65 mm. The bifurcation of the terminal ICA into the MCA and ACA serves as a reference landmark for the remainder of the study. When using a large sample volume size (5 to 10 mm), the ACA and MCA are frequently seen simultaneously as a bidirectional signal as long as they are oriented on the same axis. The M-mode display will also show bands of color, red at shallower depths and past the TICA bifurcation a blue band will appear, indicating flow away from the transducer, usually the ACA. A word of caution is that at this depth, flow away from the transducer is not necessarily the ACA. If the beam is pointing slightly inferiorly the tortuous, TICA may also reveal flow away from the transducer, making it important to always know how the beam is being aimed relative to the landmark bifurcation signal (Fig. 10-9).

From the bifurcation, the ACA is identified by increasing the sample volume depth and usually aiming the transducer

### Middle Cerebral Artery

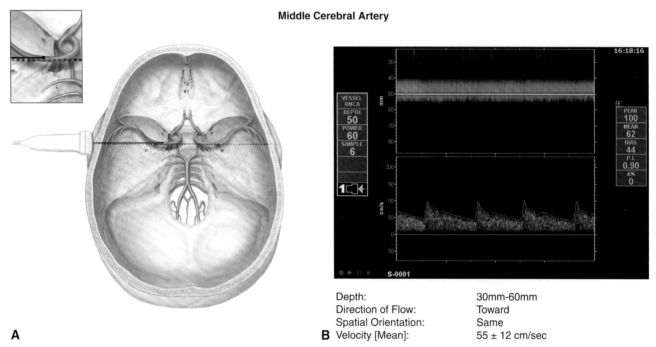

| Depth: | 30mm-60mm |
| Direction of Flow: | Toward |
| Spatial Orientation: | Same |
| **B** Velocity [Mean]: | 55 ± 12 cm/sec |

**A**

**FIGURE 10-8  A:** Temporal approach to the MCA demonstrating placement of the sample volume in the main trunk (M₁) segment. **B:** A normal spectral waveform and M-mode display illustrating band of flow toward the transducer at depths of 30 to 60 mm consistent with flow in the MCA.

### ACA/MCA Bifurcation

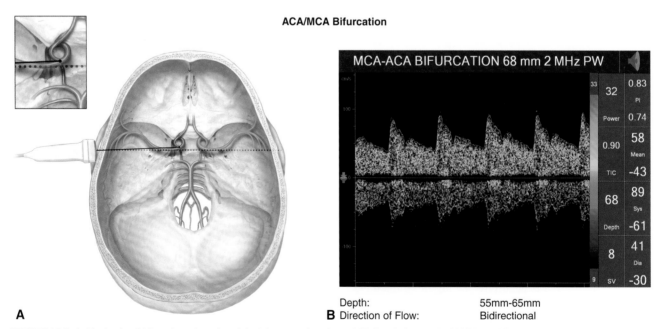

| Depth: | 55mm-65mm |
| **B** Direction of Flow: | Bidirectional |

**A**

**FIGURE 10-9  A:** The landmark bifurcation where the relatively large sample volume yields flow in the proximal MCA and ACA simultaneously. **B:** A bidirectional spectral waveform from the proximal MCA and ACA with the M-mode display showing the change of flow direction at the bifurcation depth of 55 to 65 mm.

slightly anterior and superior. The precommunicating segment of the ACA does exhibit variations in caliber with lower velocities found in hypoplastic segments. It can also vary its course and sometimes curves downward rather than upward in patients between the ages of 50 and 70 years.[2] The ACA can be traced to the midline of the brain, where again bidirectional signals may be detected related to insonation of the bilateral ACAs. The spectral waveform is normally directed away from the transducer, although it can reverse direction when acting as collateral. The M-mode display will show a narrow band of blue color at the depth appropriate to the ACA. The ACOA is not identified until it acts as a collateral channel because of its diminutive size (Fig. 10-10).

To identify the TICA, the sample volume depth is returned to the landmark bifurcation and, at the same depth, aimed directly inferior. Velocities may appear low because of the anatomic course of the TICA relative to the sound beam which tends to be perpendicular to the vessel, creating a larger angle of insonation and lower calculated velocities (Fig. 10-11).

Lastly, the PCA is located by again returning the sample volume to the ACA/MCA bifurcation, increasing the depth by 5 mm and moving the transducer slightly posterior and inferior. Only very small movements are required because it is easy to overshoot the amount of rotation used. The direction of flow in the $P_1$ segment and proximal $P_2$ segment is toward the transducer. The M-mode display will show a narrow red band representative of the $P_1$ and proximal $P_2$ at the appropriate depth, and the contralateral $P_1$ will appear blue at a greater depth. By increasing the depth to 70 to 80 mm, signals from both the right and left PCA are seen as they bifurcate from the tip of the BA, resulting in a bidirectional spectral waveform.

Once the $P_1$ segment is identified, continuing with further rotation in the same posterioinferior direction, the $P_2$ segment, flowing away from the transducer will be intersected. The PCOAs are usually not appreciated unless they are functioning as collateral pathways carrying an increased volume of blood with subsequent high velocities and turbulence (Fig. 10-12).

### Foramen Magnum Approach

The VAs and BA are studied using the suboccipital window with the transducer placed midline below the foramen magnum, the patient's head slightly flexed, and the ultrasound beam oriented upward toward the center of the patient's eyebrows. Normal direction of flow is away from the transducer but can reverse in any segment secondary to subclavian or innominate artery steals. The distal BA can also be reversed in direction because of a proximal BA occlusion. In this case, there will be anterior to posterior collateral via the PCOAs. Initially, to find the window, the sample volume depth is set at 60 mm, and by aiming minimally to the right and left, toward the orbit of the eye, an initial signal will be found. The right and left VAs are differentiated by having the signal drop out as the beam is moved from right to left and because the waveforms frequently have a different shape. It is common to have a dominant and nondominant VA, and the flow velocities will be lower in the smaller vessel, and the morphology of the waveform will have a different contour. Once the right and left vessels are differentiated, follow each from proximal to distal. In the near field around 55 mm depth, the signal becomes bidirectional as it begins to course extracranially and does so again at a depth of 65 mm where the PICA branch arises. A more lateral orientation of the transducer to the foramen magnum can also be used to identify the VAs. However, from this approach,

**Anterior Cerebral Artery**

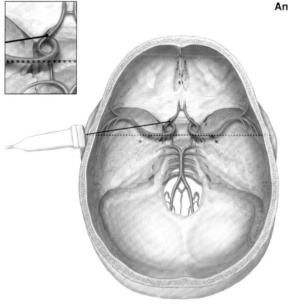

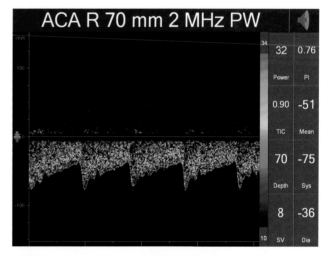

| | |
|---|---|
| Depth: | 60mm-80mm |
| Direction of Flow: | Away |
| Spatial Orientation: | Anterior/Superior |
| Velocity [Mean]: | 50 + 11 cm/sec |

**A**   **B**

**FIGURE 10-10 A:** Frequently, the ACA is located by further aiming the transducer in an anterior and superior manner. **B:** The spectral waveform demonstrates the ACA flowing away from the transducer and the M-mode display illustrating band of flow away from the transducer at 60 to 80 mm.

**Terminal Internal Carotid Artery**

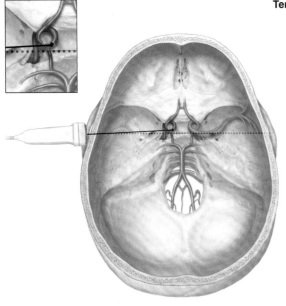

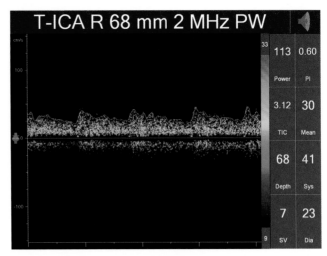

Depth: 55mm-65mm
Direction of Flow: Toward
Spatial Orientation: Inferior
**B** Velocity [Mean]: 39 ± 9 cm/sec

**A**

**FIGURE 10-11 A:** With the sample volume depth located at the landmark bifurcation and aimed inferiorly, the terminal ICA is insonated. **B:** The spectral waveform from the TICA demonstrates relatively low velocities because of the poor angle of insonation. The M-mode display of the TICA with the latter flowing away from the transducer; notice the gap between the MCA and TICA indicating they are on a different axis.

**Posterior Cerebral Artery (P1)**

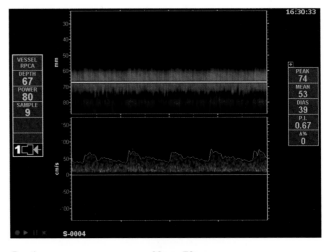

Depth: 60mm-70mm
Direction of Flow: Toward
Spatial Orientation: Posterior/Inferior
**B** Velocity [Mean]: 39 ± 10 cm/sec

**A**

**FIGURE 10-12 A:** The PCA is identified by aiming the beam posterior and inferior from the depth of the very proximal ACA. **B:** The flow direction from the P$_1$ and proximal P$_2$ segments are toward the transducer, whereas the M-mode color bands show the bilateral P$_1$ segments as the beam crosses midline.

it is possible to have the beam focused on the contralateral VA while thinking ipsilateral VA is being insonated. This is usually only problematic if the left and right VA waveforms are very similar in shape and velocity which occurs about one-third of the time. The exact confluence of the two VAs into the BA may be difficult to determine with nonimaging TCD. In some cases, as the sample volume depth increases, it begins to encompass both VAs simultaneously, and the

resultant spectral waveform will show them superimposed. The depth of the VA confluence varies with body habitus and has a range of approximately 69 ± 7 mm.[21]

The BA curves below the brainstem and courses forward and superiorly; therefore, to identify this segment, the transducer is slid slightly further down the neck and oriented somewhat higher than for the VAs. This artery is relatively long (33 ± 6 mm) and may need to be traced for 3 to 4 cm in order to capture the distal segment.[19] Both the VAs and BA give off cerebellar branches, and when these are intersected, the signal becomes temporarily bidirectional (Fig. 10-13).

## TCDI Scanning Technique

The use of duplex ultrasound instrumentation to examine the intracranial circulation has both advantages and limitations. Accurate vessel identification and decreasing the learning curve time are two significant contributions of TCDI technique. Disadvantages include a larger transducer footprint that may limit access to small or difficult windows and an inability to apply this technology to monitoring applications where the transducer is attached to a head frame and arteries are continually monitored over time. TCDI uses low-frequency broadband phased array sector transducers with Doppler frequencies in a range of 2 to 3 MHz and imaging frequencies up to 5 MHz.

### Orbital Approach

Ultrasound energy passes through the orbit of the eye prior to penetrating the skull when using the transorbital window, and the Food and Drug Administration has lowered the maximum acoustic output allowable for this approach. This is in concern for potential bioeffects to the eye, and most instruments have an orbital power setting that automatically limits the output.

The patient is placed in a supine position with both eyes gently closed. Instruct the patient to keep eyes shut until the orbital examination is complete and the acoustic gel has been removed. The transducer orientation marker is pointed medial for both the right and left sides, and the probe is gently set upon the center of the closed eyelid. The hand holding the transducer can be stabilized by placing it on the patient's cheek for support. Do not apply any pressure to the eye.

B-mode image orientation will show medial to the left of the screen, lateral to the right. The globe of the eye will appear in the near field as a round echolucent structure. With the transducer in a true anterior/posterior orientation, the optic nerve shadow will extend from the distal rim at the center of the globe. With the color box set at the back of the globe and extending to include the proximal optic nerve shadow, the central retinal artery and vein, lacrimal artery as well as the long and short posterior ciliary arteries can frequently be observed. These are all branches of the OA and supply blood flow to various parts of the eye.

### Ophthalmic Artery

To locate the main branch of the OA angle the transducer 15% to 20% aiming medially. This will distort the round shape of the globe, and the optic nerve shadow may disappear. Place the color box at a depth of 40 to 60 mm, and lower the color scale (normal velocities are 21 ± 5 cm/s). Normal flow direction is toward the transducer (red), and the path of the artery should be from lateral to medial as it courses across the optic nerve. Signals taken too shallow or too lateral may represent flow in the lachrymal artery branch. Place the spectral Doppler sample volume in the color box. The waveform will have a low velocity with high resistance similar to the extracranial ECA. Flow direction may reverse, velocity increase, and pulsatility decrease when the OA functions as a collateral channel in severe stenosis or occlusion proximally in the ICA (Fig. 10-14).

### Carotid Siphon

There are no specific B-mode landmarks surrounding the cavernous carotid artery. Using the same transducer orientation as for the OA, the color box is placed at a depth of 60 to 75 mm and the color scale increased (normal velocity is 47 ± 14 cm/s). This tortuous section of the ICA may present

**Vertebral Artery**

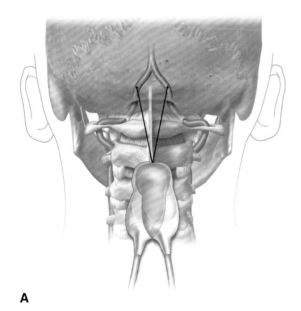

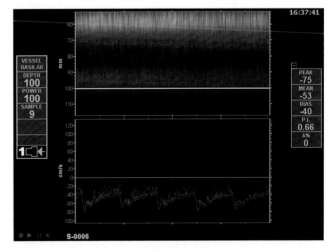

Depth: 60mm-90mm
Direction of Flow: Away
**B** Velocity [Mean]: 38 ± 10 cm/sec

**A**

**FIGURE 10-13 A:** Using the foramen magnum window to identify the intracranial VAs from a midline approach. **B:** Spectral waveforms and M-mode display and spectral waveform from the BA; notice the distance over which the BA travels.

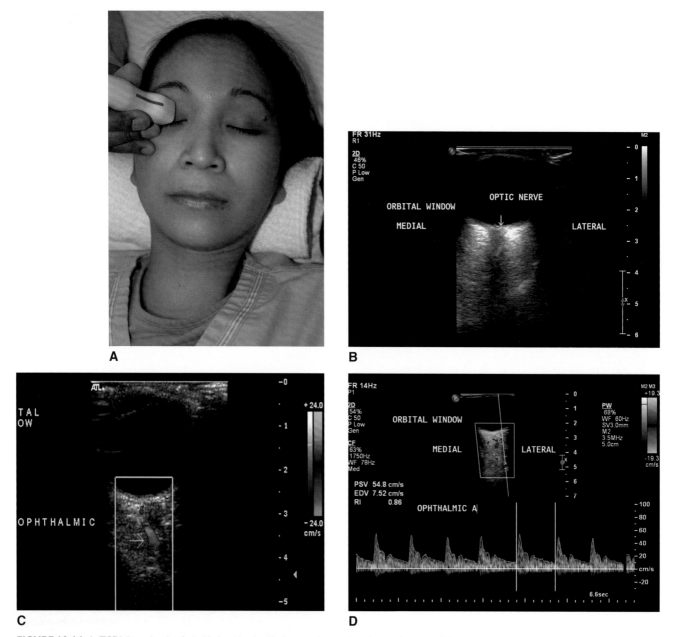

**FIGURE 10-14 A**: TCDI through using the orbital approach with the transducer orientation marker toward the patient's nose (medial). **B**: B-mode image of the globe and optic nerve (*arrow*) with the transducer in a true anterior posterior position. **C**: Color Doppler of the OA (*arrow*). **D**: Spectral Doppler waveform from the OA.

as flow toward, away, or both. Spectral Doppler waveforms are obtained from each segment (Fig. 10-15).

### Temporal Approach

Begin the examination at maximum power to facilitate finding the acoustic window. Once the window is established, reduce the power following the ALARA principle, especially if the patient has a hemicraniectomy and the bone is absent.

The temporal window provides access to multiple arteries that, along with their branches, supply all lobes of the cerebrum. It is conventional to study the left and right hemispheres from the left and right temporal windows, respectively, even in patients with good windows so that spectral Doppler strength and angles of insonation are optimal.

The transducer is positioned in cross section with the orientation marker facing anteriorly or toward the patient's nose (Fig. 10-16). The grayscale image presents a cross-sectional view of the brain. Superficial shows the ipsilateral cerebral hemisphere, whereas deep shows the contralateral cerebral hemisphere. Anterior is to the left of the screen and posterior to the right.

### Identifying the Window Using B-mode Landmarks

Apply a generous amount of gel over the temporal region of the head. Place the transducer just superior and parallel to the zygomatic arch. Set the field of view to at least 15 cm. If there is an adequate window, bright reflections are seen forming a crescent shape at a depth of around 5 cm.

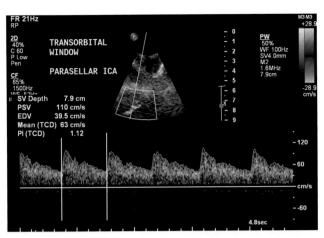

**FIGURE 10-15** Color Doppler signals seen at depths corresponding to the CS.

This bright landmark arises from the lesser wing of the sphenoid bone (anterior) and the petrous ridge of the temporal bone (posterior). Tilting the transducer slightly caudad, directly below the tip of the sphenoid wing is the anterior clinoid process. If these reflections are absent, slide or tilt the transducer forward, backward, up, and/or down, using very slow, small motions until they appear. If all B-mode reflections are homogeneous, there is no ultrasonic bone window (Fig. 10-17).

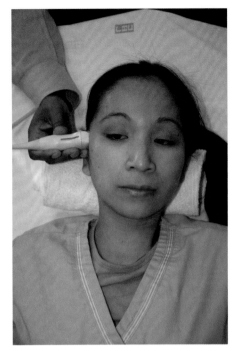

**FIGURE 10-16** Temporal approach with transducer oriented in a cross-sectional plane and the orientation marker toward the nose.

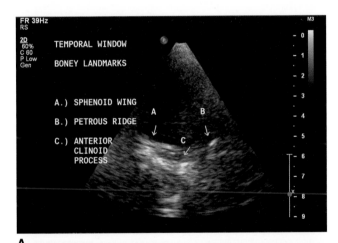

**A**

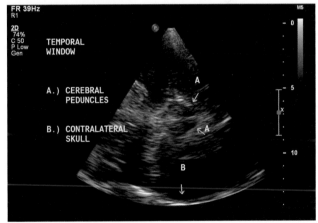

**B**

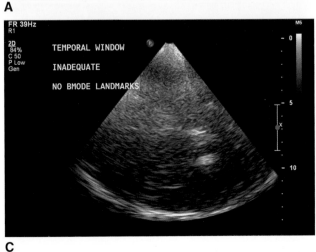

**C**

**FIGURE 10-17** Temporal approach grayscale landmarks. **A:** Bright reflections returning from the sphenoid wing and petrous ridge and anterior clinoid process bone landmarks in the near field. **B:** Parenchymal landmark, including the cerebral peduncle. **C:** Homogenous B-mode image with no landmarks consistent with mainly or totally absent temporal window.

Tilt or slide the transducer slightly cephalad above the bright reflections coming from the boney structures identified at the base of the brain and identify the following structures: (1) contralateral skull (note the depth of the inner table), midline of the brain will be at one half this depth; (2) falx cerebri, seen as a bright, thin line produced by the reflection from the double layer of dura in the interhemispheric fissure at midline; and (3) midbrain seen at midline and slightly posterior to the center of the screen image appearing as an echolucent butterfly or heart-shaped structure.

### Terminal Internal Carotid Artery

Decrease the field of view to 8 cm if the window is suboptimal. Relocate the boney landmarks, and place the color box on the anterior clinoid process around which the ICA courses. A small circle of color will appear; change the transducer orientation obliquely toward coronal, and the color image will assume an "S" shape. This is the TICA that is tortuous at this location and will appear both blue and red although flow is normally antegrade. Sample with spectral Doppler and save the highest velocity. The angle of insonation for this segment of the ICA is not optimal, and velocities will be lower than if sampled at zero degrees (Fig. 10-18).

### Middle Cerebral Artery

The MCA is slightly above and parallel to the lesser wing of the sphenoid bone. From the TICA, move the transducer cephalad using deliberate, small, and slow motions. The main trunk of the MCA, flowing toward the transducer, is red. Branches coming off the distal MCA are often seen curving upwards toward the Sylvian fissure and are blue. To see MCA branches better, aim the beam upward. Sample the branches with spectral Doppler then sample the main trunk sequentially in at least 5 mm increments obtaining flow velocities distal, mid, and proximal. Turn the color scale up if there is color aliasing or down if there is poor color visualization (Fig. 10-19).

### Anterior Cerebral Artery

The short segment of the ACA can be challenging to identify with color flow, especially when the vessel is not oriented axially to the MCA. If not seen in tandem with the MCA, the following transducer adjustments are helpful (1) twist the front end of the probe upward, (2) slide the probe upward, (3) tilt the probe upward, and (4) twist the probe downward but do not mistake the TICA for the ACA. The ACA is not

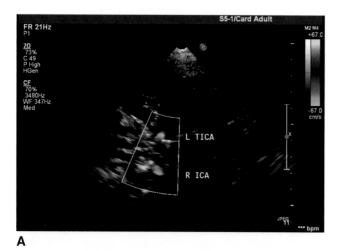

A

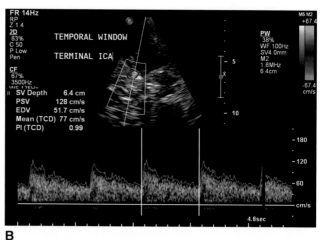

B

**FIGURE 10-18 A:** Color box placed over the anterior clinoid process bilateral TICAs. **B:** Spectral waveform from the TICA

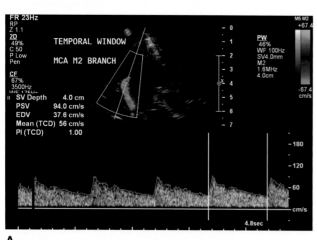

A

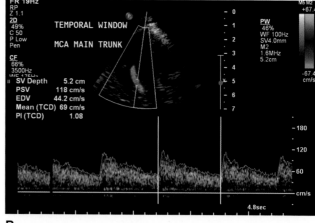

B

**FIGURE 10-19** Color and spectral Doppler signals from (**A**) M₂ branches of the MCA and (**B**) main trunk of the MCA.

surrounded by bone and the B-mode image will not display the bright boney reflections seen surrounding the TICA. The precommunicating segment of the ACA is short and ends at midline. The proximal postcommunicating segment can often be seen coursing toward the left of the screen (anterior). The ACA is blue on color Doppler but can change direction when acting as collateral. When this occurs, it is easy to cross midline and mistakenly get signals from the contralateral hemisphere. Therefore, it is important to always know the depth of midline. Take spectral Doppler waveforms in 5 mm increments. If the color box does not fill, try using the spectral Doppler at the anticipated location for the ACA (Fig. 10-20).

The ACA has a high incidence of anatomic variation and may be hypoplastic or atretic, and most often exhibits asymmetries in the caliber between the right and left sides. When functionally absent, the crossover collateral ability (from one hemisphere to the other via the ACAs and ACOA) can be severely limited or absent.

### Posterior Cerebral Artery

Locate the hypoechoic, butterfly-shaped midbrain using B-mode, and place the color box around the midbrain,

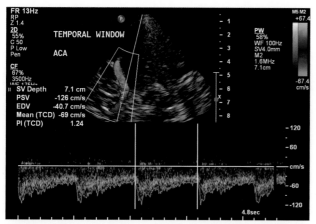

**FIGURE 10-20** Color and spectral Doppler signals from the ACA (A$_1$ segment); notice the surrounding B-mode image is not bright because the ACA courses above the boney processes.

which is encircled by the PCAs. The P$_1$ will be flowing toward the transducer (red) as will the proximal P$_2$. Twist the transducer to open up the curving vessel. As the PCA curves around the midbrain, the flow orientation is away from the transducer (blue), and this represents the postcommunicating or P$_2$ segment.

To differentiate between the P$_1$ and P$_2$ segments, set the color box to include the TICA simultaneously with the PCA. Draw an imaginary line between these two vessels, and it will represent the PCOA. This artery can frequently be seen with color flow if the scale setting is low enough, even when it is not functioning as collateral. Flow in the ipsilateral PCA deeper than the imaginary line is the P$_1$ segment, superficial to it is the P$_2$ segment. Obtain spectral Doppler signals along the PCA, and document the highest velocity in the P$_1$ and P$_2$ segments (Fig. 10-21).

In normal anatomy, the PCA originates from the BA, but in 18% to 27% of patients, it originates from the TICA, either exclusively or in combination with the BA.[6] This is referred to as a fetal origin and can frequently be seen with TCDI. Fetal origin is highly suggested when there is no communication between the BA and the PCA evidenced when color or spectral Doppler signals can be obtained from the short P$_1$ segment and a large vessel, originating from the TICA and coursing posteriorly can be seen with color Doppler. A fetal origin PCA can have a significant clinical impact on patients with ICA stenosis and/or vertebro basilar disease and should be noted in comments and on the interpretation.

### Foramen Magnum Approach

The foramen magnum is a large median opening penetrating the occipital bone. Place the transducer 1.25 inches below the skull base, aiming the beam toward the nasion. There are bright reflections from the occipital bone, and the window appears as an anechoic circular shape in the near field of the image (depth of about 5 cm). In order to find the best acoustic window, the transducer may be moved from one side or the other of the foramen magnum and twisted into an oblique or sagittal orientation. Turn the color Doppler on. Place the color box at a depth of 55 to 65 mm. The VAs appear as flow away from the transducer (blue) and may exhibit a high degree of tortuosity. In the near field, around

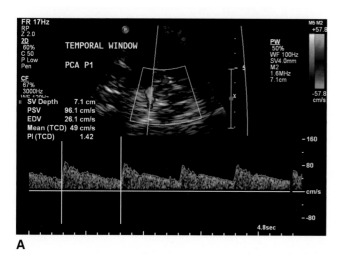

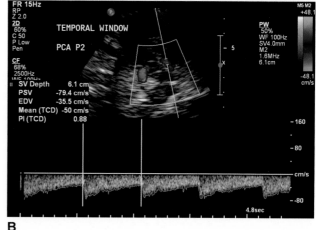

**A**     **B**

**FIGURE 10-21 A:** Hypoechoic cerebral peduncle and P$_1$ segment of the PCA. **B:** P$_2$ segment of the PCA.

50 to 55 mm depth, the color flow will be bidirectional which is caused by the vessel changing course as it travels from the atlas through the foramen magnum and into the $V_4$ segment.

Follow the two VAs to their confluence where they join to form the basilar. Sample each VA at 5 mm increments and obtain spectral waveforms. Document the highest velocity from each vessel. The VAs are often of unequal size with one or the other dominant in 74% of the population.[7] The PICA arises from each distal VA and will appear as a branch usually directed toward the transducers. At their confluence between 70 and 90 mm, the two VAs will join to form the BA that looks like a Y shape on the screen. Narrow the color box for a better frame rate and increase the depth of its placement.

The BA is 3 to 4 mm long and in some patients may extend to depths as great as 120 mm. Using TCDI, the mid and distal parts of the artery may be difficult to visualize with color flow, but the spectral Doppler sample volume can be placed to follow the trajectory of the BA, enhancing signal acquisition at greater depths. Obtain spectral Doppler waveforms at 5 mm increments and document the proximal, mid, and distal BA (Fig. 10-22).

### Submandibular Approach

The retromandibular, extradural ICA is routinely obtained in patients with abnormalities requiring calculation of the Lindegaard ratio, including SAH, head trauma, intracranial stenosis, and arteriovenous malformations. This ratio defined as the MCA/SM—ICA is important for differentiating vasospasm and stenosis of the MCA from hyperdynamic flow.[13,22] If the patient has >50% extracranial stenosis, the ratio calculation may be invalid and should not be used. Locating the ICA using this technique is also useful in determining distal arterial narrowing often associated with carotid dissection or fibromuscular dysplasia.

Set the power low and place the transducer at the angle of the jaw with the orientation marker facing up and aim slightly medial and posterior. The ICA will appear on the screen moving from right (more superficial) to left (deeper) flowing away (blue) from the transducer. Place the sample volume at the depth providing the best zero degree angle, usually around 4 to 5 cm and obtain a single spectral waveform with the highest obtainable velocity (Fig. 10-23).

## Technical Considerations

About 10% of geriatric patients will have hyperostosis of the temporal bone, and because of high attenuation of the ultrasound, no signals will be obtained through the temporal bone window. Hyperostosis occurs both unilaterally and bilaterally. Suboptimal windows provide some degree of penetration, but the numbers of arteries that can be

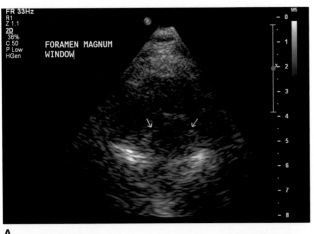

**A**

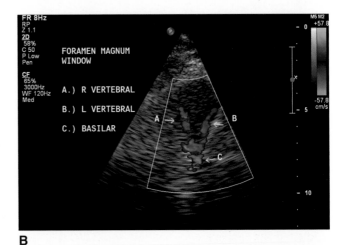

**B**

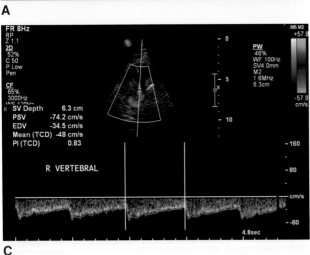

**C**

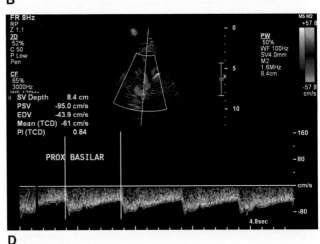

**D**

**FIGURE 10-22 A:** Grayscale showing the foramen magnum (*arrow*) surrounding by bright reflections from occipital bone. **B:** Bilateral VAs entering the cranium and coursing medially to form the BA. **C:** Spectral waveform taken from the VA. **D:** Spectral waveform taken from the BA.

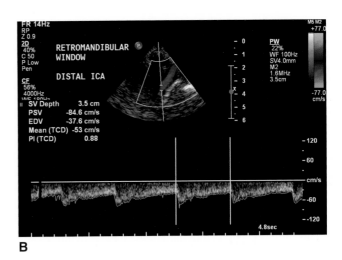

**FIGURE 10-23 A:** Transducer placement for the submandibular approach to the ICA. **B:** Color and spectral Doppler taken from the submandibular ICA.

identified are often limited. In patients without temporal access, a limited study using the transorbital and foramen magnum windows is performed.

Although a very light touch is used when the transducer is placed over the eye and care is taken to avoid applying any pressure, in order to avoid unintentional abrasion do not perform the transorbital approach sooner than 6 weeks postoperative for a recent eye surgery.

There are significant anatomic variations of the circle of Willis causing challenges for accurate vessel identification especially using nonimaging TCD. Anatomic anomalies include differences in the origin, caliber, and course of arteries. Problem areas include confusing the TICA with the PCA$_1$ differentiating the right from the left VAs and the level of their exact confluence. Accuracy is low in the distal third of the BA because of the great depths required for its insonation and tortuosity.

## Pitfalls

The accuracy of TCD findings is operator dependent. The learning curve is significant, requiring a minimum 6 months' testing experience and at least 100 abnormal studies with correlations for proficiency.

The calculation of velocity from the Doppler shifted frequencies depends on the angle of insonation. Using nonimaging technique, a zero degree angle is assumed by the equipment, but any variation from zero is not measured and is dependent on the operator's skill in obtaining the

signal with the highest audible pitch and therefore the highest velocity.

Patient cooperation is required to obtain an accurate study, and some patients may be agitated and unable to remain still and quiet.

In the setting of severe stenosis, vasospasm, collateral flow, and hyperemia, there can be very high velocities. Aliasing of the pulsed wave Doppler can occur and should be recognized.

## DIAGNOSIS

Both TCD and TCDI rely on the Doppler spectral waveforms for interpretation of normal and abnormal examinations. Normal Doppler spectral values have been established for each arterial segment. TCD interpretation requires a solid understanding of flow dynamics, systemic physiologic variables that impact the cerebral circulation and strong pattern recognition skills (see Table 10-3). The primary diagnostic features of the signals include (1) alteration in velocity; (2) deviations from laminar flow; (3) changes in pulsatility; and (4) changes in the direction of flow. Adjacent artery ratios, side to side and extracranial to intracranial indices, have been developed to help differentiate various findings.

The spectral waveform parameters include:

- Velocity: This is usually expressed in cm/s. Spectral analysis allows the quantification of the PSV, EDV, and TAP-V (commonly referred to as simply "mean velocity"). The mean velocity is the primary diagnostic feature used in TCD and TCDI.

- Pulsatility: In adults, this is expressed as Gosling's PI which is calculated as:

$$PI = \frac{(PSV - EDV)}{TAP\text{-}V}$$

- Disturbed or turbulent flow: This is represented in the spectral waveform as high-amplitude, low-velocity signals and flow velocities near and below the zero baseline. It is also apparent as a disruption of the smooth contour of the waveform outer envelope.
- Systolic upstroke: This is the initial slope of the peak velocity envelope during the acceleration phase of systole.
- Lindegaard ratio: This is calculated as the MCA mean velocity divided by the submandibular ICA mean velocity. This ratio is useful in differentiating increased volume flow from decreased diameter when high velocities are encountered in the MCA or intracranial ICA.
- Sviri ratio: This ratio is similar to the Lindegaard ratio for determining vasospasm from hyperdynamic flow in the posterior circulation. The bilateral VA mean velocities taken at the atlas loop are added together and averaged. This averaged velocity is then divided into the highest BA mean velocity (Fig. 10-24).

## APPLICATIONS FOR INTRACRANIAL CEREBROVASCULAR EXAMINATIONS

There are multiple applications for intracranial cerebrovascular examinations which, as technology has advanced, have expanded over the years.

Pathology Box 10-1 lists some of the common abnormalities observed during TCD or TCDI examinations.

## TCD Findings in Extracranial Carotid Artery Disease—Collateral Flow

When an extracranial carotid artery stenosis reaches hemodynamic significance, the brain will compensate through the mechanisms of collateral flow and autoregulation. TCD is useful in identifying and assessing the presence and adequacy of collateral circulation and improves understanding of the individual cerebral circulatory function and status. TCD assessment of cerebral collateralization also helps predict hemodynamic consequences of cross clamping during carotid endarterectomy. There are three primary collateral patterns that can be accurately determined using TCD, and the diagnostic criteria for each collateral type are listed below (Fig. 10-25).

### External Carotid to Internal Carotid Through a Reversed OA[23,24]

- Direct evidence of carotid artery disease
- Retrograde flow in the OA
- Decreased pulsatility and increased velocity in the OA
- Obliteration, diminishment, or reversal of flow in the OA with compression of the branches of the ECA (superficial temporal, facial, or angular arteries)

### Crossover Collateral Through the ACOA

- Direct evidence of carotid artery disease
- Retrograde flow in the ACA, $A_1$ segment ipsilateral to the carotid disease
- Increased flow velocities in the contralateral ACA (ACA mean velocity/Ipsilateral MCA mean velocity >150%).

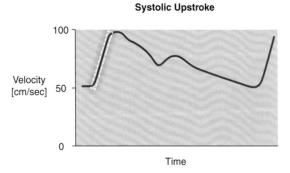

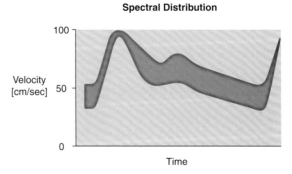

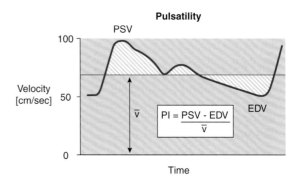

**FIGURE 10-24** Diagnostic features of spectral waveforms for interpretation of TCD studies: mean velocity, pulsatility index, systolic upstroke, and distribution of the amplitude within the waveform.

**PATHOLOGY BOX 10-1**
*Common Pathology Observed on TCD or TCDI Examinations*

| Pathology | Examination Findings |
|---|---|
| Stenosis | • Focal increase in velocity<br>• Poststenotic turbulence<br>• Use prestenotic/stenotic ratio<br>• Refer to Table 10-3 for complete criteria |
| Occlusion (acute, total) | • Absent flow on color imaging and Doppler<br>• High-resistance signal proximal to occlusion |
| Vasospasm (severe) | • MCA velocity ≥200 cm/s<br>• Lindegaard ratio ≥6.0<br>• Can be present in more than one artery<br>• Temporal changes |
| Emboli | • Brief signal lasting <300 ms<br>• M-Mode high-power tracks sloping in flow direction<br>• Amplitude at least 3 dB above background<br>• Unidirectional signal<br>• Signal has snap, chirp, or moan sound |

The increase in velocity is related to the increase in volume flow as well as the diameter of the vessel carrying that increased volume. In individual cases, there can be crossover collateral with normal ACA velocities because of the large diameter of the ACA.

• There are usually very high velocities detected at midline in the small ACOA

The accuracy of TCD in the identification of intracranial crossover collateralization through the ACOA in experienced laboratories has a sensitivity of 93%, specificity of 100%, and accuracy of 98%.[23,24]

**Posterior to Anterior Collateral Through the Posterior Communicating Artery**

• Direct evidence of carotid artery disease
• Increased flow velocities in the ipsilateral PCA, $P_1$ segment (PCA mean velocity/Ipsilateral MCA mean velocity >125%)
• In individual cases, there can be PCOA collateral with lower velocities because of the large diameter and capacity of the collateral vessel.
• Velocities in the PCOA, when detected, are usually quite high

The accuracy of TCD in the identification of posterior to anterior collateralization through the PCOA has been shown to have a sensitivity of 87%, specificity of 96%, and accuracy of 92%.[23,24]

**Leptomeningeal Collateralization**

Ipsilateral to a hemodynamically significant stenosis or occlusion of the main trunk of the MCA high velocities may be observed in the ACA and PCA because of leptomeningeal collateralization.

## Intracranial Stenosis and Occlusion

Intracranial arterial narrowing is a complicated subject with multiple causative factors and resultant complex pathophysiology. In general, stenoses and occlusions can be caused by

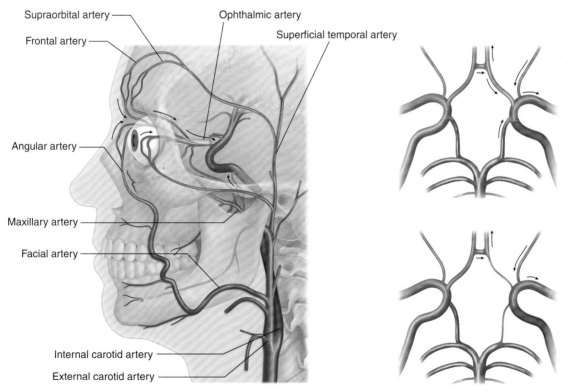

**FIGURE 10-25** Changes in flow direction seen with collateralization through the circle of Willis include reversal of the ophthalmic artery and reversal of the ACA ipsilateral to the stenosis/occlusion in the ICA.

intrinsic conditions and thromboembolic phenomena. TCD is useful for detection of >50% intracranial stenoses and occlusions.[25] It is a reliable diagnostic tool for finding disease, if limitations and sources of error are carefully considered.

There are multiple conditions that produce intrinsic narrowing of the cerebral arteries, the most common being thromboembolic and atherosclerotic disease. Additional uncommon noninflammatory conditions include dissection, fibromuscular dysplasia, radiation-induced vasculopathy, and Moyamoya disease. There are also a host of inflammatory vasculopathies and hematologic causes of stroke that may affect the basal cerebral vessels, including temporal arteritis, meningitis, toxin-related vasculitis, and SCD.

## Atherosclerosis

Approximately 9% or between 70,000 and 90,000 strokes in the United States every year result from intracranial atherosclerosis (ASO).[26] The effect of this disease is more significant for African Americans, Asians, and Hispanics,[25,27,28] and the incidence of recurrent stroke in this population is high, reported to be up to 15% per year.[29-31]

ASO of the intracranial arteries involves the cavernous ICA, MCA, ACA, VA, BA, and PCAs. The four known factors that increase the risk of large artery atherosclerotic stenosis are hyperlipidemia, arterial hypertension, cigarette smoking, and diabetes mellitus.[32] Intracranial lesions may cause microemboli, which migrate into distal vascular territories causing ischemia, and/or progress to significant severity or occlusion, which may result in perfusion failure, most notably in the absence of adequate collateral capacity. The latter may be a function of the site of the lesion, especially if it is located distal to the circle of Willis, or because of anatomic anomalies.

## Posterior Circulation

In the past, anterior circulation disease was better understood than posterior circulation. Caplan et al. developed a Posterior Circulation Registry (PCR) for patients with posterior circulation TIA's or stroke. In their analysis, the incidence of intracranial VA stenosis was equal to that of the extracranial segments.

In the PCR, intracranial VA stenosis was present in 32% of patients, some bilaterally, and 2% had BA disease. Embolism was the most common mechanism of posterior circulation stroke with a preponderance of cardiac-origin embolism versus artery-to-artery. Additionally, poor outcomes were associated with cardiogenic embolism.[33]

## Criteria for Intracranial Stenosis

As early as 1990, TCD criteria for stenosis and occlusion of the CS and MCA were reported in a large group of patients with TIA and stroke. In this seminal report by Ley-Poso and Ringelstein, 133 patients had TCD studies and conventional angiograms. Using multiple criteria, including focal velocity increases at the site of stenosis, side to side velocity differences in analogous arteries, and the downstream hemodynamic effects shown in the spectral waveforms, good results were achieved. The overall diagnostic accuracy for any lesion was 95.7% with a sensitivity of 91.7% and a specificity of 96.5%.[34] Subsequent studies have defined higher threshold criteria of 100 to 120 cm/s for the MCA and 110 cm/s for the vertebral and basilar vessels. Similar to the common carotid to internal carotid ratio used to classify extracranial disease, a stenotic velocity to prestenotic velocity ratio is used for the intracranial MCA, VA, and BA.[26,35]

Interpreting spectral waveforms requires knowledge of normal and abnormal values, appreciation of the changes in waveform morphology proximal to, at the site of and distal to a stenosis, and a good understanding of the complex and sometimes confounding physiologic variables that coexist in any individual patient at any point in time. The criteria put forth in Table 10-4 are useful as preliminary measurements.[26,35,36] It is important to understand the diagnostic criteria to differentiate high-velocities resultant from collateral flow prior to making the interpretation of intracranial stenosis. There are multiple systemic factors that significantly influence velocities and need to be factored, including age, heart rate, blood pressure, hematocrit, fever, and $CO_2$ levels (Table 10-4).

## Embolic Stenosis and Occlusion

The most common cause of occlusion beyond the circle of Willis is embolism, accounting for 15% to 30% of strokes, most of which occur in the territory of the MCA.[37] Several types of cardiac disease lead to cerebral embolism causing

| Segment | Depth (MM) | Mean Velocity cm/s | Stenotic/Prestenotic Ratio | Waveform Characteristics (Poststenotic) |
|---|---|---|---|---|
| TABLE 10-4   **Stenosis Criteria for the MCA (Middle Cerebral),[26,35] ICA (Terminal), ACA/A₁ (Anterior Cerebral), PCA/P₁ (Posterior Cerebral),[36] Vertebral and Basilar Arteries[35]** | | | | |
| MCA proximal | 50–65 | 100<br>120 | >2 = >50%<br>>3 = >70% | Turbulence, slow systolic upstroke, co-vibrations |
| ICA (siphon) | 55–65 | 90 | N/A | Turbulence, slow systolic upstroke, co-vibrations |
| ACA (A₁) | 65–75 | >90 | ACA > MCA | Turbulence, slow systolic upstroke, co-vibrations |
| PCA | 56–65 | >80 | PCA > ACA/ICA | Turbulence, slow systolic upstroke, co-vibrations |
| Basilar | 75–110 | 110 | | Turbulence, slow systolic upstroke, co-vibrations |
| Vertebral | 40–75 | 110 | | Turbulence, slow systolic upstroke, co-vibrations |

Velocities represent mean values.

stenosis and occlusion, including cardiac arrhythmias, ischemic heart disease, valvular disease, dilated cardiomyopathies, atrial septal abnormalities, and intracardiac tumors. Other sources of emboli include aortic arch atheroma, extracranial carotid and VA plaque, and crossing of a venous thrombus into the arterial tree in patients with patent foramen ovale.[31]

The use of cerebrovascular ultrasound in acute stroke requires a modified protocol that allows rapid insonation of the affected territory, supply arteries, and quick interpretation of the data. TCD can provide significant information regarding thrombus in acute intracranial arterial occlusion, often a dynamic process which can involve recanalization. A TCD flow grading system was developed by Demchuk to predict the success of intracranial clot lysis and short-term improvement after ischemic stroke. Thrombolysis in brain ischemia (TIBI) measures residual flow around the clot and, in general, a larger amount of residual flow predicts the success of the thrombolysis.[38] For acute thrombosis, the TIBI scale is used to classify changes that can occur rapidly with recanalization and re-occlusion in acute stroke (Table 10-5).

## Vasospasm

SAH, one of the most devastating types of stroke, accounts for 5% to 15% of all strokes and is fatal or disabling in about 60% of patients.[26,35,36] These patients suffer the initial effect of an intracranial bleed, the risks and complications associated with surgical or interventional treatments, and the sequelae of a host of medical complications. One of the most significant causes of delayed ischemic neurologic deficits (DINDS) is the development of cerebral vasospasm during the first 2-week period following the initial bleed. The pathophysiology, diagnosis, prevention, and treatment of vasospasm continue to be topics of intense investigation aimed at improving clinical outcomes for these patients.

Cerebral vasospasm is the transient, delayed narrowing of the basal cerebral arteries following SAH, and the exact cause remains the subject of intense study. It is mainly seen in the large skull base arteries and less frequently in the distal branches of these vessels, and it is responsible for the significant morbidity and mortality seen in this population. The onset of arterial contraction, as demonstrated by angiography, begins 3 to 4 days following the initial bleed; peak narrowing develops at 6 to 8 days; and resolution

occurs at 2 to 7 weeks following SAH.[36] The incidence of angiographic vasospasm after SAH is greater than 50% with symptomatic vasospasm affecting one-third of all aneurismal SAH patients.[37] Neurologic deficits caused by cerebral vasospasm may resolve or progress to infarction or death in spite of maximal therapy.

The medical management of cerebral vasospasm relies on hemodynamic therapy to improve CBF; calcium channel antagonists are widely used and have been shown to reduce poor outcomes. In patients with clinically significant vasospasm that does not respond to maximal medical therapy, balloon angioplasty has been shown to be effective, improving neurologic deficits. The timing of angioplasty is significant, and patients need to be treated before cerebral infarction occurs.

In 2004, the American Academy of Neurology published a special article addressing the use of TCD and TCDI for diagnosis of multiple intracranial vascular abnormalities according to a rating system. They gave TCD the highest rating (Type A, Classes I to II evidence) when used for the detection and monitoring of angiographic vasospasm in the basal segments of the intracranial arteries, especially the MCA and BA.[38]

The goals of TCD in the setting of SAH are to detect elevated blood velocities that indicate cerebral vasospasm and identify patients as risk for DINDS. These patients are studied daily, for detection of the onset, location, degree, and resolution of vasospasm for approximately 2 weeks following their initial bleed.

When using TCD or TCDI to detect vasospasm after SAH, patients will be in the hospital receiving care in the ICU or on neurologic care floors. Studies are usually done serially, as often as every 24 hours for 2 or more weeks. Depending on treatment, open surgery and clipping, or coil embolization and/or stent placement, emboli monitoring may also be ordered.

The medical history will be obtained from the medical record; however, changes in the patient's clinical status between examinations should be noted and may correlate with vasospasm. Complications and physiologic changes, which influence blood flow velocity, may occur, including increased intracranial pressure, fever, decreasing hematocrit, changing blood pressure, and variations in arterial carbon dioxide. These variables should be recorded daily and will facilitate interpretation of the waveforms (Table 10-6).

| TABLE 10-5 | TIBI Scale for TCD Detection of MCA Recanalization during and Following Thrombolytic Therapy | |
|---|---|---|
| TIBI Score | MCA Flow (DSA) | TCD Signal Description |
| 0 | Occluded with no residual flow | Absent, no flow signal |
| 1 | No antegrade residual flow | Low systolic only velocity signal |
| 2 | Subtotal occlusion with sluggish antegrade flow | Low velocity, damped systolic, and diastolic signal, with slow systolic acceleration, with a PI <1.2 |
| 3 | Subtotal occlusion with sluggish antegrade flow | High PI >1.2, systolic dominant signal with >30% decrease in velocity compared with contralateral MCA |
| 4 | Stenotic with recanalization | Increased velocity of >80 cm/s or >30% higher than contralateral MCA |
| 5 | Normal flow with total recanalization | Velocity comparable to contralateral MCA with <30% difference and similar PI |

| TABLE 10-6 **Additional Documentation for Patients with SAH** | |
|---|---|
| **SAH Patient** | **Record Physiologic Data Daily** |
| • Date of SAH | • Heart rate (HR) |
| • Location of aneurysm(s) | • Blood pressure (MAP) |
| • Treatment type and date (clip/coil/stent) | • Fever |
| • Number of days postbleed (PBD) | • Intracranial pressure when monitored (ICP) |
| • Glasgow Coma Scale (GCS) | |
| If emboli monitoring is performed: | • Cerebral perfusion pressure especially in trauma patients, calculated as MAP minus ICP |
| • Number of emboli | |
| • Location of emboli | |
| • Rate per hour | |
| • Treatment | |
| | • Hematocrit (HCT) |
| | • Carbon dioxide ($CO_2$) |

The physiologic parameters are recorded on worksheet and final report. These variables can influence velocity and are taken into consideration when making a final interpretation.

| TABLE 10-7 **Vasospasm Criteria for Each Arterial Segment** | | |
|---|---|---|
| **Vasospasm Criteria** | **Velocity (cm/s)** | **Lindegaard or Sviri Ratio** |
| **MCA AND ICA** | | |
| Mild | 120–149 | >3.0 |
| Moderate | 150–199 | >3.0 |
| Severe | >200 | >6.0 |
| Hyperdynamic flow | >80 | <3.0 |
| **ACA** | | |
| Vasospasm (not graded) | >130 | |
| Vasospasm vs. collateral flow | >130 | With the presence of MCA and/or ICA vasospasm |
| **PCA** | | |
| Vasospasm (not graded) | >110 | |
| Vasospasm vs. collateral flow | >110 | With the presence of MCA and/or ICA vasospasm |
| **VA** | | |
| Vasospasm | >80 | |
| **BA** | | |
| Possible vasospasm | 70–84 | >2.0 |
| Moderate/severe vasospasm | >85 | >2.5 |
| Severe vasospasm | >85 | >3.0 |

Accuracy of TCD is dependent on the expertise of the sonographer doing the studies. Interpretation is complicated by a set of potentially changing factors such as intracranial pressure, blood pressure, hematocrit, arterial $CO_2$, collateral flow, autoregulation, and responses to therapeutic interventions. TCD results in the anterior circulation are most reliable in the MCA. Mean flow velocities in the MCA of ≥200 cm/s, a rapid daily rise in flow velocities, and a hemispheric ratio ≥6.0 predict the presence of significant (>50% diameter reduction) angiographic MCA vasospasm.[39–42]

TCD may be used in combination with CBF to facilitate treatment decisions. CBF studies measure perfusion to the brain territory affected by vasospasm. Often, the clinical examination on SAH patients is imprecise because of the severity of their condition. Complimentary TCD and CBF data inform the clinician in determining the appropriate treatments and their timing during the 2-week period when patients are at risk for a secondary ischemic insult from vasospasm.

More research is needed to better define exact velocity criteria for each arterial segment, and by far, the MCA has the highest correlative accuracy against cerebral angiography, and more prospective studies are warranted to determine the predictive value for the posterior circulation (Table 10-7).[14]

## Emboli Monitoring

TCD is used to monitor for emboli in patients suffering or at risk for TIA and stroke. It is also used for neurovascular monitoring during invasive procedures, including carotid endarterectomy, carotid stenting, cardiac procedures and

following coil and stent treatment of intracranial aneurysms. A headband is used to secure the TCD transducer in place for continuous monitoring. Typically, the MCA is the vessel monitored for emboli. Most manufacturers have software within the TCD systems that will automatically count the number of microemboli. Microembolic signals have also been referred to as HITS (Fig. 10-26). They have four characteristic components: (1) the signal is very short or brief, usually lasting for less than 300 ms; (2) the amplitude of the TCD signal must be at least 3 dB above the background signals; (3) the signal is mainly unidirectional within the spectral waveform; and (4) the signal will produce a characteristic audible sound which has been described as a "snap," "chirp," or "moan."[43]

Embolic signals have been shown to predict stroke risk in acute stroke, symptomatic carotid disease and post operatively after carotid endarterectomy. The presence and rate of emboli in patients at risk for stroke is useful in guiding and assessing therapies.[44]

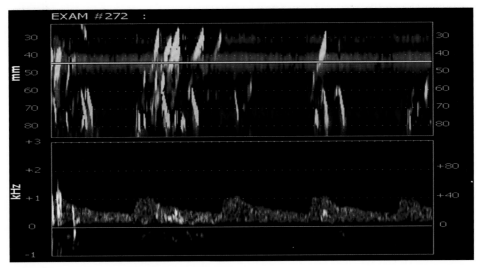

**FIGURE 10-26** Example of a TCD signal illustrating the presence of microemboli.

## Detection of Cardiac Shunts

TCD can be used to detect the presence of a patent foramen ovale or other right to left cardiac shunts.[45] The technique, often referred to as a bubble study, involves the intravenous injection of agitated saline mixed with air. A cardiac shunt is confirmed when there are HITS detected while monitoring the MCA using TCD. The more HITS detected, the more severe the cardiac shunt.

## Cerebral Circulatory Arrest

Brain death is a clinical diagnosis made using established clinical criteria. In 2010, the American Academy of Neurology published an evidence-based guideline confirming the use of TCD as an ancillary test to support the diagnosis of cerebral circulatory arrest (CCA). Other such tests used include an electroencephalogram, single-photon emission computed tomography with the tracer $^{99m}$Tc-HMPAO (hexamethylpropylene amine oxime) and cerebral angiography. In a meta-analysis, TCD was found to have a sensitivity of 89% and a specificity of 98% for the confirmation of CCA.[46]

The development of CCA begins distally in the arterial circulation and progresses proximally. Therefore, distal resistance increases as cerebral edema develops. When the intracranial pressure is equal to the diastolic pressure, the TCD waveforms have no diastolic flow, but forward flow remains in systole; this pattern does not correlate with CCA. When there is no longer perfusion, TCD shows an oscillating pattern with equal antegrade systolic and retrograde diastolic velocities consistent with a net flow of zero. This finding correlates with CCA as demonstrated on angiography. As CCA progresses, short-duration and low-velocity systolic spikes are seen, and finally no flow signal can be detected.[47]

Once the clinical prerequisites for CCA have been established, TCD can be used as a confirmatory test as long as ventricular drains and/or decompressive craniectomies are not present. Technical guidelines require obtaining and documenting spectral waveforms from bilateral intracranial (ICA and MCA) and extracranial (CCA, ICA, and VA) arteries

on two examinations that are a minimum of 30 minutes apart (Fig. 10-27). In a meta-analysis, TCD was found to have a sensitivity of 89% and a specificity of 98% for the confirmation of CCA.[48,49]

## Sickle Cell Disease

SCD is a genetic disorder that mostly occurs in people of African, Hispanic, Middle Eastern, and Asian Indian lineage. It impacts red blood cells by causing them to develop a sickle shape and become rigid, the viscosity of the blood lowers, and flow to limbs and organs decreases. It has been reported that 11% of patients with homozygous SCD have a stroke by 20 years of age.[50]

TCD and TCDI play a vital role in evaluating children with SCD. The Stroke Prevention Trial in Sickle Cell Anemia (STOP) study demonstrated that early detection of abnormal MCA and ICA velocities by TCD and subsequent initiation of a blood transfusion program was successful in reducing

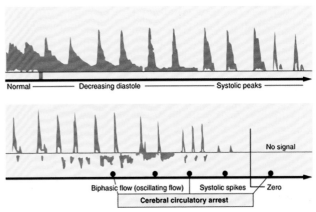

**FIGURE 10-27** Progression of MCA temporal waveform changes from normal to CCA. Increasing pulsatility and decreasing diastole reflect increased ICP and decreased CCP (upper picture). CCA corresponds only when the forward and reversed spectral waveforms are equal. The blood pumped out by the heart meets very high resistance in the brain and shunts the blood back toward the heart in diastole.

**TABLE 10-8  Head Diameter and Vessel Depth[52]**

| Head Diameter (cm) | MCA Distal | MCA Proximal | ICA Bifurcation | ACA | PCA | Top of Basilar |
|---|---|---|---|---|---|---|
| 12 | 30–36 | 30–54 | 50–54 | 50–58 | 40–60 | 60 |
| 13 | 30–36 | 30–58 | 52–58 | 52–62 | 42–66 | 65 |
| 14 | 34–40 | 34–63 | 56–64 | 56–68 | 46–70 | 70 |
| 15 | 40–46 | 40–66 | 56–66 | 56–72 | 50–70 | 75 |

**TABLE 10-9  Velocity Criteria for Sickle Cell[53]**

| Artery | Normal | Conditional | Abnormal | Inadequate |
|---|---|---|---|---|
| MCA, T-ICA, intracranial bifurcation | <170 cm/s | ≥170–199 cm/s | ≥200 cm/s | Inability to obtain information bilaterally |

STOP criteria using the time-averaged mean of the maximum (TAMM) velocity.

the rate of first time stroke by 90%.[51] Based on this trial and because the highest risk of stroke is in childhood, it is recommended that patients between the ages of 2 and 16 years should have annual TCD screening.

Sonographers doing these studies should be certified in the STOP technique prior to initiating a service in order to assure competency. Strict adherence to examination protocols must be followed, and careful attention is necessary to obtain the highest velocities; inaccurate measurements can cause incorrect stroke risk prediction. Examinations need to be done when the patients are clinically stable and to confirm abnormal findings two studies, 2 weeks apart are performed.

A child's head circumference changes as they grow so calipers are used to measure the distance between temporal windows. Caliper tips are put in front and above the zygomatic arch, and the diameter is measured and documented. Based on this, the expected depth of the intracranial arteries is established (Table 10-8).[52]

### Diagnostic Criteria

Annual TCD studies are indicated for pediatrics with normal TCD findings and repeat scans every 3 to 6 months if initial results are conditional. If abnormal, the examination is repeated in 2 to 4 weeks, and transfusion therapy may be recommended if the second study is also abnormal or if a single study is 220 cm/s or greater (Table 10-9).[53]

Clinical guidelines for treating SCD with transfusion therapy to decrease stroke are based on velocity criteria validated using nonimaging TCD. Comparisons of duplex imaging (TCDI) with nonimaging TCD have been made, and most studies showed slightly lower velocities when using TCDI. The difference is most likely because of the technique of using the color Doppler image to obtain the highest velocity. This may be improved by using the technique of finding the highest audible Doppler frequency as done when performing nonimaging TCD.[54] Angle correction is generally not recommended for this type of examination.

### The Use of TCD within Acute Stroke

There has been increasing use of thrombolytic agents in patients with acute stroke. TCD plays an important role in patient selection as well as monitoring of these patients during and following these procedures. With constant TCD monitoring during the infusion of a thrombolytic agent, changes in MCA velocities can be immediately observed and provides an accurate and noninvasive tool to assess the recanalization procedure.[55]

A more recent expansion for the role of TCD includes its utilization to enhance the effect of thrombolytic agents. The success of a thrombolytic agent relies on the ability of the agent to come in contact with the thrombus. The more the agent can permeate a thrombus, the faster the lysis will occur. Ultrasound can provide mechanical energy to the thrombus interfaces and stagnant flow areas. Ultrasound can disaggregate portions of the fibrin stands, moving them slightly which will promote flow through the area and aid in the delivery of the lytic agent.[56] Extensive research continues in this application for TCD.

## SUMMARY

- Intracranial cerebrovascular examinations with TCD techniques can provide a vast amount of anatomic and physiologic data.
- The examination of the intracranial vessels requires extensive knowledge of anatomy and meticulous attention to technique.
- Various disease states can be evaluated with TCD or transcranial imaging.
- A thorough understanding of the intracranial vessels will aid in the successful evaluation of patients presenting with suspected intracranial vascular disease.

## CRITICAL THINKING QUESTIONS

1. A TCD needs to be performed on a hospital inpatient who cannot be placed in a lateral decubitus position. Can the VAs and BA still be insonated and if so how?

2. While reviewing images from a TCD exam, should one expect to observe low-resistance or high-resistance signals?

3. When scanning via the transtemporal approach, two vessels are observed which appear to have branches. In order to determine which vessels are in view, what additional information needs to be taken into consideration.

4. A patient will require continuous monitoring of MCA velocities. Which type of ultrasound probe would be best for this application and why?

## MEDIA MENU

Student Resources available on **thePoint** include:

- Audio glossary
- Interactive question bank
- Videos
- Internet resources

## REFERENCES

1. Aaslid R, Markwalder T-M, Nornes H. Noninvasive transcranial Doppler ultrasound recording of flow velocity in cerebral arteries. *J Neurosurg.* 1982;57:769–774.
2. von Reutern G-M, von Budingen HJ. *Ultrasound Diagnosis of Cerebrovascular Disease.* New York, NY: Thieme Medical Publishers; 1993.
3. Gabrielsen TO, Greitz T. Normal size of the internal carotid, middle cerebral and anterior cerebral arteries. *Acta Radiol Diagnosis.* 1970;101:68–87.
4. Lang J. *Neurokranium, orbita, kraniozervikaler ubergang. Klinische anatomie des kopfes.* Berlin/Heidelberg/New York: Springer; 1981.
5. Riggs HE, Rupp C. Variation in form of circle of Willis: the relation of the variations to collateral circulation: anatomic analysis. *Arch Neurol.* 1963;8:24–30.
6. Hodes PJ, Campy F, Riggs HE, et al. Cerebral angiography: fundamentals in anatomy and physiology. *Am J Roentgenol.* 1953;70:61–82.
7. Taveras JM, Wood EH. *Diagnostic Neuroradiology.* Baltimore, MD: Williams and Wilkins; 1976.
8. Alexandrov AV, Sloan MA, Tegeler CH, et al. Practice standards for transcranial Doppler Ultrasound Part II—clinical indications and expected outcomes. *J Neuroimaging.* 2012;22:215–224.
9. Alexandrov AV, Sloan MA, Wong LKS. Practice standards for transcranial Doppler ultrasound: Part I—test performance. *J Neuroimaging.* 2006;17:11–18.
10. Alexandrov AV, Demchuk AM, Wein TH, et al. The yield of transcranial Doppler in acute cerebral ischemia. *Stroke.* 1999;30:1605–1609.
11. Spencer MP, Whisler D. Transorbital Doppler diagnosis of intracranial arterial stenosis. *Stroke.* 1986;17:916–921.
12. Aaslid R, ed. *Transcranial Doppler Sonography.* Wien, New York: Springer-Verlag; 1986.
13. Arnolds BJ, von Reutern MG. Transcranial Doppler sonography. Examination techniques and normal reference values. *Ultrasound Med Biol.* 1986;12:115–123.
14. Lindegaard KF, Nornes H, Bakke SJ, et al. Cerebral vasospasm diagnosis by means of angiography and blood velocity measurements. *Acta Neurochir.* 1989;100:12–24.
15. Lindegaard KF. The role of transcranial Doppler in the management of patients with subarachnoid haemorrhage: a review. *Acta Neurochir.* 1999;72:59–71.
16. Soustiel JF, Shik V, Shreiber R, et al. Basilar vasospasm diagnosis: investigation of a modified "Lindegaard Index" based on imaging studies and blood velocity measurements of the basilar artery. *Stroke.* 2002;33:72–77.
17. Sviri GE, Ghodke B, Britz GW. Transcranial Doppler grading criteria for basilar artery vasospasm. *Neurosurgery.* 2006;59:360–366.
18. Grolimund P. Transmission of ultrasound through the temporal bone. In: Aaslid A, ed. *Transcranial Doppler Sonography.* Wien, New York: Springer-Verlag; 1986:10–21.
19. Ringelstein EB. A practical guide to transcranial Doppler sonography. In: Weinberger J, ed. *Noninvasive Imaging of Cerebrovascular Disease.* New York, NY: Alan R. Liss; 1989:75–121.
20. Martin PJ, Evans DH, Naylor AR. Transcranial color-coded sonography of the basal cerebral circulation reference data from 115 volunteers. *Stroke.* 1994;25:390–396.
21. Alexandrov Av, Demchuk AM, Burgin WS. Insonation method and diagnostic flow signatures for transcranial power motion (M-mode) Doppler. *J Neuroimaging.* 2002;12:236–244.
22. Kellermann M, Babava DG, Csiba L, et al. Visualization of the basilar artery by transcranial color-coded duplex sonography: comparison with postmortem results. *Stroke.* 2000;31:1123–1127.
23. Newell DW, Winn HR. Transcranial Doppler in cerebral vasospasm. *Neurosurg Clin N Am.* 1990;1:1–28.
24. Lindegaard K, Bakke S, Grolimund P. Assessment of intracranial hemodynamics in carotid artery disease by transcranial Doppler ultrasound. *J Neurosurg.* 1985;63:890–898.
25. Fujioka KA, Nonoshita-Karr L. The effects of extracranial arterial occlusive disease. *J Vasc Tech.* 2000;24(1):27–32.
26. Felberg RA, Christou I, Demchuk AM, et al. Screening for intracranial stenosis with transcranial Doppler: the accuracy of mean flow velocity thresholds. *J Neuroimaging.* 2002;12:9.
27. Sacco RL, Kargman DE, Gu Q, et al. Race—ethnicity and determinants of intracranial atherosclerotic cerebral infarction; the Northern Manhattan Stroke Study. *Stroke.* 1995;26:14–20.
28. Wityk RJ, Lehman D, Klag M, et al. Race and sex differences in the distribution of cerebral atherosclerosis. *Stroke.* 1996;27:1974–1980.
29. Feldmann E, Daneault N, Kwan E, et al. Chinese-white differences in the distribution of occlusive cerebrovascular disease. *Neurology.* 1990;40:1541–1545.
30. Jiang WJ, Wang YJ, Du B, et al. Stenting of symptomatic M1 stenosis of middle cerebral artery, an initial experience of 40 patients. *Stroke.* 2004;35:1375–1380.
31. Chimowitz MI, Kokkinos J, Strong J, et al. The Warfarin-aspirin symptomatic intracranial disease study. *Neurology.* 1995;45:1488–1493.
32. The Warfarin-Aspirin Symptomatic Intracranial Disease (WASID) Study Group. Prognosis of patients with symptomatic vertebral or basilar artery stenosis. *Stroke.* 1998;29:1389–1392.
33. Chaves CJ, Jones HR. Ischemic Stroke. In: Jones HR, ed. *Netter's Neurology.* Teterboro, NJ: Icon Learning Systems; 2005:195–199.
34. Caplan LR, Wityk RJ, Glass TA, et al. New England medical center posterior circulation registry. *Ann Neurol.* 2004;56:389–398.

35. Zhao L, Barlinn K, Alexandrov AV, et al. Velocity criteria for intracranial stenosis revisited, an international multicenter study of transcranial Doppler and digital subtraction angiography. *Stroke.* 2011;42(12):3429–3434.

36. Zhao L, Sharma VK, Tsivgoulis G, et al. Velocity criteria for intracranial stenosis revisited: a multicenter study of transcranial Doppler (TCD) and digital subtraction angiography (DSA). *Stroke.* 2010;41:e233–e234.

37. Ley-Pozo J, Ringelstein EB. Noninvasive detection of occlusive disease of the carotid siphon and middle cerebral artery. *Ann Neurol.* 1990;28:640–647.

38. Bederson J, Awad IA, Wiebers DO, et al. Recommendations for the management of patients with unruptured intracranial aneurysms. *Circulation.* 2000;102:2300–2308.

39. Bederson JB, Awad IA, Wiebers DO. Recommendations for the management of patients with unruptured intracranial aneurysms: a statement for healthcare professionals from the Stroke Council of the American Heart Association. *Stroke.* 2000;31:2742–2750.

40. Weir B, Grace M, Hansen J, et al. Time course of vasospasm in Man. *J Neurosurg.* 1978;48:173.

41. Dorsch NWC, King MT. A review of cerebral vasospasm in aneurismal subarachnoid haemorrhage: I. Incidence and effects. *J Clin Neurosci.* 1994;1:19.

42. Sloan MA, Alexandrov AV, Tegeler CH, et al. Assessment: transcranial Doppler ultrasonography: report of the therapeutics and technology assessment subcommittee of the American Academy of Neurology. *Neurology.* 2004;62:1468–1481.

43. Consensus Committee of the Ninth International Cerebral Hemodynamic Symposium. Basic identification criteria of Doppler microembolic signals. *Stroke.* 1995;26:1123.

44. King A, Markus HS. Doppler embolic signals in cerebrovascular disease and prediction of stroke risk, a systmeatic review and meta-analysis. *Stroke.* 2009;40:3711–3717.

45. Blersch WK, Draganski BM, Holmer SR, et al. Transcranial duplex sonography in the detection of patent foramen ovale. *Radiology.* 2002;225:693–699.

46. Chang JJ, Tsivgoulis G, Katsanos S, et al. Diagnostic accuracy of transcranial Doppler for brain death confirmation: systematic review and meta-analysis. *Am J Neuroradiol.* 2016;37:408–414.

47. Hassler W, Steinmeerz H, Pirschel J. Transcranial Doppler study of intracranial circulatory arrest. *J Neurosurg.* 1989;71:195–201.

48. Ducrocq X, Hassler W, Moritake K, et al. Consensus opinion on diagnosis of cerebral circulatory arrest using Doppler-sonography. Task Force Group on cerebral death of the Neurosonology Research Group of the World Federation of Neurology. *J Neurol Sci.* 1998;159:145–150.

49. Monteiro LM, Bollen CS, Van Huffelen AC, et al. Transcranial Doppler ultrasonography to confirm brain death: a meta-analysis. *Intensive Care Med.* 2006;32(12):1937–1944.

50. Yawn BP, John-Sowah J. Management of sickle cell disease: recommendations from the 2014 expert panel report. *Am Fam Physician.* 2015;92(12):1069–1076.

51. Adams R, McKie V, Nichols F, et al. The use of transcranial ultrasonography to predict stroke in sickle cell disease *N Engl J Med.* 1992;(326):605–610.

52. Nichols FT, Jones AM, Adams RJ. Stroke Prevention in Sickle Cell Disease (STOP) study guidelines for transcranial Doppler testing. *J Neuroimaging.* 2001;11:354–362.

53. Enninful-Eghan H, Moore RH, Ichord R, et al. Transcranial Doppler ultrasonography and prophylactic transfusion program is effective in preventing overt stroke in children with sickle cell disease. *J Pediatr.* 2010;157(3):479–484.

54. Padayachee ST, Thomas N, Arnold AJ, et al. Problems with implementing a standardized transcranial Doppler screening program: impact of instrumentation variation on STOP classification. *Pediatr Radiol.* 2012;(42):470–474.

55. Rubiera M, Cava L, Tsivgoulis G, et al. Diagnostic criteria and yield of real-time transcranial Doppler monitoring of intra-arterial reperfusion procedures. *Stroke.* 2010;41:695–699.

56. Alexandrov AV. Ultrasound enhancement of fibrinolysis. *Stroke.* 2009;40:S107–S110.

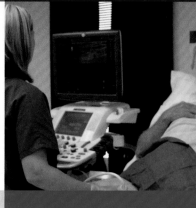

# PART FOUR

# PERIPHERAL ARTERIAL

## Indirect Assessment of Arterial Disease

TERRY NEEDHAM

## CHAPTER 11

## OBJECTIVES

- Describe the types of indirect testing, including systolic pressure measurements, Doppler waveforms, and plethysmography
- Identify normal and abnormal continuous wave and plethysmographic waveforms
- Define the various signs and symptoms associated with peripheral arterial occlusive disease
- List the indirect testing techniques employed in the evaluation of upper extremity

## KEY TERMS

**ankle-brachial index**

**claudication**

**photoplethysmography**

**rest pain**

**volume plethysmography**

## GLOSSARY

**Allen test** A series of maneuvers testing the digital perfusion of the hand while compressing and releasing the radial and ulnar arteries

**ankle-brachial index** The ratio of ankle systolic pressure to brachial systolic pressure

**claudication** Pain in muscle groups brought on by exercise or activity which recedes with cessation of activity; can occur in the calf, thigh, and buttock

**photoplethysmography** An indirect physiologic test that detects changes in backscattered infrared light as an indicator of tissue perfusion

**plethysmography** An indirect physiologic test that measures the change in volume or impedance in a whole body, organ, or limb

**Raynaud's disease** Vasospasm of the digital arteries brought on by exposure to cold; can be caused by numerous etiologies

**rest pain** Pain in the extremity without exercise or activity, thus "at rest," can occur in the toes, foot, or ankle area

**thoracic outlet syndrome** Compression of the brachial nerve plexus, subclavian artery, or subclavian vein at the region where these structures enter or exit the thoracic cavity

Indirect (nonimaging) testing modalities can be reliable for detecting the presence of peripheral arterial occlusive disease (PAOD) affecting the extremities and for categorizing its overall severity. The most common symptom of PAOD affecting the lower extremities is leg discomfort caused by activity, but which abates with cessation of the activity. This is termed intermittent claudication. Patients may describe the sensation of intermittent claudication as fatigue, or as a cramping, aching, or tiredness sensation, usually starting in the calf, perhaps progressing to the thigh and/or buttocks, according to the site and severity of the disease (Table 11-1). The amount of activity that produces the symptoms can remain fairly reproducible for long periods, unless there is accelerated progression of the PAOD. The site of the symptoms indicate the site(s) of the disease, because they occur distal to the disease process, so claudication limited to the calf is

| TABLE 11-1 | **Variations in Leg Pain** | | |
|---|---|---|---|
| **Condition** | **Location** | **Associated with Exercise?** | **Relieved By?** |
| Intermittent claudication | Buttock, thigh, hip, calf | Always | Stopping |
| Spinal stenosis | Buttock, thigh, hip, calf | Yes, but also with standing | Sitting; flexing, and moving spine |
| Herniated disc | Radiates down leg | Variable | Varies; aspirin or anti-inflammatories |
| Osteoarthritis | Hips, knees, ankles | Variable, not always produced | Varies; aspirin or anti-inflammatories |

associated with superficial femoral/popliteal or tibial artery disease, thigh symptoms with iliofemoral artery disease and buttock claudication with either ipsilateral iliofemoral (if unilateral) or aortoiliac disease when bilateral.

It is important to distinguish between the causes of leg discomfort resulting from activity, especially for the mechanism(s) which results in the loss of symptoms, postactivity.[1] Cessation of symptoms with quiet standing corresponds to true ischemic intermittent claudication, whereas correction requiring sitting and/or spinal flexure is more associated with spinal stenosis (see Table 11-1). Claudication distances will decrease and symptom recovery time will increase as PAOD progresses, sometimes being accompanied by the signs of thickening of toenails and loss of toe hair. At the most severe levels of PAOD, the skin may become discolored and scaly, and forefoot pain may be constant with claudication distance less than 50 feet. At these severe levels, with the patient recumbent, raising the leg a foot or so above heart level will usually cause blanching of the skin on the foot, but which becomes red with dependency—this is called elevation pallor/dependent rubor. Blueness of the toes, perhaps unilateral, can be the first indication of aneurysmal disease. This happens with embolization of aneurysm contents into distal segments of the limb and can progress to gangrene. The most common site for a peripheral aneurysm is at popliteal level, although these are associated more with sudden occlusion rather than with embolization.

PAOD in the upper extremity is encountered in <5% of all cases.[2] Typically, it is restricted to numbness, aching or tiredness associated with positional extrinsic compression in the shoulder girdle, or to cold-related vasospasm. Approximately 95% of all extrinsic compression related symptoms have neurovascular origins, with only 3% to 4% from venous compression and arterial compression in only 1% to 2%.[3] This spectrum of symptoms are grouped as thoracic outlet syndromes (TOS).

Cold sensitivity is intense episodic vasospasm related to cold exposure or to emotional stress.[4] It is generally referred to as Raynaud's phenomenon. It comprises both Raynaud's disease (also known as primary Raynaud's phenomenon) and Raynaud's syndrome (or secondary Raynaud's). The cause of primary Raynaud's is idiopathic. Secondary Raynaud's is associated with an underlying process such as scleroderma or trauma. The primary condition is usually bilateral, involving most of the digits (although the thumbs may be spared), whereas secondary causes may be unilateral, perhaps even affecting a single digit.

The various types of nonimaging tests that are commonly used to detect the presence of PAOD include measurement of systolic pressure, Doppler waveforms, volume

plethysmography, and photoplethysmography. These tests help determine overall limb perfusion and, thus, serve as an indicator of the functional status of a limb. However, they are less specific when PAOD occurs at multiple levels, because moderate to severe disease proximally can reduce flow energy distally, masking the presence of distal PAOD. This chapter will describe these indirect testing modalities, applications for such testing, and their diagnostic criteria.

## EXAMINATION PREPARATION

Although there are various types of indirect vascular tests, all have similar preparations which are needed prior to the start of testing. Proper patient preparation and positioning are required for results adequate for diagnosis.

### Patient Preparation

The study starts with confirming the identity of the patient and verifying that the study ordered is appropriate to the patient's signs and/or symptoms. The nature of the study should be explained to the patient and/or an accompanying adult, and an understanding of the explanation can be documented as part of a departmental quality assurance plan.

A relevant PAOD history for the lower extremities should include:

- the clinical problem, signs/symptoms, onset/duration, and whether they are stable, improving, or deteriorating
- site and extent of intermittent claudication, time for the symptoms to abate following the symptom-producing activity
- coexisting clinical conditions such as stroke/transient ischemic attack, carotid artery disease, heart attack, coronary artery disease, hypertension, diabetes, and lipid disorder(s)
- smoking history
- family's cardiac/peripheral vascular history
- exercise activity

For the upper extremities, a similar history to that for the lower extremity should be obtained excluding intermittent claudication but including:

- symptoms related to positional causes of arm fatigue/numbness/aching
- symptoms related to cold sensitivity

### Patient Positioning

The examination table should be low enough for the patient to access safely, preferably without using a step stool. The ideal height for this is 22 to 24 inches, although this will then be too low for the comfort of the technologist (if standing throughout the test), so the examination table should be able to be elevated. Table width should be sufficient to avoid danger of the patient falling if rolled to a lateral decubitus position (which facilitates access at groin level, according to body habitus). For lower extremity testing, the patient should be supine and the head raised slightly upon a pillow—comfortable, but not so high that the heart level is elevated. The legs should be rotated outward slightly, with the knees flexed, allowing access for the Doppler transducer to the popliteal artery.

When using volume plethysmography, the legs should be supported by placing a pillow under the heel, to prevent the cuffs being compressed by the bed, but being careful not to elevate it above heart level. To avoid artifacts from the effect of hydrostatic pressure, systolic pressures should be measured with the point of measurement at the same (horizontal) level as the heart.

For upper extremity testing, the patient position is similar to that for a lower extremity exam, but a pillow behind the knees will reduce back strain and enhance patient comfort. The arm should be abducted *slightly*, supported upon a pillow to ensure muscle relaxation, but maintained at the heart level—this is particularly important when measuring systolic pressures.

Once the patient has been positioned appropriately, the working height of the examination table should be adjusted (usually, between 28 and 32 inches) in accordance with the height of the technologist. Table height can be lower when the examination is carried out with the technologist or sonographer in a sitting position, and this is an acceptable way of reducing back strain for the technical staff. To avoid positional injury to the staff when sitting throughout the study, the equipment should be able to be used without twisting or straining to reach a control. Using a remote control to adjust equipment settings can enhance good ergonomics and may speed obtaining results—although the technologist or sonographer will benefit from changing positions, during and following the study.

## SYSTOLIC PRESSURES

The measurement of systolic blood pressures in the limbs was one of the earliest noninvasive vascular studies performed.[5] Since these early determinations, it was understood that relationships exist between pressure measurements recorded at various points along the arms and legs. Systolic pressures obtained correspond to the pressure in the vessels at site of the blood pressure cuff and not to the vessels at the level of the transducer recording the pressure signals.

### Examination Technique

The test starts after 10 to 15 minutes of rest, with the patient recumbent. This resting period allows the patient's blood pressure to normalize in cases where the patient is initially anxious upon entering the examination room. The resting period also ensures that peripheral blood flow will be at a resting level and not increased due to any hyperemia that may have resulted from walking into the testing facility. During this period of time, the appropriate documentation is obtained, as mentioned previously.

Blood pressure cuffs are placed around the arms and legs. An appropriate cuff size is important in order to accurately measure blood pressure. The width of the cuff should be at least 20% wider than the diameter of the underlying limb segment.[6] If the cuff is too narrow, a falsely elevated pressure will be measured. Conversely, if the cuff is too wide, a falsely lower pressure can be recorded. Using 12 cm cuffs for the brachial measurements is adequate in most patients, but the cuff may need to be wider according to body habitus. The same applies to the ankle level, where 10 cm cuffs are usually appropriate. For the measurement of an ankle-brachial index, cuffs are placed around the ankle level and around both upper arms. For a multilevel lower extremity examination, cuffs are placed around both upper arms and at the thigh, calf, and ankle levels. For upper extremity evaluations, cuffs are placed around the upper arm, forearm, and wrist levels.

Measurement of a systolic pressure begins with obtaining an arterial Doppler signal distal to the cuff. Figure 11-1 illustrates the correct positioning for insonating pedal Doppler signals. Care must be exercised not to compress the underlying artery with the Doppler transducer (Fig. 11-2), particularly at the posterior tibial artery (PTA), dorsalis pedis artery (DPA), and radial artery, because each courses just above an adjacent bone. While listening to the Doppler signal, the pressure in the cuff is inflated until the audible signal is no longer heard. If the Doppler signal output is also being displayed on a monitor or a strip-chart recorder, this will be seen as a pulsatile waveform (when a Doppler signal is audible) and thus change to a flat line (once the Doppler signal is no longer audible). The pressure should continue to be inflated 20 mm Hg above this point. The cuff is then deflated slowly at a rate of approximately 3 mm Hg/s. The pressure at which the audible Doppler signal (or the pulsatile Doppler waveform) returns is the systolic pressure at the level of the cuff. An incorrect pressure measurement can be recorded when a patient is arrhythmic. In patients with arrhythmias, several measurements should be made from which to calculate an average of the varying systolic pressure.

### Ankle Brachial Indices

The association between reduced limb systolic pressures (measured using plethysmography) and PAOD affecting the lower extremities was explained in the 1950s.[5] The ratio of Doppler systolic pressures at the brachial level to those at the ankle was described first in 1969,[7] and was termed the ankle systolic pressure index—now known as the ankle/brachial index (ABI). Another less commonly used name for this ratio is the ankle arm index (AAI). ABI indicates the overall severity of PAOD between the heart and the ankle level.

An ABI is calculated by dividing the highest systolic pressure at the ankle level measured at either the PTA or the DPA/distal anterior tibial artery (ATA) by the higher of the two brachial systolic pressures. An example of an ABI calculation is:

|  | Right | Left |
|---|---|---|
| Brachial artery | 152 | 146 |
| Posterior tibial artery | 112 | 158 |
| Dorsalis pedis artery | 108 | 154 |
| **ABI** | **0.74** | **1.0** |

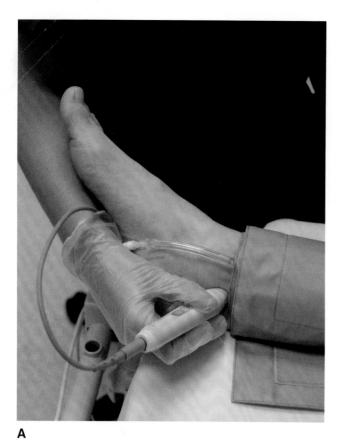

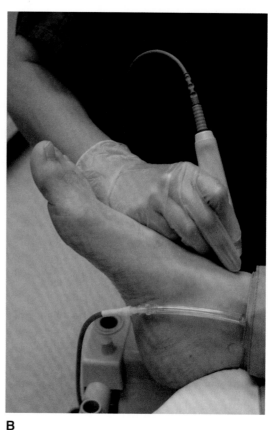

**A**

**B**

**FIGURE 11-1** Correct transducer position for the insonation of pedal Doppler signals. **A:** Insonation of the posterior tibial artery. **B:** Insonation of the dorsalis pedis artery.

The right ABI was derived by dividing the highest ankle systolic pressure (PTA pressure, 112 mm Hg) by the higher of the two brachial artery pressures (152 mm Hg). The left ABI was calculated by dividing 158 mm Hg by 152 mm Hg. An ABI worksheet should document systolic pressures from both brachial arteries and both PTA and DPA/ ATA at the ankle level.

### Diagnosis

Although there is variability in the published interpretation criteria, those in Table 11-2 are accepted widely. Whatever criteria are used when interpreting repeat studies, an ABI must be alter by at least 0.15, before such a change is considered significant.[8]

There is a normal drop of approximately 10 mm Hg in *mean* arterial pressure as blood flows from the heart to distal segments of the lower extremity.[9] However, there is a corresponding increase in the *amplitude* of distal pulse waveforms (i.e., the systolic pressure increases while diastolic pressure decreases). This results from the increased

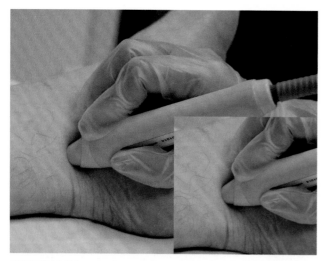

**FIGURE 11-2** Inappropriate transducer pressure is applied to this pedal artery. Such pressure may compress the artery.

| TABLE 11-2 Resting Ankle-Brachial Indices Related to the Severity of Peripheral Artery Occlusive Disease | |
| --- | --- |
| **Ankle-Brachial Index** | **Severity of PAOD** |
| >1.30 | Incompressible |
| 0.90–1.30 | Normal |
| 0.75–0.89 | Mild |
| 0.50–0.74 | Moderate |
| <0.50 | Severe |
| <0.35 | Tissue threatening |

peripheral resistance (PR) and arterial elastic recoil distally in the extremity. Thus, normal resting ankle systolic pressures tend to be higher than those in the brachial artery—although they can be slightly lower and still be regarded as normal (see Table 11-2). Initially, the lower limit of a normal resting ABI was reported as 1.0,[7] but subsequently this was modified to be 0.9,[10] especially in patients with hypertension or hypotension.

If the ABI appears to be abnormal, the higher brachial should be measured again to ensure that blood pressure has not systemically dropped enough for it to have been higher artifactually when calculating the ABI. At the ankle level, the PTA usually has a higher systolic pressure than either the DPA or the distal ATA.

A significant limitation of the noninvasive measurement of systolic pressure arises in those patients with calcific vessels. Systolic pressures are invalid when the underlying artery is calcified and incompressible,[11] so interpretations must then rely solely upon pulse waveforms and toe systolic pressures (to be discussed later in this chapter). Indication that the underlying artery is calcified occurs when a Doppler signal does not reappear at a clearly defined pressure and that it increases in amplitude with further cuff deflation. Also, the artifactually elevated pressure will not necessarily correspond with the pulse waveform. However, even when medial calcification renders the wall of an ankle artery to be noncompressible, the influence of a *negative* hydrostatic effect (lower extremity raised above heart level) can be used to indicate a minimum systolic pressure. The systolic pressure at the ankle level will be at least 50 mm Hg, if Doppler signals can still be heard, or plethysmographic waveforms remain even slightly pulsatile when the ipsilateral foot is raised 26 to 27 inches above heart level, as shown in Figure 11-3.

## Segmental Limb Systolic Pressures

As stated earlier, an abnormal ABI indicates the overall severity of PAOD, but not necessarily the site(s), especially when it is at more than one level. This multisite limitation occurs when PAOD proximally causes a significant reduction in flow energy into more distal segments—which may have additional disease. In this situation, abnormal drops in systolic pressure may not be exhibited in the distal segments, although differences in pulse waveforms may be discerned. To some degree, this can be remedied by measuring systolic pressures segmentally at two or three levels more proximally, in addition to comparing waveforms. Following measurement at the ankle level, segmental systolic pressures can then be measured at the calf and then thigh levels.

When measuring segmental pressures, choice must be made whether to use one wide cuff (17 or 19 cm) or two narrower cuffs (10 or 12 cm) above the knee (Fig. 11-4). This is often referred to as a 3-cuff versus 4-cuff method. The 3-cuff method uses a single wide, contoured thigh cuff, a calf cuff, and an ankle cuff. The 4-cuff method uses two narrower thigh cuffs, one placed high on the thigh around the most proximal segment and the second placed lower, just above the knee, plus calf and ankle cuffs. Having two cuffs along the thigh allows an interpreter to further define the level of disease by separating iliofemoral disease from superficial femoral artery disease. For the sonographer or vascular technologist, two cuffs above the knee present

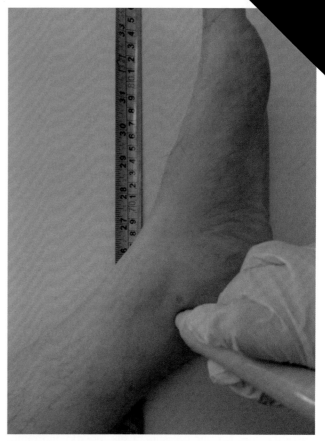

**FIGURE 11-3** When medial calcification renders the wall of an ankle artery to be non-compressible, the influence of a negative hydrostatic effect can be used to estimate the minimum systolic pressure by raising the foot above the heart level.

some practical problems. Often, the thigh may not be long enough to comfortably fit two cuffs side by side along the cuff—there is simply not enough room. In these cases, one cuff is usually removed, or the protocol is changed to a 3-cuff method. In addition, the use of the narrow 10 or 12 cm wide cuffs at the thigh levels require a higher inflation pressure to exert the same compression on the underlying tissue, to obtain a systolic pressure measurement. The patient should

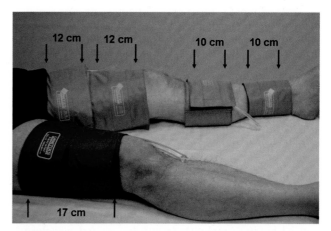

**FIGURE 11-4** Cuff placements for lower extremity segmental pressure determinations. One leg illustrates a 4-cuff technique, whereas the other leg illustrates the single contoured thigh cuff used for the 3-cuff technique.

igh will be squeezed tightly during
ient and be also reassured that this
a normal or near normal limb. The
or both measuring segmental systolic
e plethysmography studies, provided
ction tubing does not invalidate the
tion of the plethysmograph.

## Examination Technique

The technique for measuring segmental systolic pressure measurements is similar to that described earlier for measuring ABIs. Following measurement at the ankle level, segmental systolic pressures are then measured at the calf and then thigh levels. Although two sites are used to record the ankle pressures (the PT and DP), the technologist or sonographer typically selects the vessel with the greater pressure to insonate when measuring more proximally. In the case when no Doppler signals have been detected at the ankle, one can move higher up the limb to obtain a Doppler signal. With the calf cuff remaining in place, the ankle cuff is removed and a Doppler signal from a tibial vessel can be attempted at the mid-calf level. If no arterial Doppler signal is detected at the mid-calf level, a signal from the popliteal artery at the popliteal fossa level is attempted.

Segmental systolic pressures from the arms can be measured with cuffs positioned around the upper arm, forearm, and wrist. Usually, Doppler signals are obtained from both the radial and ulnar arteries, and wrist pressures are measured from both sites. The higher of the two pressures is used to record systolic pressure at the forearm and upper arm. As with the legs, if Doppler signals are not audible distally (at the wrist level), the Doppler transducer can be placed more proximally over the brachial artery to record the pressure in the upper arm cuff.

## Diagnosis

Table 11-3 lists interpretation criteria for the lower extremity and Table 11-4 for the upper extremity. Systolic pressures usually increase as blood flows distally along the lower extremity, although there can also be a slight drop (Table 11-3d). However, any reduction in distal pressure should be <30 mm Hg between adjacent segments (thigh level to calf, calf to ankle). (Table 11-3i)[12] with drops greater than this being associated with the presence of obstruction proximally.

The width of the thigh cuff(s) changes the criteria when interpreting the thigh pressure(s). Normal systolic pressure measured from a single large thigh cuff (17 or 19 cm width) should be equal to the higher of the two brachial pressures (Table 11-3f). Narrower cuffs (10 or 12 cm width) require a higher inflation pressure, so the normal systolic pressure at high thigh level (using a narrow cuff) needs to be 30 mm Hg or so above the higher brachial pressure (Table 11-3g).

PAOD is less common in the upper extremity compared with the lower extremity but, when present, it is found most commonly in the subclavian and proximal axillary arteries. Table 11-4 lists interpretation criteria for the upper extremity. A ≥75% diameter reduction in either of these arteries will cause a 15% to 10% mm Hg difference between brachial systolic pressures. Typically, these situations are accompanied by abnormal supraclavicular arterial waveforms. Segmentally, there should not a >20 mm Hg difference between above- and below-elbow levels.

---

### TABLE 11-3   Normal Interpretation Criteria for Lower Extremity

a. Resting Doppler waveforms proximal to knee are triphasic/biphasic and bidirectional

b. Plethysmography waveforms exhibit a dicrotic notch

c. Pulse waveforms have a well-defined peak

d. Resting and postexercise ABIs are 0.90–1.30

e. Resting and postexercise toe-brachial indices are >0.80

f. Single (wide) above-knee cuff systolic pressure equal to higher brachial

g. High thigh (narrow) cuff systolic pressure ≥30 mm Hg above higher brachial

h. All pulse waveforms have short (<135 ms, if able to be measured) systolic upstroke

i. Difference between adjacent limb segments is ≤30 mm Hg

j. Difference between brachial systolic pressures is ≤20 mm Hg

## Exercise Testing

Exercise testing is used primarily to investigate patients with symptoms of intermittent claudication who have normal to near normal (≥0.8) ABIs at rest. The exercise stress can be graduated on a motorized treadmill or by using reactive hyperemia.

A typical treadmill workload ranges from level to 10% grade and 1 to 2 miles/hr, for a maximum of 5 minutes (or earlier, if limited by symptoms). The degree of work is on a patient by patient basis. Even if an exercise component is suggested by a normal or near normal ABI, not all patients should be exercised, unless they are monitored by a physician or an appropriately qualified health professional. With neither of these persons present, treadmill exercise in the peripheral vascular department may be contraindicated for patients with:

- chest pain
- arrhythmias
- postmyocardial infarction/cardiac procedure and not cleared by their cardiologist
- unsteadiness
- hypertension >180 mm Hg

---

### TABLE 11-4   Normal Interpretation Criteria for Upper Extremity

a. Resting Doppler waveforms are triphasic/biphasic and bidirectional

b. Plethysmography waveforms exhibit a dicrotic notch

c. Pulse waveforms have a well-defined peak

d. Resting and postexercise digit-brachial indices are ≥0.90

e. ≤20 mm Hg systolic pressure gradient between above- and below-elbow levels

f. Gradient between brachial systolic pressures is ≤20 mm Hg

g. Pulse waveform and temperature recovery time ≤10 min

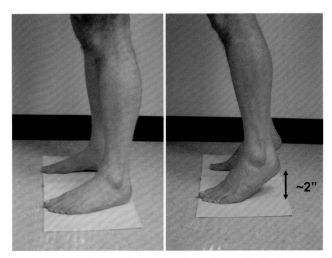

**FIGURE 11-5** An exercise study can be conducted using heel raises.

Walking at the patient's own pace and heel raising are valid alternatives to treadmill exercise, but the workload is less reproducible. Due to the variability in workload, Medicare will not reimburse these additional maneuvers. The sonographer or technologist should accompany a patient being exercised at their own pace, walking slightly behind to note onset of any symptoms and deciding when the patient should return to the study room. The effects of heel raising (Fig. 11-5) may be limited in the patient with arthritis and, because of the minimal effort from the thigh muscles, any postexercise drop in ankle systolic pressure is likely to be more transient.

### Examination Technique

Assuming that the patient is cleared for exercise, following the resting pressures measurements the cuffs can be left on (and secured with tape) or can be removed. The patient is placed on the treadmill. If the patient seems unsure, anxious, or unsteady, the initial speed can be set to "slow" and the inclination adjusted to minimum, then both can be increased to the protocol setting as the examination proceeds. If the patient is unable to perform the treadmill study because of the treadmill settings, a reduced setting may be used. This variation in protocol must be recorded. Exercise is terminated after 5 minutes or sooner if the patient shows any signs of distress (chest pain, unsteadiness, or difficulty breathing) or if the patient's leg symptoms become too painful to continue. The patient is immediately placed back on the examination table, ankle cuffs are quickly reapplied if they had been removed, and the immediate postexercise ankle pressures are obtained. Only the higher brachial artery systolic pressure needs to be measured postexercise. Typically, the ankle and higher brachial pressures are repeated every 2 minutes until they return to baseline values or for a specific time (10, 15, or 20 minutes) according to the laboratory protocol.

### Diagnosis

The lowest value of postactivity ABI categorizes functional severity (using Table 11-2), and the time to return to the preactivity level suggests whether PAOD is single or multilevel. An ABI which returns to the preexercise level in 5 minutes or less is associated with single-level disease, and an ABI taking >10 minutes to return is associated with disease at multiple levels.[13]

## DOPPLER WAVEFORMS

Typically, nonimaging-based arterial testing modalities use a continuous wave (CW) Doppler. This is usually the same Doppler transducer used to record systolic pressure measurements.

### Examination Technique

The CW Doppler beam is positioned to exclude interference from an adjacent vein; however, this is largely subjective. The patient can be requested to hold their breath for a few cardiac cycles to reduce venous flow and thus venous interference. For the lower extremity, Doppler waveforms are recorded from the common femoral artery, superficial femoral artery, popliteal artery, distal PTA, and DPA. For the upper extremity, Doppler waveforms are recorded from the subclavian, axillary, brachial, distal radial, and distal ulnar arteries. The Doppler transducer is placed over the general area of the underlying vessel. It is then slowly moved both medially and laterally until an arterial signal is obtained. The transducer is then adjusted so that an angle of approximately 45 degrees with the skin is achieved. This is varied slightly to improve the Doppler shift so that an accurate waveform with a maximum deflection is achieved.

### Diagnosis

Interpretation of extremity Doppler waveforms is limited to their shape (Tables 11-3 and 11-4a) because nonimaging modalities do not permit angle correction for calculating blood velocity. There have been ongoing discussions in the medical community concerning the terminology used to classify Doppler waveforms. These concerns have been raised for both duplex ultrasound-derived spectral waveforms and CW Doppler waveforms. Although this is still unresolved, the classic designations for CW waveforms that remain in use by most laboratories are as follows:

A. Triphasic
B. Biphasic: bidirectional
C. Biphasic: unidirectional
D. Monophasic: moderate/severe
E. Monophasic: severe/critical

Normal Doppler waveforms are bidirectional and exhibit a degree of flow reversal in late systole/early diastole, as shown in Figure 11-6A and B.[14] Waveform B does not exhibit a net return to forward flow. This waveform is seen frequently in older patients or in those whose feet are cold and is not regarded as abnormal. Waveforms C and D are seen when PAOD progresses from mild/moderate to severe, and Waveform E indicates that disease is now at a critical stage. Each of these three waveform types (C, D, and E) are unidirectional.

Figure 11-7 depicts CW waveforms from the upper extremity which are normal on the right and abnormal on the left. The abnormal waveform at the left subclavian level suggests proximal disease. The lower extremity waveforms in Figure 11-8 are abnormal on the right, suggesting iliofemoral disease. The left common femoral artery waveform is normal with abnormal waveforms distally. This is suggestive of femoropopliteal disease. In both of these upper and lower examples, systolic pressure measurements correlate

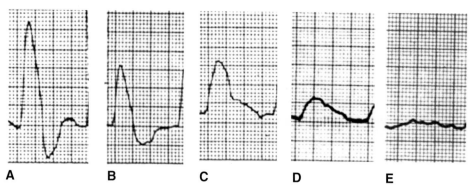

**FIGURE 11-6** Various Doppler waveforms: (**A**) triphasic, (**B**) biphasic: bidirectional, (**C**) biphasic: unidirectional, (**D**) monophasic: moderate/severe, and (**E**) monophasic: severe/critical.

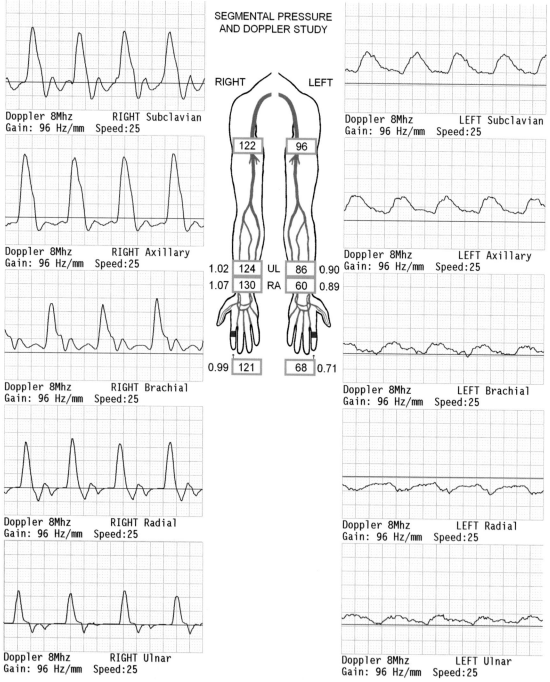

**FIGURE 11-7** Doppler waveforms from the upper extremity showing the right to be normal and the left abnormal, suggesting left proximal disease. (Image courtesy of Robert Scisson, RVT FSVU, Toledo, OH.)

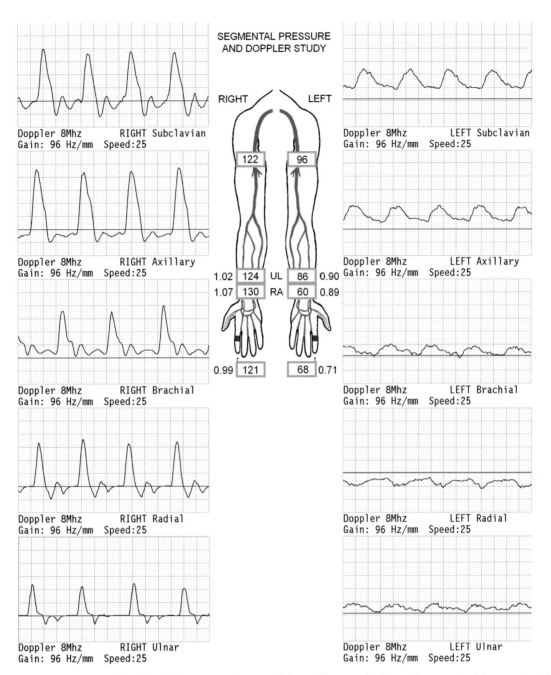

**FIGURE 11-8** Abnormal Doppler waveforms from the lower extremity suggest iliofemoral disease on the right and femoropopliteal disease on the left. (Image courtesy of Robert Scisson, RVT FSVU, Toledo, OH.)

with the CW waveform findings. Although it is possible to measure systolic rise time (from onset of systole to peak) and pulsatility index without imaging, this is now exclusively a duplex function (Table 11-3h).

Other than from an artery feeding a well-functioning dialysis fistula or graft, flow reversal at rest indicates the level of PR in the arteriolar bed, where more reversal relates to greater resistance to flow (ignoring the effects of flow reversal through an incompetent aortic valve) and less—or no reversal—relates to lower resistance. The normal progression of PAOD reduces flow energy distal to the lesion(s) which, without a corresponding reduction in PR, would

result in lowered blood flow. However, with a PR that has reduced by the same degree as the flow energy, the volume blood flow at rest does not change. At a critical stage, the arteriolar bed cannot dilate further, and blood flow into the affected segment(s) begins to drop, whereupon the patient may start to experience forefoot pain at rest, especially when lying horizontally. Thus, a resting arterial Doppler waveform with no flow reversal (i.e., it is unidirectional) is abnormal and indicates that the PR is reduced, probably relating to the presence of PAOD. (Note: Flow reversal will be absent immediately following exercise in a normal extremity, but will reappear within 2 to 5 minutes. Flow reversal may be absent in the recently successfully revascularized extremity or, as stated previously, from the artery supplying a functioning dialysis fistula or graft.)

## PLETHYSMOGRAPHY: PULSE VOLUME RECORDING (PVR) OR VOLUME PULSE RECORDING (VPR)

Air plethysmography (PVR or VPR) is a modality with a shorter learning curve than Doppler ultrasound and can give more consistent results in a vascular department with a low workload for this type of study (less than 1 week). This modality reflects the total perfusion in the underlying segment of the extremity, because the cuff encircles the whole limb but, unlike Doppler ultrasound, this testing modality does not identify specific arteries. Although it does not indicate the direction of blood flow, PVR has an advantage when the underlying arteries are not compressible because the waveform is relatively unchanged.

### Examination Technique

PVR techniques use either one cuff or two cuffs above the knee (see Fig. 11-4 and Tables 11-3 and 11-4b,c), plus one each at calf and ankle levels. These are the same cuffs used for segmental pressure examinations. Some protocols also include a cuff placed across the metatarsal level of the foot. Digital studies can performed as well, which will be discussed within the section dealing with digital evaluations.

Once in place, each cuff is inflated to 55 to 65 mm Hg, usually with a record of the inflation volume to indicate cuff tension, because inconsistent wrapping can change the waveform.[15] At this pressure, the venous outflow within the segment of the limb under the cuff is restricted. The only volume changes occurring under the cuff are those because of arterial inflow. With each cardiac cycle, a volume of blood enters the limb, and this volume change produces a pressure change under the cuff. The pressure change is converted to a waveform, which is displayed graphically. The overall height of the waveform is adjusted by a gain control. The gain should be set to produce a waveform that is straightforward to visualize with the entire contour easily evaluated. Some protocols set the gain by first recording waveforms from the calf (these usually have the greatest amplitude when compared with the other segments) and then record the remaining segments at the same gain setting. The gain used for digital studies is usually higher owing to the small volume changes occurring at this level of the vascular tree.

### Diagnosis

PVR waveforms relate to the moment-to-moment changes in (limb) volume, which is the difference between arterial inflow and venous outflow. Normal limb volume increases rapidly during systole, so the normal PVR waveform should exhibit a brisk upstroke with a well-defined peak (Fig. 11-9A; also see Tables 11-3 and 11-4b,c). A normal resting PVR waveform usually shows a "notch" on the downstroke in early diastole, which then returns to the baseline in a concave fashion (bends toward the baseline) before the onset of the next cardiac cycle. The notch may be smaller in the

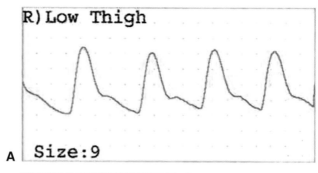
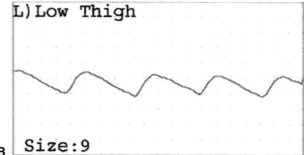

**FIGURE 11-9  A:** A normal PVR waveform from the right low thigh level exhibiting a brisk upstroke with a well-defined peak. **B:** The left low thigh level PVR in this same patient illustrates moderate to severe PAOD changes in the waveform, causing a delayed onset to peak, which is more rounded.

presence of a reduced PR, such as when the patient is warm or in the artery feeding a dialysis fistula. This notch is often termed the dicrotic notch and is the result of the reflected wave normally occurring in healthy vessels. As previously described, the normal high PR arterial bed will demonstrate a brief period of reverse flow in early diastole. This reverse flow component is also known as the reflected wave. The reverse flow component adds a small volume of blood under the cuff which produces the dicrotic notch observed on the PVR recordings. Moderate to severe PAOD changes the waveform, causing a delayed onset to peak, which is more rounded (Fig. 11-9B) as is seen also in an abnormal Doppler waveform. Additionally, the diastolic phase becomes convex as POAD progresses toward the severe category.

Figure 11-10 illustrates four general categories used to grade PVRs.[12] Because the waveforms are qualitative representations of perfusion, their interpretation is somewhat subjective. Many laboratories use a grading system of normal, mild, moderate, and severe. The waveforms become more broadened, and the peaks flatten with disease progression. With the most severe disease, waveforms may be virtually flat with very low amplitude.

Lower extremity PVR waveforms shown in Figure 11-11 illustrate normal findings for the right and abnormal on the left. The right PVR waveform exhibits a brisk systolic upstroke and a concave (bows toward the baseline) shape in diastole. Each of those from the left extremity exhibit a delayed systolic upstroke and a convex diastolic component (bows away from the baseline), with no dicrotic notch. On the left, these findings are compatible with stenosis (or occlusion with collateralization) in the iliofemoral segment. Digit waveforms are also asymmetrical, with those from the left showing slight delay in the upstroke and a more rounded appearance.

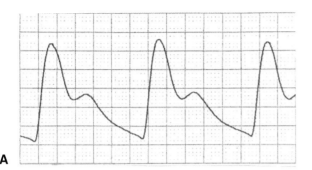

A

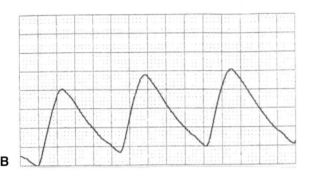

B

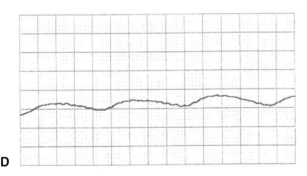

C

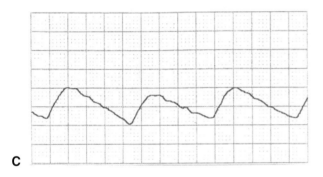

D

**FIGURE 11-10** Examples of general PVR waveform categories: (**A**) normal, (**B**) mild, (**C**) moderate, and (**D**) severe.

One of the main pitfalls in the interpretation of PVR waveforms and physiologic data is the inability to differentiate between stenosis from occlusion. Because these indirect tests do not visualize specific arteries, vessel occlusion cannot be determined. An occlusion with significant collateral flow may provide results similar to a high-grade stenosis. Thus, the term "occlusion" should never be used in interpretation of indirect testing results.

# DIGITAL EVALUATIONS

Digital evaluations can include both pressures and waveforms. Waveforms can be recorded using either air plethysmography (PVR) or photoplethysmography (PPG), although it is PPG which is used most commonly. There are various diseases impacting the vascular system that can be diagnosed with an examination of digital blood flow. The following section will review some of the techniques employed in digital evaluations as well as specific applications.

## Examination Technique

In terms of measuring digit systolic pressures, these can be recorded in a manner similar to other pressure measurements. Digital cuff widths vary slightly but usually are 1.9 to 2.5 cm. PPG is the most convenient modality for measuring digit pressures, but PVR is an alternative. It is not easy to maintain the Doppler ultrasound beam (which is typically only 1 to 2 mm wide) within the lumen of a digital artery.

PPGs are not true plethysmographic instruments because they cannot be calibrated in volume terms, but they are convenient for recording arterial pulse waveforms. They operate by transmitting infrared light into tissue and detecting variations in the light reflected from underlying blood flow, from a depth of 1 to 3 mm. PPGs can be maintained in contact with the skin with double-sided tape (Fig. 11-12A), with a Velcro strap or with a clip-style device (Fig. 11-12B). PPG is placed on the digit and after a brief period of 1 to 2 seconds, the sensor on the unit detects the reflected infrared light. This is displayed as a waveform. PPG and PVR instruments provide comparably shaped waveforms and as such are interpreted similarly, with normal characteristics being a brisk systolic upstroke, a well-defined peak, plus a concave shape as the shape returns to the baseline during diastole (see Fig. 11-10A).

In addition to recording arterial pulse waveforms, PPGs can be used to measure digital systolic pressures. The waveforms are recorded using a slow chart or sweep speed, adjusting the gain to give an amplitude approximately one-third of the chart width (Fig. 11-13). Limb or digit movement can intrude to confuse the point at which the waveforms return, if the recording has greater amplitude. The cuff is inflated until pulsatility is abolished, then deflated until waveforms are seen. Hands or feet can be warmed to increase waveform amplitude. This can be accomplished by heating a small towel in a microwave, for a minute. The towel can be wrapped around each hand or foot while the history is being documented. Having the recording with an enhanced waveform amplitude enables the point of waveform return to be determined with greater confidence.

## Diagnosis

A toe pressure can be used to calculate a toe/brachial index (TBI), which should be ≥0.8 to be reported as normal (see Table 11-3e).[16] This is similar to measuring an ankle pressure for calculating an ABI. TBIs are particularly useful when the ankle vessels are noncompressible and can be substituted for ABIs when assessing the response to exercise. Toe pressures may also be expressed directly in mm Hg. To indicate the likelihood of healing following a

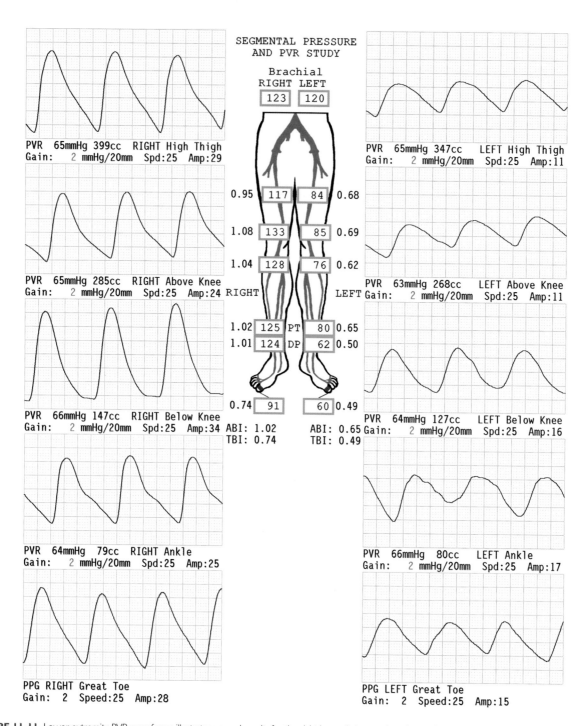

**FIGURE 11-11** Lower extremity PVR waveforms illustrates normal results for the right leg and abnormal results on the left leg consistent with left iliofemoral disease. (Image courtesy of John Hobby, RVT, Pueblo, CO.)

vascular procedure in the forefoot/toe segment, 50 mm Hg is regarded as adequate even in the presence of diabetes.

Upper extremity digit pressures are important in the workup prior to creation/revision of dialysis fistulas and grafts, plus for assessing steal from the hand by the fistula/graft. The absolute pressure indicates present or potential ischemia of the hand, or it can be used to calculate a digit/brachial index (DBI), similar to ABI and TBI. The normal value for the DBI is ≥0.9 (Table 11-4d).[17] In dialysis patients who are symptomatic for fistula steal, the digit pressures should double when the outflow side of the fistula is compressed.

## Thoracic Outlet Syndrome

Neurovascular compression affecting the upper extremity—TOS—is common and, to some degree, can be found in up to 60% of persons without necessarily causing any symptoms.[18] Symptoms result from compression by structures in the shoulder girdle, and usually they can be reproduced with the upper extremity in a specific position or when carrying out a particular activity.

The most convenient method to test for TOS is to record PPG digit waveforms with the patient warm, sitting, and

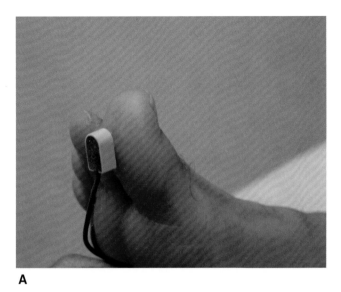
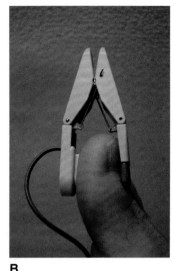

**A**                                                                                      **B**

**FIGURE 11-12** PPG probe placement (**A**) using double-sided tape to maintain contact with the skin and (**B**) with a clip-style device.

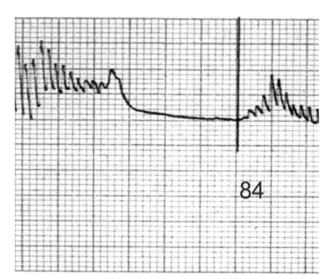

84

**FIGURE 11-13** PPG recording illustrating the use of PPG to record digital systolic pressure. The beginning of the tracing demonstrates normal pulsatile flow; pressure in an occluding cuff is increased until the pulsatile signal is obliterated; pressure is slowly released until the pulsatile signal returns; the point at which flow resumes is the systolic pressure which in this example is indicated at 84 mm Hg.

with arms resting comfortably in the lap (Figs. 11-14 and 11-15). Waveforms are then recorded with arms:

- resting in the lap
- elbows to the rear and arms almost upright, palms to front (military position)
- elevated above the head
- abducted rearward
- straight out to the sides (abducted) with the head ahead, and then turned fully to the left and then to the right (Adson maneuver)
- any other position that elicits symptoms.

Finally, waveforms should be recorded with arms resting in the lap, to document that waveforms are present at the completion of the study. If any position causes the

waveform to become flattened, maintain this position for approximately 30 seconds to establish whether the patient develops symptoms (the patient may require assistance to maintain the position). Remember, up to 60% of persons can demonstrate a compression without necessarily developing symptoms. For a TOS study to be reported as positive, the systolic pressures/pulse waveforms must be significantly affected by the maneuvers—plus the patient must develop symptoms.

## Cold Sensitivity

As mentioned earlier, Raynaud's disease is classified as primary or secondary, and a careful history can suggest one rather than the other. Secondary Raynaud's is associated with symptoms involving one or more digits or hand, with the symptoms or signs being asymmetrical. These patients often will present with some tissue loss as well. The patients tend to be older, and this can affect both men and women. The etiology of secondary Raynaud's is trauma, from the use of vibratory tools or equipment (jackhammers, riding motorcycles, etc.), injury such as using the hand as a hammer (ulnar hammer syndrome) or severe frostbite. Other causes may include underlying medical problems such as scleroderma.

When secondary Raynaud's is suspected, the patient should *not* have their hands immersed in ice water, to avoid causing increased injury. Confirmation of Raynaud's, in addition to a careful history, is to record digital waveforms and digital pressures (as in recording toe pressures, PPG being the easiest method). The presence of dampened waveforms and/or abnormal pressures (DBI lower than 0.90) should alert the technologist of this possibility prior to water immersion.

The onset of primary Raynaud's is typically seen in the late pre-teen or early teen years, and females tend to be more affected than males. In this instance, the hands will change color symmetrically when exposed to cold. The progression of this color change is white, changing to blue and then

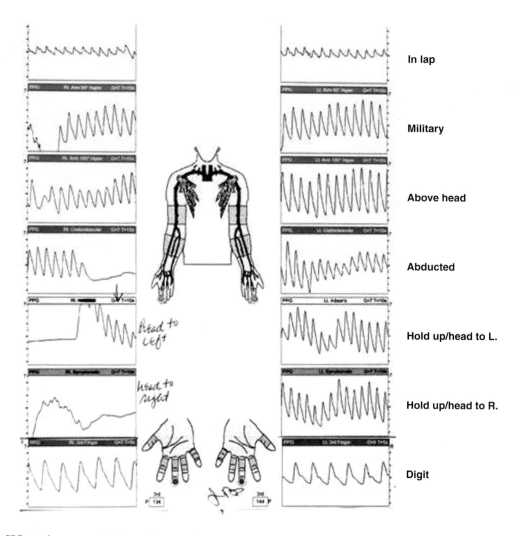

**FIGURE 11-14** PPG waveforms recorded during various postural maneuvers.

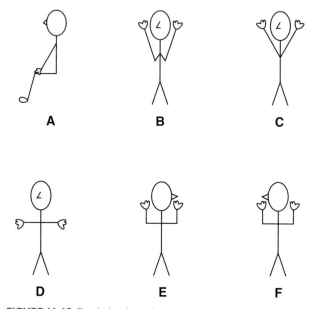

**FIGURE 11-15** Sketch showing patient positions used during thoracic outlet testing: (**A**) neutral, resting; (**B**) arms up with elbows bent at 45 degrees; (**C**) arms raised overhead; (**D**) arms abducted straight out, 90 degrees; (**E**) Adson with head to the left; (**F**) Adson with head to the right.

red, when the hands are warmed. These symptoms can occur consistently when picking up a cold item, such as a glass of ice water, evoked by emotional stress or can also be seen when the entire body is slightly cooled, such as with seasonal changes in outside temperature. In this situation, the cool mornings in the spring or fall result in the wearing of lighter clothing, then the vasospastic response triggers the autonomic sympathetic system to constrict. This is an overreaction in those with primary Raynaud's resulting in the color changes. This reaction can be reduced by dressing warmer than usual.

Testing for primary Raynaud's can be accomplished using waveform analysis of the digital tracings and/or a digital temperature monitoring device (Fig. 11-16). The digital waveform should be taken prior to immersion in ice water, and it may appear normal or exhibit a "peaked pulse" on the anacrotic (systolic) portion (Fig. 11-17) seen frequently in primary Raynaud's.[19] There are several *"Stress Level Meters"* or *"biofeedback monitors"* available which are accurate to <0.1°C and are not expensive (usually less than US$50). Prior to beginning the testing and challenge by immersion into ice water, the hands should be warmed to a minimum of 28°C. Immerse the hands in warm (not

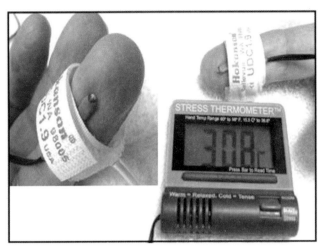

**FIGURE 11-16** A digital temperature monitoring device used for Raynaud's testing.

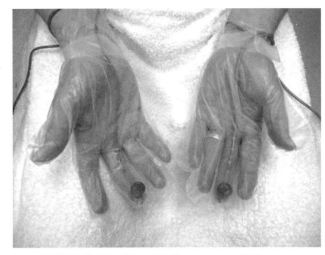

**FIGURE 11-18** The use of disposable gloves to protect PPG sensors uses during cold-sensitivity testing.

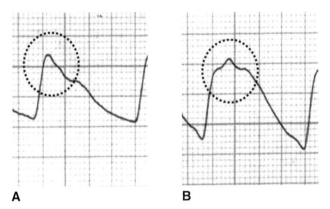

**A**          **B**

**FIGURE 11-17** Digital PPG waveforms: (**A**) a normal waveform and (**B**) a "peaked pulse" waveform frequently in primary Raynaud's.

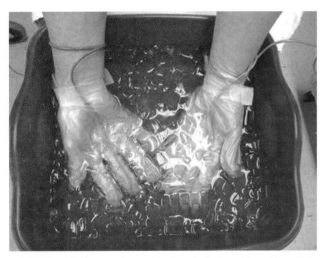

**FIGURE 11-19** Proper patient position in an ice bath used for cold-sensitivity testing.

hot) water for several minutes, until they feel warm to the touch. In addition, the testing room should be comfortably warm (74 to 76°F, 23 to 24°C), so the patient is not cooled by the environment.

For this exam, the patient sits comfortably in a chair (one having a back will facilitate comfort) with a towel placed over the lap. This will avoid water getting on the patient when the hands are removed from the water. Resting waveforms (and/or temperatures) are recorded from all digits. Digit blood pressures are measured, if indicated, or a component of individual protocols. The PPG should be secured to the wrist to avoid "pulling" of the probe away from the digit. Securing the probe to the digit with double stick tape will provide a clean tracing. If a thermometer is used, again the sensing probe should be secured to the digit with a Velcro strap and secured at the wrist as with the PPG probe.

It is helpful to place the hands in large disposable latex gloves (if no latex allergy) and secure the glove at the wrist with a strip of tape (Fig. 11-18). This will prevent the hands from getting wet and alleviate the need to dry the hands when removed from the ice water. The hands should be

immersed into the ice water, to just below the top of the gloves (Fig. 11-19). A large container is needed for the hand immersion, and a "bath basin" as used routinely in hospital settings, works very well. Placing the basin on a small table, in front of the patient, facilitates immersion and prevents accidental spills.

Cold immersion should be for no more than 30 to 40 seconds, followed by immediate removal of the hands from the water and removal of the gloves. If the hands do get water on them directly, they should be "patted" dry rather than rubbed briskly. Digital waveforms (Fig. 11-20) and/or temperatures should be measured immediately and at 2, 5, and 10 minutes. If the waveforms and/or digit temperatures are not recovered after 10 minutes, continue recordings at 15, 20, and 25 minutes. Normal digital tracings and/or temperatures should return to preimmersion status within 10 minutes to be categorized as normal (Fig. 11-21; also see Table 11-4g), with >10 minutes being consistent with cold sensitivity.

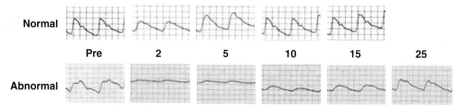

**FIGURE 11-20** Normal and abnormal digital PPG waveforms recorded during cold sensitivity testing. Pre indicates initial waveforms recorded at room temperature. The numbers 2, 5, 10, 15 and 25 indicate the minutes after removal from an ice water bath.

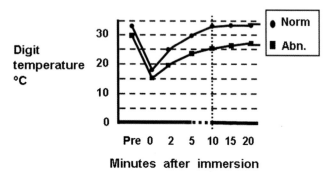

**FIGURE 11-21** Normal and abnormal temperature measurements following cold-sensitivity testing using ice water immersion. A normal response is one where temperatures return to baseline measurements within 10 minutes following removal from the cold stimulus.

| Time (min) | PPG Waveform | Digital Temperature (°C) |
|---|---|---|
| Immediately | Reduced amplitude | ≤20 |
| 2 | Increase in amplitude | 20–25 |
| 5 | Sharp peak returning | 28–30 |
| 10 | Return to preimmersion | 30–33 |

If the study is abnormal, the waveform and/or temperature should be verified prior to releasing the patient.

## The Allen Test

An application of the Allen test uses PPG waveforms to indicate adequacy of hand perfusion from the radial and ulnar arteries, combined and individually. It is necessary to establish the contribution to digital perfusion from each of these arteries prior to certain surgical procedures. These procedures include the creation of a dialysis fistula or graft and radial artery harvest prior to coronary bypass procedures. The PPG transducer is affixed to the middle finger or the forefinger, and waveforms are recorded. The radial and ulnar arteries are compressed sequentially, to verify whether or not waveforms are maintained (Fig. 11-22). The intent is to detect that the waveform amplitude is not abolished when the ulnar artery is compressed as shown in Figure 11-22. This confirms that flow into the hand will not be interrupted if the radial artery is used to feed the fistula or graft or harvested for bypass.

Pathology Box 11-1 summarizes some of the common arterial pathology observed in the lower and upper extremities. It also lists the indirect testing results associated with these abnormalities.

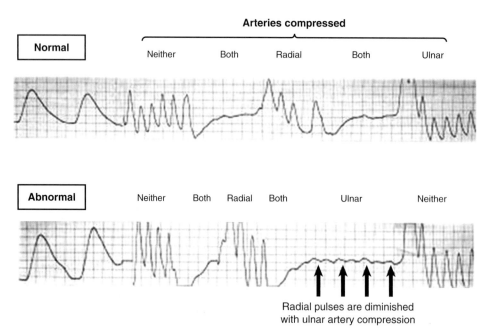

**FIGURE 11-22** PPG waveforms recorded during an Allen test. Normal and abnormal responses are indicated with compression of the radial and ulnar arteries.

## PATHOLOGY BOX II-I
### Lower and Upper Extremity Arterial Pathology

| Pathology | Indirect Testing Results |
|---|---|
| Peripheral arterial occlusive disease | • ABI < 0.9<br>• Pressure gradient >20–30 mm Hg between diseased segments<br>• Loss of reflected wave (dicrotic notch) on PVRs<br>• Loss of reverse flow component on Doppler waveform |
| Digital ischemia:<br>Lower extremity | • TBI < 0.8<br>• Diminished digital waveforms |
| Digital ischemia:<br>Upper extremity | • DBI < 0.9<br>• Diminished digital waveforms |
| Thoracic outlet syndrome | • Diminished or flat digital PPG waveforms during provocative arm/shoulder maneuvers and the development of symptoms |
| Raynaud's disease | • Diminished PPG waveforms at rest<br>• DBI < 0.9<br>• "Peaked Pulse" may be present on PPG or PVR waveforms<br>• Digital waveforms return to baseline >10 min following cold challenge |
| Incomplete palmar arch<br>(radial/ulnar dependency) | • Positive Allen test with diminished digital waveforms during manual compression of radial or ulnar arteries |

ABI, ankle-brachial index; DBI, digit-brachial Index; PPG, photoplethysmography; PVR, pulse volume recording; TBI, toe-brachial index.

## SUMMARY

- Indirect arterial testing is a valuable asset when examining patients with suspected PAOD.
- Additionally, there are several other appropriate indications for the indirect testing of the extremities.
- The combination of systolic pressures and pulse waveforms produces both quantitative and qualitative information on extremity blood flow.
- The nonimaging techniques described provide an assessment of global perfusion and thus the functional status of a limb.

## CRITICAL THINKING QUESTIONS

1. What are two important concerns about patient position for physiologic exams?
2. You perform a segmental pressure evaluation on a patient with relatively short legs. There is not enough room to place both a high thigh and low thigh cuff. You use a single contoured thigh cuff. What affect do you think this will have on your results and why?
3. You have been asked to examine the status of the common femoral artery. You can perform a PVR, CW Doppler waveform, or segmental pressure examination. Which test would you select and why?
4. Digital evaluations are commonly used to evaluate patients with TOS and Raynaud's disease. What vessels are impacted by these pathologies and why are digital studies used?

## MEDIA MENU

Student Resources available on thePoint® include:
- Audio glossary
- Interactive question bank
- Videos
- Internet resources

## REFERENCES

1. LaPerna L. Diagnosis and medical management of patients with intermittent claudication. *J Am Osteopath Assoc.* 2001;100:S10–S14.
2. Edwards JM, Porter JM. Evaluation of upper extremity ischemia. In: Bernstein EF, ed. *Vascular Diagnosis.* 4th ed. St. Louis, MO: Mosby; 1993:630–640.
3. Sanders RJ, Hammond SL, Rao NM. Diagnosis of thoracic outlet syndrome. *J Vasc Surg.* 2007;46:601–604.
4. Herrick AL. Pathogenesis of Raynaud's phenomenon. *Rheumatology.* 2005;44:587–596.
5. Winsor TA. Influence of arterial disease on the systolic blood pressure gradients of the extremity. *Am J Med Sci.* 1950;220:117–126.
6. Daigle RJ. *Techniques in Noninvasive Vascular Diagnosis.* 2nd ed. Littleton, CO: Summer Publishing; 2005:142.
7. Yao ST, Hobbs JT, Irvine WT. Ankle systolic pressure measurements in arterial disease affecting the lower extremities. *Br J Surg.* 1969;56:676–679.
8. Baker JD, Dix DE. Variability of Doppler ankle pressures with arterial occlusive disease: an evaluation of ankle index and brachial-ankle pressure gradient. *Surgery.* 1981;89:134–137.
9. Strandness DE Jr, Sumner DS. *Hemodynamics for Surgeons.* New York, NY: Grune & Stratton; 1975:228.
10. Stein R, Hrljac I, Halperin JL, et al. Limitation of the resting ankle-brachial index in symptomatic patients with peripheral arterial disease. *Vasc Med.* 2006;11:29–33.
11. AbuRahma AF. Segmental doppler pressures and doppler waveform analysis in peripheral vascular disease of the lower extremities. In: AbuRahma AF, Bergan JJ, eds. *Noninvasive Vascular Diagnosis.* London, UK: Springer; 2000:213–229.

12. Gerhard-Herman M, Gardin JM, Jaff M, et al. Guidelines for non-invasive vascular laboratory testing: a report from the American Society of Echocardiography and the Society of Vascular Medicine and Biology. *J Am Soc Echocardiogr*. 2006;19:955–972.

13. vanLangen H, vanGurp J, Rubbens L. Interobserver variability of ankle-brachial index measurements at rest and post exercise in patients with intermittent claudication. *Vasc Med*. 2009;14:221–226.

14. Scissons R, Comerota A. Confusion of peripheral arterial doppler waveform terminology. *J Diagn Med Sonogr*. 2009;25:185–194.

15. Daigle RJ. *Techniques in Noninvasive Vascular Diagnosis*. 2nd ed. Littleton, CO: Summer Publishing; 2005:151.

16. Carter SA, Lezack JD. Digital systolic pressures in the lower limbs in arterial disease. *Circulation*. 1971;43:905–914.

17. Rumwell C, McPharlin M. *Vascular Technology*. 4th ed. Pasadena, CA: Davies Publishing; 2009:110.

18. Gergoudis R. Thoracic outlet arterial compression: prevalence in normal persons. *Angiology*. 1980;31:538–541.

19. Mclafferty RB, Edwards JM, Porter JM. Diagnosis and management of Raynaud's syndrome. In: Perler BA, Becker GJ, eds. *Vascular Intervention: A Clinical Approach*. New York, NY: Thieme; 1998:239–247.

# Duplex Ultrasound of Lower Extremity Arteries

NATALIE MARKS | ANIL P. HINGORANI | ENRICO ASCHER

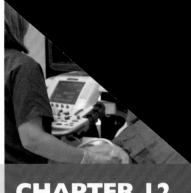

**CHAPTER 12**

## OBJECTIVES

- Describe the ultrasound techniques used to image lower extremity arteries
- Define normal image and Doppler characteristics of peripheral arteries
- Identify peripheral arterial abnormal images and waveforms
- Describe the utilization of ultrasound with arterial revascularization procedures

## GLOSSARY

**aneurysm** A localized dilation of an artery involving all three layers of the arterial wall

**contrast arteriography** A radiologic imaging technique performed using ionizing radiation and intravascular contrast material to provide detailed arterial system configuration and pathology information

**duplex arteriography** Ultrasound imaging of the arterial system performed to identify atherosclerotic disease and other arterial pathology and establish a detailed map of the arterial system evaluated

**plaque** The deposit of fatty material within the vessel walls which is characteristic of atherosclerosis

## KEY TERMS

**aneurysm**

**arterial occlusion**

**arterial stenosis**

**arterial thrombosis**

**contrast arteriography**

**duplex arteriography**

**peak systolic velocity**

**peak systolic velocity ratio**

**plaque**

Contrast arteriography (CA) has been utilized for decades as the gold standard imaging tool to evaluate the peripheral arterial system particularly prior to lower extremity revascularization procedures. It is well known that CA is associated with systemic and local complications and the media-educated patients of today are demanding less invasive alternatives. Current technical advances in ultrasonographic imaging equipment have motivated a number of authors to investigate the prospect of duplex arteriography (DA) to replace standard CA in the arterial system assessment.[1-13] Many authors have demonstrated a promising association between arteriography and DA,[1-9] whereas others received less enthusiastic results and therefore continue to promote preoperative or pre-procedure arteriography.[10-13] There are several factors contributing to this difference in results such as: (1) insufficient experience, technical skills and knowledge of anatomy and hemodynamics by the vascular sonographers, (2) lack of commitment of time and effort to perfect the technique, (3) outdated duplex equipment with poor image quality, (4) surgeons and interventionists unwilling to give up the visual effect of a complete arteriography and

incorporate a perception of duplex imaging, and (5) heavy vessel calcification and other local obstacles preventing adequate insonation in some patients.

It has been the experience of these authors to preferentially use DA for arterial imaging since 1998. At first, the efficacy of DA was explored for purely diagnostic purposes in patients undergoing lower extremity revascularizations.[14-17] Over the last 12 years, DA has been applied not only for diagnostic use but also to guide various endovascular interventions such as duplex guided angioplasties.[18-21] The utilization of intraoperative and postendovascular arterial ultrasound is discussed in subsequent chapters of this textbook. This chapter explores the DA value in the diagnosis of the lower extremity arterial system disease.

## INDICATIONS

Signs and symptoms of arterial disease, which are described in the preceding chapter on indirect arterial testing, also apply to a patient presenting for lower extremity arterial duplex ultrasound examination. These are classic symptoms arterial insufficiency or ... claudication, rest pain, ... ne. There can be some ... hair loss, nail thickening, ... such as pallor, pulseless- ... intense pain are indicative ... ipheral arterial aneurysms ... palpation a pulsatile mass ... popliteal regions. Peripheral ... ined for aneurysmal disease ... abdominal or thoracic aortic aneurysm. ... d aneurysmal diseases are the primary pathologies suspected in most individuals. There are less frequently encountered arterial diseases as well as traumatic and iatrogenic injuries, which may require DA for their diagnosis.

Although arterial disease is not an indication for testing by itself, many of the patients will present with one or more comorbid risk factors. These risk factors include diabetes, hyperlipidemia, hypertension, history of tobacco use, coronary artery disease, and chronic renal insufficiency. Additional risk factors for arterial disease are obesity, sedentary lifestyle, heredity, gender, and age.

## SONOGRAPHIC EXAMINATION TECHNIQUES

### Patient Preparation

The patient should have the test procedure explained to them. They should remove all clothing from the waist down, except for undergarments and be given a gown or appropriate drape.

### Patient Positioning

The patient is placed in supine position with mild knee flexion and thigh abduction for visualization of the common, superficial, and deep femoral arteries (Fig. 12-1). The same patient position can be used to examine the above-knee popliteal artery segment from a medial approach and the behind-knee and below-knee segment from a posterior approach. A medial approach is also used to insonate the posterior tibial artery and its plantar branches. By placing the patient in lateral decubitus position opposite to the side of interest with slight ipsilateral knee and hip flexure, the tibioperoneal trunk and peroneal artery can be examined (Fig. 12-2). By placing the transducer just posteriorly to the proximal fibula, the origin of the anterior tibial artery can be assessed. The remainder of the anterior tibial artery is visualized by positioning the transducer between the tibia and the fibula at the lateral proximal calf. Lastly, the dorsalis pedis artery and its metatarsal branches are insonated with the patient in the supine position.

### Scanning Technique

A complete evaluation for lower extremity arterial disease includes an ultrasound examination of the aortoiliac segment as well as the measurement of ankle pressures for ankle-brachial index calculation. Some laboratories include multilevel physiologic testing such as pulse volume recordings,

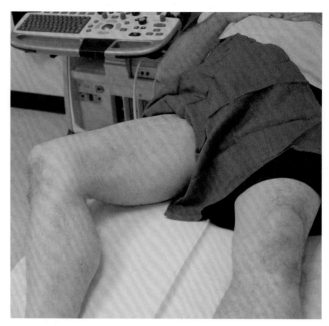

**FIGURE 12-1** A patient positioned for a lower extremity arterial ultrasound examination with the hip externally rotated and the knee slightly flexed.

continuous-wave Doppler waveforms, or segmental pressures as part of a routine lower extremity examination. The duplex ultrasound examination of the aortoiliac segment is discussed in Chapter 23, whereas the measurement of ankle pressures is described in Chapter 11.

A variety of transducers are utilized to obtain high-quality B-mode, color, and power Doppler images as well as reliable velocity spectra. Curvilinear 5 to 2 MHz and phased array 3 to 2 MHz probes are typically used for aortoiliac scanning, but these lower frequency probes may be needed to insonate deeper lower extremity vessels in heavier limbs. Linear 7 to 4 MHz transducers are used for visualization of the femoral, popliteal, and tibial vessels. High resolution of compact linear 15 to 7 MHz transducer allows for better visualization of superficial arteries on the ankle and foot.

The duplex ultrasound examination of the infrainguinal vessels begins at the groin. At this position, the distal portion of the external iliac artery and the entire common femoral artery (CFA) can be identified. The transducer is moved slightly down the leg to next identify the bifurcation of the CFA into superficial femoral artery (SFA) and

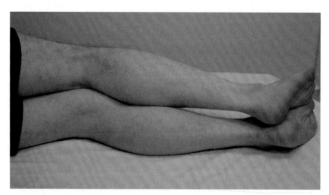

**FIGURE 12-2** A patient positioned in the left lateral decubitus position to examine the popliteal artery, tibioperoneal trunk, and peroneal artery.

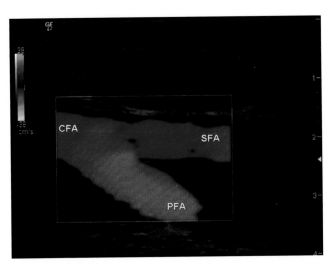

**FIGURE 12-3** The common femoral artery (CFA) bifurcating into the superficial femoral artery (SFA) and deep femoral or profunda femoris artery (PFA).

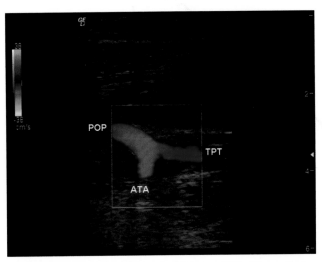

**FIGURE 12-5** The origin of the anterior tibial artery (ATA) off the popliteal artery (POP). The tibioperoneal trunk (TPT) is also shown.

deep femoral artery (DFA) or profunda femoris artery (PFA) (Fig. 12-3). Most laboratory protocols require only the first few centimeters of the PFA to be scanned. After a short distance, the PFA courses deeper in the thigh, giving rise to multiple branches. The SFA is then followed through its entire course using a medial approach. In the lower thigh, the SFA passes through the adductor canal also known as Hunter's canal. Once through the canal, the SFA becomes the popliteal artery, which is now assessed along the posterior aspect of the leg. This can be viewed by moving the transducer posteriorly to the knee joint and following the vessel proximally onto the lower thigh. Combining both medial and posterior approaches, the full course of the SFA and above, behind, and below the knee popliteal artery can be appreciated.

The popliteal artery is examined as it courses through the popliteal fossa. There are multiple small branches, including the gastrocnemius arteries (also referred to as the sural arteries), which can be noted (Fig. 12-4). In a complete examination, all three tibial arteries are followed throughout the calf. The anterior tibial artery can be observed with a posterior approach branching off the popliteal artery

(Fig. 12-5). As this vessel courses lower in the calf, it can be followed with an anterolateral approach. After anterior tibial artery takeoff, the tibioperoneal trunk can be found and assessed. It is slightly smaller in diameter than popliteal artery and is about 3 to 5 cm long. The tibioperoneal trunk bifurcates into peroneal and posterior tibial arteries. The posterior tibial artery can be followed through the calf with a medial approach. Depending on its depth, peroneal artery can be followed with a medial approach or using a posterolateral approach (Fig. 12-6). Often, the lower extremity examination includes the dorsalis pedis artery. Care should be taken when insonating the distal posterior tibial, distal anterior tibial, and dorsalis pedis arteries. These vessels are very superficial and can easily be partially compressed with the transducer if too much pressure is applied.

Individual laboratory protocols vary but typically include documentation of the grayscale image, color-flow image, and spectral waveforms. These images should be recorded over every major segment evaluated. Proximal, mid, and distal images of the SFA and tibial vessels are also usually

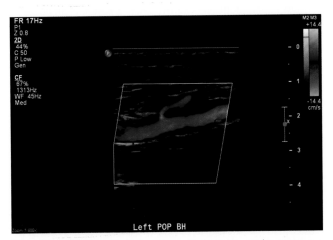

**FIGURE 12-4** The popliteal artery along with the gastrocnemius artery.

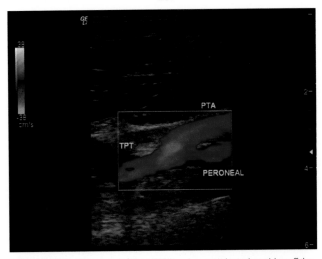

**FIGURE 12-6** The posterior tibial (PTA) and peroneal arteries arising off the tibioperoneal trunk (TPT).

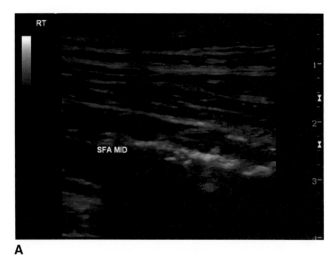

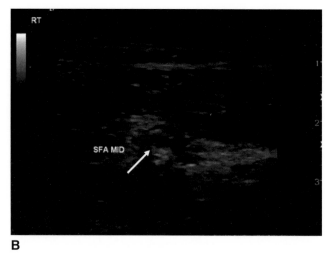

**FIGURE 12-7  A:** A sagittal scan of an artery with atherosclerotic plaque. **B:** A transverse view of the same plaque (*arrow*).

recorded. The grayscale image may be documented in sagittal and transverse planes (Fig. 12-7). In the presence of pathology, it is important to document the full extent of the disease. If aneurysmal disease is suspected, diameter measurements should be recorded along the area of concern as well as just proximal to this region.

In general, color and power Doppler are used primarily to assist with localization and tracking the course of the vessels. Color can provide a rapid assessment of the flow dynamics. Color is very useful in identifying flow abnormalities associated with arterial plaque (Fig. 12-8). Color is also helpful in guiding the placement of the Doppler sample volume at the area of the of the greatest velocity shift. Power Doppler should be used whenever very low flow states are encountered or when vessel occlusion is suspected.

Velocity spectra are used as the primary tool to categorize disease. The peak systolic velocity (PSV) is recorded along all the major vessels. In the areas of narrowing, the PSV should be recorded proximal to the stenosis, at the area of maximum velocity shift in the stenosis and just distal to the stenosis (Fig.12-9). The distal waveform usually demonstrates poststenotic turbulence associated with hemodynamically significant stenoses. The PSV at the stenosis is divided by

the PSV just proximal to the stenosis to calculate the velocity ratio ($V_r$). The $V_r$, in addition to the PSV, is used to estimate the degree of stenosis.

Because the status of the branches of the arteries can also add valuable data for the surgeon, visualization of as many tibial and pedal branches as possible, including maleolar, plantars, tarsals, deep plantar arteries, and branches of the named vessels is also performed during DA. A high-frequency transducer (15 to 7 MHz) can be especially useful in this portion of the protocol.

A precise evaluation of arterial size, length, and degree of narrowing as well as plaque characteristics is performed for a single focal lesion or sequential lesions suitable for balloon angioplasty and/or stent placement. It is important for the sonographer or vascular technologist to possess as much information from the referring physician as possible so that all the ultrasound data required for patient management decisions can be obtained. The referring physician may be planning a specific procedure or an intervention at a specific level and require pertinent data to plan the most appropriate procedure and approach. Whenever an occlusion is encountered, it is helpful to note the site where the vessel is reconstituted by collateral flow.

A color-coded map of the arterial tree is drawn to facilitate reading by the surgeon in order to select optimal inflow and outflow anastomotic sites for bypasses or potential angioplasty sites (Fig. 12-10). This drawing can contain comments about the vessel walls, velocity data, and vessel size.

## Technical Considerations

Over the years, there has been progression of preoperative DA as an integral part of revascularization procedures. In this author's institution, DA is used for procedure planning, intraoperatively and postoperatively as the first option for routine, urgent, or emergent imaging tool. This utilization versatility stems at large from duplex scanner's portability. Because DA examinations can be performed at the bedside, in the operating room or in the holding area, time and personnel used for patient transport are significantly reduced. Additionally, there is no delay associated with performance and interpretation, which can be the case

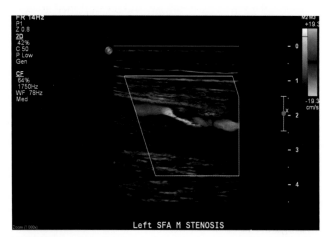

**FIGURE 12-8** Color-flow imaging identifying flow abnormalities associated with hypoechoic arterial plaque.

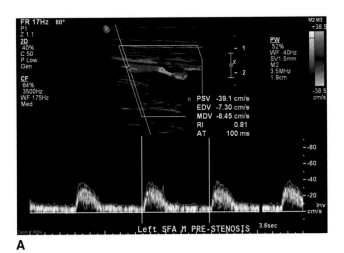

A

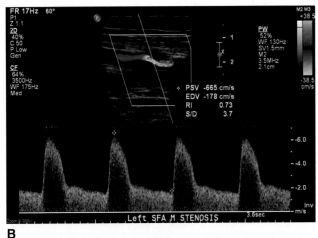

B

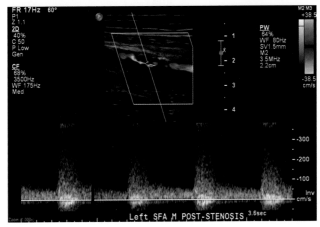

C

FIGURE 12-9  **A**: A Doppler waveform taken proximal to a stenosis. **B**: A Doppler waveform taken at the area of maximum velocity shift within a stenosis. **C**: A Doppler waveform taken distal to a stenosis documenting poststenotic turbulence.

with CA or magnetic resonance angiography (MRA) for a severely ischemic limb in a debilitated patient. With DA, once the patient is identified to need urgent revascularization, the ultrasound system and sonographer or vascular technologist can be brought to any part of the hospital for an abbreviated, targeted, or full examination.

Because DA is not just a luminal technology, it is essential in the assessment of the vessel wall. High-frequency duplex imaging can measure the luminal diameter and thickness of the wall with incredible precision of approximately one-tenth of a millimeter. This feature is very important because biplanar arteriography is not routinely used for the entire arterial tree, and therefore, eccentric arterial lesions may go undetected by CA.

Another unique advantage of DA as compared to other imaging tools is its ability to identify the softest portion of the vessel wall, which can then be marked on the skin before the intended procedure. Extensive calcification in a vessel makes suturing difficult, so an area that is compliant with no plaque or calcification is preferred. Skin marking of the most suitable site for outflow anastomosis, particularly for infrapopliteal segments, may limit incision size and eliminate extensive arterial dissection in search of a soft arterial segment (Fig. 12-11).

One of the strongest advantages of DA is its application in the setting of acute arterial ischemia.[22] Current management of acute lower limb ischemia has evolved from simple

embolectomies under local anesthesia to challenging arterial reconstructions. This dramatic change involves a more aggressive approach at limb salvage in the elderly patient by well-trained vascular surgeons. On the other hand, many of these patients presenting with acutely ischemic limbs will have underlying multisegmental occlusive arterial disease rather than a simple embolus obstructing a healthy vessel (Fig. 12-12). Although the clinical diagnosis of an ischemic leg can often be made without difficulties, the anatomic pattern of the inflow, the outflow, and the occluded arterial segment may at times be impossible to ascertain by standard preoperative imaging modalities.

Finally, during the course of a lower extremity examination it may be necessary to evaluate other vascular segments. Routinely, venous mapping can also be performed during DA to identify usable veins for harvest. The examination of the subclavian–axillary segments may be performed as a possible inflow source for debilitated patients with severe aortoiliac disease. This is accomplished without the risk of an additional thoracic aortogram or the time needed for an additional thoracic MRA.

## Pitfalls

Investigators have clearly demonstrated the feasibility and multiple advantages of DA and as with any technology, it is important to appreciate its limitations. Overall, the most

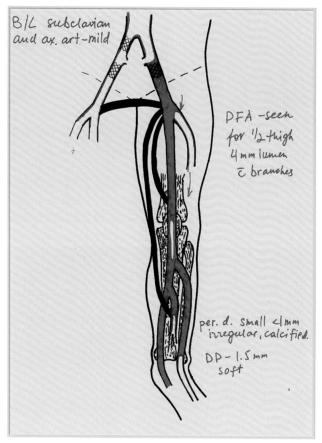

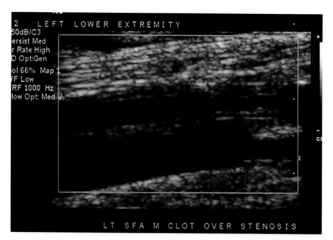

FIGURE 12-12 Color Doppler image of an occluded SFA with acute thrombus overlying severe chronic arterial disease.

FIGURE 12-10 An arterial map drawing of a patient with multiple failed PTFE bypasses.

common problem with DA has been with arterial wall calcification. However, some techniques can be used to obtain the necessary information even within severely calcified vessels such as using multiple insonation planes, increasing color and Power Doppler gain, increasing sensitivity and persistence, or using SonoCT imaging mode.

When an extremely low flow situation is encountered (PSV < 20 cm/s), DA can be unreliable, and alternative imaging modalities may need to be employed. However,

lowering the Doppler pulse repetition frequency (PRF) to 150 to 350 Hz and using the lowest wall filter setting, the highest persistence and highest sensitivity for the color-flow, duplex scanners are able to detect flows as low as 2 cm/s, which is significantly lower than the threshold for other imaging modalities such as MRA, computerized tomographic angiography (CTA), or even CA (Fig. 12-13).[23] At times, distal compression can augment arterial flow and demonstrate patency of nonthrombosed tibial vessels with absent spontaneous flow, especially in the acute ischemia setting.

Some of the obstacles encountered during DA scans may necessitate very specific approaches. When patients experience severe ischemic pain that precludes the completion of this at times extensive exam, premedication with analgesics can be helpful. Additionally, because the examination does take the cooperation of the patient, having a family member present during the examination of a confused elderly patient can comfort them and can help them tolerate the examination better. Visualization of the iliac arteries can be better accomplished by having the patient fast. Leg elevation for 24 to 48 hours prior to nonemergent DA test usually decreases calf edema and provides for adequate visualization of the tibial vessels.

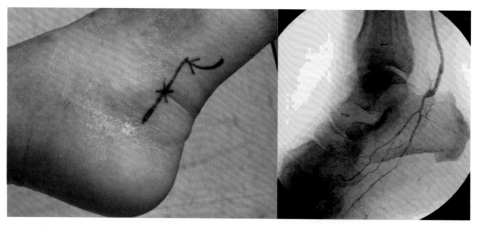

FIGURE 12-11 *Left:* Distal posterior tibial artery segment and a large inflow branch are marked preoperatively on the skin. *Right:* Intraoperative completion angiogram of the newly created vein bypass demonstrated a normal distal anastomosis to the distal posterior tibial artery and preserved large collateral branch on the same patient.

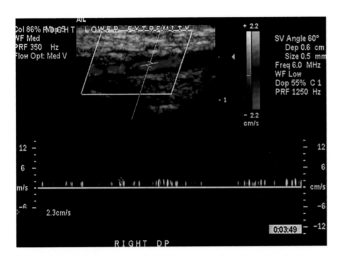

**FIGURE 12-13** Very low velocity (PSV = 2.3 cm/s) registered by duplex ultrasound in the dorsalis pedis artery (appeared occluded on diagnostic contrast arteriogram).

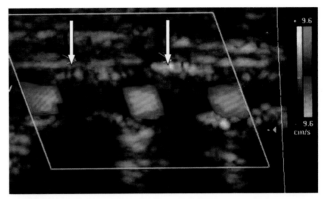

**FIGURE 12-14** Color Doppler image of a distal posterior tibial artery with segmental heavy calcifications (*arrows*) creating shadows obscuring the arterial lumen.

The depth of the tibioperoneal trunk, origin of the proximal peroneal and posterior arteries, and the SFA at Hunter's canal may necessitate the use of a lower frequency transducer for visualization. However, this tends to sacrifice resolution details and can make significant findings in these areas difficult to interpret.

Although insonation in the area of open ulcers or excessive scarring may not be possible, this also would not be a suitable area for anastomosis. Therefore, even in those patients with poor skin condition, severe obesity, or edema (resulting in excessive vessel depth), sufficient information can sometimes still be obtained to complete the needed intervention. For example, if a claudicant is found to have a patent popliteal artery and one vessel runoff, but the other tibial vessels were not fully assessed, then this information will be sufficient to perform femoropopliteal bypass regardless of the condition of other tibial vessels. If a diabetic with gangrene is found to have a patent dorsalis pedis artery and an adequate conduit, but the anterior tibial artery is too calcified to visualize, one may choose to perform a bypass to the dorsalis pedis because the anterior tibial artery would not be an optimal site for the distal anastomosis anyway.

The length of time to perform a complete DA has always been listed as one of its disadvantages and has often been criticized. However, is it necessary to visualize all of the vessels from the aorta to the pedal vessels in every case? For example, the need to scan all tibial vessels for a patient with claudication, severe iliac disease, and no significant femoral disease may be questioned if the surgeon is only planning on iliac angioplasty procedure. Thus, the DA protocol may need to be tailored for each case because a complete examination may not be absolutely necessary or additional examinations may need to be performed in certain types of patients depending on the clinical approach of the operating team.[24] With experience, DA time can be as short as 25 minutes in many simple cases.

### Training Methods

To successfully achieve these results is to establish the training method for sonographers/technologists and surgeons interpreting the results and planning revascularization strategy. In an attempt to develop a training period at the author's institution, the first 25 examinations completed by any new sonographer or vascular technologist are prospectively confirmed with CA or repeated DA examination by an established staff technical member. In an effort to facilitate the advancement of the DA protocol, every completion angiogram is reviewed with the staff member who performed the examination, as are the iliac angioplasties. The characteristics of the proximal and distal arteries, vein conduit, or tibial vein in the case when an adjunctive arteriovenous fistula is performed are discussed, and any discrepancies are reviewed as a quality assurance measure. The technical staff visits the operating room to witness the intraoperative findings firsthand. In this manner, the constant feedback becomes the cornerstone for the continual improvement in the quality of the DA exams.

## DIAGNOSIS

### Grayscale Findings

Normal arterial walls appear smooth and uniform. As atherosclerotic disease progresses, the vessel walls will thicken. Calcification may be present and will produce acoustic shadowing, thereby limiting complete evaluation of the vessel. Vessel wall thickness and degree of calcification are reported to aid in the choice of anastomosis sites (Fig. 12-14). As stated earlier, a surgeon will want to avoid areas of heavy calcification, because it is difficult to pass sutures through heavily calcified vessels. Plaque can be seen encroaching on the vessel lumen. Most plaque will appear heterogeneous with mixed levels of echogenicity. Occasionally, some plaque may be observed which appears homogeneous with similar echogenicity throughout the plaque. The surface characteristics of a plaque should be reported when possible, particularly if the plaque appeared irregular. Irregularly surfaced plaques may represent ulcerative lesions; however, many laboratories avoid reporting a plaque as "ulcerative" and simply state "irregular." High-resolution DA much more clearly visualizes ulcerated and irregular plaques with potential of embolization, their surface and characteristic flow disturbance (Fig. 12-15).

DA has the ability to more accurately assess the age of the occlusion. It is possible to differentiate between an

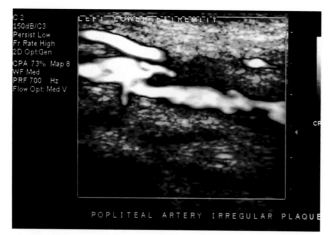

**FIGURE 12-15**  Power Doppler image of severely diseased behind-the-knee popliteal artery with very irregular ulcerated plaque surface with high embolization potential.

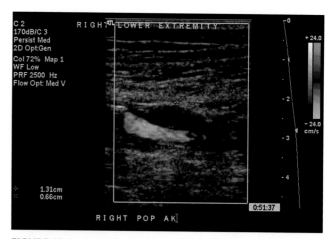

**FIGURE 12-16**  Power Doppler image of a small (13.1 mm) behind-the-knee popliteal artery aneurysm with near-wall mural thrombus (thrombus thickness is measured 6.6 mm).

isolated chronic SFA occlusion and an acute embolism with little underlying disease or acute thrombosis with severe underlying atherosclerotic disease. The adjacent vessel walls should be closely examined to determine if atherosclerotic disease is present.

Vessel size is another component of information obtained from the grayscale image. In addition to detecting atherosclerotic disease, aneurysmal disease is another finding observed during lower extremity arterial evaluations. It is well known that aneurysmal disease can be bilateral and multilevel. Table 12-1 illustrates diameters and velocities for lower extremity arteries.[25] A vessel is considered aneurysmal if the diameter is 1.5 times greater than the adjacent more proximal segment. The presence or absence of mural thrombus within an aneurysm should also be documented, because this thrombus poses an embolic risk. Aneurysmal vessels with partial thrombosis may have little to no luminal dilatation and may be completely undetectable by CA (Fig. 12-16).[26]

## Color-Flow Imaging

Normal color-flow imaging will completely fill the vessels. With proper equipment settings of gain and scale, the color will appear uniform and be limited to just the lumen. In areas of disease, color aliasing will be apparent, the color-flow

channel within the lumen will be reduced, and a color bruit may be present within the surrounding tissue.

## Spectral Analysis

Although the color and grayscale image are important, the PSV is the primary measurement obtained during DA which is used to determine the degree of stenosis. Table 12-1 lists values for normal velocities within the lower extremity vessels. There are some variations observed in PSV, and therefore, the $V_r$ is used for grading the stenosis. A PSV $V_r \geq 2$ to 2.5 usually reflects a stenosis of $\geq 50\%$, a PSV $V_r \geq 3$ to 3.5 is used to confirm a severe stenosis of $\geq 70\%$ (Fig. 12-17). The arterial segments are classified as normal or mildly diseased ($<50\%$), moderately diseased (50% to 69%), severely diseased (70% to 99%), and occluded or not visualized (Table 12-2).

The hemodynamic information obtained using DA may greatly influence patient's management. Velocity ratios can help assess whether the visualized lesion is hemodynamically significant and determine whether repair of the lesion may be beneficial. For example, a poorly visualized plaque

| TABLE 12-1 **Duplex Ultrasound Mean Arterial Diameters and Peak Systolic Velocities (PSVs)[25]** | | |
|---|---|---|
| **Artery** | **Diameter ± SD (cm)** | **PSV ± SD (cm/s)** |
| External iliac | 0.79 ± 0.13 | 119 ± 22 |
| Common femoral | 0.82 ± 0.14 | 114 ± 25 |
| Superficial femoral (proximal) | 0.60 ± 0.12 | 91 ± 14 |
| Superficial femoral (distal) | 0.54 ± 0.11 | 94 ± 14 |
| Popliteal | 0.52 ± 0.11 | 69 ± 14 |

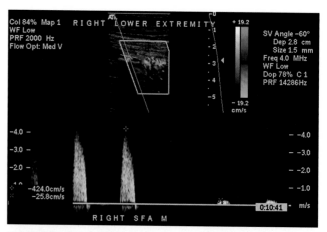

**FIGURE 12-17**  Doppler spectral analysis of a severe mid-SFA stenosis confirmed by a PSV ratio step-up of 16.4 (PSV of 424 cm/s at the stenosis over PSV of 25.8 cm/s prestenosis).

| TABLE 12-2 | **Arterial Disease Classification Based on $V_r$** | |
|---|---|---|
| **Description** | **Percent Stenosis** | **Peak Systolic Velocity Ratio, $V_r$** |
| Normal or mildly diseased | <50 | <2.0 |
| Moderately diseased | 50–69 | ≥2.0–2.5 |
| Severely diseased | 70–99 | ≥3.0–3.5 |
| Occluded | Occluded | No flow |

with low PSV ratios (<2) may not be of clinical significance, whereas calcified lesions with a high PSV ratio step-up (≥2) suggest a hemodynamically significant obstruction. Other luminal imaging modalities such as CA, MRA, or CTA do not provide objective hemodynamic information and significance of lesions is often judged rather subjectively.

Waveform configuration should also be noted. Normally, the peripheral arterial bed is high resistance, which results in a multiphasic waveform (Fig. 12-18). There is a sharp upstroke to peak systole, a rapid deceleration, a reflected wave displayed as retrograde flow below the baseline, and often a small brief wave of antegrade flow in diastole. In situations where the peripheral resistance is lowered, constant forward flow through diastole may be observed. In the cases of a distal arteriovenous fistula, trauma, or cellulitis, or in the postexercise patient, antegrade flow will be observed throughout diastole (Fig. 12-19). However, in these cases a normal sharp upstroke to peak systole will be maintained. In the event of significant arterial disease or an occlusion, the vessels distal to this disease will display a low-resistance signal with antegrade flow through diastole, but there will be a delayed rise time to peak systole (Fig. 12-20). Lastly, when scanning vessels proximal to an occlusion or near occlusion, the spectral waveforms can display a very high-resistance pattern with only an antegrade flow component during systole and no flow during diastole (Fig. 12-21).

Pathology Box 12-1 lists the duplex ultrasound findings with lower extremity arterial disease. Gray-scale, spectral Doppler, and color imaging results are summarized.

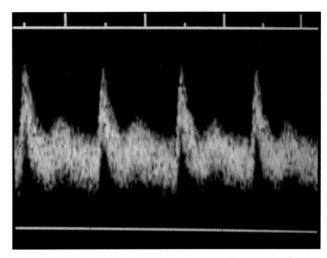

**FIGURE 12-19** A waveform displaying a normal systolic upstroke with constant forward flow through diastole. This can be observed immediately after exercise or in the presence of a distal arteriovenous fistula, trauma, or cellulitis.

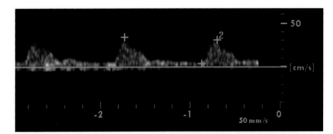

**FIGURE 12-20** An abnormal waveform illustrating constant forward flow throughout the cardiac cycle in addition to a delayed upstroke. This is observed distal to a high-grade stenosis or occlusion.

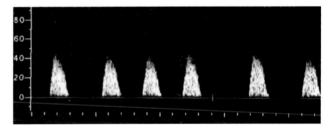

**FIGURE 12-21** An abnormal high-resistance waveform with only antegrade flow through systole. This is observed proximal to a near occlusion, or occlusion.

## OTHER IMAGING PROCEDURES

Standard percutaneous preoperative CA can be obtained when DA is not able to provide adequate imaging of arterial segments essential for limb revascularization or is severely disadvantaged by poor runoff. In a review of 1,023 cases at this author's institution, 112 cases (10%) were found to require CA. This was because of severe arterial calcifications present in 71 cases (63%), severe edema or morbid obesity in 23 cases (21%), extremely limited runoff with no treatment options as concluded by DA in 20 cases (18%), extensive skin wounds in 9 cases (8%), extremely low flow in 8 cases (7%), and patient's intolerance in 7 cases (6%). Of these 112 patients, 18 (16%) had undergone multiple prior revascularization attempts.

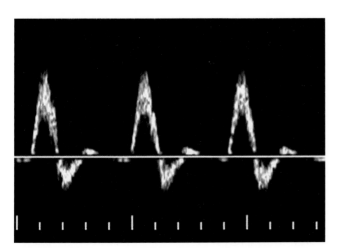

**FIGURE 12-18** A normal multiphasic waveform taken from SFA.

## PATHOLOGY BOX 12-1
*Lower Extremity Arterial Ultrasound Findings*

| | Grayscale | Spectral Doppler | Color Imaging |
|---|---|---|---|
| Normal | • Walls smooth and uniform | • No focal areas of increased PSV<br>• Slight change in PSV across segments of arterial tree<br>• Multiphasic waveform with reverse flow component | • Uniform color filling |
| Stenosis | • Wall thickening<br>• Calcification<br>• Plaque encroaching into vessel lumen | • Focal increase in PSV<br>• Poststenotic turbulence<br>• $V_r \geq 2.0$<br>• Monophasic waveform distally with no reverse flow and continuous flow in diastole | • Focal area of aliasing<br>• Turbulence distally |
| Aneurysm | • Increased diameter 1.5 times larger than adjacent more proximal segment | • Turbulence within dilated area | • Turbulence in dilated area |
| Occlusion | • Echogenic material completely filling lumen<br>• No patent lumen identified | • No flow identified<br>• Increased resistance noted in waveform proximally | • No color filling |

Factors associated with an increased need to obtain CA included diabetes ($p < 0.001$), infrapopliteal calcification ($p < 0.001$), older age ($p = 0.01$), and limb-threatening ischemia ($p < 0.001$). Factors not associated with the need to obtain CA included the sonographer or vascular technologist performing the examination and history of prior revascularization procedures.

Invasive CA has several limitations particularly when compared to duplex ultrasound: (1) it delineates the patent arterial lumen only; (2) it misses thrombosed popliteal aneurysms; (3) it fails to visualize an outflow and inflow sources in very low flow situations; (4) it requires potentially nephrotoxic agents; (5) it requires the use of ionizing radiation; and (6) it delays prompt treatment. Furthermore, avoidance of nephrotoxic agents and radiation, visualization of low flow arteries and a more expeditious examination are some of the advantages of DA that are particularly important in this often sick subset of patients presenting with acute lower limb(s) ischemia.

A well-performed DA offers several practical advantages over CA in this subset of patients: (1) it is noninvasive; (2)

it does not require nephrotoxic agents; (3) it is portable, and it can be done expeditiously; (4) color-flow and waveform analysis provide a better estimation of the hemodynamic significance of occlusive disease; (5) it allows for direct visualization of the entire artery and not only of the lumen, thus enabling plaque characterization; (6) with color-flow and power Doppler techniques, it is possible to identify patent arteries subjected to very low flow states; and (7) it can detect occluded arterial aneurysms, thereby avoiding unnecessary attempts at thromboembolectomies.

The key difference between using DA and preoperative CTA or MRA is that during DA the sonographer or vascular technologist can identify the arterial segments where adequate visualization was not achievable and alert the surgeon that results are unreliable. In contrary, the factors that suggest when CTA or MRA are no longer supplying reliable data have yet to be identified.[27–30] Based upon the present experience of the authors, about 90% of lower extremity revascularization procedures can be performed based upon preoperative DA alone.

## SUMMARY

- Duplex ultrasound can be efficiently used for evaluation of the lower extremity arteries and is particularly helpful in patients being evaluated for lower extremity revascularization.
- It is a highly operator-dependent test that demands constant optimization of the image by an operator who has mastered ultrasound technology, hemodynamics understanding and has a deep knowledge of pertinent anatomy.
- The multiple advantages, few limitations, and promising results of the technique may potentially significantly improve with the use of exceptional quality imaging provided by contemporary ultrasound instruments.

## CRITICAL THINKING QUESTIONS

1. You are asked to scan the dorsalis pedis artery in a patient prior to a bypass graft. What are the two technical elements of the examination that should be taken into consideration?
2. What is the most significant pitfall in imaging the lower extremity arteries, how can it be overcome, and why is it important to pay attention to this in the region of a distal anastomosis?
3. In addition to the $V_r$ calculated from the PSV, what is another component of spectral imaging that can help identify a stenosis and what changes are expected?

## MEDIA MENU

Student Resources available on thePoint® include:
- Audio glossary
- Interactive question bank
- Videos
- Internet resources

## REFERENCES

1. Sensier Y, Hartshorne T, Thrush A, et al. A prospective comparison of lower limb colour-coded Duplex scanning with arteriography. *Eur J Vasc Endovasc Surg.* 1996;11:170–175.
2. Ligush J Jr, Reavis SW, Preisser JS, et al. Duplex ultrasound scanning defines operative strategies for patients with limb-threatening ischemia. *J Vasc Surg.* 1998;28:482–490.
3. Sensier Y, Fishwick G, Owen R, et al. A comparison between colour duplex ultrasonography and arteriography for imaging infrapopliteal arterial lesions. *Eur J Vasc Endovasc Surg.* 1998;15:44–50.
4. London NJ, Sensier Y, Hartshorne T. Can lower limb ultrasonography replace arteriography? *Vasc Med.* 1996;1:115–119.
5. Polak JF, Karmel MI, Mannick JA, et al. Determination of the extent of lower-extremity peripheral arterial disease with color-assisted duplex sonography: comparison with angiography. *AJR Am J Roentgenol.* 1990;155:1085–1089.
6. Moneta GL, Yeager RA, Antonovic R, et al. Accuracy of lower extremity arterial duplex mapping. *J Vasc Surg.* 1992;15(2):275–283.
7. Wilson YG, George JK, Wilkins DC, et al. Duplex assessment of run-off before femorocrural reconstruction. *Br J Surg.* 1997;84(10):1360–1363.
8. Karacagil S, Lofberg AM, Granbo A, et al. Value of duplex scanning in evaluation of crural and foot arteries in limbs with severe lower limb ischaemia—a prospective comparison with angiography. *Eur J Vasc Endovasc Surg.* 1996;12:300–303.
9. Koelemay MJ, Legemate DA, de Vos H, et al. Can cruropedal colour duplex scanning and pulse generated run-off replace angiography in candidates for distal bypass surgery. *Eur J Vasc Endovasc Surg.* 1998;16:13–18.
10. Cossman DV, Ellison JE, Wagner WH, et al. Comparison of contrast arteriography to arterial mapping with color-flow duplex imaging in the lower extremities. *J Vasc Surg.* 1989;10(5):522–528.
11. Larch E, Minar E, Ahmadi R, et al. Value of color duplex sonography for evaluation of tibioperoneal arteries in patients with femoropopliteal obstruction: a prospective comparison with anterograde intraarterial digital subtraction angiography. *J Vasc Surg.* 1997;25:629–636.
12. Lai DT, Huber D, Glasson R, et al. Colour duplex ultrasonography versus angiography in the diagnosis of lower-extremity arterial disease. *Cardiovasc Surg.* 1996;4:384–388.
13. Wain RA, Berdejo GL, Delvalle WN, et al. Can duplex scan arterial mapping replace contrast arteriography as the test of choice before infrainguinal revascularization? *J Vasc Surg.* 1999;29(1):100–107.
14. Mazzariol F, Ascher E, Salles-Cunha SX, et al. Values and limitations of duplex ultrasonography as the sole imaging method of preoperative evaluation for popliteal and infrapopliteal bypasses. *Ann Vasc Surg.* 1999;13:1–10.
15. Ascher E, Mazzariol F, Hingorani A, et al. The use of duplex ultrasound arterial mapping as an alternative to conventional arteriography for primary and secondary infrapopliteal bypasses. *Am J Surg.* 1999;178(2):162–165.
16. Mazzariol F, Ascher E, Hingorani A, et al. Lower-extremity revascularization without preoperative contrast arteriography in 185 cases: lessons learned with duplex ultrasound arterial mapping. *Eur J Vasc Endovasc Surg.* 2000;19:509–515.
17. Ascher E, Hingorani A, Markevich N, et al. Lower extremity revascularization without preoperative contrast arteriography: experience with duplex ultrasound arterial mapping in 485 cases. *Ann Vasc Surg.* 2002;16(1):108–114.
18. Ascher E, Marks NA, Schutzer RW, et al. Duplex-guided balloon angioplasty and stenting for femoral-popliteal arterial occlusive disease: an alternative in patients with renal insufficiency. *J Vasc Surg.* 2005;42(6):1108–1113.
19. Ascher E, Marks NA, Hingorani AP, et al. Duplex guided balloon angioplasty and subintimal dissection of infrapopliteal arteries: early results with a new approach to avoid radiation exposure and contrast material. *J Vasc Surg.* 2005;42(6):1114–1121.
20. Ascher E, Marks NA, Hingorani AP, et al. Duplex-guided endovascular treatment for occlusive and stenotic lesions of the femoral-popliteal arterial segment: a comparative study in the first 253 cases. *J Vasc Surg.* 2006;44(6):1230–1237.
21. Ascher E, Hingorani AP, Marks NA. Duplex-guided angioplasty of lower extremity arteries. *Perspect Vasc Surg Endovasc Ther.* 2007;19(1):23–31.
22. Ascher E, Hingorani A, Markevich N, et al. Acute lower limb ischemia: the value of duplex ultrasound arterial mapping (DUAM) as the sole preoperative imaging technique. *Ann Vasc Surg.* 2003;17(3):284–289.
23. Ascher E, Markevich N, Hingorani A, et al. Pseudo-occlusions of the internal carotid artery: a rationale for treatment on the basis of a modified carotid duplex scan protocol. *J Vasc Surg.* 2002;35(2):340–345.
24. Ascher E, Markevich N, Schutzer RW, et al. Duplex arteriography prior to femoral-popliteal reconstruction in claudicants: a proposal for a new shortened protocol. *Ann Vasc Surg.* 2004;18(5):544–551.
25. Jager KA, Risketts HJ, Strandness DE Jr. Duplex scanning for the evaluation of lower limb arterial disease. In: Bernstein EF, ed. *Noninvasive Diagnostic Techniques in Vascular Disease.* St. Louis, MO: CV Mosby; 1985:619–631.
26. Ascher E, Markevich N, Schutzer RW, et al. Small popliteal aneurysms: are they clinically significant? *J Vasc Surg.* 2003;37(4):755–760.
27. Hingorani A, Ascher E, Markevich N, et al. A comparison of magnetic resonance angiography, contrast arteriography, and duplex arteriography for patients undergoing lower extremity revascularization. *Ann Vasc Surg.* 2004;18(3):294–301.
28. Hingorani A, Ascher E, Markevich N, et al. Magnetic resonance angiography versus duplex arteriography in patients undergoing lower extremity revascularization: which is the best replacement for contrast arteriography? *J Vasc Surg.* 2004;39(4):717–722.
29. Soule B, Hingorani A, Ascher E, et al. Comparison of magnetic resonance angiography (MRA) and duplex ultrasound arterial mapping (DUAM) prior to infrainguinal arterial reconstruction. *Eur J Vasc Endovasc Surg.* 2003;25(2):139–146.
30. Hingorani A, Ascher E, Markevich N, et al. A comparison of magnetic resonance angiography, contrast arteriography, and duplex arteriography for patients undergoing lower extremity revascularization. *Ann Vasc Surg.* 2004;18(3):294–301.

# Duplex Ultrasound of Upper Extremity Arteries

OLAMIDE ALABI | GREGORY L. MONETA

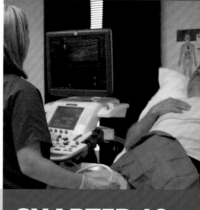

## CHAPTER 13

## OBJECTIVES

- List the blood vessels imaged during an upper extremity ultrasound examination
- Identify normal and abnormal spectral Doppler waveforms
- Describe the scanning techniques used to properly insonate upper extremity vessels
- Define diseases that impact upper extremity arteries

## GLOSSARY

**Raynaud's syndrome** A vasospastic disorder of the digital vessels

**Takayasu's arteritis** A form of large vessel vasculitis resulting in intimal fibrosis and vessel narrowing

**thoracic outlet** The superior opening of the thoracic cavity that is bordered by the clavicle and first rib; the subclavian artery, subclavian vein, and brachial nerve plexus pass through this opening

**vasospasm** A sudden constriction of a blood vessel that will reduce the lumen and blood flow rate

## KEY TERMS

**axillary**

**brachial**

**radial**

**Raynaud's syndrome**

**subclavian**

**Takayasu's arteritis**

**thoracic outlet**

**ulnar**

Upper extremity arterial examination utilizes components of the history and physical examination in conjunction with noninvasive and, sometimes, invasive vascular studies.

Duplex ultrasound examination is a key diagnostic modality when evaluating upper extremity arterial disease. Upper extremity arterial disease occurs much less frequently than lower extremity ischemia, accounting for only about 5% of extremity ischemia. Its low-incidence and highly variable etiology may cause considerable confusion in clinical practice. Causes of upper extremity symptoms related to arterial disease include mechanical obstruction at the thoracic outlet, embolism, trauma, digital artery vasospasm, and digital artery occlusion. A thorough history and physical, in conjunction with a duplex ultrasound examination, is often sufficient to determine definitive management and minimize the use of arteriography. This chapter will review the arterial anatomy of the upper extremities, identify important anatomic variants that may be encountered, and common clinical applications of upper extremity arterial duplex ultrasound scanning. Both normal and abnormal duplex ultrasound findings, some of which are unique to insonation of the upper extremities arteries, are presented.

A stepwise process for duplex ultrasound examination of the upper extremity arteries is also presented.

## ARTERIAL ANATOMY

Arterial duplex ultrasound examination of lower extremity arteries is more commonly performed compared to evaluation of the upper extremity arteries. As such, many sonographers and physicians are less comfortable with upper extremity arterial anatomy. Understanding the normal arterial anatomy of the upper extremities, along with common anatomic variants, will facilitate examination of the upper extremity arteries with duplex ultrasound (Fig. 13-1).

The subclavian arteries originate in the chest usually arising from the innominate (also known as the brachiocephalic) artery on the right and directly from the aortic arch on the left. The innominate artery is the first major branch of the aortic arch and divides into the right common carotid artery and the right subclavian artery. Infrequently, however, the right subclavian artery may originate directly from the aorta distal to the left subclavian artery in what is frequently a retroesophageal subclavian artery, or a so-called aberrant

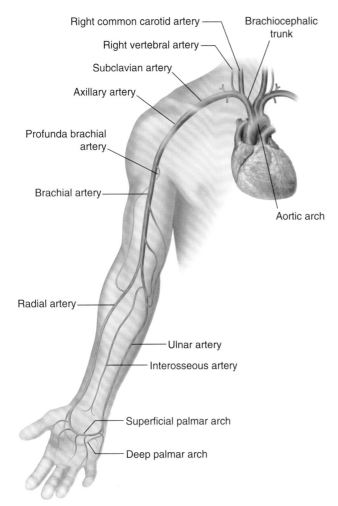

Right common carotid artery
Brachiocephalic trunk
Right vertebral artery
Subclavian artery
Axillary artery
Profunda brachial artery
Brachial artery
Aortic arch
Radial artery
Ulnar artery
Interosseous artery
Superficial palmar arch
Deep palmar arch

**FIGURE 13-1** Schematic drawing of the principle arteries of the upper extremity.

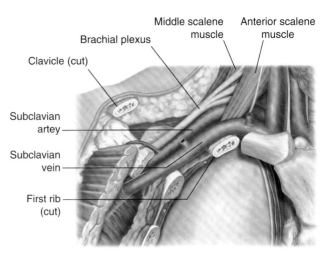

Middle scalene muscle　Anterior scalene muscle
Brachial plexus
Clavicle (cut)
Subclavian artery
Subclavian vein
First rib (cut)

**FIGURE 13-2** Anatomy of the thoracic outlet. The subclavian artery passes over the first rib between the anterior and middle scalene muscles.

subclavian artery. This aberrant right subclavian artery often arises from a dilated segment of the proximal descending aorta known as a Kommerell's diverticulum. While most patients are asymptomatic, some may have difficulty with swallowing from compression of the esophagus (dysphagia lusoria) by the abnormally positioned subclavian artery. Palsy of the recurrent laryngeal nerve can also occur and is called Ortner's syndrome.

The left subclavian artery takes its origin directly from the aortic arch as the third major branch following the left common carotid artery. The vertebral arteries are the first major branches of both the right and left subclavian arteries. The left vertebral artery, however, may originate directly from the aortic arch in 4% to 6% of patients.[1]

Also arising from the subclavian arteries are the thyrocervical and costocervical trunks. These arteries can be distinguished from the vertebral arteries by their multiple branches and lower end-diastolic flow velocities.

The subclavian arteries exit the chest through the thoracic outlet (Fig. 13-2).

In the course of the subclavian artery, there are three distinct sites for potential compression. The first is when the subclavian artery passes over the first rib between the anterior and middle scalene muscles through the scalene triangle. (The subclavian vein passes superficial to the anterior scalene muscle and bypasses the scalene triangle.) The costoclavicular space is bound by the clavicle and first rib and is the second area of possible compression. It is traversed by all three components of the neurovascular bundle. The third (most lateral) space is the pectoralis minor space. It is infrequently involved in symptomatic arterial compression.[2] Upper extremity arterial symptoms may be caused by impingement within the thoracic outlet. The effects on the subclavian artery may include stenosis, aneurysmal dilatation, laminar thrombus, and dynamic compression with arm abduction. The subclavian artery is renamed the axillary artery at the lateral margin of the first rib. The axillary artery lies deep to the pectoralis major and minor muscles. Within the axilla, it is found deep to the axillary fat pad.

The axillary artery transitions to the brachial artery at the level of the inferolateral border of the teres major muscle. This muscle cannot be routinely identified by duplex ultrasound. Here, the artery assumes a more superficial course in the medial arm between the biceps muscle anteriorly and the triceps muscle posteriorly. The deep brachial artery is visualized in the upper arm passing posterior to the humerus. The deep brachial, radial, and ulnar recurrent arteries are important sources of collateral blood flow at the elbow. The most common anatomic variant at this level is a so-called "high takeoff" of the radial artery, where the radial artery originates in the mid to upper arm instead of distal to the antecubital fossa. An accessory or duplicated brachial artery is seen with a prevalence as high as 19% of some angiographic series. Less commonly, the ulnar artery may originate in the upper arm in 2% to 3% of the population.

At the elbow level, the brachial artery passes obliquely from medial to lateral, dividing into the radial, ulnar, and interosseous arteries. The radial artery continues to the wrist deep to the lateral flexor muscles of the forearm (flexor carpi radialis and brachioradialis) before taking a more superficial course at the wrist between the flexor carpi radialis tendon and the radius. This is where the radial artery is readily palpated by physical exam. At the wrist, the radial artery divides into two branches. The superficial branch passes anterior to the thumb where it anastomoses with the superficial palmar arch. The main branch of the radial artery courses posterior to the thumb where it becomes the deep palmar arch.

The ulnar artery gives origin to the interosseous artery in the proximal forearm before passing deep to the medial forearm flexor muscles (flexor digitorium sublimis and flexor carpi ulnaris). The interosseous artery continues to the wrist as the median artery in 2% to 4% of patients.[3] The ulnar artery then courses toward the wrist adjacent to the flexor carpi ulnaris tendon before crossing the wrist where it then passes deep to the hook of the hamate bone. It terminates as the superficial palmar arch. The hamate is an important landmark. Traumatic injury to the ulnar artery in this region can lead to arterial degeneration, thrombus formation, and potential occlusion. This describes the hypothenar hammer syndrome.

Branches from the superficial palmar arch, and to a lesser extent the deep palmar arch via communicating vessels, give origin to the metacarpal arteries. These continue to the digits forming paired digital arteries.

## CLINICAL INDICATIONS

### Raynaud's Syndrome

Many patients presenting with upper extremity ischemia demonstrate a clinical syndrome of intermittent digital ischemia from cold exposure or emotional stimuli. Primary Raynaud's syndrome is a condition of abnormal digital artery vasospasm resulting in pain and a characteristic pallor of the digits followed by cyanosis and hyperemia upon rewarming. Anatomically, the digital arteries appear normal. Primary Raynaud's syndrome generally has a benign prognosis, but Raynaud's type symptoms may be the first manifestations of an underlying systemic disease. When there is an underlying disease process responsible for the symptoms, the terms secondary Raynaud's syndrome, or Raynaud's phenomenon, are used.

The most common systemic condition resulting in secondary Raynaud's syndrome is the autoimmune disorder scleroderma. Other systemic conditions associated with digital artery occlusion include mixed connective tissue disease, systemic lupus erythematosus, rheumatoid arthritis, drug-induced vasospasm, and cancer. Patients with secondary Raynaud's syndrome tend to develop occlusive lesions of the upper extremity digital arteries. Even though patients with primary Raynaud's may present with a dramatic history of transient ischemic changes, they infrequently develop tissue necrosis beyond occasional mild erosions. However, in patients with Raynaud's symptoms, as a result of fixed occlusive lesions of the upper extremity digital arteries, tissue necrosis can develop. The large majority of digital artery occlusive disease originating distal to the wrist is a result of a systemic disorder. Only an important minority of patients have digital occlusion secondary to embolization from a proximal source. Such patients have potentially curable lesions that include subclavian artery aneurysms, aneurysms of branch arteries of the axillary artery, stenotic lesions of the upper extremities arteries, as well as fibromuscular disease of forearm arteries. Duplex ultrasonography can play a role in diagnosis of anatomic abnormalities of the subclavian, axillary, brachial, and forearm arteries.

## Thoracic Outlet Syndrome

Impingement of components of the neurovascular bundle as they traverse the confines of the thoracic outlet can cause symptoms related to the compression of the brachial plexus or vascular structures, but rarely both at the same time. Compression of structures in the thoracic outlet may be secondary to cervical ribs, anomalous first ribs, abnormal fibrous bands, and, possibly, hypertrophy of scalene muscles. Large cervical ribs, or traumatic clavicular, or first rib abnormalities can also compress and damage the subclavian artery. This can result in a poststenotic subclavian artery aneurysm, or stenosis, or occlusion of the subclavian artery. All these abnormalities can be the source of acute or chronic distal embolization to forearm, digital, and palmar arteries. This can lead to occlusion of forearm and digital and palmar arteries and, in more advanced cases, even occlusion of the brachial and axillary arteries, all of which can be detected by arterial duplex ultrasound scanning.

Symptoms of pure neurogenic thoracic outlet syndrome (TOC) may consist of pain, weakness, and muscle atrophy. A definitive diagnosis is made by appropriate history and physical combined with electromyography (EMG) or nerve conduction studies. Demonstration of positional subclavian artery occlusion with arterial duplex ultrasound is often used as "supportive evidence" of neurogenic TOC because impingement of the subclavian artery is thought to suggest impingement of the adjacent neural tissues at the thoracic outlet. However, these provocative maneuvers are not specific, and subclavian artery occlusion can be demonstrated in up to 20% of normal individuals.[4] There is no convincing evidence that arterial duplex ultrasound can or should be used to confirm or suggest a diagnosis of neurogenic TOC.

Venous TOC is another variant of TOC. Patients present with swelling of the arm due to venous obstruction and/or thrombosis. Chapter 18 discusses the use of venous duplex ultrasound in the upper extremity venous system.

Major arterial TOC occurs primarily in younger patients. Repeated trauma to the artery occurs most often in the setting of a bony abnormality that over time leads to stenosis, ulceration, and possible aneurysm formation. Ulcerated lesions or aneurysms can cause thrombus formation and be a source of distal embolization.

Arterial duplex ultrasound or plethysmographic findings suggestive of unilateral digital artery occlusion should prompt a search for a proximal embolic source. Duplex ultrasound can readily identify subclavian artery aneurysms and significant occlusive lesions. However, emboli can also result from seemingly trivial lesions and small aneurysms of branches of the axillary artery. Slight areas of luminal irregularity and branch artery aneurysms are not definitively excluded by arterial duplex ultrasound scanning. When there are unilateral digital artery occlusions and negative proximal arterial duplex ultrasound studies, arteriography or intravascular ultrasound (IVUS) is indicated to definitively rule out a proximal arterial source of emboli.

Some patients with positional occlusion or stenosis of the subclavian artery may be quite symptomatic with activity, especially when working with their arms overhead. In such cases, the subclavian artery is compressed between the clavicle and first rib when the arms are abducted for overhead activity. Duplex ultrasound or plethysmographic techniques can be used to demonstrate positional changes in distal arterial waveforms. It is uncommon for this so-called "arterial minor" form of TOC to result in damage to the arterial wall or cause distal embolization. Treatment, consisting of first rib resection without arterial reconstruction, is only indicated in severely symptomatic patients.

## Blunt and Penetrating Trauma

Currently, the standard of care for identifying clinically significant vascular injuries is catheter-based or computed tomographic (CT) arteriography or direct surgical exploration. There is benefit in performing screening arterial duplex ultrasound examinations in patients with a normal physical exam with a history of blunt or penetrating trauma distal to the axillary crease. One study evaluated 198 patients with 319 potential vascular injuries to the neck or extremities. The mechanism of injury was gunshot wounds in 62%, stabbings in 17%, and blunt trauma in 21%. All patients were hemodynamically stable without a clinically obvious arterial injury. Arterial duplex ultrasound studies correctly diagnosed 23 vascular injuries with two false negative studies, neither of which required intervention, giving a sensitivity of 95% and a specificity of 99%.[5]

Another study evaluated upper extremity trauma patients with an indication for arteriography (with or without clinical signs of arterial injury). Fifty-one injuries were evaluated with both duplex ultrasound and arteriography with an ultrasonographic sensitivity of 90.5% and specificity 100%.[6]

A study of nearly 200 consecutive patients with 225 injuries was also performed to compare ultrasound with angiography or operative exploration.[7] Duplex ultrasound diagnosed 18 injuries, 17 these were confirmed by correlation with angiography and/or surgery. This study gives further evidence that duplex ultrasound serves as an effective means of evaluating for occult upper extremity arterial injury. If immediate operative repair is not indicated, positive findings can be followed up with arteriography and/or serial examinations as clinically appropriate. A well-performed normal arterial duplex ultrasound examination essentially rules out clinically significant injuries of the upper extremity arteries distal to the axillary crease.

## Cardiogenic Arterial Embolism

Duplex ultrasound can be useful in the workup of patients with cardiogenic embolism to the upper extremities and, furthermore, provides a useful modality for successful preoperative revascularization planning. In a retrospective review comparing duplex ultrasonography to CT angiography and contrast angiography, it was noted that the use of duplex ultrasound for preoperative evaluation in patients with upper extremity arterial emboli hold similar surgical outcomes and survival when compared to CT angiography or contrast angiography when utilized for preoperative planning.[8]

## Arterial Occlusive Disease

Clinically important upper extremity atherosclerosis in the absence of renal failure or diabetes is generally confined to the proximal subclavian artery. This is more often seen in the left subclavian artery and is typically an extension of atherosclerotic involvement of the aortic arch. Proximal subclavian artery stenosis, however, can, although infrequently, produce significant upper extremity symptoms. If there are symptoms, they typically manifest as exertional pain in the forearm. Progression to rest pain, ischemic ulceration, or gangrene in the absence of embolization is unusual. Atherosclerosis proximal to the origin of the vertebral artery can result in an anatomic subclavian steal syndrome with reversal or bidirectional flow in the ipsilateral vertebral artery. In order for there to be a true subclavian steal syndrome, there must be posterior circulation symptoms attributable to inadequate blood flow. On duplex ultrasonography, the upper extremity arterial anatomy of an anatomic subclavian steal syndrome is seen as stenosis or occlusion of the subclavian artery as manifested by blunted proximal subclavian artery velocity waveforms along with reversed or staccato flow in the vertebral artery (Fig. 13-3). One study evaluated 7,881 extracranial vessels with duplex ultrasound and found that the greater the blood pressure differential, the greater the likelihood of subclavian steal as demonstrated on duplex ultrasound as flow reversal or staccato flow in the ipsilateral vertebral artery.[9]

Takayasu's arteritis, an autoimmune disorder, affects the arteries of the aortic arch, visceral abdominal aorta, and pulmonary arteries. The disease most commonly affects women in their 20s and 30s. Variants of Takayasu's disease are defined by the arteries involved, which are typically proximal stenoses and occlusions of the great vessels.[3] The classification scheme is based on angiographic arterial involvement. The six types include Type I, branches of the aortic arch; Type IIa, ascending aorta, aortic arch and its branches; Type IIb, ascending aorta, aortic arch and its branches, and thoracic descending aorta; Type III, thoracic descending aorta, abdominal aorta, and/or renal arteries; Type IV, only the abdominal aorta and/or renal arteries; and Type V, combined features of Types IIb and IV. Aortic valve insufficiency and pulmonary hypertension

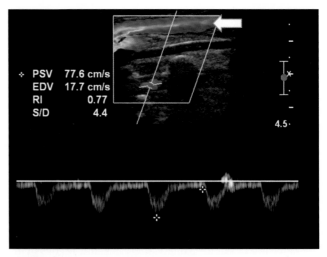

**FIGURE 13-3** Duplex ultrasound color-flow image of a vertebral artery with flow reversal. The flow in the vertebral artery is below the baseline in the Doppler display. Note that with color-flow analysis, the flow in the vertebral artery (*cursor*) is in the same direction as the flow in the internal jugular vein (*white arrow*).

occur in advanced cases involving the proximal ascending aorta and pulmonary arteries, respectively.[10] In the acute phase, Takayasu's arteritis is associated with fever, malaise, arthralgias, and myalgias. Laboratory studies demonstrate an elevated erythrocyte sedimentation rate and C-reactive protein levels. Steroids and immunosuppressive medications are the primary treatment. Arterial duplex ultrasound can be used to monitor response to therapy. After the acute inflammation has subsided, patients who have not responded to medical intervention and have ongoing ischemic symptoms may benefit from vascular reconstruction.

Giant cell arteritis generally affects Caucasian women who are over 40. Takayasu's arteritis and giant cell arteritis are histologically similar; however, the clinical presentation and distribution of lesions are different. Giant cell arteritis can involve the ophthalmic artery as well as the subclavian and axillary arteries. In the acute phase of giant cell arteritis, ultrasound findings of the axillary artery consist of a thickened, hypoechoic arterial wall due to edema in addition to evidence of flow restriction. Anti-inflammatory and immunosuppressant medications are the mainstay of treatment. Following resolution of the acute phase, B-mode images may demonstrate a hyperechoic, fibrotic arterial wall.[11]

Thromboangiitis obliterans, or Buerger's disease, primarily involves the small vessels of the hands and feet. This condition is seen in cigarette smokers typically under the age of 50. Duplex ultrasound is useful to rule out proximal occlusive lesions, but a definitive diagnosis requires exclusion of other underlying causes as well as angiography. It is important to rule out the two most common causes of extremity ischemia, atherosclerosis, and autoimmune disorders, with the available noninvasive vascular studies as well as a battery of serologic laboratory tests prior to determining a diagnosis of Buerger's disease. Most patients will improve with cessation of tobacco use and local wound care therapies.[12]

## SONOGRAPHIC EXAMINATION TECHNIQUES

### Patient Preparation

An explanation of the procedure and obtaining a pertinent history are the initial steps in upper extremity arterial duplex ultrasound scanning. Clothing covering the area to be examined should be removed, and a gown or drape should be provided. Any jewelry, including necklaces, chains, bracelets, and watches, should be removed.

### Patient Positioning

The patient is positioned supine with the head elevated (Fig. 13-4). The evaluation of the axillary artery can be conducted with the arm in the "pledge position" with the arm externally rotated and positioned at a 45 degree angle from the body.

### Scanning Technique

Blood pressures at the brachial artery level are obtained and documented for each arm. Each extremity is examined sequentially to include the subclavian, axillary, brachial, radial, and ulnar arteries. The peak systolic velocities (PSVs) are documented point to point in each major vessel utilizing an optimal 45 to 60 degree transducer angle in the longitudinal plane. When irregularities are noted, Doppler signals are obtained using a "stenosis profile" consisting of a prestenosis PSV, PSV at the stenosis, and documentation of poststenotic turbulence. When an aneurysm is encountered, measurements are obtained in the transverse view of the proximal, mid, and distal site in both the anterior–posterior and lateral orientations. An attempt is made to visualize intraluminal thrombosis. It is important to visualize the

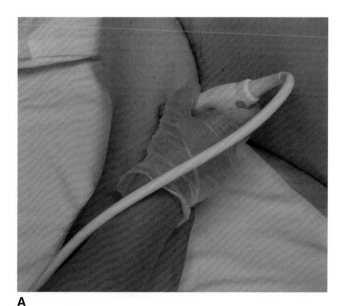

**A**

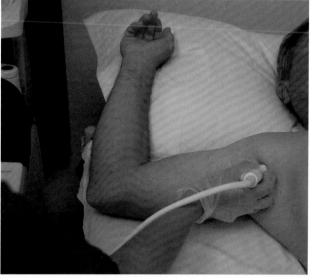

**B**

**FIGURE 13-4** Patient position for upper extremity arterial duplex ultrasound examinations. **A:** The patient is positioned supine with the head of the bed slightly elevated. **B:** Evaluation of the axillary artery can be conducted with the arm in the "pledge position."

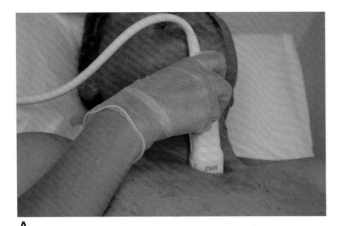

A

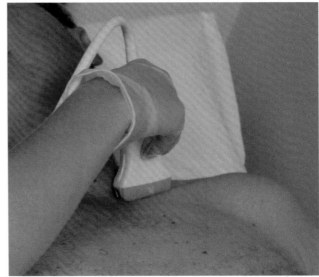

B

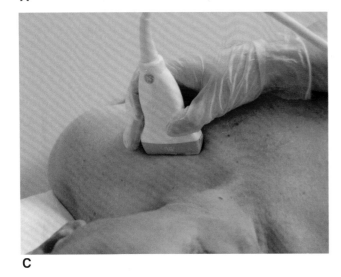

C

**FIGURE 13-5** The windows for the duplex ultrasound assessment of the proximal subclavian artery include (**A**) the sternal notch, (**B**) the supraclavicular approach and (**C**) the infraclavicular appoach.

vessel in a true axial plane so as to not falsely overestimate aneurysm diameter with an oblique view.

Examination of the subclavian artery can generally be accomplished with a 5 MHz transducer. The windows for insonation of the origin of the subclavian artery include the sternal notch, supraclavicular, and infraclavicular approaches (Fig. 13-5A–C).

Obese patients may require a lower MHz transducer. Using the sternal notch window, a recent study found 48 out of 50 right subclavian artery origins and 25 of 50 left subclavian artery origins could be examined.[13] To use the sternal notch approach, a small footprint 3 to 5 MHz transducer is used. The artery may be identified in the transverse view with the assistance of color Doppler. Once the artery is identified, the transducer is rotated 90 degrees to obtain a longitudinal view (Fig. 13-6).

The subclavian artery is followed as it crosses under the clavicle and over the first rib. The axillary artery is identified in an anterior approach deep to the pectoralis major and minor muscles. In the axilla, it is seen deep to the axillary fat pad. The axillary artery becomes the brachial artery after crossing the teres major muscle. There is normally no difference noted in the artery as the subclavian artery becomes the axillary artery. The brachial artery assumes a more superficial course in the medial arm between the biceps muscle anteriorly and the triceps muscles posteriorly.

Views of the proximal, mid, and distal brachial, radial, and ulnar arteries are obtained. Any areas of stenosis, occlusion, or aneurysmal enlargement are documented, as previously described.

Even though upper extremity arterial duplex ultrasound is not clearly indicated to confirm or rule out neurogenic

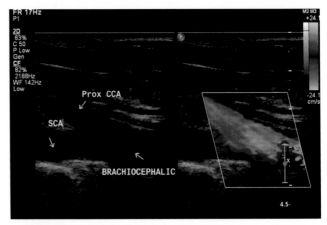

**FIGURE 13-6** Longitudinal color-flow image of the brachiocephalic artery giving rise to the right common carotid artery (CCA) and the right subclavian artery (SCA).

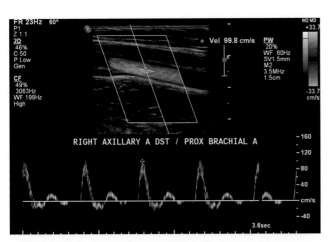

**FIGURE 13-7** A normal high-resistance upper extremity arterial waveform. This triphasic (multiphasic) waveform demonstrates a rapid systolic upstroke and an end systolic flow reversal with minimal or no flow at the end of diastole.

TOS, provocative maneuvers in an attempt to elicit vascular compromise as supportive evidence for possible neurogenic TOS are widely practiced. Patients are examined with a series of provocative positional changes in an attempt to provoke and, therefore, detect subclavian artery compromise. Other noninvasive vascular lab techniques, including segmental pressures with pulse volume recordings (PVR) and/or digital photoplethysmography (PPG) may also be used with these maneuvers. Chapter 11 discusses the utilization of PPG in patients with suspected TOC and also describes these provocative maneuvers. When significant changes are encountered by these noninvasive tests, the subclavian velocities and waveforms should be recorded with duplex ultrasound.

## Pitfalls

Potential impediments to the examination are noted and include the presence of wounds/dressings, intravenous access, and orthopedic fixation devices. Multiple approaches must be used to maximize visualization around these obstacles.

## DIAGNOSIS

The normal upper extremity artery waveform is multiphasic with a sharp systolic peak followed by a brief period of diastolic flow reversal and then minimal continued forward flow in diastole. This is characteristic of normal high-resistance peripheral arteries (Fig. 13-7).

The normal PSVs range from 80 to 120 cm/s in the subclavian arteries and 40 to 60 cm/s in the forearm arteries, with similar velocities in radial and ulnar arteries. Stenosis results in increased PSVs with loss of end systolic reverse flow, poststenotic turbulence, and dampened distal arterial waveforms (Fig. 13-8). There are no generally accepted velocity criteria to determine the degree of stenosis in the upper extremity arteries.[14] General guidelines are listed in Table 13-1.

Arterial duplex ultrasound was performed in 57 patients to evaluate 578 arterial segments in 66 upper extremities

| TABLE 13-1 Duplex Ultrasound Criteria for Evaluation of Upper Extremity Arterial Stenosis | |
|---|---|
| **Condition** | **Characteristics** |
| Normal | Uniform waveforms; biphasic or triphasic (multiphasic) waveforms; clear window beneath systolic peak |
| <50% diameter reduction | Focal velocity increase; spectral broadening; possibly triphasic or biphasic flow |
| >50% diameter reduction | Focal velocity increase; loss of triphasic or biphasic velocity waveforms; poststenotic flow (color bruit) |
| Occlusion | No flow detected |

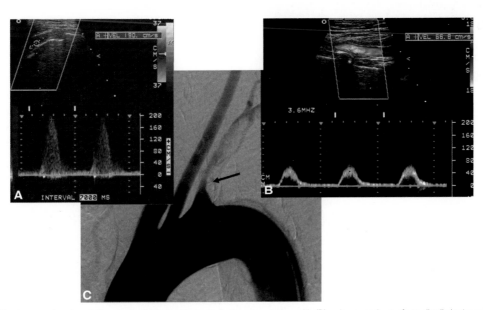

**FIGURE 13-8** **A:** The increased peak systolic velocity (190 cm/s) in a subclavian artery lesion with **(B)** a dampened waveform distally in the subclavian artery suggest the patient's exercise induced arm pain is likely related to the subclavian stenosis. **C:** An angiogram illustrating proximal left subclavian artery stenosis.

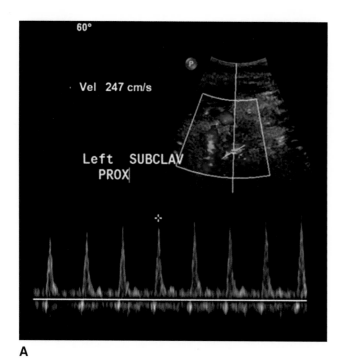
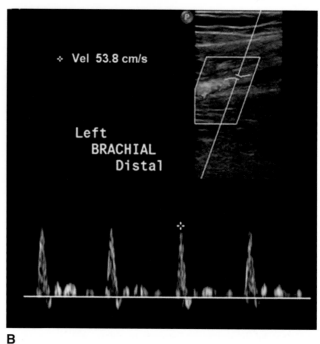

A

B

**FIGURE 13-9** A normal duplex ultrasound examination of the left subclavian and brachial arteries. Angles of insonation can be difficult to determine at the origins of the subclavian arteries. In this case, the elevated left proximal subclavian peak systolic velocity of 247 cm/s (**A**) may not indicate a hemodynamically significant lesion because the distal brachial artery has a normal triphasic Doppler waveform (**B**).

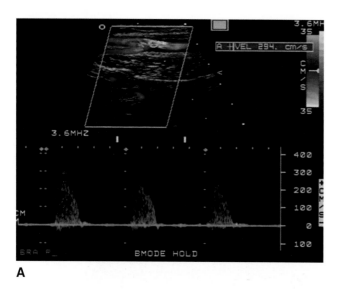

A

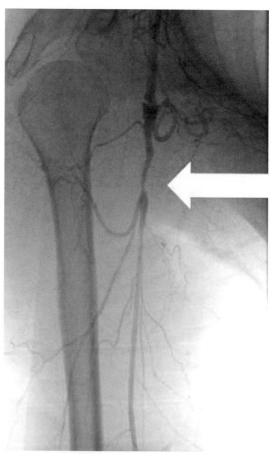

B

**FIGURE 13-10** Duplex ultrasound color-flow image and velocity waveform in a patient with brachial artery stenosis and symptomatic arm ischemia secondary to a crutch injury. **A:** Note the loss of the end systolic reverse flow component of the arterial waveform. **B:** Corresponding angiogram with brachial artery stenosis (*arrow*).

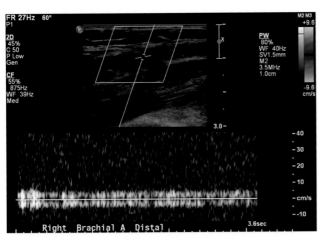

**FIGURE 13-11** Occluded brachial artery with no flow on spectral Doppler or color-flow imaging.

to determine the clinical utility of velocity criteria to detect a >50% stenosis. The criteria utilized for >50% stenosis was a PSV ratio of greater than 2, relating the narrowed segment to that of the artery immediately proximal to the lesion. All of the extremities underwent intra-arterial digital subtraction angiography. Duplex ultrasound correctly identified 15 of 19 hemodynamically significant stenoses, giving a sensitivity of 79% and a specificity of 100%.[15] In another comparison study of duplex ultrasound and angiography loss of diastolic flow reversal was the earliest sign of significant arterial stenosis in 21 patients with ischemic upper extremities when compared to controls.[16] The angle of insonation can be difficult to determine when examining the proximal brachiocephalic arteries. False elevations of PSV, therefore, may occur. The true hemodynamic significance of the stenosis may, however, be inferred from examination of more distal arterial waveforms. A triphasic waveform distal to a high PSV may indicate a falsely elevated proximal PSV (Fig. 13-9), whereas monophasic distal waveforms suggest the proximal lesion is indeed hemodynamically significant. Like in the lower extremity, stenosis in the upper extremity arteries distal to the subclavian artery is primarily diagnosed by focally elevated PSVs with loss of end systolic reverse flow, poststenotic turbulence, and monophasic distal arterial waveforms (Fig. 13-10). Measurement of bilateral brachial artery pressures is also useful to help sort out the hemodynamic significance of an elevated proximal PSV in the subclavian, axillary, or proximal brachial arteries.

## Occlusions

Occlusions are documented by demonstrating the absence of flow within the lumen of the artery by color imaging and spectral Doppler (Fig. 13-11). Power Doppler can also be used to confirm the absence of flow. Care must be taken to properly adjust equipment settings to increase sensitivity to detect low flow states.

In the forearm, there are multiple structures, including tendons, nerves, and muscle fascicles, that may be mistaken for occluded arteries. Fortunately, the arterial anatomy of the forearm is generally constant. The relatively superficial location of the arteries facilitates the vascular sonographer's ability to follow these structures proximally and distally. Although rarely necessary, exercise or warming the extremity can assist in the examination by increasing blood flow.

## Aneurysms

Aneurysms, by definition, are a permanent localized dilation resulting in a 50% increase in the diameter of the artery compared to the diameter of the normal adjacent artery. Several regions of the upper extremity arteries deserve consideration. First, aneurysms of the subclavian artery often occur in association with arterial TOC, accounting for 16/38 (42%) of subclavian artery aneurysms in one series.[17] Arterial TOC is not commonly associated with neurologic or venous symptoms of TOC.

The duplex ultrasound evaluation of subclavian aneurysms can be challenging because of their subtle fusiform nature and location in proximity to the bony landmarks of the thoracic outlet. Examination for outer wall measurement and documentation of mural thrombus are important determinants of aneurysms and can be accomplished with B-mode ultrasound (Fig. 13-12). Atherosclerosis and trauma are also well-known

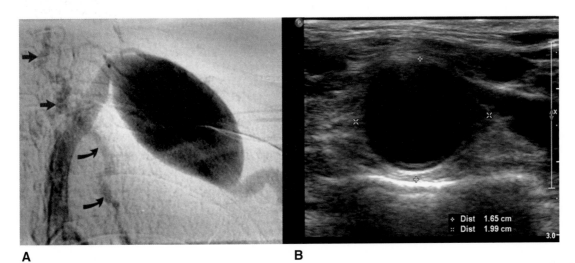

**A**                    **B**

**FIGURE 13-12** Left subclavian artery aneurysm as demonstrated by **(A)** arteriogram and **(B)** duplex ultrasonography.

**PATHOLOGY BOX 13-1**
*Upper Extremity Arterial Pathology*

| Pathology | B-Mode Findings | Doppler Findings | Color/Power Doppler Findings |
|---|---|---|---|
| Atherosclerotic stenosis | Plaque evident along vessel walls producing narrowed vessel lumen | Focal increase in PSV; loss of multiphasic waveform | Focal color aliasing with distal turbulence |
| Occlusion | No visible patent lumen | Absent spectral Doppler signal; high-resistance waveforms proximally | No color or power Doppler signals |
| Aneurysm | A localized dilation with a 50% increase as compared to the adjacent vessel | Turbulence in the dilated region | Turbulence in dilated region; dilated lumen visible on color |
| Raynaud's syndrome | Digital artery occlusion | Diminished digital waveforms on spectral Doppler or PPG | Poor or no color filling of digital vessels |
| Arterial thoracic outlet syndrome | Subclavian artery aneurysm, stenosis, ulceration, thrombus, or occlusion | Focal increase in PSV of subclavian artery or no flow seen with occlusion; Spectral waveforms or PPG changes with provocative maneuvers | Reduced flow lumen at subclavian artery; no color filling seen with occlusion |
| Trauma | Intimal tear or dissection; vessel thrombosis or occlusion | Focal increase in PSV; turbulence in waveforms at site or distally | Poor color filling or turbulent pattern; no color filling with occlusion |

PPG, photoplethysmography; PSV, peak systolic velocity.

etiologies of aneurysms of the axillary, brachial, radial, and ulnar arteries. However, these lesions are infrequent. When encountered, they may present with a pulsatile mass, thrombosis, or embolization. The characterization of these aneurysms is facilitated by the ease of insonation of these arteries.

As discussed previously, the ulnar artery passes deep to the hook of the hamate bone in the hand. This is a site of arterial degeneration which can result from repeated use

of the palm of the hand as a hammer, possibly in conjunction with underlying fibromuscular disease, resulting in the so-called hypothenar hammer syndrome. Patients may present with symptoms of finger ischemia from embolization to digital and palmar arteries.

Pathology Box 13-1 summarizes the diagnostic features of some of the more commonly encountered pathology of the upper extremity arterial system.

## SUMMARY

- A wide range of upper extremity arterial conditions can be evaluated by duplex ultrasound reliably and effectively.
- Pathology of the upper extremity arteries includes stenosis, occlusion, aneurysms, Raynaud's syndrome, arterial TOC, and trauma.
- Combined with the history and physical, as well as other noninvasive vascular laboratory techniques, duplex ultrasound can play a key role in the diagnosis and management of patients with upper extremity arterial disease.

## CRITICAL THINKING QUESTIONS

1. When examining the subclavian artery and its branches, what are two ways you can distinguish the vertebral artery from the other subclavian branches?
2. You are examining the left subclavian artery and obtain a PSV of 270 cm/s within the most proximal segment you

can insonate. What should you do to confirm whether this is a flow-limiting stenosis?
3. You are asked to examine the upper extremities of a 28-year-old female who does not smoke. Her chief complaint is pain in the second and third digits of her right hand. What diagnostic test or tests would you perform and why?

## MEDIA MENU

Student Resources available on thePoint® include:
- Audio glossary
- Interactive question bank
- Videos
- Internet resources

## REFERENCES

1. Rose SC, Kadir S. Arterial anatomy of the upper extremity. In: Kadir S, ed. *Atlas of Normal and Variant Angiographic Anatomy.* Philadelphia, PA: WB Saunders; 1991:55–95.
2. Sanders RJ, Cooper MA, Hammond SL, et al. Neurogenic thoracic outlet syndrome. In: Rutherford R, ed. *Vascular Surgery.* 5th ed. Philadelphia, PA: WB Saunders; 2000:1184–1200.
3. Kaufman JA, Lee MJ. Upper-extremity arteries. In: Kaufman JA, ed. *The Requisites, Vascular and Interventional Radiology.* Philadelphia, PA: Mosby; 2004:144.
4. Longley DG, Yedlicka JW, Molina EJ, et al. Thoracic outlet syndrome: evaluation of the subclavian vessels by color duplex sonography. *AJR Am J Roentgenol.* 1992;158(3):623–630.
5. Bynoe RP, Miles WS, Bell RM, et al. Noninvasive diagnosis of vascular trauma by duplex ultrasonography. *J Vasc Surg.* 1991;14(3):346–352.
6. Kuzniec S, Kauffman P, Monar LJ, et al. Diagnosis of limbs and neck arterial trauma using duplex ultrasonography. *J Cardiac Surg.* 1998;6(4):358–366.
7. Fry WR, Smith RS, Sayers DV, et al. The success of duplex ultrasonographic scanning in diagnosis of extremity vascular proximity trauma. *Arch Surg.* 1993;128:1368–1372.
8. Crawford JD, Annen A, Azarbal AF, et al. Arterial duplex for diagnosis and operative planning of peripheral arterial emboli. *J Vasc Surg.* 2015;61(6):29S–30S.
9. Labropoulos N, Nandivada P, Bekelis K. Prevalence and impact of the subclavian steal syndrome. *Ann Surg.* 2010;252(1):166–170.
10. Hata A, Noda M, Moriwaki R, et al. Angiographic findings of Takayasu arteritis: new classification. *Int J Cardiol.* 1996;54:S155–S163.
11. Schmidt WA, Kraft HE, Borkowski A, et al. Color duplex ultrasonography in large-vessel giant cell arteritis. *Scand J Rheumatol.* 1999;28(6):374–376.
12. Mills JL, Taylor LM, Porter JM. Buerger's disease in the modern era. *Am J Surg.* 1987;154:123–129.
13. Yurdakul M, Tola M, Uslu OS. Color Doppler ultrasonography in occlusive diseases of the brachiocephalic and proximal subclavian arteries. *J Ultrasound Med.* 2008;27:1065–1070.
14. Jager KA, Phillips DJ, Martin RL, et al. Noninvasive mapping of lower limb arterial lesions. *Ultrasound Med Biol.* 1985;11:515–521.
15. Tola M, Yurdakul M, Okten S, et al. Diagnosis of arterial occlusive disease of the upper extremities: comparison of color duplex sonography and angiography. *J Clin Ultrasound.* 2003;31:407–411.
16. Taneja K, Jain R, Sawhney S, et al. Occlusive arterial disease of the upper extremity: colour Doppler as a screening technique and for assessment of distal circulation. *Australas Radiol.* 1996;40(3):226–229.
17. Bower TC, Pairolero PC, Hallett JW Jr, et al. Brachiocephalic aneurysm: the case for early recognition and repair. *Ann Vasc Surg.* 1991;5:125–132.

# Ultrasound Assessment of Arterial Bypass Grafts

PETER W. LEOPOLD | ANN MARIE KUPINSKI

**CHAPTER 14**

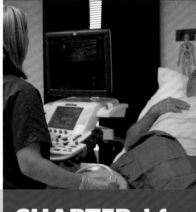

## OBJECTIVES

- Describe the types of common arterial bypass grafts
- Define the essential components of an arterial bypass scan, including grayscale, color, and spectral Doppler requirements
- Describe the normal hemodynamic profiles of arterial bypass grafts
- List the diagnostic criteria employed for identifying a bypass stenosis, occlusion, and other pathology

## GLOSSARY

**anastomosis** A surgically created joining of two vessels that were formerly not connected

**arteriovenous fistula** A connection between an artery and a vein that was created as a result of surgery or by other iatrogenic means

**bypass** A channel that diverts blood flow from one artery to another, usually done to shunt flow around an occluded portion of a vessel

**graft** A conduit that can be prosthetic material or autogenous vein used to divert blood flow from one artery to another

**hyperemia** An increase in blood flow. This can occur following exercise. It can also occur following restoration of blood flow following periods of ischemia

**in situ bypass** The great saphenous vein is left in place in its normal anatomical position and used to create a diversionary channel for blood flow around an occluded artery

## KEY TERMS

**arteriovenous fistula**

**autogenous vein**

**bypass**

**distal anastomosis**

**graft**

**hyperemia**

**in situ bypass**

**orthograde vein bypass**

**prosthetic graft**

**proximal anastomosis**

**reverse vein bypass**

Duplex ultrasound evaluation of arterial bypass grafts has become a well-recognized fundamental component in postoperative follow-up and management. Careful monitoring of patients with infrainguinal bypasses has clearly shown to improve long-term patency rates.[1] There are several noninvasive methods that can be used to evaluate bypass function, including clinical assessment, indirect assessment with systolic pressure measurements and plethysmographic waveforms, and lastly direct assessment with ultrasound. Clinical assessment of patient symptoms and physical examination of the limb often fails to identify problems early. Prior studies have shown that ultrasound can detect significant pathology in asymptomatic patients and before a measureable change in physiologic testing results.[2] However, there is a complementary role for ultrasound and indirect physiologic testing. Combining duplex ultrasound with physiologic testing provides both direct assessment of the bypass conduit itself and indirect assessment of global limb perfusion. This chapter will focus on the use of duplex ultrasound to evaluate lower extremity bypass grafts. Using these methods, disease can be detected early, prior to bypass graft thrombosis, and thus aid the long-term maintenance of graft patency.

## TYPES OF BYPASS GRAFTS

The types of bypass grafts can be categorized by the components of the graft and the surgical techniques employed. There are two main types of bypass graft materials. Prosthetic (synthetic) bypass grafts are made of various manufactured materials, including polytetrafluoroethylene (PTFE) and woven composites such as Dacron. The preferred bypass graft material is autogenous vein, and this chapter will focus primarily on this type of graft. The great saphenous vein, small saphenous vein, cephalic vein, and basilic vein can all be used as bypass conduit. Vein grafts have better long-term patency than synthetic grafts by being less thrombogenic than their synthetic counterparts.[3-7] Although vein grafts are the preferred bypass of choice, they have the potential for early failure, and early surveillance is recommended.[8] PTFE grafts have a low potential for early technical failure and ultrasound-detected abnormalities. However, these PTFE grafts have a distinctly worse long-term success rate because of progressive stenoses, usually at the inflow or outflow arteries, which will be detectable on ultrasound usually later in the grafts' history. Another type of bypass graft is a cryopreserved human allograft. This type of material is not commonly used for lower extremity bypasses; however, ultrasound evaluation of these graft types would be similar to those outlined in this chapter.

## In Situ Bypass Grafts

Because bypass grafts using autogenous vein can be constructing using various surgical techniques, these grafts are further described based on the surgery employed. An in situ bypass graft is performed using the great saphenous vein left in place or in situ within its natural tissue bed. Tributaries of the vein are ligated, and the valves within the vein are lyzed. This allows a downward flow of blood without the need to reverse the vein and allows the larger end of the great saphenous to be anastomosed to the larger artery proximally (inflow artery) and the smaller end to be anastomosed distally, usually to a smaller artery such as a tibial artery (outflow artery). This provides a conduit where one end can then be sutured to an artery proximal to the site of disease (the inflow artery) and the other end of the vein conduit is sutured to an artery distal to the distal (the outflow artery). There is often a preference for this type of orientation when the proximal and distal vein sizes match more closely the size of the arteries at the anastomotic sites.

## Orthograde and Retrograde Bypass Grafts

The great saphenous vein and other autogenous veins can also be used as a free vein graft where the vein is completely dissected free from it natural position in the body. This conduit can be placed in an orthograde position where the proximal portion of the vein is used for the proximal anastomosis and the distal portion of the vein is used at the distal anastomosis. In this position, the valves with the vein will need to be lyzed so that blood can flow freely. A free vein graft can also be placed in a retrograde (reversed) position where the vein now has the smaller distal end of the vein anastomosed to the inflow artery and the larger proximal end of the vein is anastomosed to the outflow artery. Essentially, the vein is flipped or reversed so the valves leaflets do not need to be removed, and there is no barrier to blood flow.

## Bypass Graft Placement

The actual position of a bypass is determined by the level of arterial disease. The proximal anastomosis is commonly performed using the common femoral or superficial femoral artery as the inflow artery (Fig. 14-1). Less commonly, the popliteal can be used as the inflow artery. Rarely, the profunda femoral artery is used as the inflow artery. The surgeon will pick an inflow artery that is free of disease and proximal to the stenosis or occlusion that needs to be bypassed. The distal anastomosis is generally constructed below the level of the most distal site of arterial disease. Thus, the outflow artery can be the popliteal artery (either the above-knee or below-knee portions), the tibioperoneal trunk, or any of the tibial-level vessels (anterior tibial, posterior tibial, or peroneal arteries). Occasionally, the distal anastomosis of a bypass may be to the dorsalis pedis artery. Given the options for conduit type, orientation, and anatomical position, it can save a great deal of time if the sonographer or technologist refers to an operative note when examining a bypass graft.

## MECHANISMS OF BYPASS GRAFT FAILURE

When performing ultrasound examinations on bypass grafts, it is important to have a firm understanding of normal bypass findings, but equally important is knowing the types of problems that may exist. There are distinct problems that arise at specific time periods during the lifetime of a bypass graft.

During the first 30 days following surgery, ultrasound scanning will identify technical problems that can lead to

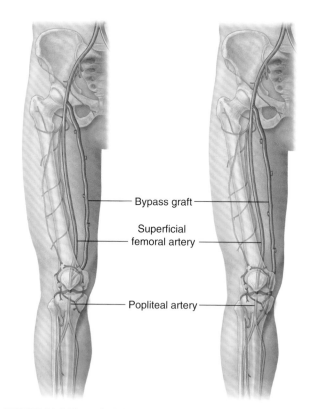

**FIGURE 14-1** Types of vein bypass grafts. The inset on the left illustrates a common femoral to popliteal bypass, while on the right the bypass is from the common femoral artery to the tibioperoneal trunk.

bypass failure. There may be a retained valve or valve leaflet, an intimal flap caused by the surgical instrumentation of the vein conduit, problems at the anastomotic sites because of suture placement, or possible graft entrapment because of improper positioning of a free vein graft. Additionally, a bypass may thrombose because of the use of an inadequate venous conduit or limited runoff bed. Occasionally, early thrombosis can also occur in some patients with a hypercoagulable state. Perioperative bypass graft failure accounts for one-fourth of all failures.[9]

Between months 1 and 24, myointimal hyperplasia can develop, leading to a bypass stenosis. This is not atherosclerotic plaque and has a different ultrasound appearance. A stenosis can occur at any point within the conduit, but often a stenosis develops at a valve site. A stenosis can also occur at either the proximal or distal anastomoses. Of all, 11% to 33% bypasses will have these types of stenoses occur and often they appear within the first year, causing 75% of all revisions performed during this postoperative period.[10]

After 24 months, progression of atherosclerotic disease occurs within the inflow or outflow vessels. It is important to pay close attention to spectral waveform characteristics within the bypass itself because changes in these waveforms may help identify disease in native vessels remote to the bypass graft itself. Loss of diastolic flow is routinely seen within vein bypasses within the first few weeks of surgery, particularly when carried out for critical limb-threatening ischemia. However, significant changes in diastolic flow after this early phase, in addition to a possible increase in rise time and or decreases in peak systolic velocity (PSV), can all be signals of development of pathology elsewhere. Aneurysmal dilation of the venous conduit or at the anastomotic sites can develop during this late time period necessitating graft revision.[11] These aneurysmal dilations are rare but can result in late bypass graft thrombosis if not corrected.

## SONOGRAPHIC EXAMINATION TECHNIQUES

Without any specific indications, duplex ultrasound scanning is performed on bypass grafts at routine intervals as part of standard postoperative care. There are instances where duplex ultrasound can be performed which do not follow the routine surveillance schedule. If a patient presents with acute onset of pain, diminished or absent pedal pulses, persistent nonhealing ulcers or a recent history of loss of limb swelling (normally found in most successful vein bypass grafts) suggestive of graft failure and ischemia, a duplex ultrasound scan can be performed. Poor physiologic testing results, including an ankle-brachial index which falls by greater than 0.15, would also be an appropriate indication for a duplex ultrasound scan.

A routine surveillance protocol can consist of an ultrasound performed early in the postoperative period, usually within the first 3 months. Subsequent ultrasounds can be performed at 3-month intervals for the first year, every 6-month for the second postoperative year, and then annually thereafter. In most laboratories, direct ultrasound scanning is performed in conjunction with indirect physiologic testing, including ankle pressures and plethysmographic waveforms. Pulse volume recordings can be safely performed over bypass grafts because the cuff pressures are low enough not to occlude the grafts. Many laboratories choose to avoid measuring

systolic pressures at levels where cuffs are placed over the grafts. In cases of grafts with distal tibial or pedal outflow vessels, toe pressures and waveforms can be recorded. At a minimum, an ankle-brachial index measurement should accompany an ultrasound examination of a bypass graft.

There are patients in whom surveillance should be more intense. Patients who have undergone an intraoperative revision, early postoperative thrombectomy or revision, and patients with limited venous conduits, should be scanned more frequently. Many surgeons will choose to follow these patients at 2-month intervals.

The surveillance of prosthetic bypass grafts is less common. Many laboratories may follow these patients with physiologic testing and clinical evaluation. It has been shown that duplex ultrasound is more sensitive in determining prosthetic grafts failure than an ankle-brachial index or clinical examination.[12]

### Patient Preparation

As with any examination, the procedures should be explained to the patient, taking into consideration the age and mental status of the patient. If relatives or caregivers are present, they can be used to assist with the explanation if necessary.

As noted earlier in this chapter, another consideration prior to the beginning of the ultrasound is review of the patient's operative notes. An operative note provides important information about the specific course and composition of the bypass graft that can be used as a guide to facilitate bypass graft imaging.

### Patient Positioning

The patient should be positioned supine with the head of the bed slightly elevated. The limb to be examined should be externally rotated at the hip, and the knee slightly bent. In those patients with various joint conditions such as arthritis, a small pillow may be placed under the knee to avoid joint pain. The patient should be resting comfortably for a few minutes prior to the recording of any velocity measurements.

### Equipment

Various transducer frequencies can be used to image bypass grafts. For superficial in situ bypass grafts, a transducer with imaging frequencies of 10 to 12 MHz will provide optimal near-field imaging. For deeper bypass grafts, imaging frequencies of 5 to 7 MHz will be needed. The technologists and sonographers must remember that many of the ultrasound transducers commonly used today have multiple grayscale imaging, color imaging, and Doppler frequencies. These frequencies can and should be adjusted if the course of the bypass is such that various tissue depths are encountered.

### Required Documentation

Individual laboratory protocols vary slightly; however, there are several essential elements that need to be documented. The following lists the minimum suggested documentation; however, additional images are often necessary. Grayscale images should be recorded of the inflow artery, proximal anastomosis, mid graft, distal anastomosis, and outflow artery. At each of these locations, a spectral Doppler waveform

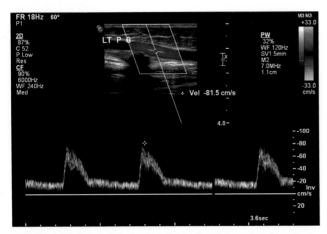

**FIGURE 14-2** Appropriate placement of the Doppler sample volume (center stream) and alignment of the Doppler angle (parallel to the walls of the vessel).

should also be recorded with the PSV measured. If color-flow imaging is part of the protocol, color-flow images should be documented at the same sites. In the case of any abnormalities, additional documentation in grayscale, spectral Doppler, and color should be recorded. For any stenotic areas, spectral Doppler needs to noted prior to the stenotic region, at the area of greatest velocity shift, and distal to the stenotic region.

These requirements are based on current standards established by the Intersocietal Accreditation Commission-Vascular Testing (IAC VT).[13]

## Scanning Technique

The examination should begin with the selection of the appropriate transducer based on body habitus and bypass depth. The ultrasound system application preset for peripheral arterial imaging should be chosen. The ultrasound system controls for grayscale, spectral Doppler, and color should be optimized specific to each patient and adjusted as needed during the course of the examination.

Proper Doppler techniques should be followed. Spectral analysis should be recorded at approximately a 60 degrees whenever possible. Angles greater than 60 degrees should never be used. Angles less than 60 degrees may need to be used depending on the course of the vessel. If this is a follow-up examination, one should try to use the same angles previously employed to avoid additional variations in data owing to the angle of insonation. The sample volume placement should be in the center of the vessel or flow channel (Fig. 14-2). The sample volume should be small unless searching for a small jet or total vessel occlusion.

As mentioned in the preceding section, if disease is present within any portion of a vessel or graft, record the spectral analysis with the greatest Doppler shift as well as proximal and distal to this area, if possible. This is often referred to as "walking through" the stenosis. The PSV is recorded, and in some laboratories, the end-diastolic velocity (EDV) is also noted. Poststenotic turbulence should be documented. All this information is helpful for the interpreting physician to properly categorize the severity of a stenosis.

The ultrasound examination should begin within the inflow vessel. Vessels can initially be identified using transverse or sagittal views. Using a transverse view, an initial rough scan of the full length of the bypass as well as inflow and outflow vessels can help orient the vascular technologist or sonographer prior to beginning the formal scanning. Once the inflow artery is identified, the examination should be then performed using a sagittal orientation. A representative grayscale image should be recorded of the inflow artery (Fig. 14-3). Typically, the end of the vein

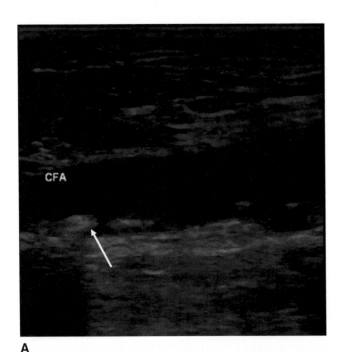

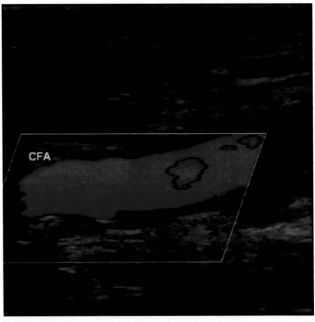

**A**　　　　　　　　　　　　　　　　　　**B**

**FIGURE 14-3 A:** A grayscale image of the common femoral artery which is the inflow source for an in situ bypass graft. A mild amount of plaque is present along the posterior wall of the vessel (*arrow*). **B:** The same portion of the vessel with color-flow imaging.

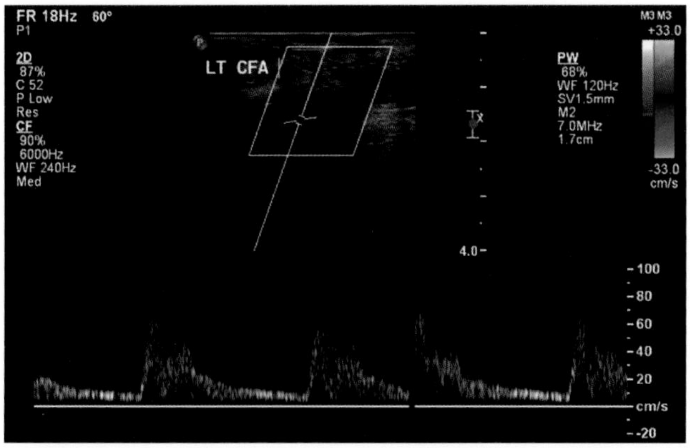

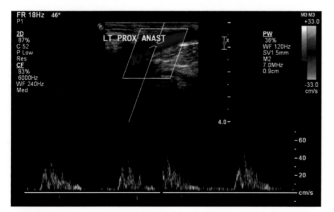

**FIGURE 14-4** A normal Doppler spectrum obtained from the common femoral artery which is the inflow source for an in situ bypass graft.

conduit is anastomosed to the side of the inflow artery. This allows for flow down the bypass conduit as well as some flow to be maintained within the native distal artery. This orientation will provide for some nutritive flow into the native arterial bed, including any collaterals which may be present. Any pathology observed should be documented in both transverse and sagittal planes. A transverse orientation is particularly helpful to identify patent tributaries of an in situ bypass graft. A spectral Doppler waveform is obtained, and the PSV is recorded (Fig. 14-4).

Color-flow imaging can be used to facilitate vessel identification and with following the course of a bypass graft. However, color will often mask small wall defects and other pathology. Color imaging should be documented at the various levels where grayscale and spectral Doppler images are recorded (see Fig. 14-3). Color-flow imaging should also be documented in stenotic areas to illustrate the disturbed flow patterns and aliasing, if present.

The scan proceeds through the proximal anastomosis. Again, at this point grayscale, color and spectral Doppler are recorded. It is not uncommon to observe some slight changes in velocity or minimal disturbed flow (Fig. 14-5). There is typically a change in caliber as one moves from the inflow artery through the anastomosis and into the proximal segment of the bypass that results in a small disruption of the laminar flow profile. This is also encountered at any point where blood flow changes direction, such

as around a bend or kink, because the various vectors of the moving blood will change around a curve. Continuing down the leg, the entire portion of each bypass graft should be examined. Simultaneous duplex mode observing both the grayscale image and spectral Doppler analysis is ideal method for looking and listening for any potential bypass problems. When a "walk through" is used, listening to Doppler signal changes is a highly sensitive tool to localize abnormalities with an increase in velocities for more careful analysis. At a minimum, grayscale, color, and spectral Doppler should be recorded in the mid-graft region; however, a more thorough protocol would include these images documented from the proximal, mid, and distal segments (Fig. 14-6).

The examination concludes with continuing to scan through the distal anastomosis and into the outflow artery (Fig. 14-7). At both of these levels, grayscale, color, and spectral Doppler are recorded. The distal anastomosis may also exhibit mild turbulence caused by the geometry of the anastomosis and the slight disruption in the laminar flow profile. One can often encounter an increase in PSV within the outflow artery because this may be a smaller caliber than the bypass conduit itself (Fig. 14-8).

The primary goal of the examination is to document anatomic and hemodynamic characteristics of the bypass graft and adjacent vessels. It is also important to use the hemodynamic information within or near the bypass to determine if additional testing is required. Abnormal waveforms may suggest pathology remote to the region, thus justifying extending the ultrasound examination further proximally or distally. These waveforms will be discussed later in the chapter.

Even though the focus of the examination is on the bypass, the scanning protocol should include documentation of incidental findings. Other pathology such as venous thrombosis, dilated lymph nodes, hematoma, seroma, abscesses, and similar structures can be encountered. Length, width, and depth of masses, cysts, nodes, or other structures should be recorded. Color-flow and spectral Doppler can be used to document the presence or absence of blood flow within an incidental finding. Multiple scanning planes should be used to fully document the additional pathology. Proximity to the bypass graft is also important to note particularly in the event of an abscess.

## Pitfalls

This examination can be slightly limited in a very obese patient. A bypass graft which is anatomically placed and tunneled deeply will necessitate the use of lower frequency transducers in order to penetrate deep enough to visualize the graft; however, this will result in poorer resolution. Dressings, skin staples, and sutures will also limit accessibility of portions of the bypass grafts to the ultrasound examination.

## DIAGNOSIS

There are three components to the analysis of the data obtained from ultrasound: the B-mode or grayscale image, the spectral Doppler waveform (which is the primary source of quantitative data used to classify disease), and the color-flow image.

**FIGURE 14-5** A Doppler spectrum taken at the proximal anastomosis of a bypass graft. Slight turbulence is present.

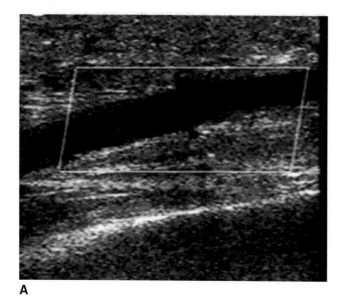

A

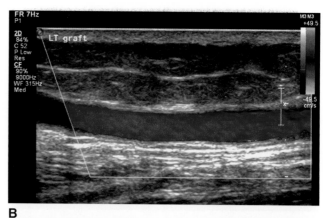

B

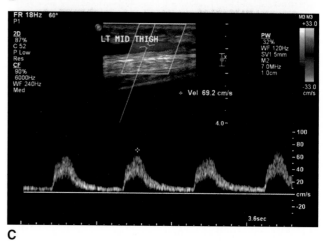

C

**FIGURE 14-6** Normal appearance of the midportion of a bypass graft. **(A)** Grayscale image, **(B)** color-flow image, and **(C)** Doppler spectrum.

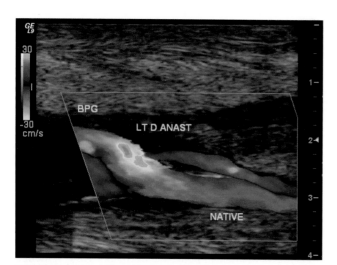

**FIGURE 14-7** An ultrasound image of a distal anastomosis to a posterior tibial artery. (Image courtesy of Phillip J. Bendick, PhD RVT, Royal Oak, MI.)

## Grayscale Findings

The B-mode or grayscale image should be closely examined for disease. The walls of a vein graft normally appear smooth and uniform. Figure 14-9 illustrates the normal grayscale appearance of a vein bypass graft and a PTFE graft. The intimal–medial layer should be clearly visible if the bypass graft is perpendicular to the ultrasound beam.

Within the inflow and outflow arteries, atherosclerotic plaque may be present. Plaque should be characterized as homogeneous or heterogeneous. Homogeneous plaques have uniform echogenicity. Heterogeneous plaques have mixed-level echoes within the plaques. Calcification, which appears as bright white echoes causing acoustic shadowing, should be noted (Fig. 14-10). If possible, the surface characteristics of a plaque should be noted. This can be described as smooth surfaced or irregularly surfaced.

Within the vein conduit itself, the two most common image abnormalities that can be observed are valves and myointimal hyperplasia. Valves or valve remnants may be present because of incomplete valve disruption during surgery (Fig. 14-11). Small remnants will have a minimal impact on flow through bypass. Larger remnants or completely intact leaflets will produce a flow-limiting stenosis (Fig. 14-12). Myointimal hyperplasia can occur along any point of the bypass conduit but typically takes place in areas where the vein has sustained injury or at the site of a valve sinus. Myointimal hyperplasia is a rapid proliferation of cells into the intimal layer of the cell wall which can result in a stenosis (Fig. 14-13).

Dissections, intimal flaps, aneurysms, or pseudoaneurysms may also be present on the ultrasound image. Intimal flaps will appear as small, confined projections into the vessel lumen made up of a segment of the vessel wall which has separated from the remainder of the wall. An intimal flap may progress and extend over several centimeters at which

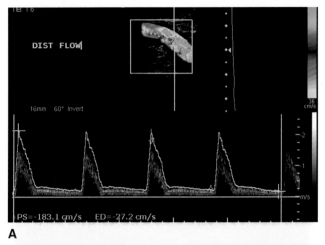

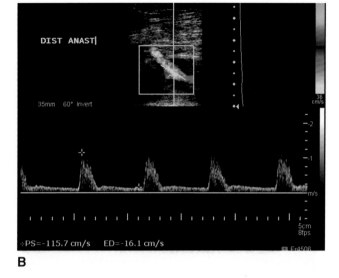

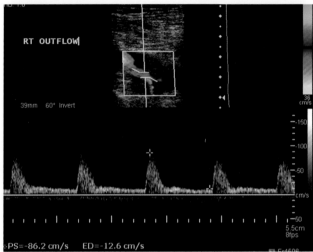

**FIGURE 14-8** Spectral Doppler tracing through a distal anastomosis. **(A)** Distal bypass, **(B)** distal anastomosis, and **(C)** outflow artery.

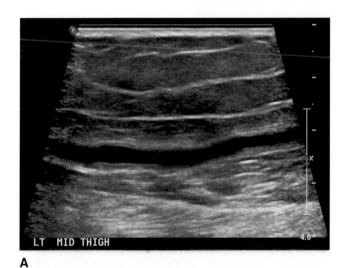

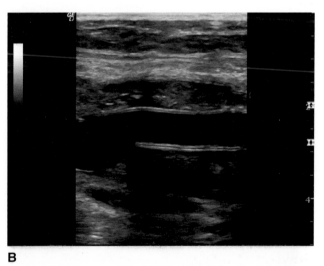

**FIGURE 14-9** Normal grayscale appearance of various types of bypass grafts. **A:** Autogenous vein. (Image courtesy of Debra Joly, RVT RDMS, Houston, TX.) **B:** PTFE. (Image courtesy of William Zang, BS RVT RDMS, GE Healthcare, Wauwatosa, WI.)

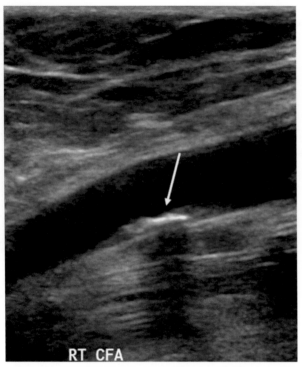

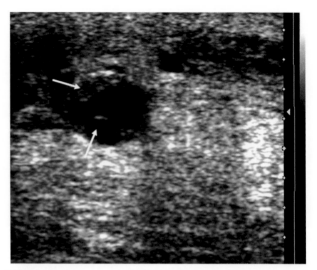

FIGURE 14-11 A transverse image of a retained valve (*arrows*) within an in situ bypass.

**FIGURE 14-10** A grayscale image of the common femoral artery proximal to a bypass graft. The image demonstrates heterogeneous calcific plaque (*arrow*) within the common femoral artery. (Image courtesy of Debra Joly, RVT RDMS, Houston, TX.)

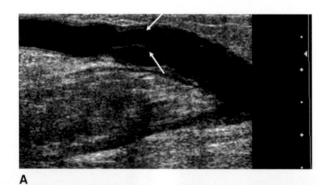

A

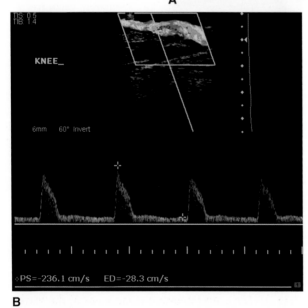

B

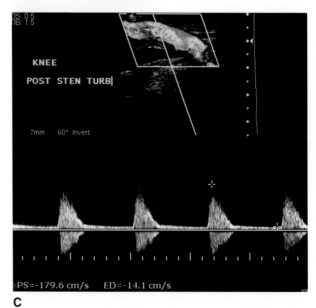

C

**FIGURE 14-12** A stenosis at a retained valve. **A:** The valve (*arrows*) shown in a sagittal view. **B:** Spectral Doppler waveform at the stenosis with a PSV of 236 cm/s. **C:** A spectral Doppler waveform illustrating poststenotic turbulence.

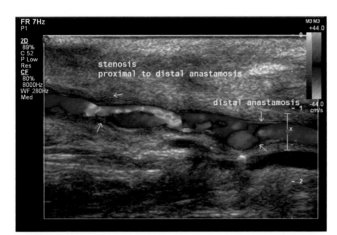

FIGURE 14-13 An image of a bypass stenosis due to myointimal hyperplasia.

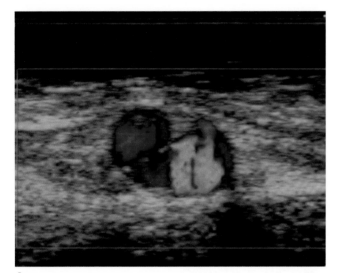

A

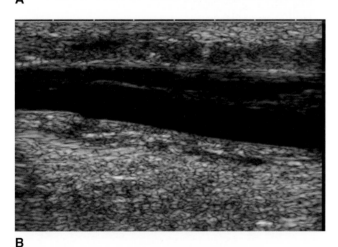

B

FIGURE 14-14 A: A transverse image of a vein bypass graft with a dissection. Color flow is observed in both the true lumen and the false lumen. B: A sagittal view of a bypass with a dissection.

point it is usually referred to as a dissection (Fig. 14-14). Intimal flaps and dissections can occur early on in the life of a bypass graft owing to technical problems which take place during surgery.

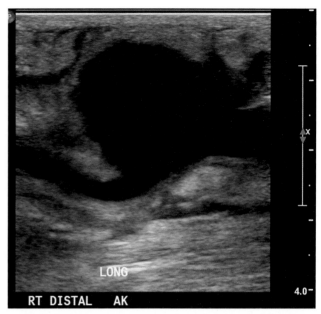

FIGURE 14-15 A sagittal image of a vein bypass graft with a focal aneurysmal dilation. (Image courtesy of Debra Joly, RVT RDMS, Houston, TX.)

Aneurysmal dilatation can sometimes be observed in the native artery near the anastomosis. This can occur adjacent to the suture line because it is thought the vessel wall may be slightly weaker at this point. Occasionally, in older bypass grafts, the vein wall itself can become weakened and dilate. Aneurysmal dilation can manifest as a focal dilation or diffuse dilation of the bypass graft over a long segment. As with aneurysmal native arteries, a dilation equal to 1.5 times the caliber of the adjacent vessel is considered aneurysmal (Fig. 14-15). Pseudoaneurysms are a rare pathology encountered and usually form at anastomotic sites. The most common site would be the common femoral artery in the groin at the outflow of a prosthetic aortofemoral or femorofemoral crossover graft.

Some findings observed on the grayscale image are not part of the bypass itself but may be contained within the tissue adjacent to the bypass. Figure 14-16A illustrates a vein bypass graft with a large perigraft fluid accumulation which was determined to be a hematoma. Figure 14-16B illustrates a transverse view of an accumulation of fluid surrounding a PTFE graft.

## Color-Flow Imaging

Color-flow imaging is considered to be an adjunctive tool in the diagnosis of bypass graft pathology. Color-flow imaging can indicate mild changes in flow profiles and slightly disturbed laminar flow patterns which are consistent with mild degrees of stenosis. As a stenosis worsens, color aliasing will be evident (Fig. 14-17). These changes in the color patterns should alert the technologist to examine the grayscale image and spectral Doppler carefully for the presence of an abnormality.

## Spectral Analysis

Normal bypass grafts should demonstrate multiphasic waveforms with a sharp upstroke and a narrow systolic peak (Fig. 14-18A). An important component of the waveform

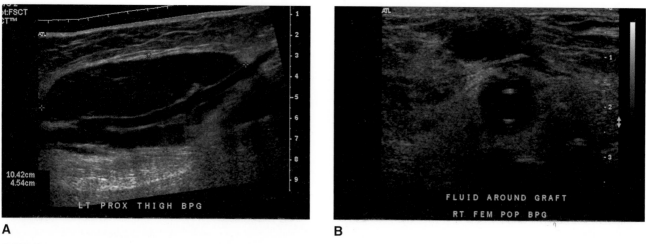

**FIGURE 14-16  A:** A sagittal view of a vein bypass graft with a fluid accumulation adjacent to the graft. **B:** A transverse view of a PTFE graft with fluid surrounding the graft. (Images courtesy of William Zang, BS RVT RDMS, GE Healthcare, Wauwatosa, WI.)

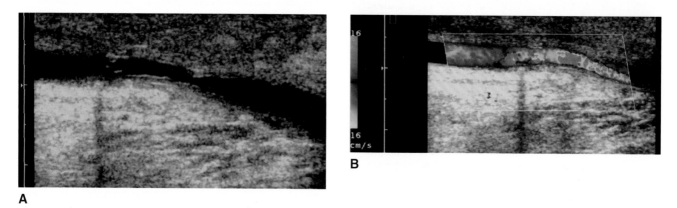

**FIGURE 14-17**  Images of a mid-bypass stenosis. **A:** The grayscale image demonstrates narrowing of the lumen with echogenic material along the bypass graft walls. **B:** The color-flow image displays normal color filling within the bypass near the left of the image then color aliasing along the region of the stenosis.

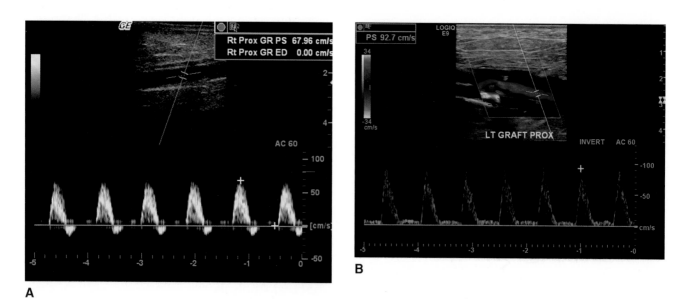

**FIGURE 14-18**  Normal multiphasic Doppler signals from vein bypass grafts: **(A)** reverse or retrograde flow in diastole and **(B)** antegrade flow through diastole.

is the reverse flow observed during early diastole. This is indicative of a normal high-resistance peripheral arterial bed. Many bypass grafts will not display a reverse flow component in diastole, particularly in the early postoperative period. These grafts will display antegrade flow throughout diastole (Fig. 14-18B). Continuous diastolic flow may be present in some bypass grafts due to hyperemia or arteriovenous fistulae. This waveform will demonstrate a normal sharp rise to peak systole with continuous forward flow in diastole, indicating a decrease in resistance distally, associated with a low-resistance outflow bed.

An arteriovenous fistula is a complication unique to in situ bypass grafts. This type of fistula occurs when a tributary of the great saphenous vein connects, directly or indirectly, via a perforator with the deep venous system and is left unligated after creation of the bypass. A perforating vein normally has valves which direct flow from the superficial to the deep venous system. Thus, once the great saphenous vein is arterialized as a bypass conduit, there is no impedance to blood flow through the bypass graft, into the perforating vein (now acting as a fistula), and into the deep venous system. This low-resistance path can divert a great deal of blood flow into the venous system. The Doppler spectrum of the bypass graft proximal to the level of the fistula will display constant antegrade flow. Distal to the fistula, the bypass graft Doppler spectrum will exhibit no or little diastolic flow.

A blunted, monophasic pattern with zero diastolic flow is abnormal. This type of waveform indicates an abnormally high resistance to flow distally (Fig. 14-19). This is often associated with a stenosis or occlusion distally within the bypass or outflow vessels. This can sometimes progress to a staccato waveform with minimal forward flow in systole.

Another type of abnormal bypass spectrum is a waveform with continuous diastolic flow and a prolonged rise to peak systole. This dampened and delayed pattern is observed distal to a high-grade stenosis (Fig. 14-20). Energy losses across a stenosis will produce lower velocities distal to a stenosis and result in a broadened peak. The physiologic affects of an arterial stenosis are discussed further in detail in Chapter 5 of this book.

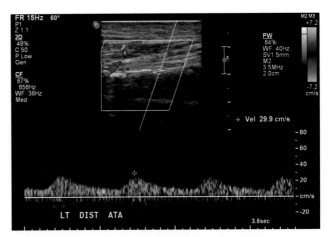

**FIGURE 14-20** An abnormal waveform with a prolonged upstroke taken from an anterior tibial artery distal to an in situ bypass with a high-grade stenosis. (Image courtesy of Debra Joly, RVT RDMS, Houston, TX.)

While pattern recognition will provide clues to the overall function of a bypass graft, categorizing a stenosis depends on the measurement of PSV. Normally, functioning bypass grafts have a wide range of velocities, but the PSV is typically less than 150 cm/s. As a stenosis develops, a focal increase is noted in the PSV. A value of PSV greater than 180 cm/s is considered to be the cutoff for an abnormality. Another useful parameter is the velocity ratio. The velocity ratio is measured by dividing the maximum PSV obtained at a stenosis by the PSV obtained just proximal to the stenosis. A doubling in PSV as compared to the adjacent more proximal segment (velocity ratio of 2.0) is consistent with a ≥50% stenosis. The PSV for a stenosis in this range is 180 to 300 cm/s. A velocity ratio of 3.5 and a PSV greater than 300 cm/s is consistent with a ≥75% stenosis[14] and associated with a high level of surgical revision.[15] A critical feature of all stenotic disease is the presence of poststenotic turbulence. Distal to a stenosis the spectral waveforms will be disrupted with extensive turbulence, and both antegrade and retrograde flow can be present. Figure 14-21 illustrates the velocity changes through a stenosis.

An additional parameter used to assess bypass graft patency is the value of mean graft flow velocity (GFV). Mean GFV is calculated by taking an average of 3 to 4 PSV values in nonstenotic segments of a bypass graft at various levels (proximal, mid, and distal). Normally, GFV is greater than 45 cm/s. A GFV of less than 40 cm/s can be present normally in large diameter grafts (>6 mm) or in grafts with limited outflow such as those to a pedal artery, isolated popliteal artery, or to an isolated tibial artery. Trends in the GFV are also helpful diagnostic indicators. A decrease in GFV of greater than 30 cm/s (compared to a previous examination) indicates that a bypass may be in jeopardy of failure.[4] This could be caused by progression of disease with inflow or outflow vessels or a stenosis within the bypass itself.

Pathology Box 14-1 summarizes the various pathologies that can be observed with bypass grafts. Grayscale, spectral Doppler, and color findings are listed.

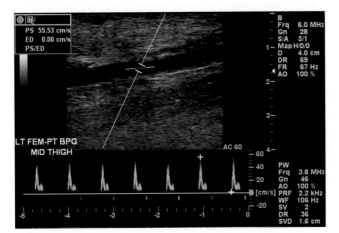

**FIGURE 14-19** An abnormal high-resistance waveform with no flow through diastole. (Image courtesy of Phillip J. Bendick, PhD RVT, Royal Oak, MI.)

**PATHOLOGY BOX 14-1**
*Bypass Graft Pathology*

| Pathology | Grayscale | Color | Doppler |
|---|---|---|---|
| | | **Sonographic Appearance** | |
| Aneurysms and pseudoaneurysms | Focal increase in diameter either along the bypass or at an anastomosis; thrombus may or may not be present | Swirling of color flow into the dilated portion; "yin-yang" appearance may be present with color changing from red to blue as flow fills the dilation | Low-velocity, turbulent, disturbed flow will be present in the dilated segment; bidirectional flow in neck of pseudoaneurysm |
| Arteriovenous fistula | A patent venous tributary will be present off the bypass graft; this tributary may be seen to communicate into the deep venous system | Color filling will be seen within the fistula, extending to the deep venous system; aliasing is likely to be present | Flow may be slightly pulsatile to continuous within the fistula; antegrade diastolic flow will be evident in the bypass proximal to the fistula |
| Dissection | Linear object seen extending for several centimeters, parallel to bypass walls | Turbulent flow; red to blue flow may be seen in either lumen | Disturbed flow with increased resistance; flow may be bidirectional |
| Intimal flap | Small projection into the vessel lumen usually less than 1 cm; not associated with a valve | Disturbed flow or aliasing may be present | Disturbed flow or aliasing may be present |
| Myointimal hyperplasia | Occurs within the bypass or along anastomotic areas; focal increase in vessel wall thickness which protrudes into the lumen | Disturbed flow or aliasing may be present | Increased velocities, turbulence or aliasing may be present |
| Thrombus | Intraluminal echoes of varying echogenicity dependent on the age of the thrombus | No flow or reduced color filling of bypass lumen | Absent Doppler signal or if present, increased resistance |
| Valve remnants | Hyperechoic structure seen protruding into bypass lumen; may be partial or complete leaflet | May demonstrate disturbed color-flow patterns or aliasing in region of valve | May demonstrate elevated velocities in region of valve |

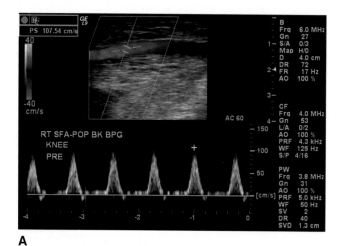

**A**

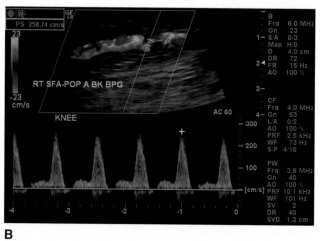

**B**

**FIGURE 14-21** A bypass stenosis (**A**) spectral analysis proximal to a stenosis with a PSV of 108 cm/s; (**B**) at the level of the stenosis the PSV increases to 259 cm/s, $V_r$ 2.4; (*continued*)

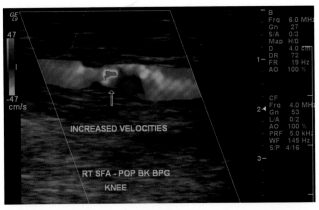

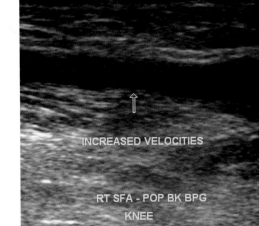

C

D

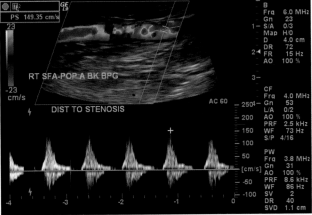

E

**FIGURE 14-21** *(continued)* **(C)** color-flow imaging at the stenosis with aliasing present; **(D)** grayscale image at the stenosis demonstrating a luminal narrowing with hypoechoic material along the walls of the graft; **(E)** distal to the stenosis poststenotic turbulence is present.

## SUMMARY

- It is important to remember that there are three components to the data obtained with modern ultrasound equipment: the B-mode or grayscale image, the spectral Doppler waveform, and the color-flow image.
- The B-mode or grayscale image will identify pathology within the bypass such as stenotic regions, retained valves, dissections, or aneurysmal dilations.
- The spectral Doppler waveform, which is the primary source of numerical data, is used to classify disease.
- The color-flow image can rapidly identify areas of disturbed flow necessitating closer evaluation.
- It is only by reviewing information from all three of these components will the best evaluation of the bypass by determined.
- Routine surveillance of bypass grafts is a standard component of postoperative patient management.
- Thorough attention to ultrasound findings and application of spectral Doppler criteria can identify failing bypasses grafts prior to occlusion thus maintaining patency.

## CRITICAL THINKING QUESTIONS

1. You are to examine a patient with a bypass graft which is 4 years old. What if anything should you pay particular attentions to and why?
2. Describe what transducer you may select to examine a femoral–popliteal PTFE graft which has been tunneled?
3. When looking for a partial retained valve or intimal tear, is color-flow imaging helpful or not? Why?

## MEDIA MENU

Student Resources available on thePoint° include:
- Audio glossary
- Interactive question bank
- Videos
- Internet resources

## REFERENCES

1. Bandyk DR, Schmitt DD, Seabrook GR, et al. Monitoring functional patency of in situ saphenous vein bypasses: the impact of a surveillance protocol and elective revision. *J Vasc Surg.* 1989;11:280–294.

2. Leopold PW, Shandall AA, Kay C, et al. Duplex ultrasound: its role in the non-invasive follow up of the in situ saphenous vein bypass. *J Vasc Technol.* 1987;11:183–186.
3. Tinder CN, Chavanpun JP, Bandyk DF, et al. Duplex surveillance after infrainguinal vein bypass may be enhanced by identification

of characteristics predictive of graft stenosis development. *J Vasc Surg.* 2008;48:613–618.

4. Gupta AK, Bandyk DF, Cheanvechai D, et al. Natural history of infrainguinal vein graft stenosis relative to bypass grafting technique. *J Vasc Surg.* 1997;25:211–225.

5. Berceli SA, Hevelone ND, Lipsitz SR, et al. Surgical and endovascular revision of infrainguinal vein bypass grafts: analysis of midterm outcomes form the PREVENT III trial. *J Vasc Surg.* 2007;46: 1173–1179.

6. Calligaro KD, Doerr K, McAfee-Bennett S, et al. Should duplex ultrasonography be performed for surveillance of femoropopliteal and femorotibial arterial prosthetic bypasses? *Ann Vasc Surg.* 2001;15:520–524.

7. Brumberg RS, Back MR, Armstrong PA, et al. The relative importance of graft surveillance and warfarin therapy in infrainguinal prosthetic bypass failure. *J Vasc Surg.* 2007;46:1160–1166.

8. Landry GL, Liem TK, Mitchell EL, et al. Factors affecting symptomatic vs asymptomatic vein graft stenoses in lower extremity bypass grafts. *Arch Surg.* 2007;142:848–854.

9. Giannoukas AD, Adrouulakis AE, Labropoulos N, et al. The role of surveillance after infrainguinal bypass grafting. *Eur J Vasc Endovasc Surg.* 1996;11:279–289.

10. Mills JL, Bandyk DF, Gahtan V, et al. The origin of infrainguinal vein graft stenosis: a prospective study based on duplex surveillance. *J Vasc Surg.* 1995;21:16–25.

11. Reifsnyder T, Towne JB, Seabrook GR, et al. Biologic characteristics of long-term autogenous vein grafts: a dynamic evolution. *J Vasc Surg.* 1993;17:97–106.

12. Calligaro KD, Musser DJ, Chen AY, et al. Duplex ultrasonography to diagnose failing arterial prosthetic grafts. *Surgery.* 1996;120:455–459.

13. Intersocietal Accreditation Commission Vascular Testing. IAC Standards and Guidelines. http://www.intersocietal.org/vascular. Accessed October 12, 2016.

14. Bandyk DF, Armstrong PA. Surveillance of infrainguinal bypass grafts. In: Zierler RE, ed. *Strandness's Duplex Scanning in Vascular Disorders.* 4th ed. Philadelphia, PA: Lippincott, Williams & Wilkins; 2010:341–349.

15. Mofidi R, Kelman J, Bennett S, et al. Significance of the early postoperative duplex result in infrainguinal vein bypass surveillance. *Eur J Vasc Endovasc Surg.* 2007;34:327–332.

# Duplex Ultrasound Testing Following Peripheral Endovascular Arterial Intervention

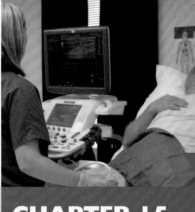

DENNIS F. BANDYK  |  KATHRYN L. PARKER

## CHAPTER 15

## OBJECTIVES

- List the types of commonly performed interventions
- Describe the pathology observed on ultrasound during postinterventional evaluations
- Define the duplex ultrasound criteria applied to lower limb arteries following angioplasty and stenting
- Identify normal and abnormal spectral Doppler waveforms obtained from arteries following angioplasty and stenting

## GLOSSARY

**angioplasty** A surgical repair of a blood vessel by reconstructing or replacing part of the vessel; balloon angioplasty is a specific type of angioplasty in which a balloon-tipped catheter is used to enlarge a narrowing (stenosis) or to open an occlusion in a blood vessel

**atherectomy** An endovascular procedure to remove plaque from an artery or a vein graft using a catheter with cutting device at the tip that cuts away the plaque to enlarge the lumen

**dissection** A tear in the artery wall that results in the splitting or separation of the plaque from the wall and or the layers of the blood vessel wall

**hyperplasia** An abnormal increase in the number of cells; myointimal hyperplasia is an increase in the number of smooth muscle cells within the intima of an artery or a stent in response to vessel injury which can produce stenosis

**stent** A circular metal structure placed inside a blood vessel to expand the lumen and provide wall support, and may be coated with drugs or be covered with vascular graft material

Vascular diagnostics are integral to the care of patients with peripheral arterial disease (PAD) prior to and following endovascular intervention.[1-3] Care of the patient with PAD includes medical treatment such as atherosclerotic risk factor reduction, antiplatelet and statin medications, exercise training, and drug therapy for claudication. In the selected patients with symptoms of disabling claudication not improved by medical treatment or signs of advanced limb ischemia, intervention by surgical reconstruction/bypass grafting or endovascular therapy is recommended.[3-6] The type of intervention depends primarily on disease location and extent which can be accurately determined using duplex ultrasound; but comorbid medical conditions and the risk–benefit ratio of the proposed intervention also influence treatment decisions. Endovascular therapy has become a preferred initial intervention with a variety of techniques available to treat lower and upper limb atherosclerotic occlusive (ASO) disease (Table 15-1).[6-13] The type of lesion repair, stenosis-free patency, and failure mode varies with intervention technique. Percutaneous transluminal angioplasty (PTA) is the most common endovascular procedure and requires passage of guidewire across a stenosis or an occlusion followed by inflation of angioplasty balloon (bare or drug coated) or deployment of stent to expand the artery lumen. Other endovascular techniques such as subintimal angioplasty, mechanical atherectomy (plaque debulking or excision), or stent graft angioplasty are used to treat more extensive (long stenotic segments, occlusion,

**TABLE 15-1　Endovascular Interventions for Lower Extremity Atherosclerotic Occlusive Disease[6-12]**

| Intervention Option | Mechanism | Lesion Anatomy | Stenosis-Free Patency at 1 yr | Failure Mode |
|---|---|---|---|---|
| Balloon angioplasty | Lumen dilation | Focal, <5 cm stenosis or occlusion | 40%–55% POBA<br>65%–80% DCB | Plaque dissection<br>Myointimal hyperplasia |
| Stent angioplasty | Lumen dilation | Focal and longer (>10 cm) stenosis or occlusion | 50%–60%<br>70%–80% DCS | Myointimal hyperplasia<br>Stent fracture |
| Atherectomy | Plaque excision | Focal and longer (>10 cm) stenosis | 40%–50% | Myointimal hyperplasia<br>Atherectomy-site thrombosis |
| Subintimal angioplasty | Lumen dilation | >10 stenosis or occlusion | 55%–60% | |
| Stent graft angioplasty | Lumen dilation | Long, >15 cm stenosis or occlusion | 60%–70% | Myointimal hyperplasia<br>Graft thrombosis |

DCB, drug-coated balloon; DCS, drug-coated stent; POBA, plain old balloon angioplasty.

multiple lesions) ASO disease.[7,9-15] Often, endovascular therapy does not restore normal peripheral pulses because of multilevel disease, especially in limbs treated for critical limb ischemia (CLI).[1,15] The outcome of endovascular intervention is largely dependent on the procedure indication (claudication vs. CLI) and lesion severity classified using Trans-Atlantic Inter-Society Consensus (TASC II) criteria based on lesion location and anatomy.[6] Endovascular intervention is a preferred therapy for focal, <5 cm length regions of stenosis or occlusion (TASC A and B lesions) with an expected 30-day technical and clinical success rates above 95%.[1,4,7-10] In claudicants, the patency of iliac angioplasty is higher (85% at 3-year) than for superficial femoral/popliteal artery angioplasty (55% at 2-year).[6,10,14,16] Treatment of CLI or TASC C and D lesions by endovascular techniques has lower stenosis-free patency rate typically in the 40% to 50% range at 1 year.[6,10,12,15] Factors associated with angioplasty failure include lesion calcification, occlusion, diseased tibial artery runoff, diabetes mellitus, smoking, and renal failure.[2,4,17,18] Approximately one-third of peripheral angioplasty sites will require reintervention to maintain stenosis-free patency during the first year, but the use of the drug-coated balloons and stent has reduced the incidence of angioplasty stenosis.[11,12]

The rationale for vascular laboratory testing following intervention is twofold: (1) to document improvement in limb perfusion was sufficient to expect symptoms (claudication and rest pain) and signs (ulcer healing) to resolve and (2) to detect angioplasty-site stenosis a harbinger of procedure failure. The duplex ultrasound identification of >70% diameter-reducing (DR) stenosis or low peak systolic velocity (PSV) in prosthetic bypass or stent graft are markers for predicting graft stenosis.[19,20] Because the patient with PAD is prone to disease progression, including myointimal hyperplasia-producing stenosis within or adjacent to the angioplasty site, duplex ultrasound is the recommended diagnostic modality. Testing can be performed during the procedure to assess for residual stenosis, suited for surveillance studies, and highly accurate in detection of angioplasty-site complications versus ASO progression. Duplex ultrasound testing can classify angioplasty stenosis severity and thus provide an opportunity to retreat high-grade occlusive lesions prior to thrombosis.[2,3,17,20-24] Reliance on the patient to recognize angioplasty failure based on symptom recurrence is inadequate, especially in the sedentary patient who does not walk sufficient distance to develop claudication.

## SONOGRAPHIC EXAMINATION TECHNIQUES

### Patient Preparation

Arterial testing after endovascular intervention mirrors surveillance used after lower limb bypass grafting.[1,19,20] Patient functional status is documented, including any new or unresolved symptoms of PAD, and limb perfusion is evaluated by physiologic testing and a duplex ultrasound scan of the angioplasty site for abnormality (Fig. 15-1). In the claudicant, initial indirect physiologic testing should verify improvement in ankle-brachial index (ABI) to a normal (>0.9) or an increased (>0.2) level sufficient that walking distance is likely to be improved. Limbs treated for CLI should have measurement of toe pressure to verify whether an increase to >30 mm Hg has been achieved. In limbs with healing foot ulcers or digit amputations, a toe pressure >40 mm Hg predicts healing.

Duplex ultrasound arterial mapping of the limb should be individualized based on whether the ABI is normal, abnormal, or the patient has calcified tibial arteries which preclude accurate ankle pressure measurement. If the ABI is normal and tibial artery velocity spectra at the ankle indicate multiphasic or triphasic artery flow, angioplasty-site imaging is not necessary.

### Patient Positioning

Scanning is performed with the patient supine and lower limb positioned with the knee bent slightly. Prone or lateral decubitus positions can be used to image the popliteal artery, tibioperoneal trunk, and peroneal arteries. Imaging can be performed with a 5 to 7 MHz linear array transducer.

### Scanning Technique

Duplex ultrasound mapping should begin at the common femoral artery (CFA) level to document the presence normal,

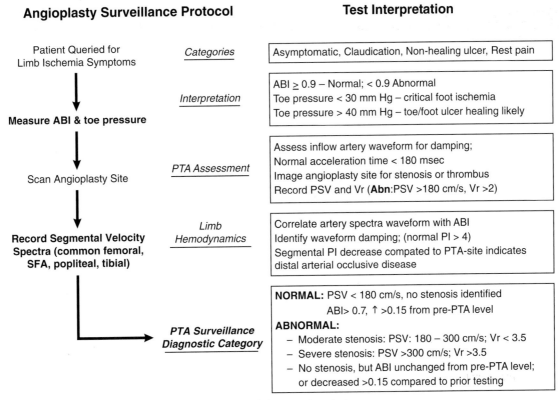

**Angioplasty Surveillance Protocol**

Patient Queried for
Limb Ischemia Symptoms

↓

**Measure ABI & toe pressure**

↓

Scan Angioplasty Site

↓

**Record Segmental Velocity
Spectra (common femoral,
SFA, popliteal, tibial)**

→

*PTA Surveillance
Diagnostic Category*

**Test Interpretation**

*Categories*

| Asymptomatic, Claudication, Non-healing ulcer, Rest pain |

*Interpretation*

ABI ≥ 0.9 – Normal; < 0.9 Abnormal
Toe pressure < 30 mm Hg – critical foot ischemia
Toe pressure > 40 mm Hg – toe/foot ulcer healing likely

*PTA Assessment*

Assess inflow artery waveform for damping;
Normal acceleration time < 180 msec
Image angioplasty site for stenosis or thrombus
Record PSV and Vr (**Abn**:PSV >180 cm/s, Vr >2)

*Limb
Hemodynamics*

Correlate artery spectra waveform with ABI
Identify waveform damping; (normal PI > 4)
Segmental PI decrease compated to PTA-site indicates
distal arterial occlusive disease

**NORMAL:** PSV < 180 cm/s, no stenosis identified
        ABI> 0.7, ↑ >0.15 from pre-PTA level
**ABNORMAL:**
  – Moderate stenosis: PSV: 180 – 300 cm/s; Vr < 3.5
  – Severe stenosis: PSV >300 cm/s; Vr >3.5
  – No stenosis, but ABI unchanged from pre-PTA level;
    or decreased >0.15 compared to prior testing

**FIGURE 15-1** Peripheral angioplasty surveillance testing protocol and study interpretation criteria.

multiphasic velocity spectra—indicating <50% proximal aortoiliac or stent stenosis (Fig. 15-2). If the CFA velocity spectra waveform is monophasic, damped compared to the contralateral CFA, or has an abnormal (>180 ms) acceleration time, duplex ultrasound assessment of the iliac segment should be performed.

Duplex ultrasound mapping then proceeds distal from the CFA to include the superficial femoral artery (SFA) and deep femoral artery origins, imaging of the SFA-popliteal arterial segment, including the angioplasty site, and recording of ankle-level, tibial artery velocity spectra. The technologist should provide sufficient duplex ultrasound images and

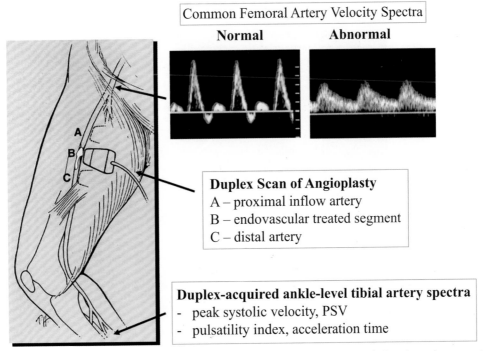

Common Femoral Artery Velocity Spectra

**Normal**        **Abnormal**

**Duplex Scan of Angioplasty**
A – proximal inflow artery
B – endovascular treated segment
C – distal artery

**Duplex-acquired ankle-level tibial artery spectra**
- peak systolic velocity, PSV
- pulsatility index, acceleration time

**FIGURE 15-2** Schematic depicting sites of duplex ultrasound scanning, including the common femoral artery, angioplasty site, and assessment of distal tibial artery hemodynamics.

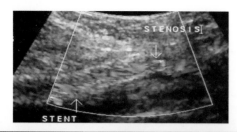

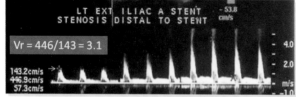

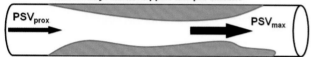

**Walk-thru of Pulsed Doppler Sample Volume**

**FIGURE 15-3** Duplex ultrasound image and velocity spectra of an external iliac stent stenosis. The color duplex ultrasound image (**top**) depicts an area of color aliasing at the stenosis (*arrow*). The pulsed Doppler (**middle**) sample volume is walked through the stenosis with measurement of peak systolic velocity proximal to (PSV$_{prox}$) and at the site of stenosis (PSV$_{max}$) for calculation of velocity ratio, $V_r$ = PSV$_{max}$/PSV$_{prox}$. A schematic drawing illustrates the stenosis and PSV measurements (**bottom**).

lumen caliber reduction, flow jets, disturbed flow identified by color or power Doppler imaging should be evaluated by pulsed Doppler spectral analysis recorded using ≤60 degree angle correction relative to the vessel/stent wall. A valuable scanning tip is to "walk" the sample volume through the region of abnormality to locate and measure PSV changes (Fig. 15-3). Measurement of PSV proximal (PSV$_{prox}$) to and within the stenosis flow jet (PSV$_{max}$) allows calculation of the stenosis velocity ratio, $V_r$, where $V_r$ = PSV$_{max}$/PSV$_{prox}$. A $V_r$ >2 indicates >50% DR stenosis. The combination of PSV$_{max}$, $V_r$, and end-diastolic velocity (EDV) at the stenosis is used to classify stenosis severity (Fig. 15-4). Duplex ultrasound findings should be recorded on a schematic of the lower or upper limb arterial tree to facilitate study interpretation and provide a comparison baseline when evaluating for stenosis progression. In the majority of the patients, duplex ultrasound testing alone provides sufficient information to inform the patient of PTA-site stenosis and decide whether to proceed to reintervention. Following prosthetic bypass grafting or stent grafting, PSV should be measured at 1 or 2 locations in the conduit. If a PSV <50 cm/s is recorded, a more careful examination for proximal or distal occlusive lesions should be performed, because low PSV has been associated with graft thrombosis.[20,23]

## Technical Considerations

The goal of peripheral arterial testing following intervention is to provide objective hemodynamic and anatomic information of functional angioplasty patency. The technologist should have information of the indication for intervention, the arterial site(s) treated, and the endovascular procedure performed. Measurement of limb pressures combined with

segmental velocity spectra recordings for study interpretation into the categories as "normal" or "abnormal."

B-mode and color Doppler imaging of the angioplasty site should be performed to document vessel/stent lumen patency, arterial plaque characteristics, and evidence of stent/stent graft deformation or intimal thickening. Sites of

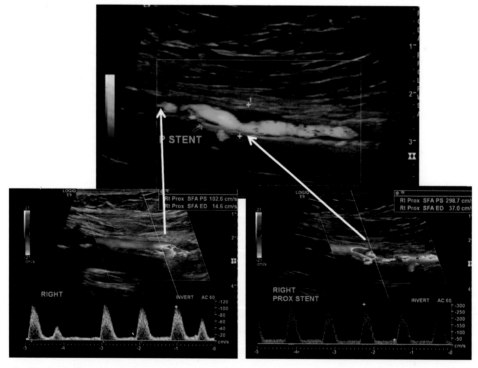

**FIGURE 15-4** Power (**top**) and color Doppler velocity spectra images of a >50% DR stent-angioplasty-site stenosis. Proximal PSV was 100 cm/s (**bottom left**) and increased to 297 cm/s at the stenosis (**bottom right**) resulting in a calculated velocity ratio of 3.

arterial duplex ultrasound scanning enables study interpretation in categories ranging from "normal," that is, stenosis-free patency, to "severe stenosis," with the latter category based on threshold criteria appropriate for reintervention. Testing immediately following an endovascular intervention confirms procedural success or failure by documenting patency and whether a residual stenosis is present. Subsequent testing is based on procedure indication; less frequent in active individuals treated for claudication, but in patients treated for CLI, surveillance should be similar following lower limb bypass graft grafting.[1,22] Duplex ultrasound surveillance after lower limb angioplasty has demonstrated >50% DR stenosis in 20% to 40% of treated limbs within 12 months of the procedure.[7,15,18] The most common etiology is development of myointimal hyperplasia within the angioplasty site regardless of endovascular therapy (balloon inflation, stent angioplasty, and atherectomy) used. Detection of >50% residual stenosis despite a completion angiogram showing adequate lumen expansion (<30% DR) can occur, predicts angioplasty, and is the rationale for performing intra- or early (<30-day) postprocedural study.[1,20] The prevalence of duplex-detected residual stenosis following femoropopliteal angioplasty is lowest after stent angioplasty or stent grafting (<5%), and higher after balloon angioplasty (15% to 20%) or atherectomy (25%). While angiogram-monitored angioplasty showing <20% to 30% residual stenosis predicts 30-day patency, that is, technical success, a duplex ultrasound of angioplasty-site hemodynamics provides more precise assessment of functional patency. Schillinger et al.[9] documented that duplex-detected >50% stenosis developed more frequently after balloon angioplasty than after Nitinol stenting in treatment of SFA occlusive disease at both 6 (45% vs. 25%, $p = 0.06$) and 12 months (63% vs. 37%, $p < 0.01$). Other techniques, including cutting or cryoplasty balloon angioplasty, atherectomy, and stent grafting, also have a high technical success rate, but similar to balloon angioplasty, angioplasty restenosis or treatment-site thrombosis has been observed in 20% to 50% of limbs depending on TASC lesion severity by 1 year.[6,10,15]

## DIAGNOSIS

Peripheral arterial laboratory testing following PTA includes interpretation of the limb pressures and duplex ultrasound findings (see Fig. 15-1). The interpretation should comment on the severity of limb ischemia (mild, moderate, or severe),

changes from preintervention values, and in patients treated from CLI whether adequate foot perfusion has been achieved, that is, a toe pressure >30 mm Hg. Duplex ultrasound findings at the angioplasty site are interpreted as showing no stenosis (<50% DR stenosis), moderate stenosis (>50% DR), severe stenosis (>70% DR), or occlusion (Table 15-2). A "normal study" interpretation should indicate that no stenosis was identified at the angioplasty site, and that the ABI is normal, or unchanged, if prior testing was performed. Duplex ultrasound detection of a >50% DR stenosis proximal to, within, or distal to the endovascular intervention is interpreted as a "new" abnormal finding.

Velocity criteria used to interpret PTA stenosis severity relies primarily on measurements of PSV and $V_r$ at the stenosis. Although a $V_r > 2$ is generally accepted to indicate a >50% DR stenosis, this interpretation should also be associated with the duplex ultrasound findings of lumen reduction, color Doppler imaging of disturbed flow, and a focal PSV increase to >180 cm/s. Under resting conditions, a stenosis with $V_r$ of 2 to 3 is associated with minimal resting systolic pressure gradient, and the ankle artery velocity spectra may demonstrate a "near-normal" multiphasic waveform. The functional significance of the stenosis can be determined by exercise testing with measurement of ABI and ankle pressure changes. Published duplex-derived criteria for classification of angioplasty site recommend use of three disease categories (<50% stenosis, >70% stenosis, and occlusion). This author's vascular group has utilized combined $PSV_{max}$ and $V_r$ threshold criteria of 300 cm/s and 3.5, respectively, to define the >70% DR stenosis (Fig. 15-5). The University of Pittsburgh group reported a PPV of >95% in predicting >50% or >80% in-stent stenosis following femoropopliteal angioplasty for TASC B and C lesions (Table 15-3).[21] In patients with developed recurrent limb ischemia symptoms and a decrease of ABI >0.15, the angioplasty-site stenosis had mean $PSV_{max} = 360$ cm/s and $V_r = 3.6$—criteria of >70% DR stenosis in both classification schemes.

The presence of plaque dissection after balloon dilation, stent geometry, and the nature of myointimal hyperplasia development can affect the significance of PSV elevation and thus accuracy in predicting stenosis severity. In general, PSV values for grading in-stent stenosis are higher than for de novo atherosclerotic stenosis where a value >125 to 150 cm/s is an "accepted" threshold for >50% stenosis. Stent angioplasty decreases artery wall compliance that elevates PSV within the stent and produces abnormal, nonuniform

**TABLE 15-2  Published Duplex Ultrasound Velocity Criteria for Classification of Angioplasty-Site Stenosis (University of California, San Diego)[18]**

| Stenosis Category | Peak Systolic Velocity (PSV, cm/s) | Velocity Ratio ($V_r$) | End-Diastolic Velocity (cm/s) | Distal Artery Waveform |
|---|---|---|---|---|
| <50% DR | <180 | <2 | NA | Normal |
| >50% DR Moderate | 180–300 | 2–3.5 | >0 | Monophasic |
| >70% DR Severe | >300 | >3.5 | >45 | Damped, monophasic, low velocity |
| Occluded | No flow detected | | | Damped, monophasic, low velocity |

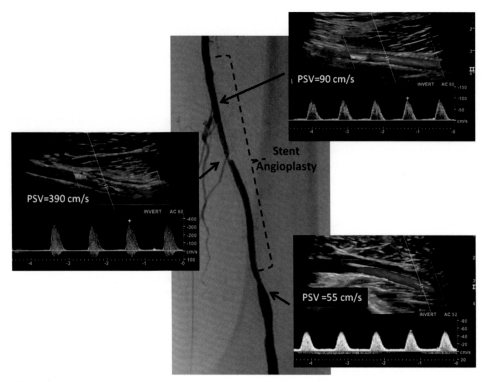

**FIGURE 15-5** Angiogram (**center**) and duplex ultrasound scan images of a focal >70% DR in-stent stenosis (PSV = 390 cm/s, velocity ratio = 390/95 = 4.1). The image at the **top right** demonstrates the PSV proximal to the stenosis (PSV 95 cm/s). The PSV of 390 cm/s at the stenosis is shown at the **left**. The dampened distal flow signal (PSV 55 cm/s) is pictured at the **lower right**. ABI had decreased from 0.92 to 0.7, and the patient complained of recurrent claudication symptoms.

TABLE 15-3   **Published Duplex Ultrasound Velocity Criteria for Superficial Femoral Artery Stenosis (University of Pittsburgh)[14]**

| Stenosis Category | Peak Systolic Velocity (PSV, cm/s) | Velocity Ratio ($V_r$) |
|---|---|---|
| <50% DR | <190 | <1.5 |
| >50% DR | 190–275 | 1.5–3.5 |
| >80% DR | >275 | >3.5 |
| Occluded | No flow detected | |

wall sheer stress at stent endpoints that potentiate the development of myointimal hyperplasia. This author's vascular group utilize the same interpretation criteria for grading both lower limb arterial bypass graft stenosis and angioplasty-site stenosis, including the threshold criteria for reintervention (PSV >300 cm/s, $V_r$ >3.5).[1,20] This allows for uniform study interpretation between vascular laboratory staff, the diagnosis of disease progression, and clinical decision-making regarding surveillance schedule or reintervention.

Angioplasty failure can manifest as an occlusion, diffuse, or multiple stenosis (Fig. 15-6), or as a focal, high-grade (see Fig. 15-5) stenosis. Duplex ultrasound findings of diffuse

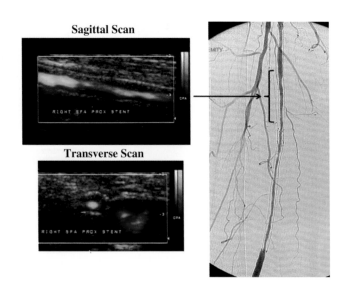

Sagittal Scan

Transverse Scan

**FIGURE 15-6** Power Doppler images (sagittal, transverse) and angiogram of a superficial femoral artery stent with diffuse in-stent stenosis. PSV ranged from 200 to 300 cm/s within the stent. Measured ABI was 0.56.

in-stent stenosis include power Doppler lumen reduction and elevated (200 to 300 cm/s) PSV values along the entire stent length. The reduction in ABI can be similar to a high-grade focal stenosis with PSV >400 cm/s and EDV >100 cm/s. An important hemodynamic feature of angioplasty failure is the presence of damped, low-velocity spectra waveform in the distal arterial tree.

## Surveillance Protocol

The frequency of endovascular intervention failure is highest within the first 6 months, especially if a residual stenosis (PSV >180 cm/s, $V_r$ 1.5 to 2.5) is identified. The rationale for surveillance testing is to identify "failing" PTA sites before thrombosis occurs; and in the medically fit patient, repair of a duplex-detected >70% angioplasty stenosis should be considered. Angioplasty failure is commonly the result of myointimal hyperplasia developing within or immediately adjacent to the treatment site. Stent fracture, a known risk factor for stenosis development and thrombosis, cannot be identified by duplex ultrasound imaging, but the presence of stent deformation or kinking is abnormal and predicts stent thrombosis, especially if associated with a >70% stenosis (Pathology Box 15-1).

Reporting standards of clinical improvement and procedure patency following endovascular therapy is identical to "open" surgical repair or bypass grafting. Intervention-site patency documented by duplex ultrasound and an ABI increase >0.15 are minimal outcome criteria for clinical improvement.[3] Clinical success requires resolution of limb ischemia symptoms or signs, and <50% DR stenosis of the arterial repair documented by duplex ultrasound or angiography. Duplex-detected >50% DR stenosis based on velocity spectra findings is an abnormal finding, and if progressive to a >70% DR stenosis is criteria for loss of "stenosis-free" patency whether repaired or selected for watch-full observation in the asymptomatic patient. An open or percutaneous secondary intervention undertaken to maintain or improve functional angioplasty changes procedural outcome to "assisted" primary patency. If the angioplasty-site thrombosed and a secondary procedure are performed to restore patency, the outcome status changes to "secondary" patency. A successful surveillance program following PTA should produce an assisted primary patency in the range of 80% to 90% at 2 years, and no significant improvement in secondary patency. Failure to identify clinically significant lesions prior to thrombosis is present if the primary and assisted primary patency rates are similar.

An abnormal or change in ABI indicates PAD, but is not diagnostic for angioplasty-site failure. In many diabetic patients, measurement of ABI is inaccurate, and limb arterial testing requires pulse volume recording and duplex ultrasound testing to evaluate limb perfusion and PTA functional patency. The application of objective criteria provided by duplex ultrasound scanning is essential for a useful surveillance program. Use of combined threshold criteria for intervention, that is, PSV >300, $V_r$ >3.5, is associated with a high (>90%) positive predictive value when compared to angiogram findings for >70% DR stenosis. Following prosthetic bypass or stent grafting, a PSV <40 to 50 cm/s is an important test result because low graft velocity has been reported as a predictor for graft thrombosis.

The initial surveillance examination should be performed within 2 weeks; ideally combined with an outpatient vascular clinic evaluation to assess the patient's activity level, ASO risk factor modifications, and review drug (antiplatelet and statin) therapy. If the initial PTA testing is "normal," follow-up testing in 3 months is appropriate for patients treated for CLI and 6 months in claudicants. Subsequent testing is individualized at 6- to 12-month intervals. If initial duplex ultrasound testing detects a residual 50% to 70% DR angioplasty-site stenosis, a repeat evaluation in 4 to 6 weeks is recommended and reliable in detection of stenosis progression. The patient should be instructed that any new limb ischemia symptoms should be evaluated in the vascular laboratory immediately. Abbreviated testing intervals, that is, 3 months, may also be appropriate during the first year following endovascular treatment of TASC C and D lesions because of the higher likelihood of failure. The incidence of reintervention is higher following balloon (30%) than stent (20%) angioplasty, and drug-coated balloons and stent further reduce the likelihood of stenosis development.

---

**PATHOLOGY BOX 15-1**
*Common Postinterventional Abnormalities*

| Abnormality | Ultrasound Findings |
| --- | --- |
| In-site stenosis | Luminal caliber reduction; color-flow jet with disturbed/turbulent color-flow distally; focal PSV increase with turbulent Doppler spectrum distally |
| Stent deformation/kinking | Irregular stent walls, may protrude into vessel lumen; may be sharply angled in normally straight vessel segment; color and spectral turbulence |
| Myointimal hyperplasia | Homogeneous tissue growth along vessel lumen at angioplasty site or across stent walls; Smooth surface contour; may appear as very thin layer along vessel or stent; may progress to in-site stenosis |
| Thrombosis/occlusion | No patent lumen detected; no color filling; no spectral Doppler signal |

## SUMMARY

- The application of duplex ultrasound surveillance following peripheral arterial interventional procedures can be useful and should be considered a part of PAD patient care.
- Reliance on the patient to recognize changes in limb perfusion is not reliable.
- Interpretation of arterial testing performed within a surveillance protocol can be challenging, and some vascular specialists are not convinced that routine duplex ultrasound surveillance is of benefit, worth the health care expense, or persuaded the vascular laboratory is competent to execute a quality surveillance program.
- Duplex ultrasound surveillance when correctly performed and interpreted should improve patency and clinical outcomes following lower limb bypass grafting and endovascular therapy—interventions with known limited functional patency and performed in a patient cohort subject to ASO disease progression.[20,22,23]
- Endovascular interventions for duplex-identified stenosis have been shown to result in similar patency to non-threatened grafts.[19,20]

## CRITICAL THINKING QUESTIONS

1. During a duplex ultrasound examination of a patient with an SFA stent, the CFA ultrasound reveals an acceleration time of 210 ms. With this information, how would you augment the examination and why?
2. A patient comes in for a duplex ultrasound examination 6 months following a balloon angioplasty and stent placement. At this time interval within the follow-up protocol, where is the most likely place along the limb where a stenosis may be present?
3. When examining a patient following balloon angioplasty and stenting, do you expect the PSV within the treated site to be similar to or different from a patient who underwent an atherectomy?

## MEDIA MENU

Student Resources available on thePoint® include:
- Audio glossary
- Interactive question bank
- Videos
- Internet resources

## REFERENCES

1. Hodgkiss-Harlow KD, Bandyk DF. Interpretation of arterial duplex testing of lower extremity arteries and interventions. *Semin Vasc Surg.* 2013;26:95–104.
2. Bandyk DF, Hodgkiss-Harlow KD. Chapter 18: Surveillance after peripheral artery endovascular intervention. In: Zierler RE, Meissner MH, eds. *Strandness's Duplex Scanning in Vascular Disorders.* Philadelphia, PA: Lippincott Williams & Wilkins; 2015.
3. Ahn SS, Rutherford RB, Becker GJ, et al. Reporting standards arterial endovascular for lower extremity. *J Vasc Surg.* 2009;49:133–139.
4. White CJ, Gray WA. Endovascular therapies for peripheral arterial disease. *Circulation.* 2007;116:2203–2215.
5. Goodney PP, Beck AW, Nagle J, et al. National trends in lower extremity bypass surgery, endovascular interventions, and major amputations. *J Vasc Surg.* 2009;50:54–60.
6. Norgren L, Hiatt WR, Dormandy JA, et al. Inter-Society Consensus for the Management of Peripheral Arterial Disease (TASC II). *J Vasc Surg.* 2007;45(Suppl S):S5–S67.
7. Grimm J, Muller-Hulsbeck S, Jahnke T, et al. Randomized study to compare PTA alone versus PTA with Palmaz stent placement for femoropopliteal lesions. *J Vasc Interv Radiol.* 2001;12:935–942.
8. Mewissen MW. Self expanding Nitinol stents in the femoropopliteal segment: technique and mid term results. *Tech Vasc Interv Radiol.* 2004;7:2–5.
9. Schillinger M, Sabeti S, Loewe C, et al. Balloon angioplasty versus implantation of nitinol stents in the superficial femoral artery. *N Engl J Med.* 2006;354:1879–1888.
10. Conrad MF, Cambria RP, Stone DH, et al. Intermediate results of percutaneous endovascular therapy of femoropopliteal occlusive disease: a contemporary series. *J Vasc Surg.* 2006;44:762–769.
11. Laird JR, Schneider PA, Tepe G, et al. Durability of treatment effect using a drug-coated balloon for femoropopliteal lesions: 24-month results of IN.PACT SFA. *J Am Coll Cardiol.* 2015;66:2329–2338.
12. Tepe G, Laird J, Schneider P, et al. Drug-coated balloon versus standard percutaneous transluminal angioplasty for the treatment of superficial femoral and/or popliteal peripheral artery disease: 12-month results from the IN.PACT SFA randomized trial. *Circulation.* 2015;131:495–502.
13. Dearing DD, Patel KR, Compoginis JM, et al. Primary stenting of the superficial femoral and popliteal artery. *J Vasc Surg.* 2009;50:542–548.
14. Schneider GC, Richardson AI, Scott EC, et al. Selective stenting in subintimal angioplasty: analysis of primary stent outcomes. *J Vasc Surg.* 2008;48:1175–1181.
15. Keeling WB, Shames ML, Stone PA, et al. Plaque excision with the Silverhawk catheter: early results in patients with claudication or critical limb ischemia. *J Vasc Surg.* 2007;45:25–31.
16. Back MR, Novotney M, Roth SM, et al. Utility of duplex surveillance following iliac artery angioplasty and primary stenting. *J Endovasc Ther.* 2001;8:629–637.
17. Westin GG, Armstrong EJ, Singh S, et al. Endovascular therapy is effective treatment for focal stenoses in failing infrapopliteal grafts. *J Vasc Surg.* 2013;58:557–558.
18. Abularage CJ, Conrad MF, Hackney LA, et al. Long-term outcomes of diabetic patients undergoing endovascular infrainguinal interventions. *J Vasc Surg.* 2009;52:314–322.
19. Bandyk DF, Schmitt DD, Seabrook GR, et al. Monitoring functional patency of in situ saphenous vein bypasses: the impact of surveillance protocol and elective revision. *J Vasc Surg.* 1989;9:286–296.
20. Barleben A, Bandyk DF. Surveillance and follow-up after revascularization for critical limb ischemia. *Semin Vasc Surg.* 2014;27:85–89.
21. Baril DT, Rhee RY, Kim J, et al. Duplex criteria for determination of in-stent stenosis after angioplasty and stenting of the superficial femoral artery. *J Vasc Surg.* 2008;48:627.
22. Oresanya L, Makam AN, Blekin M, et al. Factors associated with primary vein graft occlusion in a multicenter trial with mandated ultrasound surveillance. *J Vasc Surg.* 2014;59:996–1002.
23. Troutman DA, Madden NJ, Dougherty MJ, et al. Duplex ultrasound diagnosis of failing stent grafts placed for occlusive disease. *J Vasc Surg.* 2014;60:1580–1584.
24. Patel SD, Zymvragoudakis V, Sheehan L, et al. The efficacy of salvage interventions on threatened distal bypass grafts. *J Vasc Surg.* 2016;63:126–132.

# Special Considerations in Evaluating Nonatherosclerotic Arterial Pathology

PATRICK A. WASHKO | S. WAYNE SMITH

**CHAPTER 16**

## OBJECTIVES

- Define the clinical presentation of nonatherosclerotic arterial disease
- List the most common nonatherosclerotic arterial diseases
- Identify the ultrasound presentation of nonatherosclerotic disease
- Describe the most common cardiac pathologies associated with cardioembolic events
- Explain the importance of clinical history before performing the arterial examination

## KEY TERMS

**aneurysm**

**arteriovenous fistula**

**arteritis**

**Buerger's disease**

**iatrogenic**

**popliteal entrapment**

**pseudoaneurysm**

**Takayasu's arteritis**

**traumatic**

## GLOSSARY

**aneurysm** A dilation of an artery wall involving all three layers of the vessel wall

**arteriovenous fistula** An abnormal communication between an artery and a vein which can be the result of iatrogenic injury or trauma or may be congenitally acquired

**Buerger's disease** A type of vascular arteritis also known as thromboangitis obliterans; it affects small- and medium-sized arteries

**embolism** An obstruction or occlusion of a blood vessel by a transported clot of blood or mass or bacteria or other foreign substance

**giant cell arteritis** A type of vascular arteritis also known as temporal arteritis; is associated with the superficial temporal artery and other arteries of the head and neck

**pseudoaneurysm** An expanding hematoma; a hole in the arterial wall which allows blood to leave the vessel and collect in the surrounding tissue

**Takayasu's arteritis** A type of vascular arteritis that affects the aortic arch and its large branches

**vascular arteritis** An inflammatory disease that affects the blood vessels

Nonatherosclerotic peripheral vascular disease is relatively uncommon. In approximately 90% of patients with peripheral arterial disease (PAD), the etiology is atherosclerosis. Nonatherosclerotic arterial pathology is often recognized by a detailed history that demonstrates the absence of any risk factors for atherosclerotic disease. Some of these typical atherosclerotic risk factors include smoking, diabetes, hypertension, and hyperlipidemia. Nonatherosclerotic arterial disease is composed of many atypical diseases that may include inflammatory diseases, congenital abnormalities, and acquired diseases or injuries. Many nonatherosclerotic arterial diseases can be assessed and properly diagnosed with vascular laboratory imaging, physiologic studies, and a detailed careful history. This chapter reviews imaging and physiologic tests used to assess a variety of nonatherosclerotic arterial pathology.

## SONOGRAPHIC EXAMINATION TECHNIQUES

The sonographic examination of a patient with nonatherosclerotic arterial disease is similar to that employed when evaluating patients for suspected atherosclerosis (refer to Chapter 12). The portion of the vascular system interrogated is determined by the presenting symptoms and the disease suspected. In some instances, a combination of direct duplex ultrasound imaging techniques along with indirect physiologic testing is employed to fully characterize the disease. Specific examination details will be included within the discussion of each disease entity. Basic ultrasound techniques are described in the following section.

## Duplex Ultrasound Techniques

Generally, the grayscale image will be examined in both transverse and sagittal orientations to fully visualize any wall abnormalities or vessel defects. Images should be recorded from all major vessels examined. Additional images should be obtained from adjacent vessels when documenting wall abnormalities and compared to normal portions of vessels.

Spectral Doppler and color-flow imaging techniques should be used to evaluate the vessels for flow disturbances and stenoses. Color can be quickly used to determine general flow patterns as well as to detect turbulent flow, increased flow, flow outside a vessel, or the absence of flow. Spectral Doppler must be used to characterize the peak systolic velocity (PSV) from each vessel examined. End-diastolic velocity (EDV) may also need to be recorded, particularly if abnormally high- or low-resistance flow patterns are observed. In areas of suspected stenosis, PSV should be recorded before the area of interest, at the area of maximum PSV, and distal to this area. Poststenotic turbulence should be also documented.

## VASCULAR ARTERITIS

Vascular arteritis is a phrase used to describe several inflammatory diseases that affect the blood vessels. The etiology of arteritis is unknown but often involves an immunologic condition. The inflammatory process of arteritis is associated with the media of the cell wall becoming infiltrated with a variety of white blood cells. Muscular and elastic portions of the wall are eroded and fibrosis develops. The end result is an overall weakening of the blood vessel and necrosis within the vessel wall.[1,2]

The symptoms of arteritis can often be similar to those symptoms encountered with atherosclerosis. When an arteritis involves extremity vessels, symptoms such as claudication or rest pain can be present. Several types of arteritis can impact the upper extremities. The most common upper extremity arterial pathology seen is proximal atherosclerotic subclavian artery disease. Typically, these patients are referred to the vascular laboratory for asymmetrical blood pressures, dizziness, or syncope. If assessment demonstrates stenosis of the axillary or brachial artery segments, this finding is seldom due to atherosclerosis and may be more consistent with giant cell arteritis or Takayasu's arteritis.

## Giant Cell Arteritis

Giant cell arteritis or temporal arteritis is an inflammatory vasculitis seen in elderly patients.[3] The average age of onset is 70 years old and rarely occurs in people less than 50 years of age. Caucasians and females are more prone to the disease than males or other races. Patients are frequently referred to the vascular laboratory because of asymmetrical upper extremity blood pressures.[3] Patients may also typically present with temporal headaches, tenderness over the superficial temporal artery (a branch of the external carotid artery), decreased pulse, or a cord-like structure over the superficial temporal artery. Other symptoms may include aching or stiffness in the neck, headaches, jaw claudication, and visual disturbances. A significant risk exists of optic nerve ischemia and blindness can occur in giant cell arteritis, hence giant cell arteritis can be a medical emergency. The most common site for giant cell arteritis is in the superficial temporal artery, but there can be involvement of multiple extracranial arteries and other arteries of the head and neck. Occasionally, arteries below the aortic arch are involved. The erythrocyte sedimentation rate is often elevated as well as another inflammatory marker, C-reactive protein. The gold standard for diagnosis is a temporal artery biopsy showing mononuclear cells and giant cells infiltrating the area around the elastic lamina within the media of the cell wall.

### Scanning Technique

The sonographic examination of a patient with suspected giant cell or temporal arteritis involves imaging the region of the vascular system related to the presenting symptoms. If a patient presents with temporal pain and headaches, the temporal artery itself will be examined usually in association with a complete carotid duplex ultrasound examination. The temporal artery is the smaller of two terminal branches of the external carotid artery. It begins behind the mandible, crosses the zygomatic process, then courses along the temporal bone. It continues for about 5 cm before it divides into the frontal and parietal branches. The temporal artery is small and superficial, requiring a high-frequency transducer in order to properly insonate it.

If the patient presents with upper extremity symptoms, an upper extremity duplex ultrasound is performed paying close attention to the subclavian, axillary, and brachial arteries. The following images were obtained from a 63-year-old white female who presented with stiffness in her shoulders and upper arms. Additionally, 1 month later, she began to notice pallor in the left hand with paresthesia and a cold sensation. She also noted left upper extremity fatigability with any activity using her left arm. A physical examination revealed decreased pulses in the left upper extremity with the left brachial blood pressure 60 mm Hg lower than the right. Significantly dampened flow was noted by photoplethysmography (PPG) in all five digits of the left hand. She underwent an upper extremity arterial duplex ultrasound. A high-grade stenosis was found within the left axillary artery with a PSV of greater than 400 cm/s (Fig. 16-1A). The color Doppler image of the vessel at this level revealed an irregular lumen with mural thickening. An area of echolucency surrounding the residual lumen was observed (Fig. 16-1B). Continuing distally down the arm, the brachial artery was identified. The color imaging displayed several areas of poor filling and aliasing. Angiography was then performed (Fig. 16-1C). The giant cell arteritis lesion was identified and successfully treated with angioplasty (Fig. 16-1D and E).

A stenosis caused by giant cell or temporal arteritis will produce the typical ultrasound findings associated with any stenosis. The primary tool used to define a stenosis will be a focal increase in PSV. A PSV which is twice the value of the PSV in the adjacent more proximal vessel is indicative

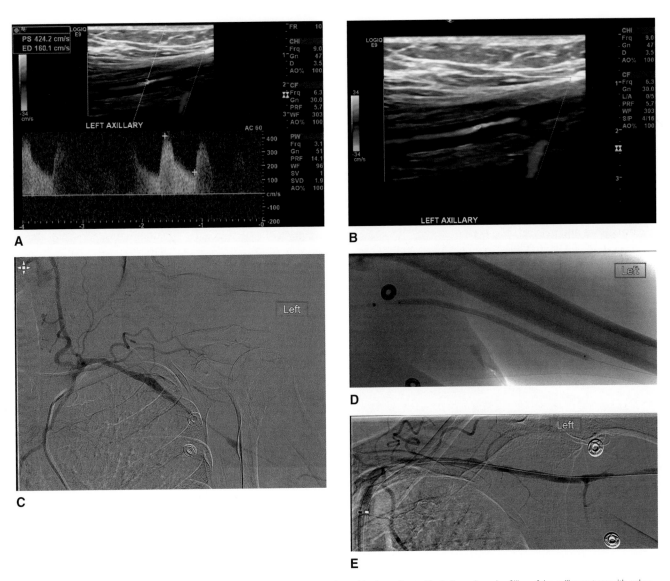

**FIGURE 16-1** **A:** A high-grade stenosis >400 cm/s of an axillary artery in a patient with giant cell arteritis. **B:** Irregular color filling of the axillary artery with color aliasing and echolucency observed surrounding the vessel. **C:** Initial angiography of axillary artery with giant cell arteritis lesion. **D:** Angioplasty of lesion. **E:** Postaxillary angioplasty of giant cell arteritis.

of at least a 50% stenosis. This criterion can be applied to most arteries. On B-mode image, giant cell arteritis often appears as a concentric wall thickening that is hypoechoic. This thickening can occur over a long segment of the vessel and lead to a tapering of the arterial lumen.[4] Additionally, an anechoic area may be present surrounding the vessel producing a "halo" around the vessel. This is thought to occur because of white blood cell infiltration. The "halo" should be present in both transverse and sagittal imaging planes.

## Takayasu's Arteritis

Takayasu's arteritis mainly impacts the aortic arch and its large branches. The subclavian arteries are involved in over 90% of the cases, whereas the common carotid arteries are involved in approximately 60% of patients.[5] As with other forms of arteritis, the inflammatory process may be part of an immune system disorder. Takayasu's arteritis involves all three layers of the vessel wall. It can lead to a

partial obstruction of the vessel lumen or complete vessel occlusion. Vessel walls may also become weakened such that aneurysm formation may occur. The disease is most common in Southeast Asia. There is an 8:1 female to male prevalence with greater than 80% of affected individuals being less than 40 years of age. The presenting symptom of patients is often an absent peripheral pulse. There may be a brachial blood pressure gradient of greater than 30 mm Hg. Lightheadedness, vertigo, amaurosis fugax, transient ischemic attacks, hemiparesis, diplopia, and upper extremity claudication may also occur. Angiography and ultrasound can be used to diagnose the presence of this disease.

### Scanning Technique

The sonographic examination of a patient with suspected Takayasu's arteritis will be similar to that employed for temporal arteritis. The portion of the vascular system interrogated is usually the carotid and subclavian vessels. The grayscale image is closely examined for evidence of wall

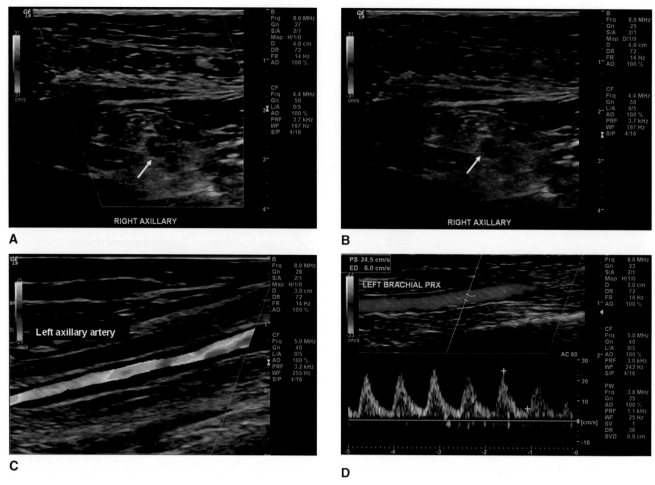

**FIGURE 16-2** Ultrasound images from a patient with Takayasu's arteritis. **A:** Axillary artery transverse image with color illustrating the reduced flow lumen (*arrow*). **B:** Axillary artery transverse colorized grayscale image highlighting the circumferential wall thickening (*arrow*). **C:** Sagittal view of the axillary artery with color filling the reduced lumen. **D:** Dampened arterial signals from the distal brachial artery.

thickening, while spectral Doppler and color imaging are used to detect a stenosis.

The ultrasound image typically reveals thickened walls with concentric narrowing. The thickened areas are usually homogeneous in appearance with adjacent segments of the vessels appearing normal and disease free (Fig. 16-2A–C). Often, the wall thickening will occur over long segments of several centimeters. The stenosis will produce elevated velocities within the segment with poststenotic turbulence present distally. In transverse view, the circumferential thickening of the vessel wall has been termed the macaroni sign.[6] Distal to areas of stenosis, dampened arterial signals will be present (Fig. 16-2D).

## Thromboangitis Obliterans (Buerger's Disease)

Thromboangitis obliterans or Buerger's disease is another nonatherosclerotic inflammatory disease. This disease affects the small- and medium-sized arteries involving the upper and lower extremities, including the digital, plantar, tibial, peroneal, radial, and ulnar arteries.[7] This disease typically manifests in patients under the age of 45 and has a 3:1 male to female distribution. Presenting symptoms can consist of ischemic digital ulcers. Ulcerations on the toes are slightly

more common than finger ulcers. Gangrene of the digits can also occur. Superficial thrombophlebitis can be seen in one-third of the patients, and one-half of the patients have symptoms involving numbness and tingling in the hands and feet. Other symptoms include claudication in the arch of the foot, and also in the arms and hands.[8] This disease is always bilateral in nature though findings may be more pronounced in one extremity than the other. Greater than 80% of patients will have involvement of the disease in three of the four extremities. Because these symptoms are similar to those produced by other diseases, autoimmune diseases, hypercoagulable states, and cardioembolic disease must be excluded. Tobacco abuse is always present in the clinical history of patients with Buerger's disease and essential to the progression of the disease. Both smoking tobacco and chewing tobacco are associated with the disease. The disease is very prevalent in India where people of low-socioeconomic class smoke homemade cigarettes made from raw tobacco.[9] Blood tests for various inflammatory markers are often normal in these patients and thus not very helpful in the diagnosis of this disease.

### Scanning Technique

Both physiologic testing and duplex ultrasound examinations are performed in order to identify Buerger's disease.

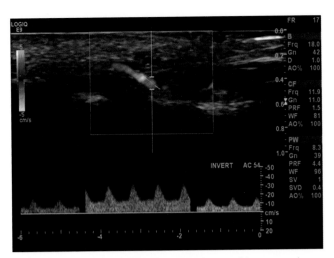

**FIGURE 16-3** Duplex ultrasound form a digital artery of the great toe in a patient with Buerger's disease.

Plethysomographic waveforms and pressures can be obtained from the arms (upper arm, forearm, and wrist) or legs (thigh, calf, and ankle) depending on the symptoms present. Digital evaluation is essential because in some patients waveforms recorded at the wrist or ankle levels are found to be normal. However, analysis of digital vessel waveforms will reveal the abnormality. Standard techniques for these studies have been previously described in Chapter 11.

Duplex ultrasound will be conducted on the suspected extremity to determine the level of arterial occlusion. Typically, in the upper extremity, this can include examination of the brachial, radial, and ulnar arteries. In the lower extremity, ultrasound can be performed distally along the tibial arteries. These duplex ultrasound images should be carefully examined to rule out the presence of atherosclerotic plaques. Digital vessels can be evaluated with ultrasound although this is not often the case. The digital vessels are small and superficial, and as such require a high-frequency transducer with a small footprint in order to be adequately examined. A stenosis can sometimes be observed using digital duplex ultrasound, providing successful insonation of the digital vessels are achieved. Figure 16-3 illustrates a duplex ultrasound image from the great toe of a patient with Buerger's disease. A focal digital artery stenosis can be noted.

The preferred method to interrogate digital perfusion is with physiologic techniques. The next series of images were taken from a 31-year-old female who presented with pain in the first and second digits of her right hand. She was postpartum and had quit smoking during the pregnancy. She recently resumed smoking. Her medical history was also significant for hypertension. Digital PPG was performed (Fig. 16-4A). The waveforms were significantly dampened within the right second digit and slightly diminished within the right first digit as compared to the right third, fourth, and fifth digits. Clinical examination revealed an abnormal demarcation on the first and second digits, with the second digit being more severe (Fig. 16-4B). Angiography demonstrated digital artery obstruction of several vessels which was consistent with the noninvasive vascular laboratory findings (Fig. 16-4C).

## Radiation-Induced Arteritis

Radiation-induced arteritis is a rare complication of radiation therapy for cancer. It results in perivascular fibrosis, inflammation, and acceleration of atherosclerosis. The radiation-induced arterial lesion may be difficult to distinguish from atherosclerosis. However, the localization, focal nature, and absence of atherosclerosis in other sites favor radiation as the etiology.[10,11] Typically, these patients present with claudication that may occur several months after completion of radiation treatment. Successful treatment with balloon angioplasty and stents has been performed for this condition.[12]

### Scanning Technique

Duplex ultrasound evaluation includes the arterial system within the radiated region as well as adjacent vessels. Gray-scale imaging is closely examined for wall irregularities and wall thickening. The appearance of these thickened areas is similar to that observed with giant cell or Takayasu's arteritis. Images from the radiated areas should be compared to those obtained from normal segments remote to the radiated area. Spectral Doppler and color waveforms are obtained from each vessel to look for evidence of stenosis. Often, physiologic tests such as an ankle-brachial index (ABI) may be performed to document global ischemia.

## EMBOLIC DISEASE

An embolism is an occlusion or obstruction of an artery by a transported clot of blood or mass, bacteria, or other foreign substance. There are many sources for the clotted blood, some of which are discussed in the following section.

The classic presentation of patients with a peripheral embolism is an abrupt onset of leg pain with no past medical history of arterial disease. Arterial embolization must be distinguished from preexisting arterial disease with thrombosis. Arterial duplex ultrasound demonstrating the absence of plaque and the absence of collateral flow strongly favor acute embolization.

The site of embolization outside the cerebrovascular system includes the following locations[13]:

| | |
|---|---|
| Upper extremity: | 14% |
| Visceral: | 7% |
| Aortoiliac: | 22% |
| Femoral: | 36% |
| Popliteal: | 15% |
| Other: | 6% |

### Cardioembolic Disease

Approximately 80% to 99% of arterial emboli are from a cardiac source. This can include atrial fibrillation, postmyocardial infarction with left ventricular thrombus, mechanical heart valves, intracardiac tumor, vegetation from endocarditis, and paradoxic emboli. Cardiac embolic disease is seen across all age spectrums. The most common underlying cardiac disease seen is chronic atrial fibrillation. Thrombus forms in the left atrial appendage because of stagnation of blood, then embolizes to a distal site. Though embolic stroke is the most common presentation, emboli can occur throughout the arterial tree. Figure 16-5 illustrates the spectral Doppler pattern in a patient with rapid atrial fibrillation.

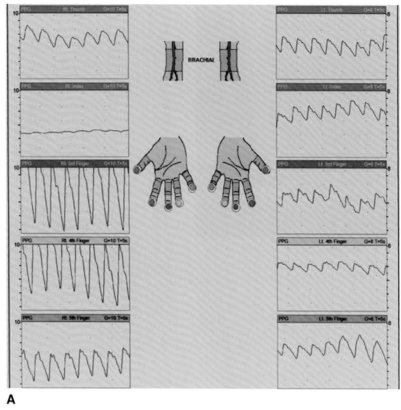

**A**

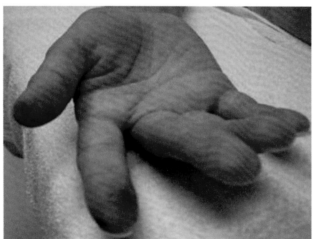

**B**

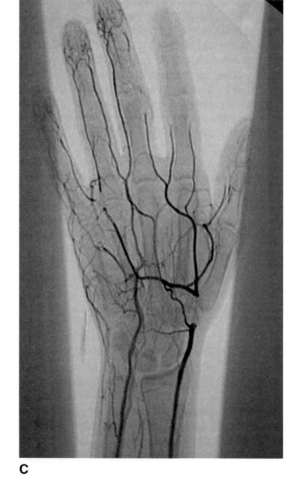

**C**

**FIGURE 16-4 A:** Digital photoplethysmography in a patient with Buerger's disease demonstrating digital ischemia. **B:** The right hand of the patient with ischemic skin changes to the first and second digits. **C:** Angioplasty revealing multiple areas of digital vessel occlusion.

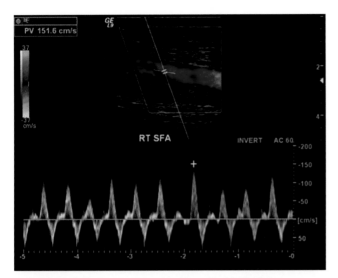

**FIGURE 16-5** Doppler spectrum of a patient with atrial fibrillation.

Another common source is paradoxic embolization secondary to an intracardiac right to left shunt (patent foramen ovale or atrial septal defect). Patients who present with an acute arterial occlusion that may have deep venous thrombosis should be considered for paradoxic arterial emboli. A typical workup for these patients may include transthoracic echocardiography or transesophageal echocardiography with agitated saline.

### Scanning Technique

The following images were obtained from a 26-year-old female. She was a nonsmoker who was taking oral contraceptives. She had recently been treated for dehydration secondary to alcohol abuse. She presented with severe right lower extremity pain, pallor, and pulselessness. She was normotensive and in normal sinus rhythm. Figure 16-6A illustrates the presenting pallor of the patient's right foot. A duplex ultrasound examination was performed on the right lower extremity. The duplex ultrasound examination revealed an abnormal common femoral artery waveform with increased resistance demonstrated by the abrupt "spike" noted in systole (Fig. 16-6B). Continuing the ultrasound distally, echogenic material was observed within the popliteal artery (Fig. 16-6C and D). No atherosclerotic disease was present within any of the vessels imaged. Sagittal and transverse projections of the popliteal vessels revealed no flow within either the popliteal artery or vein. The patient also underwent transthoracic echocardiography that demonstrated a right to left cardiac shunt. A deep vein thrombosis was present which had embolized to the heart but passed into the systemic circulation via the cardiac shunt. This embolus occluded the right popliteal artery, resulting in the acutely ischemic right leg.

### Arterial Embolic Sources

The remaining 10% to 20% of emboli arise from outside the heart. Large upper extremity arteries such as the subclavian arteries may be a source. Disease within the aorta or iliac, femoral or popliteal arteries may also result in emboli. This disease may be in the form of ulcerated plaques or mural thrombus aneurysms.

## TRAUMATIC AND IATROGENIC ARTERIAL INJURY

Various arterial injuries can result from vascular trauma or iatrogenically during another procedure. These injuries can include pseudoaneurysms, arteriovenous fistulae (AVF), vessel thrombosis, emboli, or dissection.

### Pseudoaneurysm

Owing to the increased numbers of angiographic procedures, the incidence of pseudoaneurysms has increased significantly. A pseudoaneurysm or false aneurysm is a pulsating encapsulated hematoma that communicates with the adjacent artery. This process occurs from a leakage of blood after an injury into the soft tissue. The pseudoaneurysm may cause extrinsic compression of an adjacent nerve and lead to nerve irritation with tingling or shock-like pain down the affected extremity. The pseudoaneurysm may lead to compression of the adjacent deep vein leading to extremity swelling. The most common cause of pseudoaneurysms is the use of large bore catheters required for endovascular procedures during cardiac or peripheral vascular interventions. The most common site for a pseudoaneurysm is the right common femoral artery. Blunt or penetrating trauma may also cause an injury and secondary pseudoaneurysm. Pseudoaneurysm can also be seen postsurgical bypass and may represent dehiscence secondary to graft infection. Pseudoaneurysms are also frequently seen in association with dialysis grafts.

### Scanning Technique

Most patients with a suspected pseudoaneurysm present with a pulsatile mass. This mass may be over the site of a catheterization or traumatic injury. There may be ecchymosis and pain. A duplex ultrasound examination should be performed of both the arteries and veins in the region. Figure 16-7A illustrates a pseudoaneurysm observed in a patient who had undergone a cardiac catheterization 4 days prior. There is color outside the vessel wall with a neck or tract that connects the vessel with the pseudoaneurysm sac. The color demonstrates a red-blue swirling pattern consistent with a pseudoaneurysm. This red-blue pattern often resembles the Chinese yin-yang symbol. In this particular example, there are two pseudoaneurysm sacs that while uncommon this does occur. Spectral Doppler patterns within the neck of the pseudoaneurysm will demonstrate a flow into the sac as well as flow out of the sac, which is referred to as a to-and-fro Doppler pattern (Fig. 16-7B).

### Arteriovenous Fistula

Traumatic AVF can occur following arterial trauma such as a direct stab wound, gunshot wound, or after blunt trauma. Most iatrogenic AVFs result as a complication of percutaneous femoral artery catheterization. Central venous catheterization occasionally leads to AVFs, and rarely AVFs are seen following total knee replacement or lumbosacral surgery. Patients with an AVF usually present with signs and symptoms at site of intervention or injury. Typically, a new bruit is ascultated, a thrill may be palpated, or a

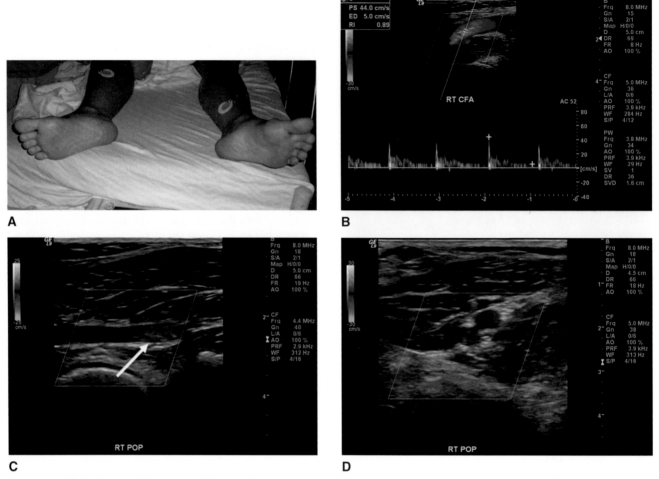

**FIGURE 16-6 A:** Right foot pallor in a patient with embolic disease. **B:** Abnormal Doppler waveforms in the common femoral artery in this patient with a popliteal artery embolus. **C:** Sagittal view of the popliteal artery embolus (*arrow*). **D:** Transverse view of the popliteal artery and vein with no flow detected in either vessel.

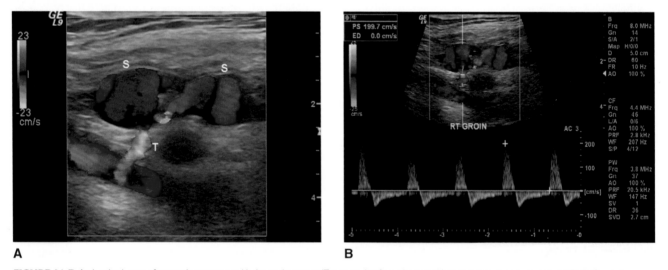

**FIGURE 16-7 A:** A color image of a pseudoaneurysm with the neck or tract (*T*) connecting from the vessel into two pseudoaneurysm sacs (*S*). **B:** Spectral Doppler patterns within the neck of a pseudoaneurysm with a classic to-and fro pattern.

hematoma is present. The patients are often referred for an ultrasound to rule out the presence of a pseudoaneurysm. Rarely, both a pseudoaneurysm and an AVF may be present at the same location.

### Scanning Technique

The gold standard to detect an AVF remains digital subtraction angiography, but duplex ultrasound is a frequently used alternative for detection of an AVF. The characteristic findings on ultrasound include:

- high-diastolic flow in an artery proximal to AVF
- high-velocity turbulent flow (arterialized venous flow) in the vein near the fistula connection
- may see a color bruit at the site near the fistula connection

The following images were taken from a 62-year-old male who presented with a palpable thrill over an arterial puncture site in the right groin. Figure 16-8A illustrates a prominent color bruit over the region of the common femoral artery. The angiography demonstrates filling of the venous system via an AVF at the common femoral artery (Fig. 16-8B). The spectral Doppler patterns in the femoral

vein at the saphenofemoral junction reveal an arterialized or prominently pulsatile Doppler signal (Fig. 16-8C).

## Arterial Occlusion

Iatrogenic arterial occlusions can occur after various interventions or cannulations. Occasionally an arterial occlusion may be seen following the deployment of an arterial closure device. These devices are commonly used following femoral arterial catheterization to aid with proper closure of the puncture site. The presentation of the patient seen with this complication is highly variable. Partial thrombosis to complete thrombosis with a cold pulseless leg may be observed.

### Scanning Technique

Duplex ultrasound can be directly performed over the puncture site. Depending on the composition of the closure device and how it was placed, it may be difficult to identify. Occasionally, only a small defect may be present in the vessel wall, or a slight change in echogenicity was noted at the site of the closure device. Figure 16-9A–C was

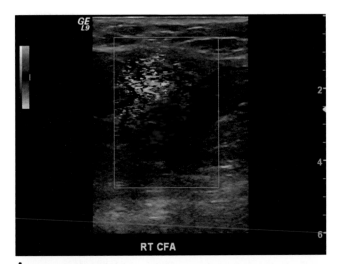

**A**

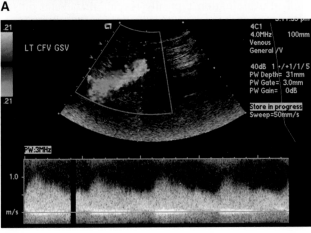

**C**

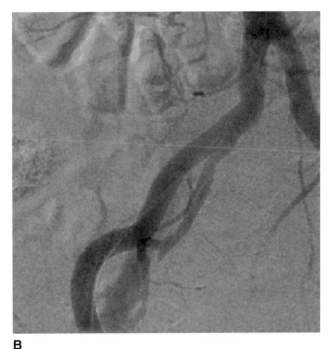

**B**

**FIGURE 16-8 A:** Color bruit of a common femoral artery arteriovenous fistula. **B:** Angiography demonstrating filling of the venous system via the common femoral artery arteriovenous fistula. **C:** The arterialized Doppler signal present within the common femoral vein at the saphenofemoral junction.

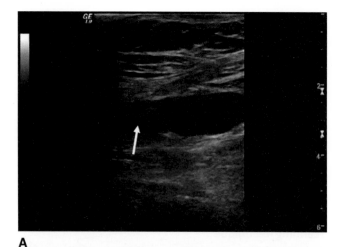

**A**

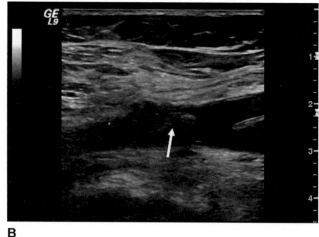

**B**

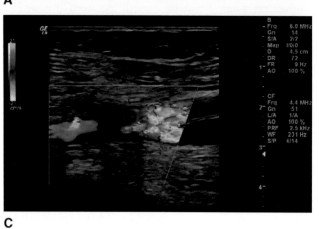

**C**

**FIGURE 16-9  A:** Sagittal ultrasound of a common femoral artery with echogenic material (*arrow*) present within the lumen consistent with an acute thrombus. **B:** Thrombus (*arrow*) in the common femoral artery just proximal to the superficial and deep femoral arteries. **C:** Color-flow imaging demonstrating poor filling around the thrombus with filling of the vessel distal to the thrombus.

taken at the common femoral artery of a patient who had a cardiac catheterization 3 days prior. A small hematoma was present in the area, and weak popliteal and femoral pulses were noted on a physical examination. Echogenic material was seen in the proximal common femoral artery consistent with vessel thrombosis. Poor color filling was noted around the thrombus.

## POPLITEAL ARTERY ENTRAPMENT SYNDROME

Popliteal artery entrapment is a difficult syndrome to diagnose. Popliteal entrapment occurs when the popliteal artery is compressed by the medial head of the gastrocnemius muscle or adjacent tendons.[14] This is the result of a congenital deformity of the muscle or tendon structures. The repeated extrinsic compression of the popliteal artery produces trauma to the vessel wall, which can lead to aneurysm formation, thromboembolism, or arterial thrombosis.

The presence of claudication symptoms in a young patient with no risk factors for atherosclerosis is suggestive popliteal artery entrapment. The onset of claudication may occur after extensive exercise (such as marathon running), may be chronic with predictable claudication, or may occur with walking but not running. Rarely, symptoms

may be acute if the popliteal artery has become occluded. Patients may also complain of numbness or paresthesia of the foot. There is a male to female incidence of 2:1. About two-third of patients may have entrapment in the contralateral limb.

### Scanning Technique

Clinical examination typically reveals that distal pulses are present at rest with the ankle in the neutral position. Pulses disappear with active plantar or dorsiflexion. Various imaging modalities can be used to aid in the diagnosis of popliteal entrapment. However, interpretation of the lower extremity vascular examination must relate to the patient's symptoms because many asymptomatic patients will partially compress the popliteal artery with provocative maneuvers.

Ultrasound can be employed to image the popliteal artery at rest and with active plantar flexion. Normal velocities at rest will become altered during the maneuver and demonstrate diminished or no flow (Fig. 16-10A and B). Digital subtraction angiography can also be performed and will demonstrate compression of the popliteal artery with active maneuvers. Figure 16-10C demonstrates angiographic evidence of a luminal irregularity in the neutral position. Figure 16-10D demonstrates significant angiographic obstruction after passive dorsiflexion being performed.

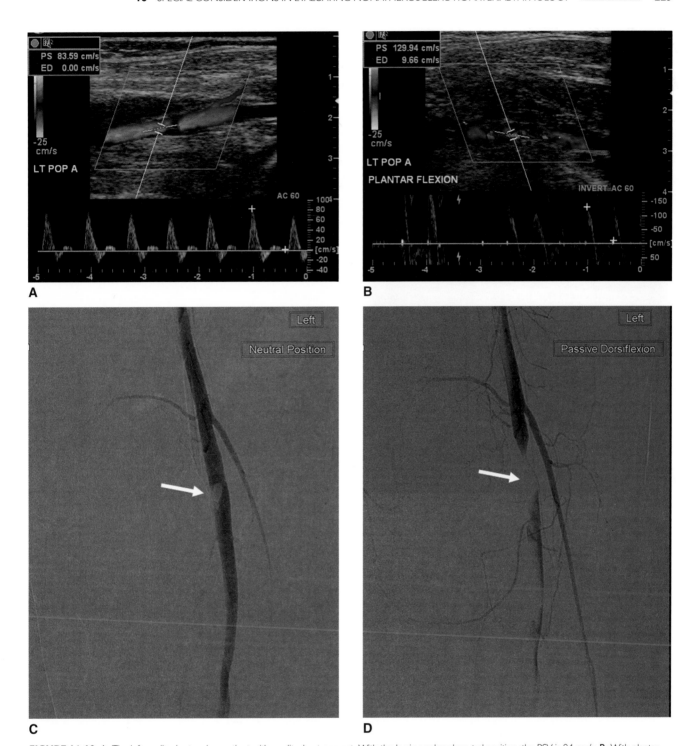

**FIGURE 16-10** **A:** The left popliteal artery in a patient with popliteal entrapment. With the leg in a relaxed neutral position, the PSV is 84 cm/s. **B:** With plantar flexion the popliteal artery velocities increase to 130 cm/s. **C:** Angiogram taken with the leg in a neutral position with a filling defect (*white arrow*). **D:** Angiogram with passive dorsiflexion demonstrating a significant obstruction (*white arrow*).

However, other imaging modalities such as magnetic resonance or computerized tomography are often employed. These other modalities will not only provide information about the vascular system but also identify the skeletomuscular features of the popliteal fossa. These anatomic details can identify those components responsible for the compression of the vessel. It can also exclude other pathology such as adventitial cystic disease of the popliteal artery.

## NONATHEROSCLEROTIC ARTERIAL ANEURYSMS

Although atherosclerosis is a major cause of aneurysm formation, there are multiple other diseases which can result in aneurysm formation. Aneurysms can be associated with various inflammatory processes such as some of the arteritis diseases discussed earlier in this chapter. Takayasu's disease

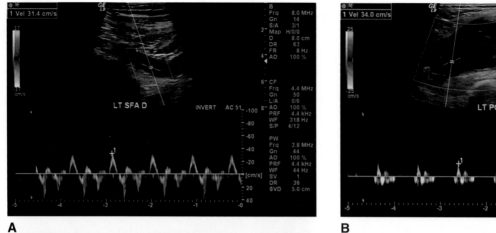

**A**

**B**

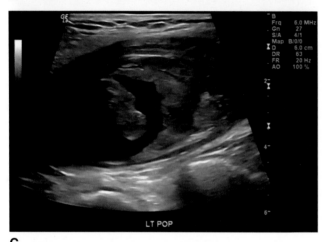

**C**

**FIGURE 16-11** **A:** Abnormal distal superficial femoral artery velocities. **B:** Staccato-type flow with the proximal popliteal artery. **C:** Thrombosed popliteal artery aneurysm.

involves large arteries and typically causes flow reducing stenosis of the aortic arch arteries. However, aneurysms are the most frequent fatal complication of Takayasu's arteritis. The reported incidence of aneurysms in these patients varies with one recent paper reporting a 45% occurrence of aortic aneurysms in these patients.[15] Other more rare inflammatory diseases, including Behcets's syndrome, polyarteritis nodusa, and Kawasaki's disease, can also be associated with aneurysms.

Aneurysms are associated with inherited matrix defects such as Marfan's syndrome. Marfan's syndrome is a connective tissue disorder that is typically associated with aortic arch aneurysms. Ehlers-Danlos Syndrome (EDS) is another well-known and often suspected cause aneurysms. Patients with EDS have a congenital defect in type III collagen, and this can lead to arterial rupture with or without an aneurysm.

## Scanning Technique

Duplex ultrasound imaging has long been used to identify arterial aneurysms. Aneurysms of the aortic arch and thoracic aorta are best identified with various types of angiography. When evaluating peripheral arteries for aneurysm formation, measurements of vessel diameter should be obtained for both proximal and distal to an area of suspected dilation. If a vessel diameter increases at least 50% as compared to the native more proximal adjacent segment of artery, this vessel is considered aneurysmal. The following images were obtained from a 51-year-old male with Marfan's syndrome. He had previously undergone an aortic arch and valve repair. He presented with left lower leg pain which had been worsening over the past 4 days. He had no history of smoking or peripheral vascular disease. Figure 16-11A illustrates grossly abnormal flow within the distal superficial femoral artery. Staccato type flow was seen in the proximal popliteal artery (Fig. 16-11B). The mid to distal popliteal artery was found to be aneurysmal and thrombosed (Fig. 16-11C). Popliteal artery aneurysms are very rare manifestations with patients with Marfan's syndrome.[16]

Pathology Box 16-1 summarizes the nonatherosclerotic pathologies discussed in this chapter. It lists the common sites and vascular test findings.

## PATHOLOGY BOX 16-1
### Nonatherosclerotic Arterial Pathology

| Pathology | Common Site Affected | Vascular Test Findings |
|---|---|---|
| Giant cell arteritis | Superficial temporal artery; extracranial arteries; occasionally aortic arch branches | • Increased PSV at stenosis<br>• Concentric wall thickening<br>• Anechoic "halo" may be present |
| Takayasu's arteritis | Aortic arch and its branches | • Increased PSV at stenosis<br>• Concentric wall thickening<br>• "Macaroni" sign<br>• Aneurysmal formation |
| Buerger's disease | Small- and medium-sized arteries; digital vessels | • Dampened digital PPGs<br>• Small vessel focal stenosis with increased PSV |
| Radiation-induced arteritis | Any artery | • Concentric wall thickening<br>• Increased PSV<br>• Normal adjacent arterial segments |
| Embolic disease | Cerebrovascular vessels; any artery | • Increased resistance in Doppler signals proximal to embolus<br>• Echogenic material within vessel<br>• No atherosclerosis in adjacent vessel |
| Pseudoaneurysm | Common femoral artery; dialysis fistulae/grafts; bypass graft anastomoses | • Color-flow outside normal vessel walls<br>• Yin-yang swirling color pattern<br>• To-and-fro signal in the neck or tract |
| Arteriovenous fistula | Common femoral artery; any artery | • Color tissue bruit<br>• Increased diastolic flow in artery proximal to AVF<br>• High-velocity, turbulent signals at fistula site<br>• Prominently pulsatile venous signals |
| Arterial occlusion/thrombosis | Any artery | • Echogenic material in vessel at puncture site<br>• Poor color filling<br>• Increased PSV with partial occlusion<br>• Increased resistance with total occlusion |
| Popliteal entrapment | Popliteal artery | • PSV normal in neutral, resting position<br>• Increased PSV with active plantar or dorsiflexion |
| Nonatherosclerotic aneurysm | Aorta; large and medium arteries | • Diameter increase of 50% as compared to adjacent proximal vessel<br>• No atherosclerosis<br>• May contain thrombus<br>• Increased resistance if completely thrombosed |

## SUMMARY

- The majority of patients presenting for a peripheral arterial ultrasound examination will likely have atherosclerosis as the disease identified.
- There are numerous other pathologies that will produce PAD.
- It is important for the sonographer or vascular technologist to be familiar with these entities and their ultrasound characteristics.
- These uncommon causes of arterial disease should be suspected particularly in patients without the standard risk factors for atherosclerosis.

## CRITICAL THINKING QUESTIONS

1. You are examining a patient with a 35 mm Hg brachial blood pressure difference with the right brachial blood pressure lower than the left. Will the spectral analysis or the B-mode image be more helpful to determine the cause of a stenosis?

2. When evaluating a patient for Buerger's disease, which noninvasive vascular tests would you perform and why?

3. What are three iatrogenic arterial pathologies that can arise following catheterization of the common femoral artery for coronary artery angioplasty and stenting? Which of these problems would most impact the common femoral vein Doppler signals?

## MEDIA MENU

Student Resources available on thePoint® include:
- Audio glossary
- Interactive question bank
- Videos
- Internet resources

_NCES

ıgberg DA, Quinones-Baldrich W. Takayasu's disease: nonspecific aortoarteritis. In: Rutherford RB, ed. *Vascular Surgery*. 6th ed. Philadelphia, PA: W.B. Saunders; 2005:419–430.

2. Thornton J, Kupinski AM. Vascular arteritis: the atypical pathology. *Vasc Ultrasound Today*. 2007;12:213–236.

3. Braunwald E. *Heart Disease*. 3rd ed. Philadelphia, PA: W.B. Saunders; 1992:1547.

4. Tato F, Hoffman U. Giant cell arteritis: a systemic vascular disease. *Vasc Med*. 2008;13:127–140.

5. Klippel JH. *The Pocket Primer on Rheumatic Diseases*. 2nd ed. London, UK: Springer-Verlag; 2010:149–164.

6. Maeda H, Handa N, Matsumoto M, et al. Carotid lesion detected by B-mode ultrasonography in Takayasu's arteritis: 'macaroni sign' as an indicator of the disease. *Ultrasound Med Biol*. 1991;17:695–701.

7. Garcia LA. Epidemiology and pathophysiology of lower extremity peripheral arterial disease. *J Endovasc Ther*. 2006;13(Suppl II):II-3–II-9.

8. Puechal X, Fiessinger JN. Thromoangiitis obliterans or Buerger's disease: challenges for the rheumatologist. *Rheumatology*. 2007;46:192–199.

9. Olin JW. Thromboangiitis obliterans (Buerger's disease). *N Engl J Med*. 2000;343:864–869.

10. Sacar M, Baltalarli B, Baltalarli A, et al. Occlusive arterial disease caused by radiotherapy. *AJCI*. 2006;1(1):42–44.

11. Modrall JG, Sadjadi J. Early and late presentations of radiation arteritis. *Semin Vasc Surg*. 2003;16:209–214.

12. Guthaner DF, Schmitz L. Percutaneous transluminal angioplasty of radiation-induced arterial stenoses. *Radiology*. 1982;144: 77–78.

13. Kasirajan K, Ouriel K. Acute limb ischemia. In: Rutherford RB, ed. *Vascular Surgery*. 6th ed. Philadelphia, PA: W.B. Saunders; 2005:974.

14. Macedo TA, Johnson CM, Hallett JW, et al. Popliteal entrapment syndrome: role of imaging in the diagnosis. *AJR Am J Roentgenol*. 2003;181:1259–1265.

15. Sueyoshi E, Sakamoto I, Hayashi K. Aortic aneurysms in patients with Takayasu's arteritis: CT evaluation. *AJR Am J Roentgenol*. 2000;175:1727–1733.

16. Wolfgarten B, Kruger I, Gawenda M. Rare manifestation of abdominal aortic aneurysm and popliteal aneurysm in a patient with Marfan's syndrome: a case report. *Vasc Endovasc Surg*. 2001;35:81–84.

# PERIPHERAL VENOUS

# Duplex Ultrasound Imaging of the Lower Extremity Venous System

STEVEN R. TALBOT  |  MARK OLIVER

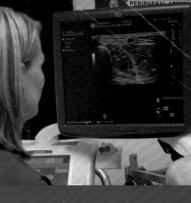

## CHAPTER 17

## OBJECTIVES

- Describe the components of the lower extremity venous system
- Define the normal image and Doppler characteristics of the venous system
- Identify the image characteristics of acute and chronic thrombi
- Describe the Doppler waveform characteristics associated with various pathologies
- List the risk factors associated with the formation of a deep vein thrombus

## KEY TERMS

**acute thrombus**

**chronic thrombus**

**deep vein**

**perforating vein**

**superficial vein**

**valve**

## GLOSSARY

**acute thrombus**  Newly formed clotted blood within a vein, generally less than 14 days old

**chronic thrombus**  Clotted blood within a vein that has generally been present for a period of several weeks or months

**deep vein**  A vein that is the companion vessel to an artery and travels within the deep muscular compartments of the leg

**perforating vein**  A small vein that connects the deep and superficial venous systems

**superficial vein**  A vein that is superior to the muscular compartments of the leg; travels within superficial fascial compartments; has no corresponding companion artery

**valve**  An inward projection of the intimal layer of a vein wall producing two semilunar leaflets, which prevent the retrograde movement of blood flow

Before the advances in ultrasound imaging that made it possible to use duplex ultrasound to look at the veins of the legs and the arms, diagnosing venous thrombosis was a complicated matter. Clinical judgment was inaccurate. The diagnostic study of choice was venography, which was painful and expensive, and carried its own set of risks.

In the 1980s, the advent of venous duplex ultrasound imaging changed all that.[1] Since that time, duplex ultrasound imaging has become the method of choice for imaging of deep vein thrombosis (DVT).[2] Occasionally, other imaging modalities may be utilized for difficult or limited duplex ultrasound examinations.[3] Duplex ultrasound has

the capability to diagnose, localize, and determine the age of a thrombus as well as follow the natural course of disease. Thus, it has become a mainstay in the management of DVT.[4] In addition, duplex ultrasound has the capability of discovering and diagnosing vascular and nonvascular incidental findings during the examination.[5]

However, venous duplex ultrasound imaging is extremely examiner dependent. Studies done improperly will be inaccurate. A patient who has been misdiagnosed with a venous thrombosis may be subjected to lengthy anticoagulant therapy with the risk and expense that go with that therapy. Conversely, a patient with an undiagnosed venous thrombosis due to an improperly performed ultrasound examination may have a life-threatening problem go undetected. This is a common tale because of the lack of standardization of qualifications for those performing venous ultrasound examinations.

The solution to this problem is to have those performing venous ultrasound examinations follow proper protocols and to have adequate supervised experience. The protocol in this chapter will assure the best likelihood of performing the venous duplex ultrasound examination utilizing techniques that will produce accurate results.

When performing venous duplex ultrasound imaging, the examiner is trying to assess three things:

1. The presence or absence of thrombus
2. The relative risk of the thrombus dislodging and traveling to the lungs
3. The competence of the contained valves

Venous duplex ultrasound is a great tool for determining each of the items listed above. The sonographer performing venous examinations must understand the venous anatomy.[6-11] Additionally, it is helpful to understand the pathophysiology, risk factors, and symptoms associated with DVT. This chapter provides a comprehensive review of information pertaining to the venous duplex ultrasound examination and DVT.

## ANATOMY

Chapter 4 of this book provides an anatomy review and diagrams of the vascular system. Continuing this discussion, a vascular technologist or sonographer needs to clearly understand the three main categories of veins that can be imaged:

1. Deep veins
2. Superficial veins
3. Perforators

### Deep Veins

The deep veins are the freeways of the venous system. They are the main conduit for blood returning to the heart and are surrounded by muscle. They accompany an artery usually of the same name. Thrombus within the deep veins is likely to be dislodged because the muscle squeezes the deep veins with each step taken. This squeezing action is the main force that propels blood out of the leg and back to the heart, but also can be the mechanism for dislodging a contained thrombus into the venous system producing a pulmonary embolism (PE). Thrombus found in a deep vein is usually larger than a thrombus found in a superficial vein. This makes the thrombus from a deep vein more likely to cause a life-threatening PE because the thrombus has the potential for becoming lodged in a larger caliber pulmonary artery branch.

### Superficial Veins

Unlike the deep veins, the superficial veins travel close to the skin, superficial to the muscle. These veins are usually smaller than their deeper counterparts and travel without an accompanying artery. They have an entirely different function than the deep veins. Their purpose is to get blood near the skin so that they can help regulate body temperature. If the body needs to get rid of heat, the superficial veins engorge and heat from the blood-filled veins escapes into the air. If the body needs to conserve heat, the superficial veins contract and shunt blood away from the skin so that the heat from the contained blood is not lost.

The traditional wisdom is that thrombi in the superficial veins do not embolize so that there is often less concern about a thrombus in the superficial system. This is not true. Thrombi from the superficial venous system do embolize and travel to the lungs. However, thrombi are generally less likely to embolize from the superficial veins because they are not surrounded by muscle similar to the deep veins. Thrombi in the superficial veins are usually smaller in caliber than a thrombus in the deep veins, but their size can vary. If a thrombus is located in a superficial vein near the junction with a deep vein (the saphenofemoral or saphenopopliteal junctions), it has a greater potential to propagate into the deep veins. Thrombi in the superficial veins must be evaluated carefully to judge its potential risk to the patient.

### Perforators

Perforators are small bridge veins that connect the deep veins with the superficial veins. Their role is to keep blood from spending too much time near the skin surface by moving blood from the superficial veins to the deep veins. They have one-way valves that insure blood moves in the proper direction. When these valves do not function, blood can pool as the patient sits or stands too long. Over time, this can lead to chronic stasis changes and the possibility of venous ulcerations.

## EPIDEMIOLOGY

Venous thromboembolism (VTE) consists of venous thrombosis (superficial or deep) and/or PE. PE is primarily a complication of DVT and a leading cause of preventable death in hospital mortality in the United States. It has been estimated that in the United States there are greater than 500,000 cases of DVT each year with more than 50% of cases unrecognized. There are also approximately 200,000 cases of fatal PE annually.[12]

In addition to acute risks from DVT, up to 30% of patients may develop symptoms of postthrombotic syndrome (pain, swelling, and ulcerations).[13] This chronic condition carries a significant morbidity.

## PATHOPHYSIOLOGY

The primary mechanism for the formation of venous thrombosis is Virchow's triad (circa 1856)[14] which includes venous stasis, vessel wall injury, and a hypercoagulable state. The balance between thrombogenesis (clotting factors), coagulation inhibitors, and the fibrinolytic system determines the formation of venous thrombus. Venous stasis being one of the components of Virchow's triad allows for the increased exposure of clotting factor, which occurs in immobility. Vessel wall injury will also affect the body's normal thrombolytic system. The vessel injury could be catheter related or injury such as that seen in trauma patients. Hypercoagulability is the last condition that can lead to thrombus formation.

| TABLE 17-1 | **Risk Factors for DVT** |
|---|---|
| Age | |
| Surgery or trauma | |
| Immobilization | |
| Past history of DVT | |
| Coagulation disorders—congenital/acquired | |
| Malignancy | |
| Septicemia | |
| Birth control pills | |
| Hormone replacement therapy | |
| Pregnancy | |
| Obesity | |
| Stroke | |
| Congestive heart failure | |
| Long distance travel | |
| Inflammatory bowel disease | |
| Varicose veins | |

| TABLE 17-2 | **Well's Criteria** |
|---|---|
| **+1 POINT EACH FOR** | |
| Active malignancy | |
| Paralysis, paresis, or recent plaster immobilization of lower limb | |
| Recently bedridden for more than 3 days or major surgery/trauma in past 4 weeks | |
| Localized tenderness along distribution of lower extremity deep veins | |
| Entire lower limb swollen | |
| Calf swelling more than 3 cm compared with asymptomatic leg | |
| Pitting edema on symptomatic leg | |
| Collateral superficial veins on symptomatic leg | |
| **−2 POINTS FOR** | |
| Alternative diagnosis as likely or more likely than that of deep vein thrombosis | |
| **PROBABILITY FOR DVT** | |
| High ≥ 3 points | |
| Intermediate 1–2 points | |
| Low ≤ 0 points | |

Hypercoagulability is associated with various diseases such as cancer and also found in patients on birth control pills and hormone replacement therapy. Patients with genetic factors such as Factor V Leiden and prothrombic gene mutations are considered hypercoagulable.

Venous thrombi very commonly begin in the soleal sinus veins in the calf or around small valve cusps in the calf because these are areas of slower flow. This slower flow may contain regions of flow stagnation—one of the features of Virchow's triad. Small thrombi can form which can continue to develop into larger occlusive thrombi.

Risk factors for DVT can generally be associated with one or more of the elements of Virchow's triad.[15] The common risk factors are shown in Table 17-1.

## SIGNS AND SYMPTOMS

The signs and symptoms of VTE are caused by venous obstruction; vascular and perivascular inflammation; and embolization of thrombi.[16] Many patients with venous thrombosis may be asymptomatic. Symptomatic patients may present with extremity pain, tenderness, swelling, venous distention, discoloration, or a palpable cord. Some patients may present with no symptoms within the extremity and only symptoms consistent with a PE such as tachypnea, chest pain, or tachycardia.

Even though the role of a sonographer or vascular technologist is to perform the venous ultrasound, it is important to be familiar with the general clinical workup of patients with suspected DVT. Many laboratories or hospitals may use clinical algorithms to assist in patient management and the scheduling of diagnostic tests such as ultrasound, particularly for after-hours studies. As mentioned at the beginning of this chapter, the clinical diagnosis of DVT is quite inaccurate with poor sensitivity and specificity. Various patient data, demographic and clinical, are often evaluated to aid in the clinical diagnosis of DVT.[17]

Different risk factors and symptoms have been combined into the scoring algorithm known as Well's criteria.[18] Table 17-2 lists the components of this algorithm.

Another useful clinical marker for DVT is the measurement of D-dimer. D-Dimer is a breakdown product of fibrin which will be elevated in the presence of DVT. It has a very high sensitivity, but low specificity. False positive and false negatives do occur. Clinical conditions such as advanced age, chronic inflammation, liver disease, malignancy, pregnancy, trauma, or recent surgery are just a few of the conditions that may result in elevated D-dimer levels. Thus, these conditions can produce a false-positive D-dimer result for the presence of DVT. False negatives may result because of the inability of the assay to measure very low levels of the fibrin fragment. D-Dimer is thought to be most useful in the setting of low probability of DVT based on clinical criteria.[18] Although D-dimer can be very useful in proper ordering (or not ordering) of a venous duplex ultrasound, it may be misused. A normal D-dimer may allow a physician to avoid ordering an unnecessary test, but this should always be coupled with a low DVT probably based on clinical criteria. However, it may be more common for a positive D-dimer to unnecessarily prompt a duplex ultrasound when there are clearly other factors that could be responsible for the increase.

## SONOGRAPHIC EXAMINATION TECHNIQUES

### Patient Preparation

The examination is explained to the patient. The patient signs and symptoms along with relevant history are obtained. Lower extremity clothing should be removed. The patient can wear undergarments, provided that the clothing allows sufficient access to the groin area. A patient gown or drape should be provided. Some departments take this time to instruct a patient how to perform a Valsalva maneuver.

## Patient Positioning

The veins of the leg in a patient lying on a flat bed are nearly closed because of low transmural pressure. This makes them extremely difficult to see. The simple solution to this problem is to tilt the bed so blood pools in the legs, thus engorging the veins. The engorged veins are large, round, and easy to see. This bed tilt maneuver is essential to doing quality venous imaging. Omitting this step is the most common reason for missing small thrombi, especially in the calf.

The entire bed should be tilted (not just elevation of the head) in a reversed Trendelenburg position. The head should be elevated in this way to an angle of about 20 degrees. In cases where the calf veins are still difficult to see because of their small size, the examiner can have the patient sit at the side of the bed (legs dangling) to further engorge the calf veins. This is extremely effective. It will however make the veins much more difficult to compress so that the examiner has to be cautious not to mistake the engorged veins for thrombus-filled veins. In this position, the veins are under greater pressure, and thus, increased transducer pressure will be required to compress the veins.

In addition to using the proper tilt, the patient must also be positioned properly on the bed. When examining the legs, this means having the patient lie flat on their back with the knee slightly bent and the hip slightly externally rotated (Fig. 17-1). This allows access to the inside of the leg and creates a nice flat imaging surface. Omitting this subtle positioning may result in potential errors. The patient should also be moved as close to the examiner as possible for ergonomic concerns.

## EQUIPMENT SELECTION

Duplex ultrasound imaging equipment quality can vary dramatically. Trying to do venous duplex ultrasound imaging with an ultrasound imager and transducers that are designed for other applications such as general or cardiac ultrasound can be extremely frustrating and potentially dangerous. Formatting imagers for venous work requires three specialized transducers:

- The workhorse transducer will be a midrange linear array transducer (5 to 10 MHz). This transducer is used for the femoral veins, the popliteal vein, and most of the calf. In the upper extremity, the midrange transducer is used to view the subclavian and larger arms.
- A second transducer, the high frequency linear array transducer is indispensable. Some institutions try to do without this transducer, but this is not the best course of action. This high frequency transducer should have a small footprint (hockey stick-type transducers are very useful). This transducer (10 to 18 MHz) is used for superficial veins such as the saphenous in the leg and for most of the arm veins. This transducer is a must for detailed reflux studies or upper and lower extremity mapping.
- The third transducer needed for venous imaging is the curved low frequency transducer (2 to 5 MHz). This transducer is useful for the inferior vena cava (IVC) and iliac veins. It is also helpful in heavy patients in whom some veins may lie deeper within the leg.

Appropriate examination presets should be selected prior to the start of the examination. Equipment settings should be optimized and adjusted throughout the examination to obtain high-quality images and waveforms.

## Scanning Technique

Changes to the names of some of the veins in the leg were adopted several years ago.[10,11] There is unfortunately some confusion regarding venous nomenclature because some laboratories have been slow to adopt the new terms and others are not aware that changes have been made. In the following sections, both terms are provided for those veins with new nomenclature. The protocol described here represents a summary of time-tested technique for properly identifying the veins and evaluating them for thrombus formation.[19-22]

### Initial Examination Position

The lower extremity venous duplex ultrasound examination begins at the groin crease. The common femoral vein (CFV) and common femoral artery (CFA) are located from a medial projection in a transverse plane. Moving above this area and above the level of the inguinal ligament, the CFV becomes the external iliac vein (EIV). Using the ultrasound transducer, gentle pressure is applied directly over the vein. Because the veins are under relatively low pressure, the walls of the vein will be seen to coapt or close together. The compression of the walls of the vein should be recorded. Remaining in a transverse plane, the compression and release technique is performed every 2 to 3 cm down the entire length of the leg, documenting the images at several locations along the leg. With each of the named vessels described as follows, these compression maneuvers are performed and recorded. The smaller the "cuts" (or spacing between compressions) used, the better the results. Spacing the cuts too far apart will allow for missing a smaller partial thrombus. After the entire vein has been imaged in a transverse plane, the examiner can then reexamine the same vein in a longitudinal

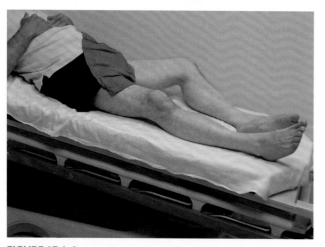

**FIGURE 17-1** Proper patient positioning for a lower extremity venous ultrasound examination for DVT.

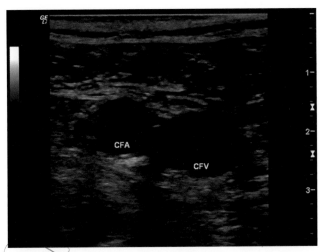

**FIGURE 17-2** A transverse view at the level of the groin. The common femoral artery (CFA) and common femoral vein (CFV) are visualized side by side.

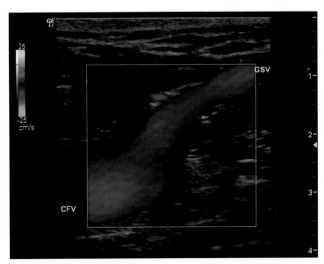

**FIGURE 17-4** A longitudinal view of the great saphenous vein (GSV) terminating into the common femoral vein (CFV) just below the level of the inguinal ligament.

plane. This will add additional information and can be used to confirm findings observed in a transverse plane. Doppler and color imaging are performed in the longitudinal plane.

It cannot be overemphasized, however, that one cannot omit the transverse view and do only longitudinal imaging. Doing so will result in missing nonobstructive thrombi. It is very easy to roll off a vein while in longitudinal plane, and therefore, compressions in a longitudinal view should never be done as a substitute for transverse imaging.

In addition to compression of the veins, spectral Doppler waveforms are usually recorded from the CFV and popliteal veins. Institutions vary at which specific veins Doppler waveforms should be obtained, but generally it is at least at two levels. For a DVT examination, Doppler waveforms are examined strictly for qualitative features such as spontaneity; phasicity with respiration; augmentation with distal compression; and cessation of flow with proximal compression.

### Common Femoral and Great Saphenous Veins

The CFV is identified next to an accompanying artery of the same name (Fig. 17-2). Just below the level of the inguinal ligament, a large superficial vein terminates into the CFV (Fig. 17-3). This vein had been traditionally called the greater saphenous or long saphenous but is now referred to as the great saphenous vein (GSV) (Fig. 17-4). The termination of the GSV into the CFV is called the saphenofemoral junction (SFJ). The GSV is the longest superficial vein in the body and travels close to the skin in the saphenous compartment. Below the SFJ, the GSV courses medial and superficial to the CFV. Below the knee, the GSV is more anterior as it courses through calf.

In the upper thigh, the CFV is formed by the junction of the femoral vein (FV) (formerly known as the superficial femoral vein) and the deep femoral vein (DFV) (also known as the profunda femoris vein) (Fig. 17-5).

### Femoral Vein and Deep Femoral Vein

The FV will be more superficial than the DFV (Fig. 17-6). They will parallel each other through most of the thigh.

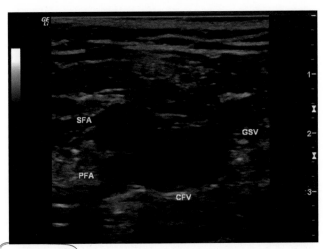

**FIGURE 17-3** A transverse view of the bifurcation of the common femoral artery into the superficial femoral artery (SFA) and deep (profunda) femoral artery (PFA), and the great saphenous vein (GSV) terminates into the common femoral vein (CFV).

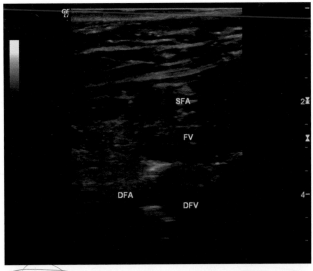

**FIGURE 17-5** A transverse view of the femoral (FV) and deep femoral vein (DFV) in the upper thigh. Also shown are the superficial femoral artery (SFA) and deep femoral artery (DFA).

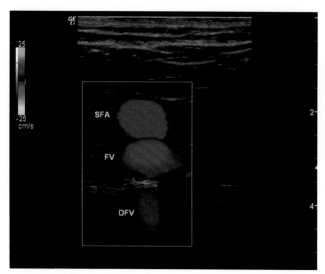

**FIGURE 17-6** A transverse view of the femoral vein (FV) and deep femoral vein (DFV) in the upper thigh with color added to assist in vessel identification. The superficial femoral artery (SFA) is also seen.

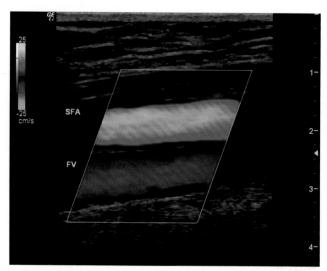

**FIGURE 17-8** A longitudinal view in color of the superficial femoral artery (SFA) and femoral vein (FV) within the mid thigh.

The FV is the main venous outflow of the calf, whereas the DFV mainly drains the thigh itself. The entire length of the FV should be examined in detail (Figs. 17-7 and 17-8) with compression images often documented in the upper thigh, mid thigh, and distal thigh. The DFV should be examined as well. Most protocols include a compression of the DFV near its terminus into the CFV. The remainder of the DFV may be too deep and has many tributaries such that a complete examination of its entire length will be difficult.

The FV through the thigh may be a bifid system (Fig. 17-9). This is fairly common and simply means that the examiner must be sure to investigate each vessel. In the case of a patient with a bifid system and venous thrombosis, it is not uncommon for one FV to be patent and the other thrombosed. At the adductor canal, the FV travels deep into the muscles of the thigh. Distal to the adductor canal, the vein is called the popliteal vein.

### Popliteal Vein

The popliteal vein is the main drainage for blood leaving the calf (Figs 17-10 and 17-11). In the upper portion of the popliteal fossa, the popliteal vein and artery are the only vessels visualized. As is the case with the FV, the popliteal vein can occasionally be bifid.

### Anterior Tibial Vein

The anterior tibial vein (ATV) terminates into the popliteal vein in the mid to upper regions of the popliteal fossa. However, this is not commonly seen on duplex ultrasound because of its depth and the angle of its termination into the popliteal vein. It empties into the popliteal vein as a single trunk. This single common ATV forms at the junction of the two ATVs in the upper calf. Although the proximal calf portion of the ATVs is hard to see, the remainder of the course of the ATVs is easily imaged from an anterolateral projection. Because thrombus formation in the ATVs is rare, imaging

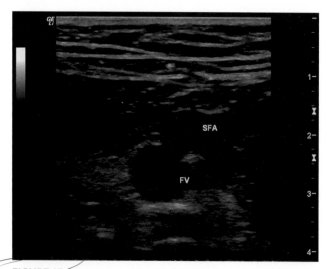

**FIGURE 17-7** A transverse view of the superficial femoral artery (SFA) and femoral vein (FV) with the medial aspect of the thigh.

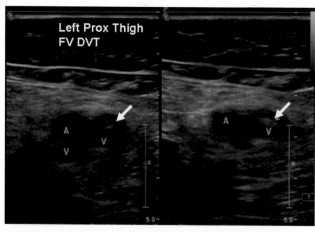

**FIGURE 17-9** Split screen view of a bifid femoral vein (V) along with the superficial femoral artery (A). Note how echogenic material is clearly seen in one of the two veins (*arrow*) in the noncompressed view (**left**). The right image shows that the thrombus-free vein is fully collapsed when transducer pressure is exerted over it. In contrast, the thrombus-filled vein (indicated at *arrow*) fails to fully compress in response to the same pressure. This is reliable evidence of the presence of a thrombus in this vein.

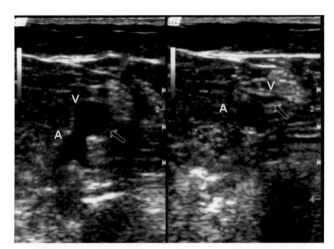

**FIGURE 17-10** A split screen transverse view of the popliteal artery (A) and vein (V). The arrow indicates the popliteal vein fully open on the right and completely compressed on the left.

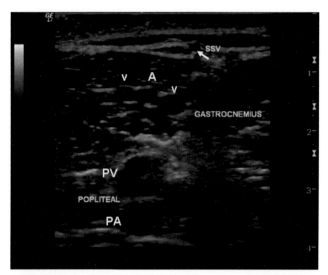

**FIGURE 17-12** A transverse view of the gastrocnemius artery (A) and veins (V) in the upper calf. Also in view are the popliteal artery (PA) and popliteal vein (PV) deep to the gastrocnemius vessels. The small saphenous vein (SSV) is indicated by the arrow superficial to the gastrocnemius vessels.

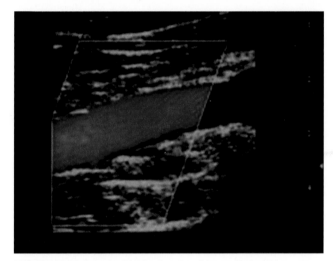

**FIGURE 17-11** A longitudinal view in color of the popliteal vein.

of these vessels is not a part of most protocols. Thrombi are rare in the ATVs because they do not communicate with the prime source of thrombi in the leg—the soleal sinus veins. Examination of the ATVs can be added to an existing protocol whenever there is an injury to this area or when a patient complains of pain or other symptoms over this region.

## Gastrocnemius Veins

The popliteal vein tributaries also include small muscular veins called the gastrocnemius veins (Fig. 17-12). There are lateral and medial paired gastrocnemius veins, each with an accompanying gastrocnemius artery. The paired veins often merge into a single trunk prior to emptying into the popliteal vein. These veins are deep veins but are not major main line deep veins of the calf. They serve to drain the gastrocnemius muscle and can be followed down the calf within the muscle.

## Small Saphenous Vein

This vein was traditionally named the lesser, small, or short saphenous vein but is now only referred to as the

small saphenous vein (SSV). This superficial vein terminates into the popliteal vein at about the same level as the gastrocnemius veins (Fig. 17-13). The terminus of the SSV into the popliteal vein is known as the saphenopopliteal junction. Sometimes, the SSV and the gastrocnemius veins share a common trunk as they enter the popliteal. The SSV courses along the posterior calf approximately in the middle of the calf. It receives tributaries from both the medial and lateral aspects of the calf with often a large tributary vein arising from the lateral malleolus. In some patients, the SSV does not terminate into the popliteal vein. Instead, it will bypass the popliteal vein and continue up the posterior thigh, eventually joining the deep system in the thigh or the GSV in the thigh. When this occurs, this extension of the SSV above the popliteal fossa is referred to as the vein of Giacomini. The currently accepted name of this vein is the "cranial extension of the Small Saphenous Vein."

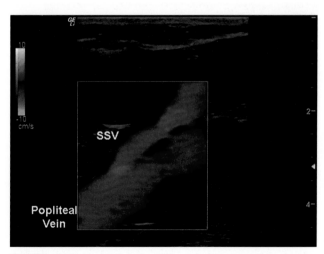

**FIGURE 17-13** A longitudinal view of the small saphenous vein terminating into the popliteal vein.

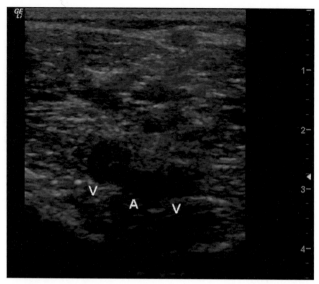

**FIGURE 17-14** A transverse view of the common posterior tibial and common peroneal trunks.

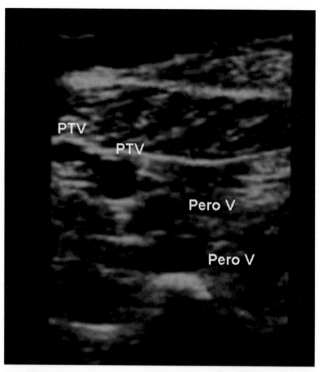

**FIGURE 17-16** A transverse view of the medial calf with the posterior tibial veins (PTV) and peroneal veins (Pero V). The large anechoic area below the peroneal veins is the fibula.

## Tibioperoneal Trunk

The tibioperoneal trunk receives blood from the posterior tibial and peroneal veins. These veins merge together in the upper calf to form the tibioperoneal trunk. The tibioperoneal trunk merges with the ATV to form the popliteal vein.

## Common Tibial and Peroneal Trunks

The specific level at which the tibioperoneal trunk forms varies somewhat, but it is usually at the distal portion of the popliteal fossa within the upper calf. The common posterior tibial and common peroneal trunks merge together to form the tibioperoneal trunk (Figs. 17-14 and 17-15). In the upper calf, the paired posterior tibial veins (PTVs) unite to form the common tibial trunk, and the paired peroneal veins unite to form the common peroneal trunk. The specific length of these two common trunks is variable.

## Posterior Tibial Veins

The PTVs will course medially in the calf near the tibia. The veins are paired following the posterior tibial artery (Fig. 17-16). They arise via tributaries between the medial malleolus and the Achilles tendon at the ankle.

## Peroneal Veins

The peroneal veins are followed deeper in the calf (Fig. 17-17) as they parallel the PTVs through most of the calf (Fig. 17-18). They travel adjacent to the fibula along with the peroneal artery.

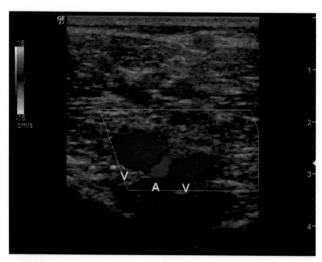

**FIGURE 17-15** A transverse view of the common posterior tibial and common peroneal trunks with color added.

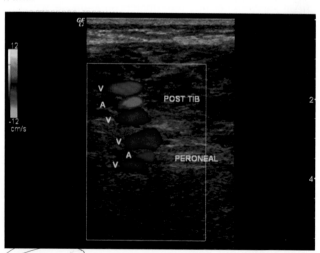

**FIGURE 17-17** A transverse view of the medial calf showing the posterior tibial (V) and peroneal veins (V) with color added. The companion arteries are also shown (A).

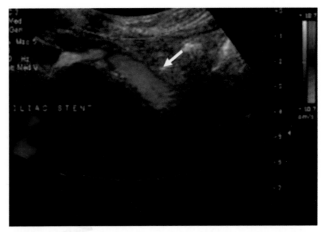

FIGURE 17-20 A longitudinal view of an iliac vein (*arrow*) that is stented.

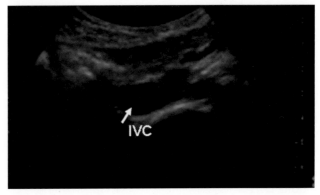

**FIGURE 17-18** A longitudinal view in color of the posterior tibial veins (PTV) and posterior tibial artery (PTA). This illustrates the parallel position of the peroneal artery (Pero A) and peroneal veins (Pero V) deep to the posterior tibial vessels. In this view, only one of the paired peroneal veins is observed.

## Soleal Sinus Veins

One of the major functions of the venous system (aside from returning blood to the heart) is to provide a storage area for blood. One of the major storage areas for blood in the calf is a network of veins called the soleal sinus veins. Because blood only moves inside these veins when the calf muscle contracts, they are a common site for thrombi formation following surgery; a long plane trip; or anytime a person sits, stands, or is in bed for extended period of time. The soleal veins communicate into the PTVs and peroneal veins. Thrombus that forms within the soleal veins can therefore easily extend into the major deep vein of the calf. These soleal veins are small and difficult to find, but when they get filled with thrombus, they enlarge and are much easier to see (Fig. 17-19).

## Imaging the Iliac Veins

In most institutions, imaging above the groin is not done unless there is a clinical indication to suggest involvement of the iliac veins or the IVC. Commonly, Doppler signals obtained at the CFVs are used to provide an indirect assessment of

the status of veins above the groin. If good phasic flow is detected in the CFV, it suggests the lack of an obstruction of the iliac veins or IVC. This is less sensitive in the case of a thrombus that is nonobstructive. When one suspects pathology in the iliac veins or IVC, the duplex ultrasound examination can be extended into the pelvic region and abdomen.

Imaging in the pelvic region and abdomen is difficult because of the depth of the vessels, bowel gas, and the fact that compression of the vessels is not likely to be accomplished. Because of the inability to compress the veins to determine if they are thrombus-free, the examiner may have to rely on more color and spectral Doppler techniques to determine patency—something that can lead to inaccurate results.

A detailed instruction of imaging of these vessels is covered in Chapter 26. Basic guidelines for imaging in the abdomen include having the patient fast if possible to reduce bowel gas and to schedule them early in the morning.

The examination of the iliac veins usually starts by following the CFV above the inguinal ligament into the pelvic region. The iliac veins will penetrate deep very quickly. The continuation of the CFV above the inguinal ligament is the EIV. At the level of the sacroiliac joints, the EIV will become the common iliac vein (CIV) as the internal iliac vein (IIV) merges with the EIV. The IIV may be difficult to insonate, so this transition level may be hard to determine. Eventually, the CIV (Fig. 17-20) is joined by the CIV from the other leg to form the IVC (Fig. 17-21).

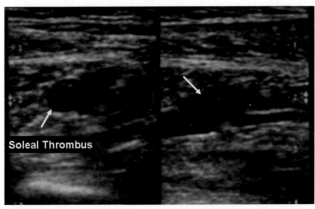

**FIGURE 17-19** A split screen view of thrombus (*arrow*) in a soleal sinus vein. The left image shows the contained thrombus (*arrow*) restricting compression of the soleal vein.

Soleal Thrombus

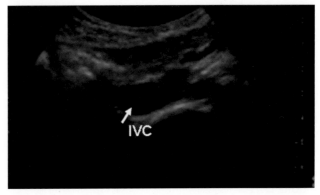

IVC

**FIGURE 17-21** A transverse view of the inferior vena cava (IVC) (indicated at *arrow*).

## Technical Considerations

Compression of the vein is an essential component to this examination. However, in the presence of a venous thrombus, caution should be used when performing compressions. This is especially important if the thrombus is nonocclusive and appears as a free-flowing tail of material within the vein lumen. There have been reports of dislodging loosely attached thrombus by ultrasound compressions and causing emboli.[23,24]

## Pitfalls

There are several pitfalls encountered with venous imaging in the lower extremities. Most issues concern the limited visualization of the veins. Body habitus can result in veins being positioned deeply in the leg. Equipment settings should be optimized for a deeper field of view, and lower frequency transducers may be utilized. For deep calf veins, various approaches including lateral and posterior approaches may result in a more complete visualization.

Compression of deeper veins is sometimes challenging. The femoral vein as it passes through the adductor canal is often difficult to compress using the transducer and applying pressure from a medial approach. At this level, the examiner should take their free hand and press up along the posterior aspect of the thigh. Pressure applied at this point will push the vein up against the muscle and transducer (Fig. 17-22). It is more easily compressed from this approach and usually more comfortable for the patient. Another solution would be to go behind the knee and follow the popliteal up doing compressions from the posterior approach until the distal femoral is viewed from this position.

There may be patients presenting for venous ultrasounds with wounds, dressings, orthopedic hardware, or surgical incisions. The veins lying under these areas may be unable to be directly assessed. Ultrasound characteristics in the veins immediately adjacent to these areas may indirectly aid in determining the patency of the veins not visualized.

## DIAGNOSIS

Until the 1980s, the diagnosis of venous thrombus in the extremities was done using venography. This was an accurate test, but it was invasive and painful, and had some inherent risks. Attempts had been made in the early vascular laboratories to find thrombus noninvasively, but the non-imaging techniques employed at that time were not acceptable. When imaging quality began to improve to the point where it became possible to see the vessels well enough to consider using ultrasound imaging to find a thrombus, attempts were made to use duplex ultrasound for this purpose. Initially, those exploring this theory were convinced to abandon the idea because the wisdom of the experts at that time was that a thrombus could not be seen on ultrasound. However, those doing the initial research quickly found that veins that were thrombus-free would collapse completely when the examiner compressed over the vein being imaged.[25] This made venous imaging possible even if one could not actually see the thrombus using the ultrasound. They also found that imaging of the thrombus was possible making this technique even more useful than its invasive counterpart because not only could one see the thrombus, but it was possible to tell if it was old or new; stable or unstable.[1]

## Normal, Thrombus-Free Veins

After initially identifying the artery and vein, the examiner uses the transducer to compress over the vessels. The thrombus-free vein will compress, whereas the artery will not. Exerting more pressure will eventually cause the walls of the artery to close as well. The compression maneuver will aid the examiner with vessel identification. It also is the first clear indicator of the presence or absence of a thrombus in the vein. If the vein being examined closes completely in response to transducer pressure (Fig. 17-23), it can be determined that the vein is thrombus-free at that location. This complete compression of the vein (where the vein walls touch each other during compression) is the key to venous imaging. In fact, some imaging professionals refer to venous imaging as "compression ultrasound." After watching the vein compress, the examiner eases up and the vein will reopen. The walls of a normal vein appear thin and smooth. Valve sinuses may be apparent as slight dilations in the vein wall.

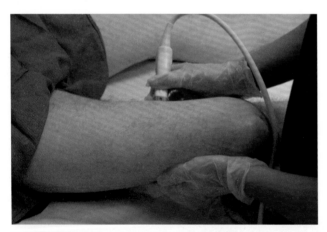

**FIGURE 17-22** Technique used to compress distal thigh portion of the femoral vein. The examiner applies pressure with his or her free hand along the posterior aspect of the thigh.

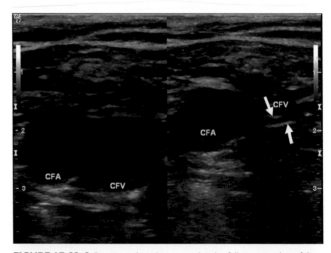

**FIGURE 17-23** Split screen view demonstrating the full compression of the common femoral vein (CFV), indicating the thrombus-free status of the vein at that location. Note how the vein walls coapt together (*arrows*). The common femoral artery (CFA) is also seen.

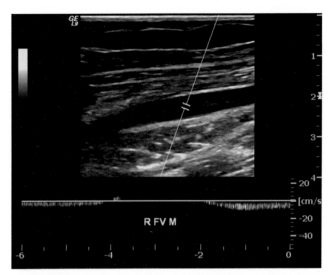

**FIGURE 17-24** A spectral Doppler waveform obtained from the mid thigh level of the femoral vein (FV) illustrating normal respiratory phasicity.

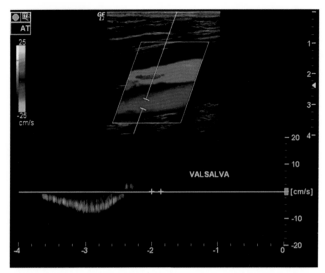

**FIGURE 17-26** A spectral Doppler venous waveform illustrating the absence of flow during a Valsalva maneuver.

Valve leaflets may be seen as thin white structures within the sinus, freely moving in the blood stream.

## Normal Color and Spectral Doppler

Spectral Doppler and color information can be added to the information gathered from visualizing the compressions of the veins. Laboratory accreditation protocols presently require spectral Doppler signals at key levels. Venous Doppler signals should display the following five characteristics. First, with modern ultrasound equipment, spontaneous Doppler signals should be present within all major vessels. Secondly, Spectral Doppler signals in a normal vein should be phasic with respiration. (Fig. 17-24) Third, compression of the leg below the level of the transducer should augment flow (Fig. 17-25). Fourth, venous Doppler signals should cease with proximal compression or Valsalva maneuver

(Fig. 17-26). Lastly, venous Doppler signals from lower extremity veins should be unidirectional, toward the heart.

Color-flow imaging should also display the same attributes as spectral Doppler. With proper equipment setting, color should be seen completely filling the vessel lumen (Fig. 17-27).

## Determining the Presence of Thrombus

A thrombus is present when echogenic material is visualized within the lumen of a vein, and the echogenic material restricts the complete compression of the vein walls (see Fig. 17-9). These two findings must occur together to definitively determine the presence of a thrombus in a vein. Too many protocols simply focus on compression ("compression ultrasound"). Failure to link compression with actual visualization of the echogenic material within the vein will result in false-positive results in cases where the vein compression is being hampered by something other than a thrombus. Examples of situations

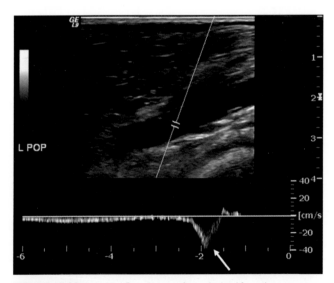

**FIGURE 17-25** A spectral Doppler waveform obtained from the popliteal vein illustrating a normal augmentation in flow (*arrow*) with a distal compression.

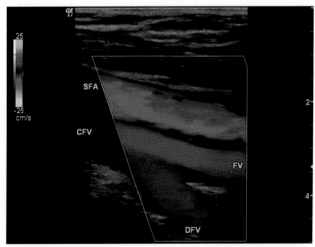

**FIGURE 17-27** A longitudinal color image of the confluence of the femoral vein (FV) and the deep femoral vein (DFV) into the common femoral vein (CFV). The superficial femoral artery (SFA) is also seen.

leading to false-positive results include a patient bearing down because of the discomfort of the compression, thus making the vein difficult to compress. In addition, the compression of the vein may be limited by adjacent structures such as bone or dense muscle bundles. The examiner may also fail to exert sufficient pressure to coapt the vein walls and thus assume a DVT is present.

There are instances when a thrombus is present, but the images are so poor that it is impossible to visually document the presence of the thrombus. In these cases, the diagnosis of thrombi within the vein can be made by pressing harder over the vessels until the accompanying artery starts to deform yet the vein walls do not compress. When this occurs, the examiner and interpreter can be assured that adequate compression has been used and that thrombus is likely present.

## Characterization of Thrombus

One of the unique benefits of venous duplex ultrasound imaging over venography is that it can be used not only to identify the presence or absence of a thrombus but also to tell the characteristic of a thrombus that may make a difference in how that it is treated. Generally, the newer the thrombus, the more likely it is to break loose and travel to the lungs. Although venous imaging does not allow one to tell the exact age of a given thrombus, there are observable clues to its age and stability that can be gleaned during venous duplex ultrasound imaging.

Characteristics usually associated with an *acute* thrombus are as follows:
1. Lightly echogenic or hypoechoic thrombus
2. Poorly attached thrombus
3. Spongy texture of thrombus
4. Dilated vein (when totally obstructed)

Characteristics usually associated with a *chronic* thrombus are as follows:
1. Brightly echogenic or hyperechoic thrombus
2. Well-attached thrombus
3. Rigid texture of thrombus
4. Contracted vein (if totally obstructed)
5. Large collaterals

### Acute Thrombus

A thrombus is simply the fluid and solid contents of the blood that has been captured in a thrombin net so that it becomes a solid mass. Therefore, a newly formed thrombus can be almost invisible by ultrasound (Fig. 17-28). The only clue to the presence of a DVT is the fact that the compression of the vein is being limited by the spongy thrombus and a faint reflection around its edges can be seen (Fig. 17-29). This faint reflection is created by the thrombin net that has recently formed to trap the blood (Fig. 17-30). The experienced examiner will spot this faint echo and investigate further. A thrombus seen at this stage will be spongy in texture and hypoechoic, and will likely be poorly attached to the vein wall (Fig. 17-31). The fact that these poorly attached acute thrombi might be more likely to embolize seems logical, although this seemingly obvious conclusion is not universally accepted.

Veins are extremely compliant and can enlarge several times their normal size. When a thrombus forms within a vein, the movement of blood through this vein back toward the heart is reduced because of the luminal restriction produced by the thrombus. As the blood flow reduces,

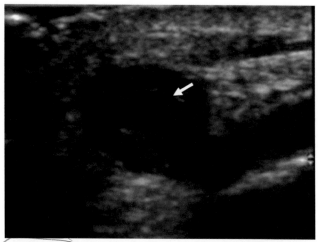

**FIGURE 17-28** Transverse view of a vein with an extremely acute thrombus (arrow) forming within it. The vein was not compressing, but no thrombus was initially seen. Gains were increased so that blood flow could be seen on grayscale. Note how the thrombus is actually less echogenic than the blood flowing around it. The faint edge of the fibrin net is also visible around the thrombus.

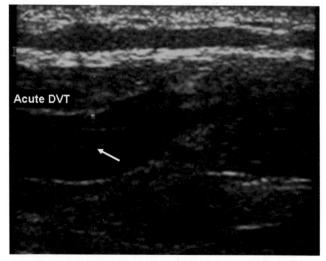

**FIGURE 17-29** A longitudinal view of an acute thrombus. Note the faint echo of the fibrin net (arrow) that surrounds the newly formed thrombus.

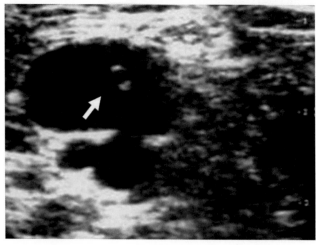

**FIGURE 17-30** A transverse view of an unstable (poorly attached) acute thrombus (arrow).

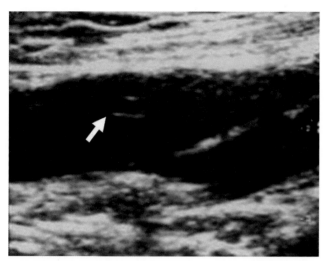

**FIGURE 17-31** A longitudinal view of the edge of a newly formed, unstable thrombus (*arrow*).

the pressure within the vein peripheral to the thrombus increases. As the pressure increases, the vein will enlarge. The thrombus usually will continue to expand until it has stretched the vein out to its maximum size (Fig. 17-32). At this point, the vein will be totally obstructed and will have a diameter much larger than the companion artery. This venous dilation that occurs during this stage of thrombus formation aids in the confirmation of acute thrombi.

## Chronic Thrombus

The human thrombolytic system is capable of dissolving a venous thrombus. In some instances, a previously completely thrombosed vein will have no residual evidence of the prior thrombus. However, often the thrombus will persist to some degree and be visible on ultrasound for several years. The thrombus that initially was relatively hypoechoic will become more echogenic as the thrombus ages (Figs. 17-33 to 17-36).

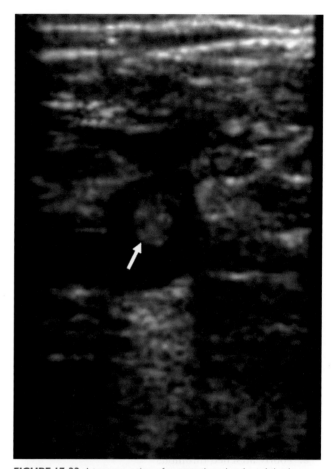

**FIGURE 17-33** A transverse view of an acute thrombus (*arrow*) that has begun to gain echogenicity making it easier to see.

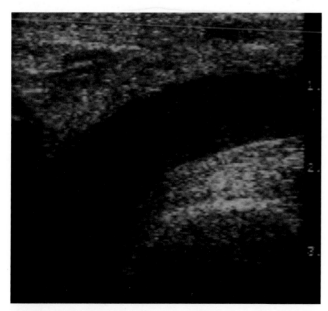

**FIGURE 17-32** A longitudinal view of an acute thrombus that has enlarged the vein.

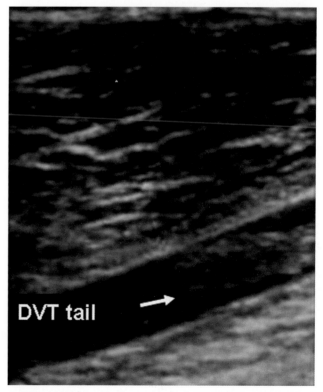

DVT tail

**FIGURE 17-34** The tip or tail of an acute thrombus (*arrow*) that has gained some echogenicity, making it easier to see.

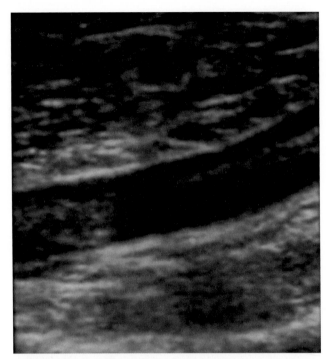

**FIGURE 17-35** The same thrombus as seen in Figure 17-34. Note how poorly attached the acute thrombus is.

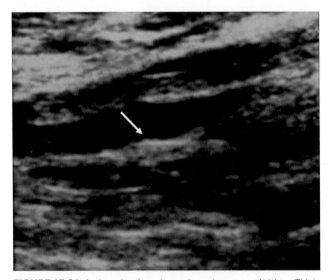

**FIGURE 17-36** As thrombus (*arrow*) ages, it continues to get brighter. This is a subacute thrombus that is not yet fully attached to the vein wall.

This increase in echogenicity aids in the identification of the vein. As the thrombus ages, the plasma or liquid component of the thrombus gets reabsorbed by the body. This results in the thrombus contracting or shrinking. The remaining material of the thrombus is more dense and composed of more solid substances such as fibrin and cellular debris (Fig. 17-37). The thrombus will now be firm, more brightly echogenic, and better attached to the vein wall (Fig. 17-38). Because of its firm attachment to the vein wall, the chronic thrombus is less likely to break loose and embolize to the lungs. Chronically thrombosed veins that have contracted may be difficult to differentiate from the surrounding tissue because the echogenicity of the vein will become similar to that of the tissue.

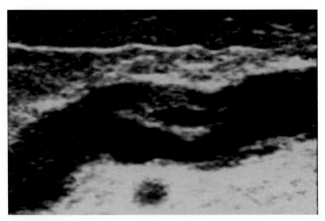

**FIGURE 17-37** As the thrombus continues to age, it will attach to the vein wall.

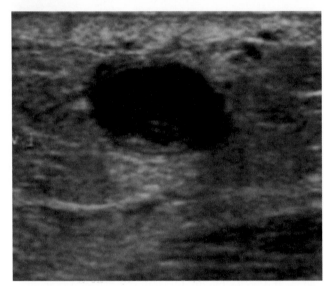

**FIGURE 17-38** A transverse view of a thrombus attaching to the vein wall.

Some chronic thrombi may not totally obstruct a vein and will appear partially attached to the vein wall. This allows blood to flow through the residual lumen (Figs. 17-39 and 17-40). The contained thrombus will continue to shrink and

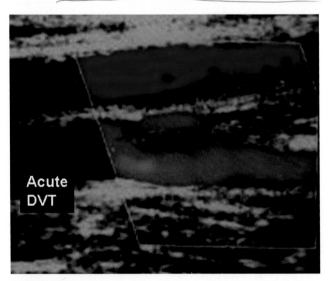

Acute
DVT

**FIGURE 17-39** A longitudinal view of color outlining an acute thrombus.

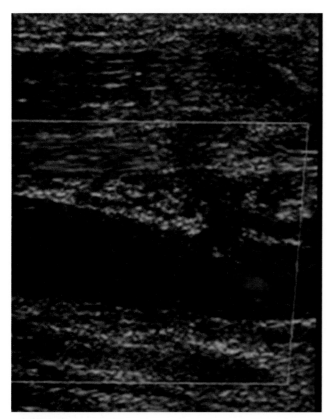

**FIGURE 17-40** A longitudinal view of a chronic residual thrombus with blood flow moving within the center of the vein.

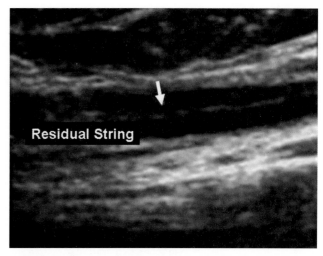

**FIGURE 17-42** A longitudinal view of an old residual "string" thrombus (*arrow*).

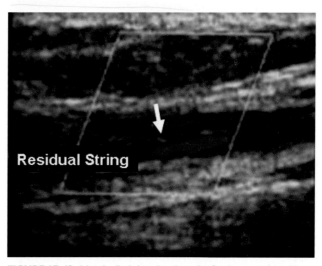

**FIGURE 17-43** A longitudinal view showing color flowing around an old residual "string" thrombus (*arrow*).

fill less and less of the vein (recanalization). Eventually, it will appear on ultrasound like a thin scar within the vein. Its borders can be irregular, and it will resemble a string inside the vein (Figs. 17-41 to 17-43). The term scar has been increasingly used to describe these chronic changes. The literature has also used terms such as "chronic changes" and "residual venous thrombosis" to describe the changes observed in a vein that has been previously afflicted with an acute thrombus.

Whenever possible, an interpreting physician should comment on the age of a thrombus because this may alter patient treatment. Any additional information that can be described and documented by the examiner will aid the physician in the rendering of the final diagnosis. As discussed, the echogenicity of the thrombus can be a useful diagnostic

indicator. However, it should be used in combination with other features such as the vein size or the deformability of the thrombus. The resolution of modern ultrasound equipment is such that in some cases various levels of thrombus echogenicity may be encountered irrespective of thrombus age. Pathology Box 17-1 summarizes the ultrasound findings associated with venous thrombosis.

## Abnormal Color and Spectral Doppler

Although image characteristics are the primary ultrasound features used to make the diagnosis of DVT, a great deal of information can be obtained by evaluating the color image and spectral Doppler waveforms. In a thrombosed vein, color-flow and spectral waveforms will be absent and along with the lack of compressibility confirm the thrombosis. In a vein that is compressible but when performing a distal compression, no color flow is observed or no augmentation is present within the spectral Doppler waveform, an obstruction to flow between the level of the transducer and the site of distal compression should be suspected. This test is less sensitive with nonocclusive thrombi.

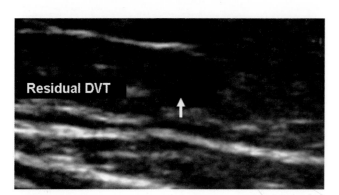

**FIGURE 17-41** A transverse view of a residual thrombus (*arrow*) creating a septum down the middle of the vein.

## PATHOLOGY BOX 17-1
### Venous Thrombosis in the Lower Extremity

| Abnormality | B-mode | Ultrasound Findings Spectral Doppler | Color |
|---|---|---|---|
| Acute thrombus | • Echogenic material within the veins (can be anechoic or hypoechoic) <br> • Veins fail to fully coapt <br> • Vein appears dilated <br> • Thrombus is poorly attached to vein wall <br> • Vein appears spongy | • No Doppler signals obtained with complete thrombosis | • No color flow present with complete thrombosis |
| Chronic thrombus | • Hyperechoic material within the veins <br> • Veins fail to fully coapt <br> • Vein appears contracted <br> • Thrombus is rigid and firmly attached <br> • Large collaterals | • No Doppler signals obtained with complete thrombosis | • No color flow present with complete thrombosis |
| Partial nonocclusive thrombus | • Echogenic material within the veins <br> • Veins will partially compress but not able to completely coapt walls | • Continuous signals <br> • Slightly phasicity may be noted <br> • Will augment with distal compression <br> • Little or no change with proximal compression or Valsalva with more central thrombus | • Color fails to fill lumen <br> • Color will outline thrombus material |

Flow that lacks respiratory phasicity and does not cease with proximal compression or Valsalva is termed continuous (Fig. 17-44). This continuous pattern is a signal that the pressure in the vein at this level exceeds the pressure changes within the abdomen during respiration. An obstruction to flow in the venous return back to the heart will produce this pattern. If continuous flow is observed unilaterally at the CFV, this is indirect evidence consistent with unilateral iliofemoral thrombus, partial thrombus, or extrinsic compression. If continuous flow is observed bilaterally at the CFVs, there is likely bilateral iliofemoral disease or an IVC thrombus, a partial thrombus, or extrinsic compression.

Flow that is spontaneous and augments with distal compression but appears pulsatile rather than phasic is also considered abnormal (Fig. 17-45). Unilateral pulsatile venous flow can be associated with arteriovenous fistulae

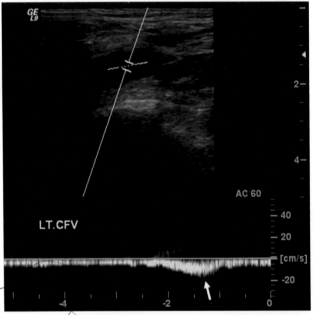

**FIGURE 17-44** A spectral Doppler waveform from a common femoral vein illustrating an abnormal continuous pattern. Note that a small augmentation in flow (arrow) is seen with distal compression.

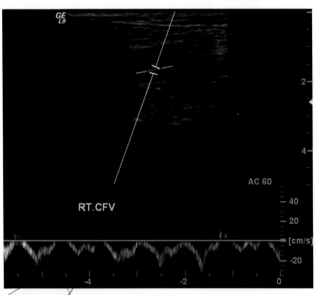

**FIGURE 17-45** An abnormal pulsatile venous Doppler waveform from a common femoral vein.

(either traumatic or iatrogenic or congenital). Bilateral pulsatile venous flow is diagnostic for systemic venous hypertension. Systemic venous hypertension can be the result of numerous cardiopulmonary pathologies including but not limited to right heart failure, tricuspid insufficiency, and pulmonary hypertension.

Flow in lower extremity veins that is both antegrade and retrograde is abnormal. As thrombus becomes attached to the vein wall, it commonly will damage the vein valves. This will result in retrograde blood flow. This condition is called venous reflux or venous insufficiency, and Chapter 20 describes in detail the techniques and criteria of venous reflux testing.

## DISORDERS

In addition to the typical venous thrombosis described above, there are some unique disorders associated with the venous system. Within the iliac venous system, May-Thurner syndrome can develop as the left CIV is compressed by the right common iliac artery. This is discussed in Chapter 26.

Two additional rare disorders arise as a result of extensive DVT, which involves the iliofemoral venous system. Phlegmasia alba dolens is a condition that is associated with marked swelling of the lower extremity, pain, pitting edema, and blanching. This has also been termed "milk leg" or white leg, and can be associated with pregnancy. There is no ischemia associated with phlegmasia alba dolens. Phlegmasia cerulean dolens is more extensive than phlegmasia alba dolens. In addition to massive swelling, cyanosis occurs, and pain is more severe. The cyanosis is produced by the extent of the venous thrombosis, which can include both deep and superficial systems. The venous outflow is completely obstructed. The extensive venous thrombosis and subsequent significant swelling may result in arterial insufficiency and venous gangrene.

### Incidental Findings

As with most types of ultrasound examinations, often incidental findings may be found when patients are referred to the vascular laboratory to rule out lower extremity DVT presenting in leg pain and/or edema. Nonvascular findings include cysts and hematomas (probably the most common), edema, abscesses, enlarged lymph nodes, and tumors. Cysts usually appear well defined and may be oval, oblong, or crescent-shaped (Fig. 17-46). A cyst will be anechoic or hypoechoic, and septations may be present. A ruptured cyst may appear as a fluid collection that dissects along the fascial planes in the limb. The ultrasound appearance of a hematoma will vary depending on the time interval between the initial injury and the ultrasound imaging. Layering of thrombus within the hematoma may be observed. Hematomas usually appear as a heterogeneous mass within a muscle or between muscle planes (Fig. 17-47). Vascular findings included aneurysms (venous and arterial), pseudoaneurysms, arteriovenous fistulas, or significant arterial disease (atherosclerotic or nonatherosclerotic). Color can be used to differentiate between vascular and nonvascular structures. It is important to report these findings so that proper patient care may be implemented.

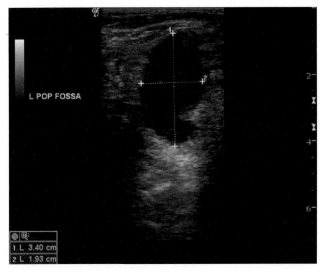

**FIGURE 17-46** A popliteal cyst measuring 3.4 cm × 1.93 cm. The interior of the cyst is relatively anechoic. Posterior enhancement of the grayscale image is seen directly beneath the cyst.

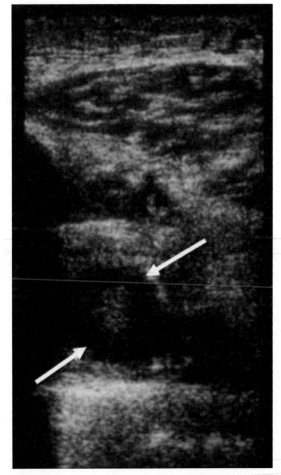

**FIGURE 17-47** A hematoma (*arrows*) within the muscle of the mid calf.

## OTHER IMAGING PROCEDURES

Although duplex ultrasound imaging is the preferred imaging technique to diagnose DVT, other modalities may occasionally be employed. Conventional contrast venography is uncommon but is still performed sporadically. Computed tomography venography (CTV) may be used to define the status of the iliac veins. CTV may be done in conjunction with computed tomography being performed to detect PE. Lastly, magnetic resonance venography (MRV) is also performed to detect DVT. This modality appears to be most useful when imaging veins above the inguinal ligament.

## TREATMENT

The treatment of DVT is not directly related to the scope of practice for the sonographer or vascular technologist. However, it is helpful to understand treatment options and to be familiar with some of the medications involved. At present, the primary treatment of acute lower extremity DVT is anticoagulation.[26] For many years, the standard treatment was heparin followed by warfarin (a vitamin K antagonist). With further developments in the field, the initial therapy became lower-molecular weight heparin followed by warfarin. New oral anticoagulants (NOACs) have recently been approved by the Food and Drug Administration and are used in the treatment of acute lower extremity DVT.[27,28] The mechanism of action for the NOACs is different from warfarin (Table 17-3). These new agents, unlike warfarin, require no monitoring of prothrombin

### TABLE 17-3   New Oral Anticoagulants

| NOAC | Action |
| --- | --- |
| Apixaban (Eliquis) | Direct factor Xa inhibitor |
| Dabigatran (Pradaxa) | Direct thrombin inhibitor |
| Edoxaban (Savaysa) | Direct factor Xa inhibitor |
| Rivaroxaban (Xarelto) | Direct factor Xa inhibitor |

time and international normalized ratio (INR). These new agents also do not have any dietary restrictions in contrast to several dietary restrictions associated with warfarin use. NOACs do have shorter half-lives, and at present an antidote to reverse the anticoagulant effect is only available for one agent. However, in the near future, antidotes will be available for the other agents.

Other treatment methods include gradient elastic stockings, which may help to reduce lower extremity symptoms and decrease the risk postthrombotic syndrome. Thrombolytic agents and thrombectomies (either catheter based or surgical) may also be used to rapidly dissolve the thrombus or physically remove it. These techniques are often limited to the larger veins of the iliofemoral region.

### SUMMARY

- Imaging of the veins of the legs is a challenging task.
- The determination of venous patency is primarily determined by the coaptation of the venous walls with compression maneuvers and the visualization of thrombus within the vein.
- Spectral Doppler waveforms and color-flow imaging also aid in the evaluation of the venous system.
- By paying attention to sound protocols and gaining clinical experience under the supervision of an experienced mentor, one can perform accurate venous duplex ultrasound examinations that will provide doctors with the information needed to safely manage their patients.

### CRITICAL THINKING QUESTIONS

1. When reviewing the relevant history of a patient, what three areas should be of the greatest concern?

2. Explain why both transverse and longitudinal imaging is used for venous DVT examinations.
3. Ultrasound is a noninvasive technique. However, venous ultrasound can have two associated negative outcomes. What are these, and how can those risks be minimized?
4. What are the three aspects of acute versus chronic thrombus that can be compared and contrasted?

### MEDIA MENU

Student Resources available on thePoint° include:
- Audio glossary
- Interactive question bank
- Videos
- Internet resources

### REFERENCES

1. Cronan JJ. History of venous ultrasound. *J Ultrasound Med.* 2003;22:1143–1146.
2. Strandness DE Jr. Diagnostic approaches for detecting deep vein thrombosis. *Am J Card Imaging.* 1994;8:13–17.
3. Meissner MH, Moneta G, Byrnand K, et al. The hemodynamics and diagnosis of venous disease. *J Vasc Surg.* 2007;46:4S–24S.
4. Oliver MA. Duplex scanning in the management of lower extremity DVT. *Vascular Ultrasound Today.* 2005;10:181–196.
5. Oliver MA. Incidental findings during lower extremity venous duplex examination. *Vascular Ultrasound Today.* 2008;13:77–96.
6. Hollinshead WH. *Textbook of Anatomy.* 3rd ed. New York, NY: Harper and Row; 1974:75.
7. Kadir S. *Diagnostic Angiography.* Philadelphia, PA: WB Saunders; 1986:541.
8. Uhl JF, Gillot C, Chahim M. Anatomical variations of the femoral vein. *J Vasc Surg.* 2010;52:714–719.
9. Blackburn DR. Venous anatomy. *J Vasc Technol.* 1988;12:78–82.
10. Caggiati A, Bergan JJ, Gloviczki P, et al. Nomenclature of the veins of the lower limbs: an international interdisciplinary consensus statement. *J Vasc Surg.* 2002;36:416–422.
11. Caggiati A, Bergan JJ, Gloviczki P, et al. Nomenclature of the veins of the lower limb: extensions, refinements and clinical applications. *J Vasc Surg.* 2005;41:719–724.
12. Park B, Messina L, Dargon P, et al. Recent trends in clinical outcomes and resource utilization for pulmonary embolism in the United States: findings from the nationwide inpatient sample. *Chest.* 2009;136:983–990.
13. Prandoni P, Lensing AW, Prins MR. Long term outcomes after deep vein thrombosis of the lower extremities. *Vasc Med.* 1998;3:57–60.

14. Virchow R. *Gesammelte Abhandlungen Zur Wissenschaftli Medizia*. Frankfurt, Germany: Medinger Sohn; 1856:719–732.

15. Meissner MH. Epidemiology of and risk factors for acute deep vein thrombosis. In: Gloviczki P, Yao JST, eds. *Handbook of Venous Disorders*. 24th ed. London: Arnold Publishers; 2009:94–104.

16. Aceno W, Squizzato A, Garcia D, et al. Epidemiology and risk factors of venous thromboembolism. *Semin Thromb Hemost*. 2006;32:651–658.

17. Dawson DL, Beals H. Acute lower extremity deep vein thrombosis. In: Zierler RE, ed. *Strandness's Duplex Scanning in Vascular Disorders*. Philadelphia, PA: Lippincott Williams and Wilkins; 2010:179–198.

18. Wells RS, Hirsh J, Anderson DR, et al. Accuracy of clinical assessment of deep vein thrombosis. *Lancet*. 1995;345:1321–1330.

19. Talbot SR. B-mode evaluation of peripheral veins. *Semin Ultrasound CT MR*. 1988;9:295–319.

20. Sullivan ED, Peters BS, Cranley JJ. Real-time B-mode venous ultrasound. *J Vasc Surg*. 1984;1:465–471.

21. Oliver MA. Duplex scanning in venous disease. *Bruit*. 1985;9:206–209.

22. Talbot SR, Oliver MA. *Techniques of Venous Imaging*. Pasadena, CA: Appleton Davies; 1992.

23. Perlin SJ. Pulmonary embolism during compression US of the lower extremities. *Radiology*. 1992;184:165–166.

24. Schroder WB, BealerJF. Venous duplex ultrasonography causing acute pulmonary embolism: a brief report. *J Vasc Surg*. 1992;15:1082–1083.

25. Talbot SR. Use of real-time imaging in identifying deep venous obstruction: a preliminary report. *Bruit*. 1982;6:41–42.

26. Kearon C, Kahn SR, Agnelli G, et al. Antithrombotic therapy for venous thromboembolic disease: American College of Chest Physicians Evidence-Based Clinical Practice Guidelines (8th edition). *Chest*. 2008;133:454S–545S.

27. Wells PS, Forgie MA, Rodger MA. Treatment of venous thromboembolism. *JAMA*. 2014;311:717–728.

28. Kearon C, Akl EA, Ornelas J, et al. Antithrombotic therapy for VTE disease: CHEST guideline and expert panel report. *CHEST J*. 2016;149:315–352.

# Duplex Ultrasound Imaging of the Upper Extremity Venous System

STEVEN R. TALBOT  |  MARK OLIVER

# PART FIVE

**CHAPTER 18**

## OBJECTIVES

- Describe the components of the upper extremity venous system
- Define the normal image and Doppler characteristics of the venous system
- Identify the image characteristics associated with acute and chronic thrombus
- Describe the Doppler waveform characteristics associated with various pathologies
- List risk factors associated with venous thrombosis in the upper extremity

## KEY TERMS

**acute thrombus**

**chronic thrombus**

**deep vein**

**superficial vein**

**valve**

## GLOSSARY

**acute thrombus** Newly formed clotted blood within a vein, generally less than 14 days old

**chronic thrombus** Clotted blood within a vein that has generally been present for a period of several weeks or months

**deep vein** A vein that is the companion vessel to an artery and travels within the deep muscular compartments of the leg or arm

**superficial vein** A vein which is superior to the muscular compartments of the leg or arm; travels within superficial fascial compartments; has no corresponding companion artery

**valve** An inward projection of the intimal layer of a vein wall producing two semilunar leaflets which prevent the retrograde movement of blood flow

This chapter discusses the venous duplex ultrasound examination of the upper extremity. The protocol techniques used in the upper extremity are similar to those discussed for the lower extremity in Chapter 17. However, there are three major differences to consider when moving from imaging of the legs to imaging of the upper extremity. They are as follows:

1. Most thrombi in the lower extremity are caused by stasis (the patient not moving). This is not true in the upper extremity. The arms do not have a counterpart to the soleal sinus veins of the legs, so there is no similar place for thrombus to spontaneously form in the arms. This is why, until modern times, thrombus in the upper extremity veins was rare. The following section on pathophysiology discusses this further.

2. The superficial veins are affected more in the arms than in the legs. Additionally, thrombus in a superficial vein in the arms may have greater clinical significance because superficial veins in the arms are commonly larger than their deeper counterparts. For instance, the basilic vein (a superficial vein) may be several times larger than the radial vein (a deep vein). Thus, a thrombus in the basilic vein may require treatment, whereas a thrombus in the radial vein may not. Veins like the axillary and subclavian, however, are large deep veins where thrombus within them is more aggressively treated than thrombus in the superficial veins.

3. Veins in the legs follow pretty reliable courses. The venous anatomy in the upper extremity can be more variable. Most of this variation occurs around the median cubital vein and how it connects with the basilic and cephalic veins.

The signs and symptoms of upper extremity venous thrombosis are similar to those described for the lower extremity venous system. These can include unilateral arm or hand swelling, a superficial palpable cord, erythema, pain, and tenderness. Some patients may present with facial swelling or dilated chest wall venous collaterals, which could be suggestive of superior vena cava thrombosis. Patients may present with indwelling catheters or a history of venous catheters.[1,2]

There may be those patients presenting for an upper extremity venous ultrasound who are asymptomatic. These may be patients in whom the central veins may be required to be examined prior to catheter placement or placement of pacemaker wires or other cardiac devices.

Upper extremity veins may also be examined in those patients with suspected pulmonary embolus. These patients may present with symptoms consistent with pulmonary embolus including chest pain, tachypnea, or tachycardia.

## PATHOPHYSIOLOGY

The pathogenesis of upper extremity thrombosis as in lower extremity venous thrombosis can be found in the components of Virchow's triad, namely, venous stasis, hypercoagulability, and vessel wall injury. Thrombosis in the upper extremity veins is now more common because of an increase in injury to the vein walls. Patients are having more frequent introduction of needles and catheters into arm veins. With a few exceptions, whenever an individual has not had a venous puncture or cannulation, the incidence of upper extremity venous thrombosis will be very low. This fact makes taking a history and selecting proper indications for study of the upper extremity veins with ultrasound much easier than with the legs. Because of the location of the subclavian and internal jugular veins, these veins are commonly used for indwelling catheters for feeding and drug administration as well as catheters used to monitor central venous pressure. Pacemaker wires are also introduced usually through the subclavian vein and are another common cause of upper extremity venous thrombosis.

Another type of venous catheter that can cause a thrombosis is a peripherally inserted central catheter (PICC). A PICC line is not inserted into one of the large veins in the neck or shoulder region but rather via a peripheral vein, often the basilic or cephalic veins. After it is inserted via one of these arm veins, the catheter is advanced to position the tip near the right atrium.

There are patients who present with upper extremity venous thrombosis without a history of venous puncture or cannulation. These patients include a unique group who present with upper extremity venous thrombosis secondary to compression of the subclavian vein at the thoracic inlet around the area of the first rib. It is thought to be the result of years of repetitive trauma and intermittent compression of the subclavian vein. This type of thrombosis is known as effort thrombosis or Paget-Schroetter syndrome. This syndrome was first described by Paget in 1875. The patients presenting with this type of venous thrombosis are young, athletic, and muscular males, but this syndrome can occur in other individuals as well.

## SONOGRAPHIC EXAMINATION TECHNIQUES

The protocols described here are a summary of tried and true protocols that will produce accurate venous duplex

ultrasound results.[3-7] The compression techniques employed in the examination of the lower extremity veins are also performed for the upper extremity veins. Using the ultrasound transducer, a gentle compression is applied directly over the vein so that the walls of the vein coapt or close together. This compression maneuver is repeated every 2 to 3 cm along the course of each vein. Spectral Doppler waveforms are recorded from all major vessels examined.

### Patient Preparation

The examination should be explained to the patient. The patient signs and symptoms along with relevant history should be obtained. Upper extremity clothing and jewelry should be removed, and a patient gown or drape provided.

### Patient Positioning

There is no need to tilt the bed for examination of the upper extremity. In fact, it is important to examine the jugular and subclavian veins with the patient lying flat. This will remove any impact of hydrostatic pressure, which will tend to collapse the veins with the patient upright. While imaging the subclavian and jugular veins, the arm is positioned at the side with the head turned in the opposite direction. Imaging of the rest of the arm veins can be done with the bed flat or with the head elevated. To view the axillary vein, the arm may be abducted to allow access to the axilla. The arm is then repositioned to a lower angle to allow access to the remaining arm veins.

### Equipment

For the examination of the upper extremity veins, at least two transducers are needed. As with the examination of the legs, a midrange transducer (5 to 10 MHz) will be commonly used to visualize the internal jugular, brachiocephalic, subclavian, axillary, deep brachial, and brachial veins. A second transducer will be needed for proper evaluation of the superficial veins of the arm (cephalic and basilic), and it is also helpful for the small forearm vessels (radial and ulnar veins). This second transducer should be a higher frequency transducer in the 10 to 18 MHz range. A high-frequency transducer is extremely valuable when mapping the superficial upper extremity veins. In some instances, a midrange (5 to 10 MHz) transducer which is not a straight linear array is helpful. A curved array transducer with a small footprint will be helpful in insonating vessels near the clavicle and sternum because it can be more easily maneuvered into these small spaces than a flat linear array transducer.

As with any ultrasound, appropriate examination-specific presets should be selected prior to the start of the procedure. Equipment settings should be optimized and adjusted throughout the examination to obtain high-quality images and waveforms.

### Scanning Technique

The complete examination of the upper extremity veins includes the multiple venous segments, as described below. As previously stated, there may be indications for a limited evaluation of specific veins, such as only the internal jugular and subclavian veins prior to central line placement.

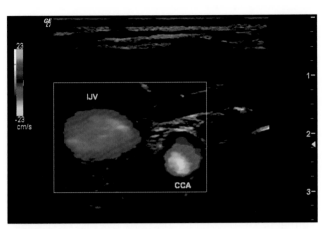

**FIGURE 18-1** A transverse view of the internal jugular vein (IJV) and the common carotid artery (CCA) with color.

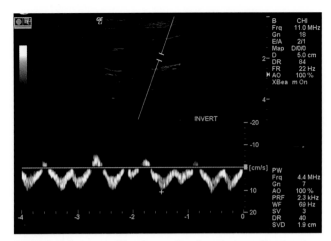

**FIGURE 18-3** A spectral Doppler waveform from the internal jugular vein.

## Internal and External Jugular Veins

Because thrombus in the veins of the arms can extend into the veins of the neck, a complete upper extremity venous duplex ultrasound examination includes evaluating the jugular veins. Thrombus may also be found isolated to the jugular veins, in particular, the internal jugular vein, as a result of a central line placement within this vessel. Lastly, the jugular veins are an important collateral pathway in the advent of upper extremity thrombosis, thus providing another reason for inclusion of these vessels in an upper extremity venous ultrasound examination.

The carotid artery is used as a landmark to find the internal jugular vein that runs alongside it (Figs. 18-1 and 18-2). The internal jugular vein will be collapsed if the patient is sitting or standing (owing to hydrostatic pressure) so this part of the examination must be done with the patient lying flat. If the examiner cannot find the internal jugular vein, the head of the patient should be lowered to determine whether the vein is collapsed. Documentation of patency of the internal jugular vein should include transverse grayscale images with the vein compressed and noncompressed. A spectral Doppler waveform should also be recorded from the internal jugular vein (Fig. 18-3).

The external jugular vein is found by lightening up on the transducer pressure and sliding posterior from the position used to view the internal jugular vein. The external jugular vein runs without an accompanying artery very close to the skin and usually terminates into the subclavian vein. This vein's patency can also be documented with transverse views of the vein compressed and noncompressed as well as with a spectral Doppler waveform. Many laboratory protocols do not include routine documentation of this vein but rather in the event of thrombosis in adjacent vessels, this vessel is then added to the examination.

## Brachiocephalic Vein

Examining the brachiocephalic veins is challenging because it is difficult to position the transducer around the bony structures in the area. As mentioned earlier, a small footprint transducer may allow for partial visualization of these veins. The brachiocephalic veins come together behind the sternum to form the superior vena cava, and this portion of these veins is not usually insonated. The beginning of the brachiocephalic veins at the confluence of the subclavian and internal jugular veins is the region of this vessel that is most often examined (Fig. 18-4). Compression of the brachiocephalic veins at this level is not able to be performed. Documentation of patency of these vessels should include a grayscale image, demonstrating the absence of thrombus.

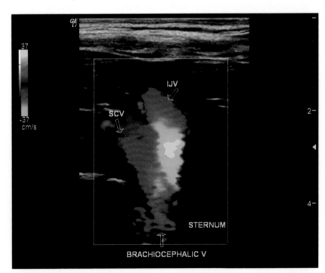

**FIGURE 18-4** Color image of the brachiocephalic vein.

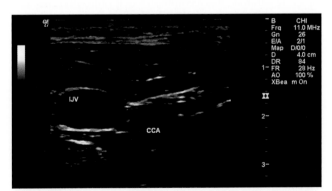

**FIGURE 18-2** A grayscale image (transverse) of the location of the internal jugular vein (IJV) alongside the common carotid artery (CCA).

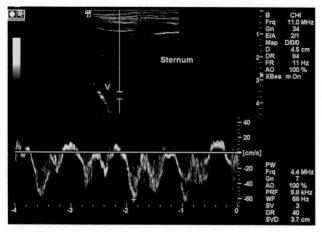

**FIGURE 18-5** Spectral Doppler waveform from the brachiocephalic vein (V).

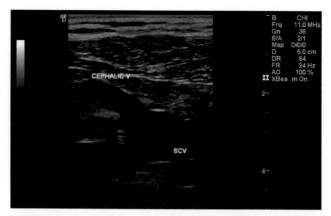

**FIGURE 18-7** A transverse view of the cephalic vein at the subclavian vein (SCV).

A color-flow image should be recorded to document full color filling of the vessel. Spectral Doppler waveforms should also be obtained because the phasicity and pulsatility observed at this level is an important diagnostic tool (Fig. 18-5). These patterns can indirectly indicate the status of the more central veins. More about these waveforms will be discussed later.

### Subclavian Vein

The subclavian vein is visualized above and below the clavicle. It accompanied by the subclavian artery (Fig. 18-6). Just after the subclavian vein passes under the clavicle as it continues toward the arm, a vessel can be seen terminating into the subclavian vein. This is the cephalic vein (Fig. 18-7). Moving distally toward the arm, beyond the terminus of the cephalic vein, the subclavian vein becomes the axillary vein. Compressing the subclavian vein to check for thrombus can be difficult because of the clavicle. The examiner can have the patient take a quick, deep, breath in through pursed lips. A similar maneuver known as the "sniff test" whereby the patient takes a quick sniff in through the nose can also be performed. If done correctly, this quick inspiration will cause the subclavian to collapse. Spectral waveforms and color images should also be documented. As noted with the brachiocephalic veins, the spectral waveforms obtained at the subclavian vein are a helpful diagnostic tool.

### Cephalic Vein

Before the cephalic vein terminates into the subclavian vein, it travels superficially near the skin line (Fig. 18-8) across

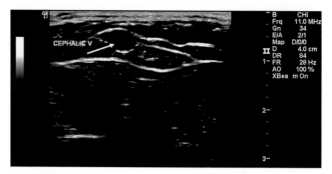

**FIGURE 18-8** A transverse view of the cephalic vein (*arrow*) in the upper arm.

the shoulder and along the arm at the anteriolateral border of the biceps muscle (Fig. 18-9). At or near the antecubital fossa, it communicates with the median cubital vein. Distally onto the forearm, there are typically two veins which will unite before the antecubital fossa. One will course along the volar aspect of the forearm to the wrist, while the other will travel along the dorsal aspect of the forearm. Compressed and noncompressed grayscale images are easily performed to document patency.

### Median Cubital Vein

The median cubital is a vein that connects the cephalic and basilic veins. It is present at in the antecubital fossa, but its pattern of connection with the basilic and cephalic veins can be quite variable. It is a common site for thrombus because

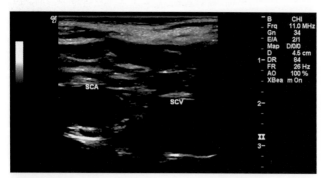

**FIGURE 18-6** A transverse view of the subclavian artery (SCA) and subclavian vein (SCV).

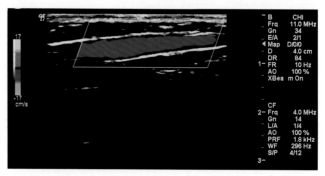

**FIGURE 18-9** A longitudinal view of the cephalic vein with color added.

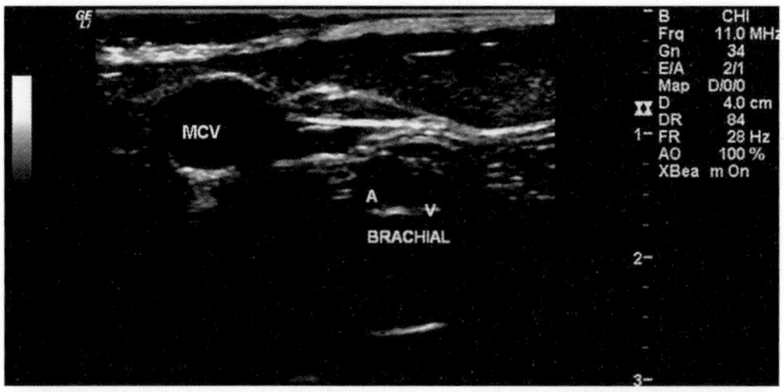

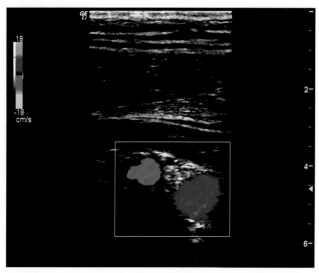

**FIGURE 18-10** A transverse view of the median cubital vein (MCV) as it passes superiorly over the brachial artery (A) and brachial vein (V).

it is a common site for venapuncture. The median cubital vein is a great landmark vein because it crosses directly over the brachial artery and vein (Fig. 18-10). Compressed and noncompressed images should be documented at this level, particularly if superficial thrombophlebitis is suspected.

### Axillary Vein

The axillary vein terminates at the junction of the cephalic and subclavian veins. This deep vein is accompanied by the axillary artery and courses deeply as it crosses the shoulder over to the axilla (Fig. 18-11). At this point, the arm is repositioned and abducted to expose the axilla. At the axilla, this vein will be seen fairly close to the skin. Usually, deep veins and their accompanying arteries are positioned side by side. In the axilla, the axillary vein and artery may not be directly adjacent to each other for a short distance (Fig. 18-12). Following the vein in the upper arm, the artery and vein will course together. Compressed and noncompressed images of the vein should be recorded along with color and Spectral Doppler waveforms. In most patients, compression of the axillary vein will be possible.

Along the medial portion of the upper arm, a large superficial vein will be observed terminating into the axillary vein. This is the basilic vein. Distally in the upper arm, below the terminus of the basilic vein, the vessel is now

**FIGURE 18-12** A transverse view of the axillary artery (in *red*) and vein (in *blue*) taken from the axilla. Note how there is spatial separation between the two vessels.

called the brachial vein. There are usually two brachial veins at this level, and each will be located on either side of the brachial artery. At this point, the brachial veins will be fairly small (Fig. 18-13).

### Brachial Vein

The brachial vein is often a bifid system. The brachial veins will accompany the brachial artery until just below the antecubital fossa. The brachial veins are formed by the junction of two radial and two ulnar veins at the level of the antecubital fossa. The patency of the brachial veins should include clear images of both brachial veins with compressed and noncompressed views. Some laboratories also choose to document venous spectral Doppler signals at this level.

### Radial Veins

The radial veins will course along the volar aspect of the forearm accompanied by the radial artery (Fig. 18-14). These vessels are very small and are not often a site for venous thrombosis. They are technically deep veins but are often not included in routine upper extremity venous examinations. Should the patient's symptoms suggest thrombosis within the forearm, the radial veins should be imaged.

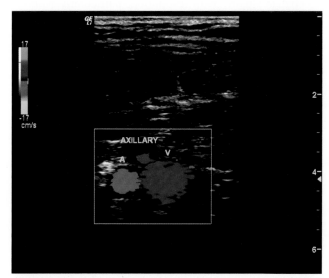

**FIGURE 18-11** A transverse view of the axillary artery (A) and vein (V) over the shoulder.

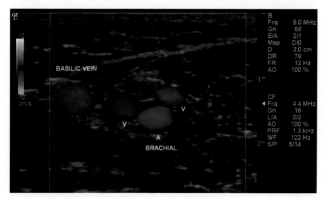

**FIGURE 18-13** A transverse view of the brachial artery (A) and veins (V) in the upper arm. The basilic vein is also noted.

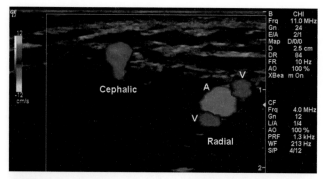

**FIGURE 18-14** A transverse view of the radial artery (A) and veins (V). The cephalic vein is also noted.

## Ulnar Veins

The ulnar veins are followed because they travel the volar aspect of the ulnar side of the forearm. Like the radial veins with their companion radial artery, the ulnar veins course on either side of the ulnar artery (Fig. 18-15). As with the radial veins, the ulnar veins are not examined unless indicated by the presenting symptoms of the patient.

## Basilic Vein

To follow the basilic vein, the examiner can begin in the upper-mid portion of the upper arm and locates the level where the basilic vein terminates into the axillary vein. The basilic vein will course medially and superficially without a companion artery and will usually be the largest vein in the region (Fig. 18-16). At a point near the antecubital fossa, the basilic vein will communicate with the cephalic vein via the medial cubital vein. Onto the forearm, the basilic vein is usually comprised of two branches. One will course mostly on the volar aspect of the forearm, while the other will extend to the dorsal aspect of the forearm.

## Pitfalls

There are several locations where compression of the veins is not possible. Compression of the brachiocephalic and subclavian veins is not usually performed because of the position of these vessels with respect to the sternum and clavicle. Spectral Doppler and color imaging are relied upon to document venous patency in those vessels where

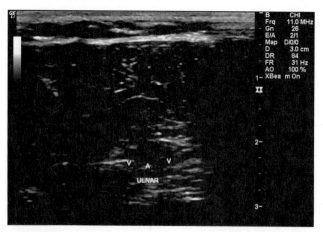

**FIGURE 18-15** A transverse view of the ulnar artery (A) and veins (V).

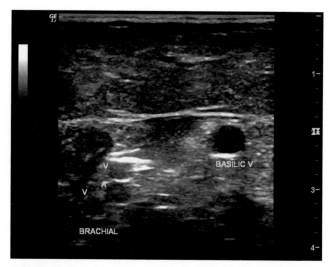

**FIGURE 18-16** A transverse view of the basilic vein in the upper arm.

compression of the vein is not possible. The patient may also present with dressings or intravenous catheters which limit direct insonation of the underlying veins. Again, in these cases, spectral Doppler and color imaging of adjacent veins are important to assist in determination of patency. If signals in adjacent vessels are normal, it is indirectly indicative of vein patency in the regions unable to be directly visualized.

## DIAGNOSIS

The diagnostic criteria for the detection of the presence or absence of thrombus, as well as distinguishing features of acute versus chronic thrombus, are the same for the upper extremity as those described for the lower extremity in Chapter 17. Briefly, normal vein walls will be able to be completely compressed together with light transducer pressure. This compression maneuver must be performed in transverse view and not in a longitudinal or sagittal plane of view. Normal vein walls appear thin and smooth on ultrasound. The vessel lumen should be hypoechoic. While in transverse view, the vein diameter may be seen to change slightly with respiration, particularly with the more central veins.

If the walls fail to coapt or completely close together, thrombus should be suspected. Echogenic material should be observed within the vein where compression fails to fully coapt the walls. There are several distinguishing characteristics associated with acute thrombus, including visualizing a poorly attached thrombus, which is spongy in texture and a dilated vein (Fig. 18-17). Chronic thrombus is often brightly echogenic, well-attached, rigid, and the vein is usually contracted (Fig. 18-18).

Superficial vein thrombus will have the same appearance as deep vein thrombosis. Depending on the degree of inflammation associated with the thrombus, hypoechoic areas may be present in the tissue immediately adjacent to the veins.

## Color and Spectral Doppler

In the upper extremity, in regions where the veins are not able to be compressed (near the clavicle and sternum), color

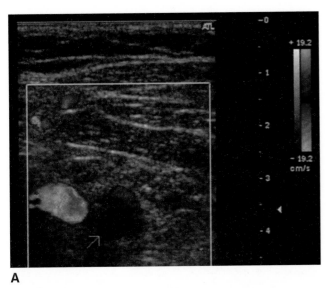
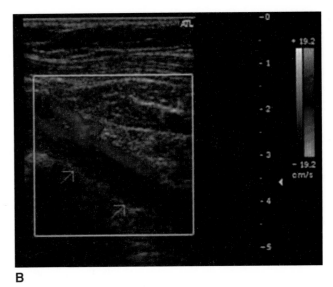

**A**          **B**

**FIGURE 18-17** An acute thrombus in the internal jugular vein: **(A)** transverse view and **(B)** sagittal view. Arrows indicate the thrombosed vein. (Image courtesy of Jean M. White-Melendez, RVT, RPhS, FSVU and William B. Schroedter, BS, RVT, RPhS, FSVU, Venice, Florida.)

and spectral Doppler characteristics are important diagnostic tools. As with normal lower extremity veins, color should be seen filling the entire vessel lumen. However, it is possible to have color overwrite grayscale information, and fill in a vessel with partial thrombus. Care should be taken to have color-priority setting on the ultrasound equipment appropriately adjusted to avoid overwriting partial thrombus with color. Additional color settings should be optimized in those vessels where the flow is diminished. In veins with partial thrombus, proper color adjustments will result in the color filling around the areas of thrombus helping to outline the extent of the disease. In completely thrombosed vessels, no color filling will be seen.

Spectral Doppler criteria are similar to those used in the lower extremity, because phasicity with respiration is expected. Compression distal to the position of the transducer should also augment flow. However, given the proximity of the more central veins to the right atrium of the heart, pronounced pulsatility is often observed (Fig. 18-19). It is common to observe pulsatile flow in the internal jugular, brachiocephalic, and subclavian veins. Respiratory phasicity is often superimposed on cardiac pulsatility. The lack of pulsatility in the internal jugular, brachiocephalic, or subclavian veins is indicative of more central pathology.[8] However, depending on the patient position, volume status, cardiac function, and respiratory status, the waveform characteristics from these vessels will be affected. Thus, it is of the upmost importance to compare the symmetry of the signal between the right and left central veins to help determine patency. As one moves further away from the

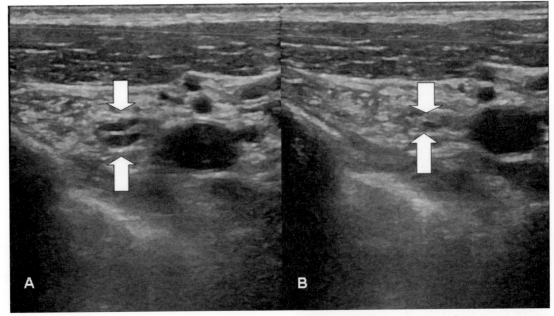

**A**          **B**

**FIGURE 18-18** A chronic thrombus in the axillary vein: **(A)** noncompressed view and **(B)** compressed view illustrating inability to fully compress the vein. Arrows indicate the outer borders of the axillary vein. (Image courtesy of Steve Knight, BSc, RVT, RDCS, Half Moon Bay, CA.)

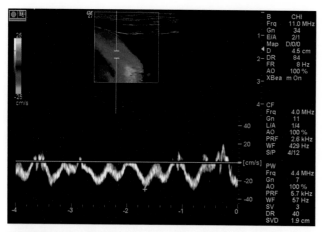

**FIGURE 18-19** A Doppler spectral waveform taken from a subclavian vein demonstrating normal pulsatile flow.

heart, the pulsatility dampens out so that a more phasic venous Doppler signal is obtained.

With complete thrombus, no spectral Doppler signals will be obtained. In veins that are partially thrombosed, the spectral Doppler will be continuous but should display augmentation with distal compression. A continuous Doppler will also be observed within veins where a more central partial thrombosis is present or where there is extrinsic compression of the more central veins. If both subclavian veins display nonpulsatile, continuous flow, disease within the superior vena cava should be suspected. It is common to observe reversal of venous flow in the presence of a central thrombus. Flow may be reversed in the internal or external jugular veins in association with an ipsilateral brachiocephalic vein thrombus. The venous outflow from the arm will pass through the subclavian vein but then move cephalad up the external or internal jugular veins. Large collateral pathways exist through various routes within the neck and shoulder region.

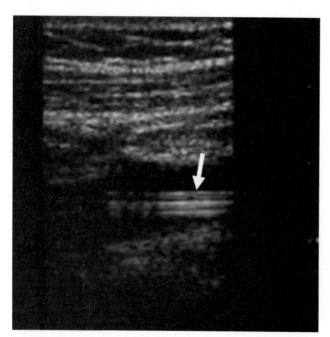

**FIGURE 18-20** A longitudinal view of a catheter (*arrow*) inside a vein.

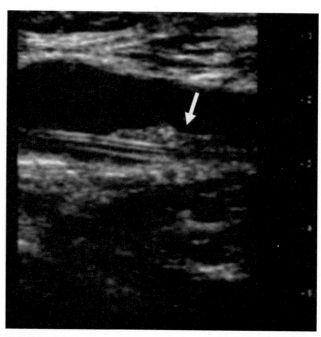

**FIGURE 18-21** A longitudinal view of thrombus (*arrow*) forming on a venous catheter.

Another type of alteration in venous Doppler signals will occur in patients with an upper extremity hemodialysis fistula or graft. This will produce pulsatile flow which displays elevated velocities throughout the cardiac cycle (low-resistance, high-diastolic flow). It may be difficult to assess respiratory variations; however, the signal will still augment with distal compression.

## Venous Catheters

Indwelling venous catheters are commonly encountered in the arm while they are rarely seen in the leg. Because the use of these catheters is so common in the arm, this can lead to the development of thrombus within the upper extremity venous system. Catheters will appear in the lumen of the vein as bright, straight, parallel echoes (Fig. 18-20). The exact appearance of these echoes will vary slightly depending on the number of lumens within the catheter. Thrombus can be seen because it forms on the catheter (Fig. 18-21) as echogenic

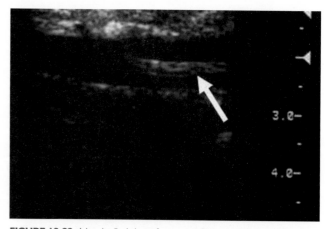

**FIGURE 18-22** A longitudinal view of a remnant fibrous sheath (*arrow*) left in the vein after removal of a catheter. Note how this appears to resemble a catheter.

**PATHOLOGY BOX 18-1**
*Ultrasound Findings with Upper Extremity Pathology*

| Abnormality | Ultrasound Findings |
|---|---|
| Acute thrombus | B-mode image: echogenic material within the veins; veins fail to fully coapt; vein appears dilated; thrombus is poorly attached to vein wall; vein appears spongy<br>Spectral and Color Doppler: no color or spectral Doppler obtained with complete thrombosis |
| Chronic thrombus | B-mode image: brightly echogenic material within the veins; veins fail to fully coapt; vein appears contracted; thrombus is rigid and firmly attached<br>Spectral and Color Doppler: no color or spectral Doppler obtained with complete thrombosis |
| Partial nonocclusive thrombus | B-mode: echogenic material within the veins; veins will partially compress but not able to completely coapt walls<br>Spectral Doppler: continuous signal; slight phasicity may be noted with lesser degrees of thrombosis; will augment with distal compression; little to no cessation of flow with Valsalva<br>Color flow: color fails to fill vessel lumen |
| Venous catheter associated thrombus | B-mode: echogenic material around brightly echogenic, straight parallel lines of catheter<br>Spectral Doppler: diminished or continuous depending on degree of thrombosis<br>Color: color filling residual lumen around thrombus |

material on the surface of the catheter. Left untreated, this thrombus may progress and fill the lumen of the vein. Color flow will outline the residual lumen, if any, surrounding the catheter. Spectral Doppler signals will be diminished and may be continuous depending on the degree of luminal reduction. Once a catheter with associated thrombus has been removed, it would be expected to observe a clear anechoic vein lumen. However, commonly there is a residual sheath of thrombus left in the vein after catheter removal that will look as if the catheter is still present (Fig. 18-22).

Pathology Box 18-1 summarizes the ultrasound findings associated with upper extremity venous pathology.

## TREATMENT

Treatment considerations for upper extremity venous thrombosis include anticoagulation, catheter removal, thrombolytic therapy, and surgical decompression of the thoracic inlet with or without venous reconstruction.[9,10] Some of these current treatment methods were described in more detail in Chapter 17. In some patients, conservative treatment may be used depending on the location of the thrombus and the condition of the patient. It is important to determine the most central extent of any thrombus because this may influence the physician's treatment choices.

## SUMMARY

- Imaging of the upper extremity veins may seem difficult at first.
- Once the examiner gets familiar with the anatomy and its variations, the upper extremity venous system becomes much easier than imaging the vein of the legs.
- Upper extremity venous imaging relies on compression of the veins where possible.
- Spectral Doppler and color imaging are performed at each major vessel imaged and are very valuable in segments where compression is not possible.
- Paying close attention to the suggestions and protocols contained in this chapter and the lower extremity chapter of this book will set the stage for accurate diagnostic imaging.

## CRITICAL THINKING QUESTIONS

1. When lower extremity veins are examined, patients can be placed in a dependent position. What position is best for an ultrasound of the subclavian and jugular veins? What is a common factor which is considered when determining the patient position for a venous ultrasound?

2. You are asked to perform an examination on a patient with a dressing in place over the subclavicular region on the shoulder. What specifically can you do to provide adequate information for the determination of the upper extremity venous system patency?

3. You are examining a patient for an upper extremity venous thrombosis. You notice several dilated chest wall veins. The spectral Doppler signals from both subclavian and internal jugular veins are antegrade but continuous. What is likely the cause of these findings?

## MEDIA MENU

Student Resources available on thePoint° include:
- Audio glossary
- Interactive question bank
- Videos
- Internet resources

## REFERENCES

1. Bernardi E, Pesavento R, Prandoni P. Upper extremity deep venous thrombosis. *Semin Thromb.* 2006;32:729–736.
2. Gaitini D, Beck-Razi N, Haim N, et al. Prevalence of upper extremity deep venous thrombosis diagnosed by color Doppler duplex sonography in cancer patients with central venous catheters. *J Ultrasound Med.* 2006;25:1297–1303.
3. Talbot SR. B-mode evaluation of peripheral veins. *Semin Ultrasound CT MR.* 1988;9:295–319.
4. Sullivan ED, Peters BS, Cranley JJ. Real-time B-mode venous ultrasound. *J Vasc Surg.* 1984;1:465–471.
5. Oliver MA. Duplex scanning in venous disease. *Bruit.* 1985;9:206–209.
6. Talbot SR, Oliver MA. *Techniques of Venous Imaging.* Pasadena, CA: Appleton Davies; 1992.
7. Hartshorne T, Goss D. Duplex assessment of deep vein thrombosis and upper limb disorders. In: Thrush A, Hartshore T, eds. *Vascular Ultrasound: How, Why and When.* 3rd ed. Edinburgh: Churchill Livingston Elsevier; 2010: 233–253.
8. Selis JE, Kadakia S. Venous Doppler sonography of the extremities: a window to pathology of the thorax, abdomen and pelvis. *Am J Roent.* 2009;193:1446–1451.
9. Qaseem A, Snow V, Barry P, et al. Current diagnosis of venous thromboembolism in primary care: a clinical practice guideline from the American Academy of Family Physicians and the American College of Physicians. *Ann Fam Med.* 2007;5:57–62.
10. Czihal M, Hoffman U. Upper extremity deep venous thrombosis. *Vasc Med.* 2011;16:191–202.

# Ultrasound Evaluation and Mapping of the Superficial Venous System

ANN MARIE KUPINSKI

## CHAPTER 19

## OBJECTIVES

- List the indications for venous mapping
- Describe the normal anatomic features of the great saphenous vein, small saphenous vein, cephalic vein, and basilic vein
- Identify pathology observed within the superficial veins
- Describe the basic techniques of venous mapping
- List the equipment necessary for vein mapping
- Define limitations encountered during vein mapping
- Describe diagnostic ultrasound criteria utilized in venous mapping

## GLOSSARY

**great saphenous vein** A superficial vein forming at the level of the medial malleolus, coursing medially along the calf and thigh, and terminating into the common femoral vein at the saphenofemoral junction

**perforating vein** A vein that connects the superficial venous system to the deep venous system

**recanalization** A vein that was previously thrombosed

**small saphenous vein** A superficial vein that courses along the posterior aspect of the calf terminating at the popliteal fossa into the popliteal vein

**varicosities** Dilated tortuous superficial veins

## KEY TERMS

**basilic**

**calcification**

**cephalic**

**great saphenous**

**mapping**

**perforator**

**planar arrangement**

**recanalization**

**small saphenous**

**varicosities**

---

Ultrasound has been used to evaluate the venous system for over 35 years. The utilization of venous ultrasound has increased greatly, and the applications have also expanded. The early application of ultrasound in the venous system had centered mainly on the detection of thrombus within the deep venous system.[1] Soon after clinicians realized the usefulness of deep venous ultrasound, they began to extend ultrasound to evaluate the superficial venous systems.[2] The superficial venous systems were of interest to assess both their competency and their suitability as a bypass conduit.[2,3] Superficial veins are used for a variety of types of bypass procedures, not the least of which is coronary artery bypass grafting. Autogenous vein is the preferred conduit of choice for lower extremity arterial bypass procedures. Lastly, continued interest in creating hemodialysis access fistulas in lieu of dialysis grafts presents yet another reason why the status of the superficial veins must be assessed.

When planning to use a segment of superficial vein for a procedure, surgeons gather as much information as possible to aid in the successful performance of these surgeries. Vein patency, position, depth, and size are some of the characteristics assessed preoperatively. These details provided by ultrasound imaging allow for the selection of the optimal vein. Proper knowledge of the anatomy of the superficial veins may alter the planned surgery as well as the surgical approach used. Information on the venous configuration will help to minimize the amount of surgical dissection needed.

This chapter describes the techniques involved in ultrasonic evaluation of the superficial venous systems. Material pertaining to the great saphenous, small saphenous, basilic, and cephalic veins is also presented. Relevant anatomy, scanning techniques, tips, diagnostic criteria, and pathologic characteristics are reviewed.

## ANATOMY

### The Great Saphenous Vein

Prior to discussing the saphenous anatomy, it is important to briefly review the nomenclature of the venous system. A multidisciplinary panel published a consensus paper in which nomenclature was revised and standardized in an attempt to avoid some commonly confused terms.[4,5] Table 19-1 lists several of the major changes regarding saphenous vein terminology. The great saphenous vein is the standard name for the vein which had been referred to as the greater or long saphenous vein. The small saphenous vein is the correct name for the vein known as the lesser or short saphenous vein. A sonographer or vascular technologist should become familiar with this revised terminology.

Most anatomy textbooks display the great saphenous vein beginning at the ankle just posterior to the medial malleolus. In the calf, it courses slightly anteriorly near the tibia and then continues up into the thigh as a single trunk coursing medially and terminating into the common femoral vein (Fig. 19-1). This is a common configuration for the great saphenous, but multiple variants exist. Extensive reviews of both ultrasound and venographic data have revealed a complex system variability in both the thigh and calf.[6,7]

The thigh portion of the great saphenous vein has been found to have five common configurations (Fig. 19-2). In about 60% of cases, this vein is a single trunk that runs medially in the thigh. It curves slightly toward the inner thigh and typically has several large tributaries which empty into the vein before it joins the common femoral vein. These tributaries include the anterior (lateral) and posterior (medial) accessory and circumflex veins.

Less commonly in only 8% of cases, the great saphenous is a single trunk that courses anteriorly and laterally in the thigh. This is likely a dominant version of the anterior accessory saphenous vein.

The remaining configurations encountered in the thigh all demonstrate the presence of multiple large tributaries that

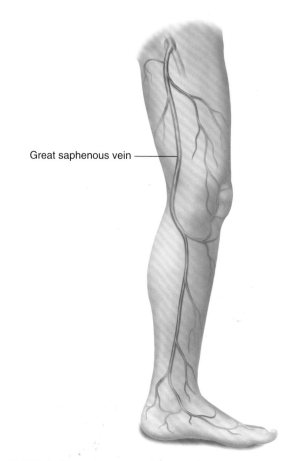

**FIGURE 19-1** Typical anatomic configuration of the great saphenous vein with a single medial dominant system in the thigh and an anterior dominant system in the calf.

Great saphenous vein

interconnect. The saphenous vein may have two separate large systems running both medially and laterally throughout the entire length of the thigh. These double systems remain separate from each other and extend below the knee. This pattern occurs in 8% of cases. Sometimes, the anteriolateral system may be slightly larger, and in others, the posteriomedial system may be larger. It is very important to identify which vein is dominant so that the surgeon can select the most appropriate vein. Even though these systems are separate, there are often small veins which communicate between the systems. Often, these duplicated systems may not course in the same anatomic plane (Fig. 19-3). One system may be superficial to the fascia (this is likely the superficial accessory great saphenous vein), whereas the other system may lie in the normal anatomic plane. Normally, the main trunk of the saphenous vein lies in what is termed the saphenous compartment bounded by the saphenous fascia superficially and deeply by the muscular fascia. The notation of planar arrangement on the ultrasound report will be discussed later in the chapter.

In approximately 7% of cases, the great saphenous vein may have a loop of tributary veins that is contained within the thigh. This closed loop system can present the vascular surgeon with particular difficulties during an in situ bypass procedure, especially if a closed vein exposure technique is used. During this form of in situ bypass, most of the thigh is kept intact (closed), and instrumentation is passed up

| TABLE 19-1 | Venous Nomenclature |
| --- | --- |
| **Current Terminology** | **Previous Terminology** |
| Great saphenous vein | Greater saphenous vein |
| | Long saphenous vein |
| Small saphenous vein | Lesser saphenous vein |
| | Short saphenous vein |
| Anterior accessory great saphenous vein | Accessory saphenous vein |
| Posterior accessory great saphenous vein | Accessory saphenous vein |
| | Leonardo's vein |
| | Posterior arch vein |
| Cranial extension of the small saphenous vein | Vein of Giacomini |

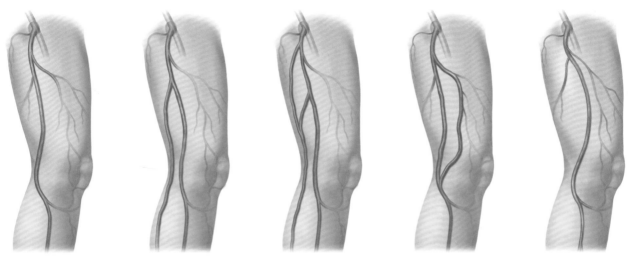

**FIGURE 19-2** Anatomic variations in the configuration of the thigh portion of the great saphenous vein.

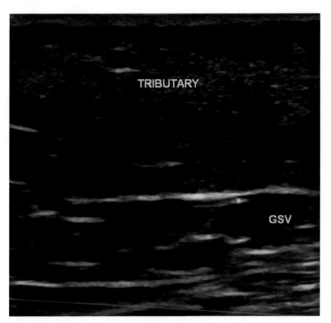

**FIGURE 19-3** Ultrasound image illustrating the planar arrangement of a double system with deep and superficial systems.

the thigh from more distal segments to disrupt valves. In the case of a closed loop, the surgeon may inadvertently pass instruments up through the smaller venous segment of the loop resulting in vein injury.

Lastly, in the remaining 17% of cases, partial double systems may be present in the thigh. Typically, there is a large posteriomedial tributary which terminates into the distal two-thirds of the thigh portion of the dominant venous system. This is the posterior accessory great saphenous vein which has been previously referred to as "Leonardo's vein" or the posterior arch vein. As with the other forms of double systems, these partial double systems may share smaller communicating tributaries.

More complex variations can occur in the thigh, but this is very rare (usually less than 1% occurrence). The so-called "triplicate systems" of three large veins with multiple communicating veins have been identified. These intricate systems

involve both anterior and posterior accessory veins and the main trunk of the great saphenous vein. Often in patients who previously had a portion or all of the great saphenous vein removed, the accessory systems in the thigh and calf dilate to accommodate venous outflow. It is important when evaluating a patient for venous conduits to always examine a leg even if a prior venous harvest, ablation or stripping has been performed. In many patients, these accessory systems are a suitable for use as a conduit.

The great saphenous vein in the calf has much less variability than the thigh portion. One of three common arrangements can be found in the calf (Fig. 19-4). In 65% of cases, the calf portion is a single dominant system, and this is almost always positioned anteriorly near the medial border of the tibia. There is often a posterior vein which is the posterior accessory great saphenous vein previously mentioned in the discussion of thigh anatomy. This is simply a smaller tributary that is typically not large enough to be used as a bypass conduit. In about 7% of patients, the posterior accessory great saphenous vein is dominant over the more anterior system of the calf.

Double venous systems in the calf can be seen in approximately 35% of cases. These double systems begin as a single vein at the ankle level and split into two veins in the lower calf. They remain as two separate systems and join back together into a single vein at the knee. Again, the more posterior system in these cases is likely the posterior accessory great saphenous vein, but it is just confined to the calf level. The anterior system is dominant in 85% of cases, whereas the posterior system in dominant in the remaining 15%. The posterior system can drain into a larger vein that will continue up the thigh to join a duplicated thigh system, or it can have tributaries which may extend further posteriorly to connect into the small saphenous vein. Table 19-2 summarizes the various anatomic distributions of the great saphenous vein.

There are multiple cutaneous tributaries of the great saphenous vein (Fig. 19-5). The exact number and level of these tributaries vary among limbs. Cutaneous tributaries are of little significance to the surgeon and are usually ligated during an open procedure. If an in situ procedure is being performed with limited vein exposure, most

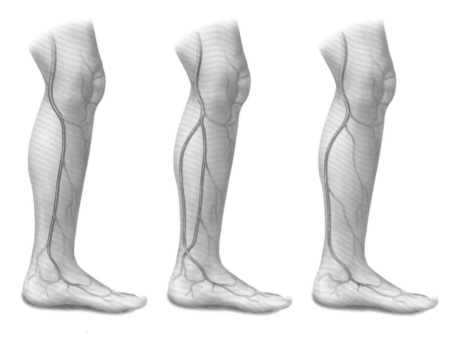

**FIGURE 19-4** Anatomic variations in the configuration of the calf portion of the great saphenous vein.

| TABLE 19-2 **Anatomic Variants of the Great Saphenous Vein** | |
|---|---|
| **Percent of Distribution** | |
| **THIGH** | |
| Single medial dominant | 60 |
| Single lateral dominant | 8 |
| Complete double system | 8 |
| Closed-loop double system | 7 |
| Partial double system | 17 |
| Triplicate/complex systems | <1 |
| **CALF** | |
| Single anterior dominant system | 58 |
| Single posterior dominant system | 7 |
| Double anterior dominant system | 30 |
| Double posterior dominant system | 5 |

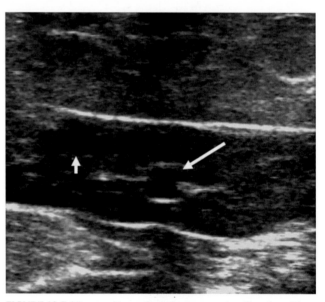

**FIGURE 19-5** Ultrasound image illustrating the normal configuration of the great saphenous vein (*large arrow*) and a cutaneous tributary (*small arrow*).

cutaneous tributaries can be simply left intact because they will spontaneously thrombose. Some cutaneous tributaries may be harvested if only a small segment of vein is needed as patch material. This keeps the main saphenous system intact for future use.

Of importance to surgeons is the location of deep perforating veins (Fig. 19-6). These perforating veins must always be identified and ligated. A perforating vein is a term reserved for a vein that perforates or penetrates the muscular fascia of the leg and connects the superficial system to the deep system. It initially can be seen as a vein that appears to be a superficial tributary emptying into the saphenous vein. However, when followed away from the saphenous vein, it will perforate the fascia and terminate into a vein of the

deep venous system (Fig. 19-7). Perforators have valves to ensure the one-way movement of blood from the superficial to the deep system. If the vein is arterialized as a bypass conduit and a perforating vein is left intact, this will create an arteriovenous fistula connecting the bypass to the deep venous system. Owing to the low resistance of the venous bed, significant blood flow can be diverted through this type of fistula. Therefore, it is important to mark the locations of these perforating veins so that a surgeon can ligate them prior to completion of the arterial bypass graft. There are several groups of perforating veins throughout the leg. Some perforating veins connect directly to the main trunk of the saphenous vein, whereas others connect to the accessory saphenous systems.

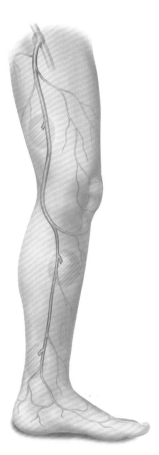

**FIGURE 19-6** Illustration of the common levels at which deep perforating veins can be observed.

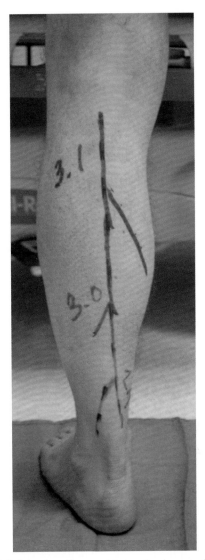

**FIGURE 19-8** Patient leg with a completed small saphenous vein mapping.

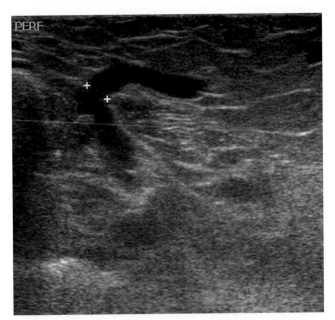

**FIGURE 19-7** Ultrasound image illustrating the orientation of a perforating vein off the main trunk of the great saphenous vein. Note how the vein penetrates the muscular fascia (between the caliper markers).

## The Small Saphenous Vein

The small saphenous vein is another superficial vein that can be mapped prior to surgery for use as a bypass conduit. The small saphenous vein courses in a fairly constant pattern along the posterior aspect of the calf (Fig. 19-8). Two smaller veins leave the foot and travel medially and laterally along the borders of the Achilles tendon. These two veins join together to form the small saphenous vein. The small saphenous is typically a single trunk that courses up the middle of the posterior aspect of the calf and terminates into the popliteal vein. In approximately 20% of limbs, the small saphenous vein continues above the popliteal fossa. This vein is referred to as the cranial extension of the small saphenous vein. In some cases, it terminates directly into the femoral vein or can end into the inferior gluteal vein. In some cases, it communicates with the great saphenous vein via the posterior thigh circumflex vein, and in this configuration is often referred to as the vein of Giacomini. The small saphenous vein also has several cutaneous tributaries as well as deep perforating veins. It is not uncommon to observe one or more intersaphenous veins connecting the small and great saphenous veins in the calf. The perforating veins may connect the small saphenous with the gastrocnemius or peroneal veins.

## The Cephalic and Basilic Veins

Venous mapping techniques have extended to the superficial veins of the arm (Fig. 19-9). This has become part of the routine preoperative assessment in patients undergoing the creation of a dialysis fistula. The cephalic vein begins at the level of the wrist, coursing along the radial aspect of the forearm and continuing through the upper arm, terminating into the subclavian vein. The basilic vein also begins at the level of the wrist, coursing along the ulnar aspect of the forearm. The basilic vein continues into the upper arm where it joins the brachial veins to form the axillary vein. The cephalic and basilic veins communicate at the antecubital fossa via the medial cubital vein. Some variability occurs with the upper extremity superficial veins. Primarily, the venous patterns at the antecubital fossa and the position of the medial cubital vein display the most variability.

## SONOGRAPHIC EXAMINATION TECHNIQUES

### Patient Preparation

Vein mapping may sometimes be limited to only the ultrasound evaluation of the superficial veins with image documentation and completion of required worksheets. Often, the procedure involves the additional step of mapping the position of suitable veins directly on the patient's skin. The patient should be instructed to avoid body lotions or powders because these will impede the marking of the skin. The actual marking devices used to create the skin map vary among laboratories that perform this technique. Because the various inks used can be messy, it is recommended to cover the ultrasound transducer with a nonsterile probe cover. Ultrasound gel should be used sparingly to allow easier skin marking. It is recommended to use limited gel directly under the transducer and mark the position of the vein in front of the transducer. Limited use of gel will also reduce the amount of cooling the patient experiences because the gel evaporates from the skin surface. The marker used should be able to easily write on the skin and resist

drying out with prolonged use. Some laboratories do not use a marker at all. These labs use a small plastic coffee stirrer or straw to place an indentation in the skin. These indentations remain on the skin for a short time to allow for a final map to be drawn when finished. A final map may be drawn on the skin with permanent marker, surgical markers, or permanent liquid ink commonly used by radiation therapy departments.

### Patient Position

Patient position is very important when performing venous imaging, particularly when dealing with small diameter veins. Venous pressure in the superficial veins should be maximized by placing the patient's limb in a dependent position. For the mapping the leg veins, the patient should be placed in a reverse Trendelenberg position with the hip externally rotated and knee slightly flexed (Fig. 19-10). This position provides adequate access to the entire length of the great saphenous vein. For the small saphenous vein, the patient may be placed on his or her side with the posterior aspect of the calf accessible to the technologist (Fig. 19-11). In cases

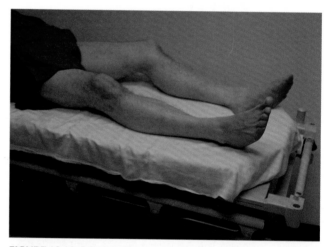

**FIGURE 19-10** Patient position for mapping the great saphenous vein.

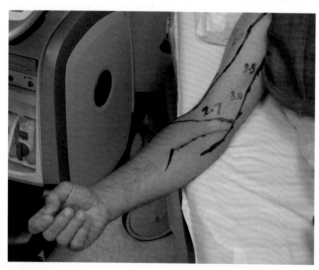

**FIGURE 19-9** Patient arm with a completed mapping of the cephalic and basilic veins.

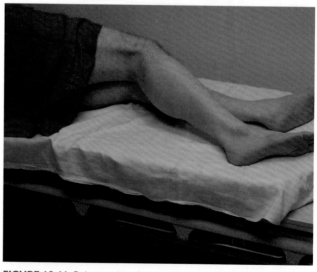

**FIGURE 19-11** Patient position for mapping the small saphenous vein.

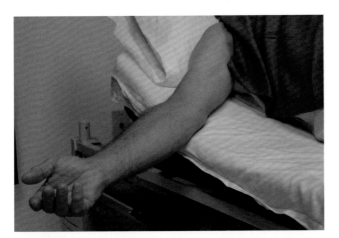

**FIGURE 19-12** Patient position for mapping the cephalic and basilic veins.

of small vein diameter, the patient can be asked to stand for brief periods of time, particularly during the measurement of vein diameter. When mapping the arm veins, the patient's arm can be extended out to the side and slightly lower than the chest level (Fig. 19-12). The arm veins can also be assessed with the patient sitting upright with their hands resting on pillow. In patients with small arm veins, tourniquets can be used to aid in dilating the veins.

The examination room should be kept warm in order to limit vasoconstriction. The patient should only expose the limb being evaluated, keeping the rest of the body covered and warm. Keeping the foot covered of the leg being examined is also helpful in reducing vasoconstriction. Warm towels can also help produce vasodilation.

## Scanning Technique

The mapping of the great saphenous vein usually begins at the groin at the saphenofemoral junction. It is important to note that very light pressure should be applied to the skin. Because these superficial veins are under low pressure, it is extremely easy to compress the vein with too much transducer pressure. With the transducer in a transverse orientation, the saphenofemoral junction is identified (Fig. 19-13A, B). The technologist can use either a sagittal or transverse transducer orientation to follow the line of the vein and map its course. The technologist must be diligent in marking the correct position of the vein given the transducer orientation. With a sagittal approach, the vein should appear to completely fill the screen from right to left in a long-axis view. The transducer should be held perpendicular to the skin surface. These techniques will assure that the vein is not being imaged obliquely but correctly being examined. A small mark is placed in front of the ultrasound transducer along the narrow edge of the transducer (Fig. 19-14A, B). If a transverse approach is used, the vein should appear circular and centered on the ultrasound screen. A skin mark is then placed exactly at the center of the long face of the transducer (Fig. 19-15A, B). It is this author's experience that following the vein in a longitudinal approach for the initial mapping of the course of the vein yields the most accurate results.8,9 Once the initial skin mark is placed, the transducer is moved slightly distally toward the foot while keeping the vein in the center of view. A new mark is placed on the skin every 2 to 3 cm. This procedure is continued to the level of the ankle. The result is a line of short dashes which mark the course of the main venous system (Fig. 19-16).

Once the main course of the great saphenous has been determined, the saphenofemoral junction is once again

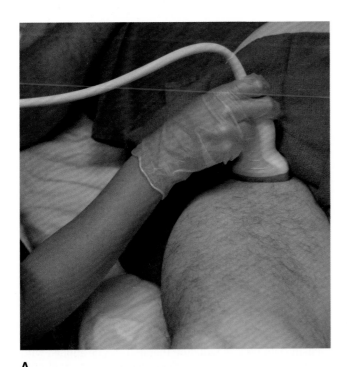

**A**

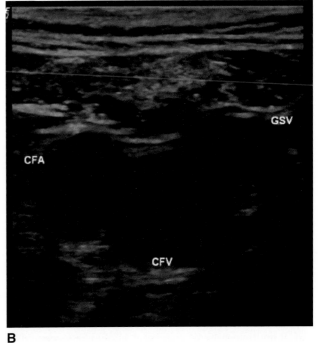

**B**

**FIGURE 19-13 A:** Transverse orientation used at the groin to identify the saphenofemoral junction. **B:** Corresponding ultrasound image at this level. CFA, common femoral artery; CFV, common femoral vein; GSV, great saphenous vein.

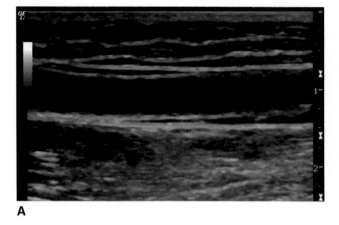

**A**

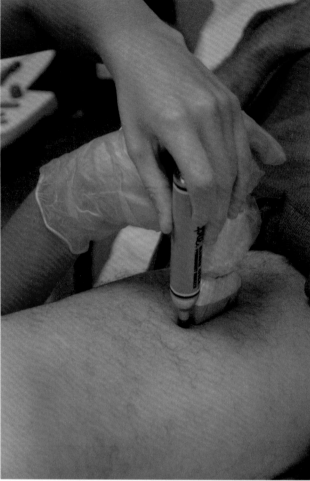

**FIGURE 19-14  A:** Longitudinal ultrasound image of the great saphenous vein. **B:** Corresponding proper position of the transducer and placement of the skin mark.

**B**

identified using a transverse orientation. Using the preliminary mark as a guide and remaining transverse to the vein, the main system is followed in order to identify tributaries and measure the vein diameter. The vein should appear circular. If it appears elliptical, then too much transducer pressure is being applied to the skin or the transducer has been moved into an oblique orientation to the vein. Two types of veins can be identified, namely, cutaneous tributaries and deep perforating veins. Each should be marked at the level they terminate into or communicate with the main system. The orientation of these veins should also be noted. Typically, anterior and posterior are used to describe the direction of tributary veins. The examiner can simply place an "A" or "P" as a key to describe the aforementioned tributary directions. However, any type of "code" system can be used as long as it results in proper placement of venous tributaries on the final skin mapping. It is especially important to follow all significant tributaries in order to identify partial loops or double systems.

The size of the saphenous vein is measured at the saphenofemoral junction; the proximal, mid, and distal thigh; the knee level; and the proximal, mid, and distal calf. If multiple systems exist, each should be measured to determine system dominance. Additional diameter measurement may be made over any segment which appears

to change in caliber. The diameter is determined using a transverse view by the placing calipers along the vein wall in an anterioposterior orientation. Because the interface between the inner vein wall and the blood is often easy to determine, many labs will measure inner to inner wall diameter (Fig. 19-17). This results in the internal diameter of the vessel being measured. Because equipment resolution has improved, the boundary between the adventitial layer of the vein wall and the surrounding tissue has become easier to discern. Thus, in some laboratories, the external diameter of the vein is measured. Surgeons should be aware of which ultrasound measurement of vein diameter is being recorded. Surgeons who choose to measure the vein at time of operation will be noting the external diameter. This will result in the internal vein diameter measurement recorded by ultrasound to underestimate the vein size as compared to the intraoperative measurements.

Once the course of the vein has been marked, the tributary and perforator locations have been noted and the vein diameters measured, the ultrasound gel can be wiped off the limb. Liquid marking ink (such as a carbol fuchsin stain used in radiation therapy) can be applied with a cotton-tipped applicator. The dashed marks originally placed can be connected to illustrate the course of the vein (Fig. 19-18). Tributary and perforator locations can

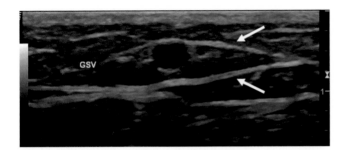

**A**

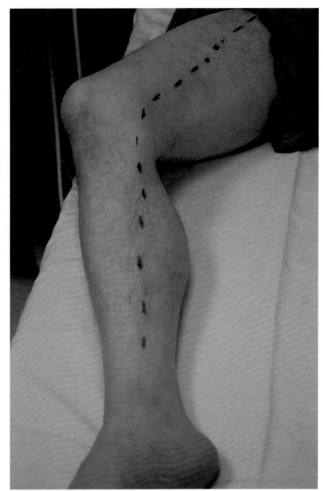

**FIGURE 19-16** Leg with the preliminary marks of a great saphenous vein mapping.

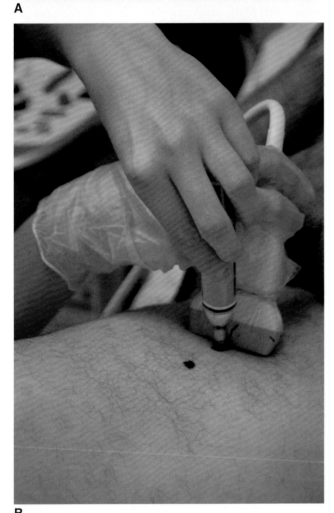

**B**

**FIGURE 19-15** **A:** Transverse ultrasound image of the great saphenous vein (GSV). Note fascial boundaries indicated by arrows. **B:** Corresponding proper position of the transducer and placement of the skin mark.

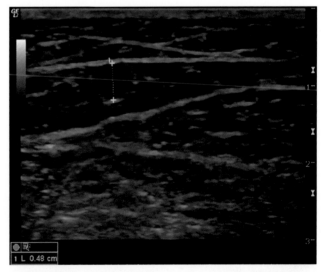

**FIGURE 19-17** Transverse ultrasound image of a vein with a diameter measurement of 0.48 cm.

be drawn in and diameters indicated at the various levels. The liquid ink requires 3 to 5 minutes to dry. During this time, a hand-drawn sketch can be made for a permanent laboratory record. This skin marking will remain on the skin for varying lengths of time depending on the type of permanent ink used. In most patients, the marks will be visible for at least 3 to 5 days.

The same scanning techniques described for the great saphenous vein can be used to map the small saphenous vein as well as the cephalic and basilic veins. The small saphenous vein should be first identified at its confluence with the popliteal vein (Fig. 19-19). It can be then followed and mapped to the lower calf level. If there is a cranial

extension of the small saphenous vein above the popliteal fossa, this can also be evaluated if the diameter meets laboratory criteria for adequacy. The small saphenous vein can often present a greater challenge to the technologist because

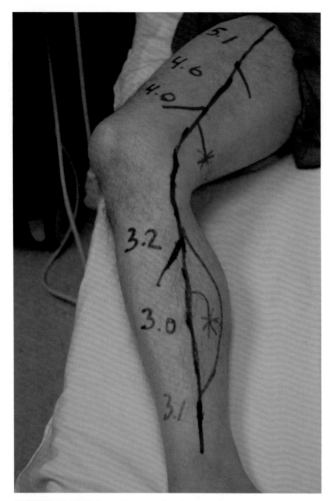

**FIGURE 19-18** Patient with a completed great saphenous vein mapping.

it is typically more superficial, yet smaller in diameter, as compared to the great saphenous vein. Vein diameters for the small saphenous vein are recorded in the proximal, mid, and distal calf.

The superficial veins of the arms are usually the easiest to identify in the upper arm where they are largest and have the least amount of tributaries. The basilic vein can be

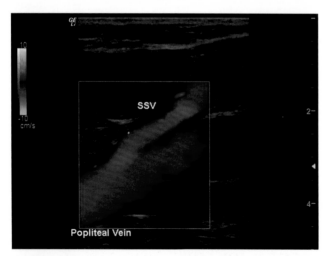

**FIGURE 19-19** Ultrasound image of the saphenopopliteal junction.

observed as it joins the brachial veins to form the axillary vein (Fig. 19-20A, B). It can be followed extending below the antecubital fossa along the ulnar aspect of the forearm and mapped from the upper arm to the wrist level. The cephalic vein will be visualized in the upper arm over the biceps muscle (Fig. 19-21A, B). The cephalic vein can be followed centrally to its termination into the subclavian vein (Fig. 19-22). The cephalic vein can be mapped from the shoulder region then followed peripherally along the radial aspect of the forearm mapping its position to the wrist level. Many surgeons also request the position of the medial cubital vein and its connections with the cephalic and basilic veins mapped. The arm veins present a challenge to the technologist because the tributaries will course over various aspects of the arm. Typically, the largest venous segments are the ones selected for mapping. The vein diameters are measured proximally and distally in the forearm and upper arm.

Table 19-3 summarizes some of the basic strategies to follow during vein mapping. These tips will help achieve accurate vein mapping results.

## Technical Considerations

It is imperative to optimize the ultrasound equipment for a venous mapping. Because the saphenous vein is a superficial structure, the equipment should be adjusted to provide a well-defined near-field image. The transmit power and focal zones should be adjusted to maximize the resolution of the near field. Ideally, the ultrasound transducer used should be at least 10 MHz, but a higher frequency of 12, 13, or 15 MHz can be used. A lower frequency transducer may be occasionally needed to image deeper veins in obese individuals. The pulsed Doppler frequency should be sufficient to detect the low-flow states in the superficial veins, and a frequency of 4 or 4.5 MHz is adequate. Pulsed Doppler is not typically employed during venous mapping examinations unless patency is in question. Occasionally, compression of small veins may be difficult to assess, and in these cases, the Doppler may be helpful. The scale or pulse repetition frequency (PRF) should be adjusted to detect low flow. Color imaging can also be used to confirm vessel patency. Color-flow settings should be adjusted to a low-flow state with increased gain and decreased scale or PRF. Vessel patency should be documented at multiple levels. In some patients with deep veins, it may also be necessary to note the vein depth from the skin surface. This can be important information prior to the creation of an arteriovenous fistula because a deeper vein may require the transposition of the vessel.

## Pitfalls

Like any ultrasound examination, there are limitations to this procedure. Patient mobility, dressings, and wounds may limit scanning access to segments of the limb. It is important to make an attempt to visualize any segments of vein that are accessible. In some cases, only short segments of vein are required as a conduit. Even a limited examination may provide enough information to select an appropriate segment of vein.

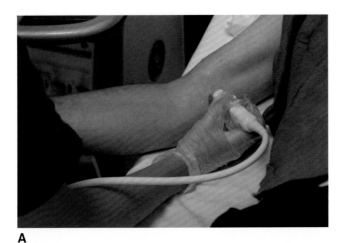

**A**

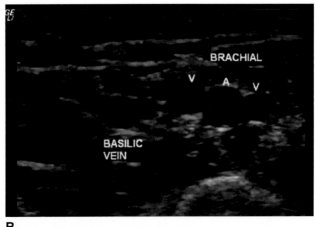

**B**

**FIGURE 19-20** **A:** Transducer position used to identify the basilic vein in the upper arm. **B:** Ultrasound image of the basilic and brachial veins.

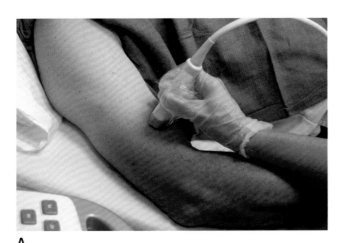

**A**

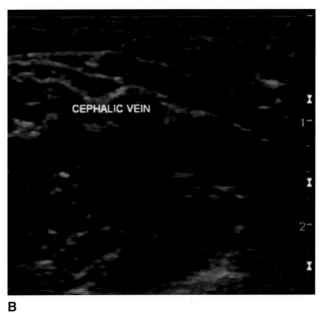

**B**

**FIGURE 19-21** **A:** Transducer position used to identify the cephalic vein in the upper arm. **B:** Ultrasound image of the cephalic vein and adjacent tissue.

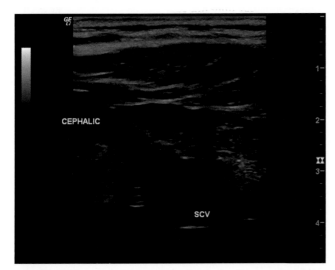

**FIGURE 19-22** Ultrasound image of the cephalic vein terminating into the subclavian vein.

| TABLE 19-3 | **Strategies for Successful Vein Mapping** | |
|---|---|
| **Action** | **Result** |
| Maximize venous pressure | Increases vein diameter |
| Keep the patient warm | Reduces peripheral vasoconstriction |
| Use light transducer pressure | Minimizes extrinsic compression of vein |
| Use gel sparingly to facilitate marking on skin | Reduces evaporation of gel and cooling of skin which can lead to vasoconstriction |
| Keep the transducer perpendicular to the skin surface | Skin mark will be most accurately placed over vein position |

## DIAGNOSIS

Vein mapping must determine much more than the presence or absence of a vein. It must also determine the suitability of that vein for use as a bypass conduit in terms of wall status, planar arrangement, and diameter.

A normal healthy vein should have smooth, thin walls (Fig. 19-23). The vein should be compliant and easily compress with minimal transducer pressure. Valve sinuses may appear elliptical, but in some smaller veins, they may be difficult to identify. If valve leaflets are visualized, they should be freely moving without any evidence of thrombus behind the leaflets.

As previously mentioned, the planar arrangement of the veins should be noted during the mapping procedure. This is of particular importance with mapping the great and small saphenous vein. Planar arrangement can easily be included within the written laboratory report. Figure 19-24 illustrates the normal orientation of the main trunk of the great saphenous vein within the saphenous compartment bounded by the saphenous fascia superficially and deeply by the muscular fascia. These layers of fascia produce what some people refer to as the "Egyptian eye" appearance of the vein. When double systems exist, often the veins travel in different anatomic planes through the thigh as shown in Figure 19-3. The dominant vein may not be the most superficial system that exists, or the larger system may not be the normal saphenous compartment. This information is important to the surgeon so that the best vein is selected. Very superficial, subdermal veins are often encountered in limbs with extensive varicosities.

Individual laboratory criteria for suitable vein diameters vary based on surgeon preference. The adequacy of a vein diameter may also vary depending on the intended use for the vein. A cardiothoracic surgeon may prefer a certain diameter vein for a coronary bypass, whereas a general surgeon may have different diameter criteria for a dialysis fistula. Generally, most surgeons will not use a vein that is less than 2.0 mm in diameter. Such small diameter veins may be prone to spasm and may be difficult to suture. Many surgeons like to select a vein that is 2.5 to 3.0 mm at

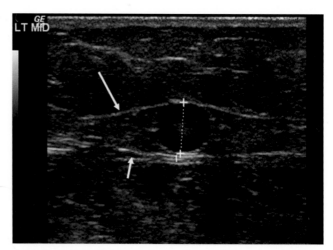

**FIGURE 19-24** Transverse view of the great saphenous vein noting the superficial fascia (*large arrow*) above the vein and the muscular fascia (*small arrow*) below the vein. This is often referred to as the "Egyptian eye" appearance of the vein.

a minimum. It is also important to instruct physicians as to whether internal or external vein diameters are measured during the ultrasound examination.

## DISORDERS

There are several commonly observed abnormalities encountered within the superficial veins. Pathology Box 19-1 provides a quick list of superficial vein pathology.

### Thrombus

Isolated segments of partial thrombus may be encountered during vein mapping. Often, patients cannot recall a prior occurrence of a superficial thrombophlebitis even though residual scarring may be present. Thrombus can be visualized adjacent to valve leaflets within the valve sinus (Fig. 19-25). Thrombus will vary in echogenicity. In some patients, acute thrombus may appear more anechoic or hypoechoic, but this is not always the case. Chronic thrombus may be hyperechoic but may also have areas of less echogenecity. Completely thrombosed veins will be noncompressible, lack any color filling, and not demonstrate a Doppler signal. Partially thrombosed veins will be partially compressible and demonstrate a reduced flow lumen. Doppler signals obtained from partially thrombosed veins will display a decrease in phasicity.

### Varicosities

Varicosities will appear as dilated, tortuous portions of the saphenous system. Varicosities are not an automatic contraindication to saphenous vein mapping. In many patients, the clinically evident varicose veins are subdermal tributaries off the main trunk (Fig. 19-26). The main system of the saphenous vein in these patients can be often found in the normal subfascial plane. It is often not dilated and can be used for bypass procedures. Even if the main system in the thigh is found to be varicose, sometimes the calf portion of the vein can be spared and vice versa. It is always

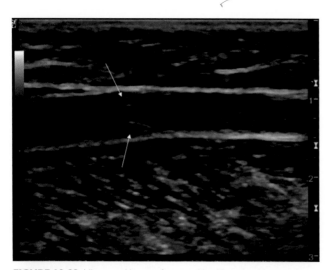

**FIGURE 19-23** Ultrasound image of a normal healthy vein with smooth, thin walls. Valve leaflets indicated by arrows.

**PATHOLOGY BOX 19-1**
*Superficial Vein Pathology*

| Pathology | Sonographic Appearance | | |
|---|---|---|---|
| | B-Mode | Color | Doppler |
| Thrombus | Intraluminal echoes of varying echogenicity | No flow or reduced color filling of lumen | Absent Doppler signal or if present, diminished phasicity |
| Varicosities | Tortuous, dilated segments of veins; | Multiple color patterns caused by changes in flow direction | May demonstrate reflux |
| Recanalization | Hyperechoic thick walls often with an irregular surface | May demonstrate a reduced flow lumen | Continuous or diminished phasicity |
| Calcification | Bright white echoes within the vessel wall with acoustic shadowing | Absent color filling in area of acoustic shadow | Absent Doppler signal in area of acoustic shadow |
| Stenotic valves | Valve leaflet protruding into vessel lumen and frozen in place | May demonstrate disturbed color-flow patterns or aliasing in region of valve | May demonstrate elevated velocities in region of valve |

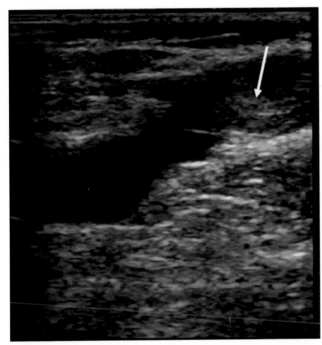

**FIGURE 19-25** Ultrasound image of a valve leaflet with thrombus (*arrow*) adjacent to it.

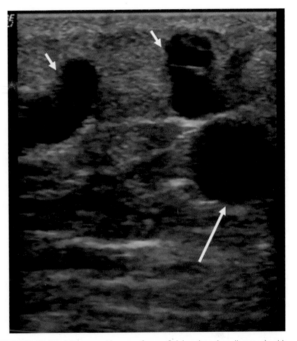

**FIGURE 19-26** Ultrasound image of superficial varices (*small arrows*) with the main saphenous (*large arrow*) system beneath the varices.

important to examine the entire length of the limb to find any suitable segments of vein.

## Recanalization

Veins presenting with an irregular intimal surface or wall thickening may indicate evidence of recanalization (Fig. 19-27). These veins are not usually considered to be adequate conduit for arterial bypasses. Description of the vein wall pathology is somewhat subjective but does alert the surgeon and aid the selection of the most appropriate vein segments.

## Calcification

Other wall pathology may include calcification. Although not as common as arterial wall calcification, venous

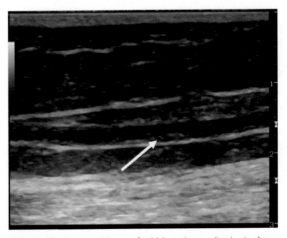

**FIGURE 19-27** Ultrasound image of a thickened recanalized vein. Arrow indicates thickened wall area.

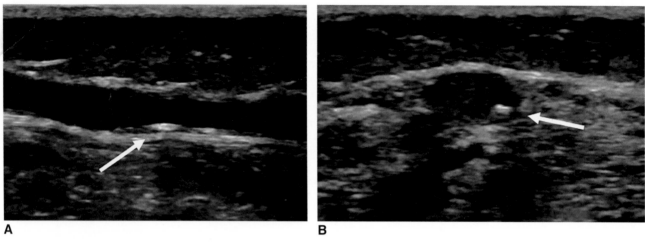

**FIGURE 19-28  A:** Sagittal view of a saphenous vein with wall calcification (*arrow*). **B:** Transverse view of a different saphenous vein with wall calcification (*arrow*).

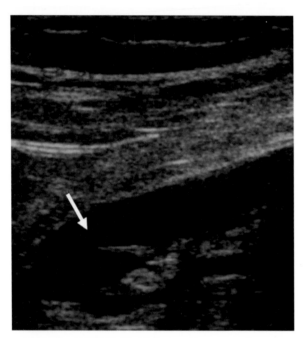

**FIGURE 19-29**  Ultrasound image of a frozen valve leaflet (indicated at *arrow*).

calcification does occasionally present in some patients. Bright echoes within the vein wall producing acoustic shadowing are the classic ultrasound appearance of calcification (Fig. 19-28). Isolated areas may not preclude the entire vein from being used as a conduit. The surgeon may simply use noncalcified segments. However, diffuse intermittent calcification renders the vein inadequate for bypass material. Venous calcification can be often observed in diabetic patients and in those with end-stage renal disease.

## Valve Abnormalities

Lastly, another pathology that can be noted on the image is a stenotic or frozen valve (Fig. 19-29). This may be encountered in a vein that was previously thrombosed. All evidence of the prior thrombus can be completed resolved, and the remainder of the vein wall may appear relatively normal. However, a valve sinus may be present that contains a valve leaflet frozen, unmoving in the blood flow stream. Again, if it is an isolated occurrence, the surgeon may simply use other healthy segments of the vein.

## SUMMARY

■ Venous mapping is a valuable component in the preoperative planning of many surgical procedures.
■ It is a highly sonographer/technologist-dependent procedure.
■ The sonographer or technologist must be familiar with venous anatomy and variants and should also be familiar with the surgical procedure being performed.
■ Proper vein mapping is highly dependent on a close working relationship between the technologist and the surgeon.
■ Preoperative mapping of the superficial venous system can provide detailed information on vein anatomy and anatomic variants can be clearly delineated.
■ Venous pathologies can be described so that diseased vein segments are avoided.

■ Careful skin marking as well as descriptive information within the vein mapping report can aid the surgeon in the placement of incisions.
■ This can minimize the need for large skin flaps and decrease operative time.
■ The details provided by ultrasound vein mapping will allow the surgeon to select the optimal vein to be used as conduit material.

## CRITICAL THINKING QUESTIONS

1. A patient presents for a bilateral lower extremity mapping of the great saphenous vein. On the right leg, there is an incision that runs from the upper thigh to the mid calf. The patient explains that he underwent a coronary

artery bypass graft several years earlier, and the surgeons used vein from his right leg. Do you alter your planned mapping procedure? Why or why not?

2. You begin a mapping procedure of the cephalic and basilic veins. In the upper arm, both veins are found to be approximately 2.0 mm in diameter. What step can you take to aid in the examination of these veins?

3. You are explaining the techniques of saphenous vein mapping to a new staff member. What aspects of the ultrasound system, including specific setting and adjustments, should you review?

## REFERENCES

1. Talbot SR. Use of real-time imaging in identifying deep venous obstruction: a preliminary report. *Bruit*. 1982;6:41–42.
2. Leopold PW, Shandall AA, Kupinski AM, et al. The role of B-mode venous mapping in infrainguinal arterial bypasses. *Brit J Surg*. 1989;76:305–307.
3. Shandall AA, Leather RP, Corson JD, et al. Use of the short saphenous vein in situ for popliteal-to-distal artery bypass. *Am J Surg*. 1987;154:240–244.
4. Caggiati A, Bergan JJ, Gloviczki P, et al. Nomenclature of the veins of the lower limbs: an international interdisciplinary consensus statement. *J Vasc Surg*. 2002;36:416–422.
5. Caggiata A, Bergan JJ, Gloviczki P, et al. Nomenclature of the veins of the lower limbs: extensions, refinements, and clinical application. *J Vasc Surg*. 2005;41:719–724.
6. Kupinski AM, Evans SM, Khan AM, et al. Ultrasonic characterization of the saphenous vein. *Cardiovasc Surg*. 1993;1:513–517.
7. Shah DM, Chang BB, Leopold PW, et al. The anatomy of the greater saphenous venous system. *J Vasc Surg*. 1986;3:273–283.
8. Chang BB, Kupinski AM, Darling RC III, et al. Preoperative saphenous vein mapping. In: AbuRahma AF, Bergan JJ, eds. *Noninvasive Vascular Diagnosis*. London: Springer-Verlag;1999:335–344.
9. Kupinski AM, Leather RP, Chang BB, et al. Preoperative mapping of the saphenous vein. In: Bernstein EF, ed. *Vascular Diagnosis*. St. Louis, MO: Mosby;1993:897–901.

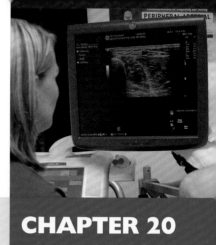

# Venous Valvular Insufficiency Testing

SERGIO X. SALLES CUNHA | DIANA L. NEUHARDT

**CHAPTER 20**

## OBJECTIVES

- To define clinical, etiologic, anatomic, and pathophysiologic conditions of chronic venous valvular insufficiency used as indicators for vascular laboratory venous testing.

- To describe both direct and indirect noninvasive vascular testing performed by vascular laboratory personnel.

- To describe protocol differences based on the objectives of testing for screening, definitive diagnosis, pretreatment mapping, peritreatment imaging, and procedure/patient follow-up.

- To define the role of duplex ultrasonography in the evaluation of patients with lower extremity venous valvular disorders.

## GLOSSARY

**anterior accessory great saphenous vein**  Superficial vein at the anterior thigh

**CEAP**  Acronym for clinical, etiologic, anatomic, and pathophysiologic classification of venous disease

**chronic venous insufficiency**  Long-lasting venous valvular or obstructive disorder

**great saphenous vein**  Superficial vein in the medial aspect of the lower extremit thigh and calf

**elastic compression**  Term attributed to the effects of stockings used to compress the leg with intent to compress the veins

**leg edema**  Leg swelling

**lipedema**  Swelling attributed to fat tissue

**lymphedema**  Swelling attributed to lymph channels or lymph node disorders

**nonsaphenous veins**  Superficial venous segments that are not part of the great and small saphenous systems. Nonsaphenous veins include gluteal, posterolateral thigh perforator, vulvar, lower posterior thigh, popliteal fossa tributaries, knee perforator, and sciatic nerve veins

**plethysmography**  Graphic presentation of pulses such as changes in volume within an organ or other part of the body such as the lower extremity

**posterior accessory saphenous vein**  Superficial vein at the posterior medial thigh

**reflux**  Reverse flow, usually in veins with incompetent valves

**reticular vein**  Superficial vein with diameter smaller than 3 mm

**spider vein**  Small clusters of veins near the skin surface that may be red, blue, or purple measuring between 0.5 and 1 mm; also known as telangiectasias

**small saphenous vein**  Superficial vein in the posterior aspect of the calf

**tributary vein**  A vein that terminates or empties into another; often larger vein

**varicose veins**  Veins with diameter equal or greater than 3 mm

**vein of Giacomini**  Superficial vein communicating the great and small saphenous vein

Chronic venous valvular insufficiency (CVVI) is a common disorder of modern era. The development of minimally invasive techniques has enhanced awareness and treatment potential of deep or superficial veins with incompetent valves and reflux. CVVI is a subset of the classic, most commonly used term "chronic venous insufficiency" (CVI). CVI includes venous obstruction and/or valvular insufficiency. This chapter focuses on valvular disorders, and not on venous obstruction, most commonly a consequence of deep venous thrombosis (DVT). Most patients presenting with CVVI do not have venous obstruction. The hypothesis is that patients with venous obstruction have characteristics distinct from those with venous valvular insufficiency, and the two groups deserve to be differentiated for appropriate diagnosis and treatment.

One of the philosophies behind the clinical, etiologic, anatomic, and pathophysiologic (CEAP) classification of CVI recommendations is to clearly specify and differentiate the types of CVI to improve understanding of distinct disorders.[1-3] This chapter reviews CVVI with summaries of relevant anatomy, prevalence of disease, signs and symptoms, classes of disorders, quality of life questionnaires, noninvasive examinations, types of treatment, and follow-up.

## ANATOMY

The sonographer must have precise knowledge of deep and superficial venous anatomy as detected by ultrasound. The anatomy of the venous system has been discussed in previous chapters. Pertinent sonographic information is provided as follows:

Current knowledge about the superficial venous system has expanded, with description of ultrasound landmarks to differentiate veins by location within the fascial layers of the tissue. Descriptive nomenclature has been globally adopted and applied specifically to the superficial system: the great saphenous vein (GSV), formerly named the greater or long saphenous, and the small saphenous vein (SSV), formerly named the lesser or short saphenous vein.[4,5] Saphenous nomenclature follows anatomic position and includes the anterior accessory great saphenous vein (AAGSV), the posterior accessory great saphenous vein (PAGSV), and the vein of Giacomini (VOG). Saphenous veins are readily identified with ultrasound,[6,7] within a compartment bordered by the deep fascia and the superficial fascia. The saphenous "eye" differentiates the saphenous compartment from the superficial and deep compartments (Figs. 20-1 and 20-2). The GSV courses medially in the thigh and leg within the saphenous compartment. Although the AAGSV is within a saphenous compartment, the "alignment sign" is the anatomic landmark for its location (Fig. 20-3). The AAGSV is aligned with the femoral artery and vein following a vertical line perpendicular to the transducer surface in cross-sectional imaging. The AAGSV and PAGSV course anteriorly and posteriorly in the thigh, respectively. The PAGSV may connect to the VOG. Tributaries are veins that drain into saphenous veins. Superficial tributaries pierce the saphenous fascia, enter into the saphenous compartment, and drain into the corresponding saphenous vein (Figs. 20-4 and 20-5). Nonsaphenous veins arise from a nonsaphenous source and describe veins draining from the pelvis or previous vein stripping, for example. Bulging varicose veins are

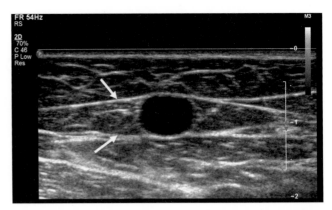

**FIGURE 20-1** A transverse ultrasound image of the great saphenous vein illustrating the normal position of the vein within the saphenous compartment. *Arrows* indicate fascia both superficial and deep to the veins.

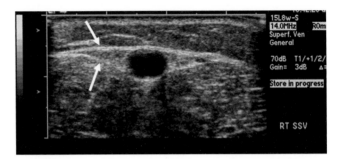

**FIGURE 20-2** A transverse ultrasound image of the SSV within the saphenous compartment distally within the leg. *Arrows* indicate fascia both superficial and deep to the veins.

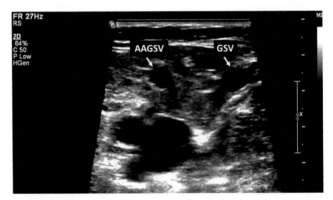

**FIGURE 20-3** The "alignment sign" with the anterior accessory great saphenous vein (AAGSV) aligned over the deep system artery and vein whereas the GSV lies more medially.

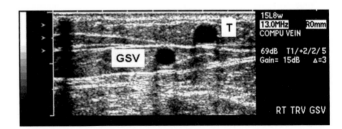

**FIGURE 20-4** A tributary vein (T) positioned outside the saphenous compartment and superficial to the GSV.

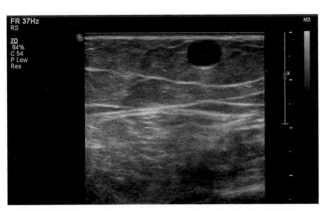

**FIGURE 20-5** A tributary vein positioned superficially outside the saphenous compartment.

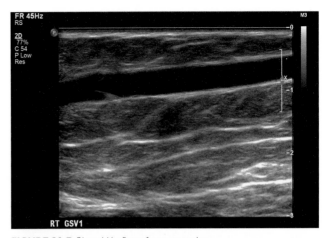

**FIGURE 20-7** Bicuspid leaflets of a venous valve.

often associated with abnormal superficial tributaries. Ultrasound identification of the GSV below the knee is aided by identification of the "angle sign" in cross-sectional imaging (Fig. 20-6). The triangular form of the gastrocnemius muscle, tibial bone, and the GSV within the fascia helps to differentiate the saphenous vein from prominent tributaries. There is some confusion regarding the interpretation of saphenous duplications. Most true duplications are infrequent and are segmental; complete duplications are rare. By strict definition, duplicated saphenous veins must follow the same path and remain parallel within the fascia. The duplication must demonstrate the beginning and end along the same path. As stated in the previous chapters, the presence of more than one large superficial venous system often represents the true GSV along with a large accessory system.

The GSV and common femoral vein confluence is referred to as the saphenofemoral junction (SFJ). The proximal GSV has two major valves. The terminal valve is at the SFJ. The preterminal valve is distal to tributaries that join the GSV at the SFJ. The junctions of these tributaries most commonly lie between the terminal and preterminal valves. The superficial epigastric vein, one of these tributaries, is a landmark for ablation treatment. The superficial external pudendal and the superficial circumflex iliac veins are other proximal draining tributaries in the junction region. Besides the SFJ, these veins may be the most proximal source of GSV reflux, raising the suspicion of pelvic CVVI.

The SSV confluence with the deep venous system is variable and ultrasonographically challenging. The SSV may terminate into (a) the popliteal vein at the saphenopopliteal junction (SPJ), (b) the gastrocnemius vein, (c) the distal

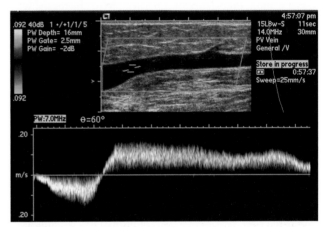

**FIGURE 20-8** A Doppler spectrum demonstrating retrograde flow or reflux (displayed above the baseline).

femoral vein of the thigh, (d) a small unnamed deep vein, (e) a perforating vein at the posterior thigh, or (f) into the GSV via the VOG. Proximal reflux sources of the SSV can be identified from an SSV thigh extension or VOG. The terminal valve of the SSV, therefore, would also be variable in location.

Venous valve leaflets are identified quite readily with B-mode imaging. The bicuspid leaflets point to the direction of normal venous drainage (Fig. 20-7). Venous valves vary in number, increasing in frequency with the distance away from the heart. Venous valves open with muscular contraction (referred to as venous systole) and close with muscular relaxation (referred to as venous diastole). Series of synchronized valves regulate blood return from the skin, to tributaries, to saphenous veins, to perforating veins or junctions, and to deep veins, toward the heart. Incompetent valves permit abnormal retrograde flow, or reflux (Fig. 20-8).

## PREVALENCE

CVVI is prevalent in many different populations, affecting both men and women. Prevalence of varicose veins varies between 2% and 56% in men and 1% and 60% in women.[8–11] Varicose veins are associated with valvular reflux, venous obstruction, or both. Valvular insufficiency can be noted despite the absence of varicose veins. Varicose

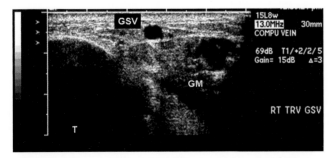

**FIGURE 20-6** The "angle sign" of the GSV below the knee. A triangle is formed by the gastrocnemius muscle (GM), the tibial bone (T), and the GSV.

veins were noted more in men (40%) than in women (32%) in a general population registered in clinics of Edinburg, United Kingdom.[12]

Screening programs funded by the American Venous Forum initially documented varicose veins in 32% and venous reflux in 40% of the subjects evaluated.[13] As the program expanded, the worst-case conditions of the subjects screened were telangiectasias (29%), varicose veins (23%), edema (10%), skin changes (9%), and ulcers (2%).[14] Telangiectasias were present in 79% of the men and 88% of the women in the Edinburg study.[15] Varicose veins have also been linked to a higher incidence of arterial disease.[16]

In another study, prevalence of reflux in veins of the lower extremity was 35% in a general population: 21% in superficial veins and 20% in deep veins.[17] Prevalence of either superficial or deep vein reflux increased with severity of the CEAP classification. Prevalence of superficial reflux increased with age. The Edinburg study described the prevalence of reflux for various segments of deep and superficial veins.[18] There was no difference among prevalence on the right or left lower extremities. The GSV had the highest prevalence of reflux.

These statistics indicate that CVVI is common and demands significant efforts and resources. Education and awareness are being promoted by the American College of Phlebology and other medical societies; investigations are being performed among diverse population groups.

## SIGNS AND SYMPTOMS

A basic concept of CVI or CVVI pathophysiology, reviewed in Chapter 6, involves the concept of venous pressure and abnormal venous hypertension. Abnormal venous pressures result in a multitude of signs and symptoms. On clinical examination, visual signs include telangiectasias (spider veins), reticular veins, varicose veins, edema, skin changes (such as pigmentation or atrophie blanche), and ulceration. Visual signs are the primary basis for the "C" of the CEAP clinical classification.

Edema is also a palpable sign and may not be visible early on. Description of symptoms associated with temporary swelling often varies from patient to patient. Feelings of temporary leg swelling at the end of a working day, after prolonged standing, or as a consequence of certain activities or leg positioning may represent what is known as phleboedema.

Differential diagnosis of edema includes sources other than venous obstruction or valvular insufficiency. Lymphatic obstruction results in enlarged hypoechoic channels in the thigh, lower leg, and foot.[19] Edema related to cardiac disease, arterial disease, sympathetic tone, or lipid disorders (lipedema) should also be suspected in the vascular laboratory.

Skin changes can vary widely. Localized redness, either with light or dark coloration, atrophie blanche (occurs after skin injury when blood supply is poor), corona phlebectatica as a cluster of veins and skin changes, hardening of the skin as lipodermatosclerosis develops and ulcerated wounds, healed or not, are observed with different frequencies, as a function of each vascular laboratory patient population. Skin changes may also be seen in patients with calf pump dysfunction, or nonuse of the calf pump while ambulating. Patients commonly describe symptoms, including heaviness,

tension, aching, fatigue, restlessness of the legs, muscle cramps (primarily nocturnal), tingling, discomfort, pain, burning, itching, skin irritation, tightness, or other variations of neurologic sensations. Restless leg syndrome can be associated to venous disease or several other nonvascular conditions. The presence of birthmarks such as port wine stains may initiate a multifaceted study to identify the presence of vascular or nonvascular malformation.

## CEAP Classification

An international committee organized by the American Venous Forum elaborated an initial and a subsequent advanced CEAP classification.[1-3] The initial, basic idea was to classify the patients in their worst-case condition. The advanced classification groups together a variety of patient conditions. C, E, A, and P is an acronym for clinical, etiologic, anatomic, and pathophysiologic classifications.

### Clinical Classification

The clinical classification has seven classes from $C_0$ to $C_6$, depending on extremity conditions as follows:
- $C_0$: no venous insufficiency signs or symptoms
- $C_1$: telangiectasias (spider veins) and/or reticular veins (<3 mm in diameter)
- $C_2$: varicose veins (≥3 mm in diameter)
- $C_3$: edema
- $C_4$: skin changes, presently subdivided into
  - $C_{4A}$: minor skin changes
  - $C_{4B}$: major skin changes such as lipodermatosclerosis
- $C_5$: healed skin ulcers
- $C_6$: open skin ulcers

The authors recommend a subdivision of $C_3$ into:
  - $C_{3A}$: intermittent, functional swelling
  - $C_{3B}$: classic, constant edema

### Etiologic Classification

The etiologic classification has the following four classes:
- Ep: CVVI is the major cause of clinical manifestations.
- Es: CVI or CVVI is secondary to DVT or other pathology.
- Ec: CVI or CVVI has a congenital origin, for example, venous malformations or lack of valves.
- En: unknown etiology, no venous etiology identified.

### Anatomic Classification

The anatomic classification has three abnormal classes or a combination of such classes and the class describing no findings:
- Ad: CVI or CVVI affects the deep veins
- As: CVI or CVVI affects the superficial veins
- Ap: CVI or CVVI affects the perforating veins
- Ads, Adp, Asp, and Adsp are multiple combinations
- An: no venous anatomy identified.

### Pathophysiologic Classification

The pathophysiologic classification describes two primary abnormalities, combined or not, and a class without apparent findings:
- Pr: reflux or reverse venous flow
- Po: chronic venous obstruction
- Pro: a pathologic combination
- Pn: no venous pathophysiology identified.

One of the changes in the revised classification was to consider varicose veins as ≥3 mm rather than ≥4 mm in diameter. Most clinical articles use at least the clinical CEAP classification to describe the patients studied; the authors recommend that statistics be conducted for each class without bundling patients with different conditions in the same group. Another recommendation is a venous segmental disease score based on the veins involved.[20]

## Clinical Severity Score

The CEAP classification is descriptive.[20] The clinical severity score attempts to determine a numerical, quantifiable index, mostly for longitudinal research comparisons. A summary of the guidelines for venous clinical severity score lists 10 attributes as follows:

- 1: pain
- 2: varicose veins
- 3: edema
- 4: skin pigmentation
- 5: inflammation
- 6: induration
- 7: number of active ulcers
- 8: duration of active ulcers
- 9: size of active ulcers
- 10: compressive therapy.

Each attribute is then scored from 0 to 3 for a maximum of 30 points as follows:

- 0: absent
- 1: mild
- 2: moderate
- 3: severe.

Note that the clinical severity score has yet to have the acceptability and common practice of the clinical CEAP classification.

## Disability Score

A summary of the guidelines for venous disability score lists the conditions of the patient as follows[20]:

- 0: asymptomatic
- 1, 2, 3: symptomatic
- 1: able to carry out usual activities without compressive therapy
- 2: able to carry out usual activities only with compressive therapy and/or leg elevation
- 3: unable to carry out usual activities even with compressive therapy and/or leg elevation

Usual activities are the activities before onset of disability because of venous disease.

## Quality of Life Questionnaires

Awareness of a dual role is growing in medicine. Clinicians are concerned not only with the provision of successful physiopathologic treatment but also that of improved quality of life.[21–25] Patients' perception of successful treatment is being analyzed with quality of life questionnaires. Such questionnaires are divided according to the objectives evaluated. There are general, overall health questionnaires such as the SF-36. The Aberdeen questionnaire examines detailed peripheral venous performance. The Chronic Venous Insufficiency Questionnarie (CIVIQ-2) is an example of a simplified peripheral venous performance questionnaire and has been used successfully in the evaluation of radiofrequency treatment.

## SONOGRAPHIC EXAMINATION TECHNIQUES

Duplex Doppler ultrasonography has become the standard technology to evaluate CVVI. Several objectives are accomplished with ultrasonography of the peripheral venous system and can include:

- screening
- definitive diagnosis
- pretreatment assessment
- peritreatment guidance and completion ultrasonography
- posttreatment follow-up
- patient follow-up

The ultrasound examination for CVVI has two major diagnostic goals. The first is to exclude deep venous obstruction or venous thrombosis. The second is to evaluate the function of the venous valves, or reflux detection.

Screening is a concise evaluation of patients at risk or high probability of having CVVI. It could be the basis for prevalence studies.

Definitive diagnosis includes evaluation of the deep veins and a segmental evaluation of valvular function. Differential diagnosis of nonvenous disease such as types of edema (e.g., lymphedema), arterial pathology (e.g., popliteal aneurysm), and masses (e.g., hematoma) are part of definitive diagnosis.

Pretreatment asssessment registers details of reflux sources (i.e., pelvic) and drainage, perforating vein competence, and vein diameters as a secondary variable.[26,27] Details of the report are often influenced by the technical thoroughness of perioperative ultrasonography. Some reports should include detailed measurements to localize source, drainage, or perforating vein precise location. Availability of perioperative ultrasonography minimizes the need for such details.

Peritreatment ultrasonography varies on the type of treatment planned. Using ultrasound guidance, some centers place skin markings with a pen or marker along the course of the vein that creates a pretreatment "mapping." Ultrasound guidance has become a standard for thermal and chemical ablation treatments. Completion ultrasonography documents patency of the deep venous system and efficacy of superficial venous ablation or eradication.

Follow-up examinations can be subdivided into two categories: (1) direct assessment of individual veins and (2) assessment of overall pathophysiologic condition. Ultrasonography is used for the direct assessment of individual veins postprocedure. Air plethysmography (APG) determines overall effects caused by pathology in virtually all veins draining the lower extremity. Photoplethysmography (PPG), in its most common, simplest form, gives a compound representation of the effects of venous reflux in the region tested. These specific techniques are described later in the chapter. Ultrasonography has become the most popular, most used, most mandatory examination to evaluate CVVI. APG, however, is likely a better indicator of treatment performance, providing a global assessment of total limb venous function.

Although invasive, venography or phlebography is another diagnostic method to detect venous thrombosis, congenital venous malformations, or valvular function. The venogram (another term is phlebography) is an X-ray of the veins after dye is injected distally (ascending) or by direct puncture and injection of the contrast into the common femoral vein or external iliac vein with the patient in a semi-erect position (descending). Less invasive methods are preferred by patients, and ultrasonography has virtually replaced venography of the lower extremity in most diagnostic settings.

## Treatment Types

It is important for the sonographer to understand the various treatments for CVVI because the use of ultrasound varies with the treatment option. Treatment options for superficial venous disease may include stripping, ligation, thermal ablation, chemical ablation/sclerotherapy, and phlebectomy (microincision). Treatment for deep venous disease may include anticoagulation, valve replacement, venoplasty/stenting, and thrombolysis or chemical/physical recanalization.

Stripping and ligation of the superficial veins have been traditional treatments for decades. Ligation alone has been associated with "neovascularization." This side effect perhaps may be better described as neodilatation of small arteries and veins as a result of injury, fresh thrombosis, and inflammation.

Endovenous thermal ablation by radiofrequency or laser energy has become a popular choice for treatment of saphenous and nonsaphenous trunk veins.[28–30] Thermal ablation has largely replaced stripping and ligation for many centers. Chapter 21 will discuss ultrasound use during venous treatment in more detail. Briefly, thermal ablation begins with distal vein access under ultrasound guidance, step-up wires and sheaths placed, and the thermal device tip positioned in the saphenous vein at a relative distance from the confluence to the deep venous system (Fig. 20-9). Anesthesia is strategically placed in the saphenous sheath and surrounding areas (Fig. 20-10). Heating of the tip of the thermal device is activated and controlled by the physician, and the device is pulled back to the insertion site at a standard rate defined for the instrument utilized. Completion of the procedure is achieved once the device is successfully removed from the vein. Owing to thermal injury inside the vein, the treated vein segment gradually shrinks and sonographically disappears

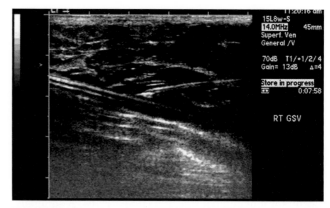

**FIGURE 20-10** Tumescent anesthesia injected around the saphenous sheath and surrounding tissue.

over 6 to 9 months. Prior to this time period, sonographic appearance of the thermally injured vein may inaccurately be termed "thrombosed" (Fig. 20-11).

Chemical ablation is the formal term for sclerotherapy, achieved with a foamed or liquid chemical (osmotic, detergent, or corrosive agent) which is injected into the vein.[31,32] A variety of superficial, saphenous and nonsaphenous, veins are amenable to sclerotherapy. Incompetent veins that are not visible from the skin are directed for injection with ultrasound guidance. Direct needle puncture into the vein and injection of the chemical is an effective treatment of small or tortuous veins, even as a complement of thermal ablation.

## Patient Preparation

An extensive clinical history and physical examination is obtained. This may be performed prior to or at the same time as the appointment for the ultrasound examination depending on the practice. The "C" of the CEAP classification is noted. The patient's gait is observed to determine whether the patient's outward signs are related to poor calf pump function (i.e., patient shuffles while walking without engaging calf pump). The patient symptoms are assessed, and the basic components of the testing procedure are explained to the patient. The patient removes clothing from the waist down except for undergarments. Some laboratories instruct the patient to bring a pair of loose fitting shorts or

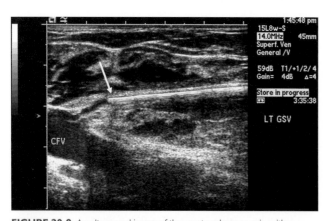

**FIGURE 20-9** An ultrasound image of the great saphenous vein with a thermal ablation device placed just distal to the SFJ (*arrow*).

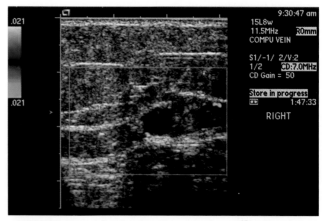

**FIGURE 20-11** A postablation ultrasound of the great saphenous vein with no flow present.

provide shorts for the patients. While standing, the patients may be provided nonslip booties. The sonographer reviews with the patient the purpose of the study. The sonographer also reviews with the patient instructions for performing a Valsalva maneuver and distal calf maneuvers prior to the beginning of the examination. A standardized Valsalva maneuver can be accomplished with the simple use of a drinking straw tied into a knot. The patient is instructed to blow into the knotted straw when assessing proximal venous valvular function. Standardized distal augmentation can be accomplished with the patient performing flexion and extension of the foot on command to assess distal venous valvular function. The flexion and extension can also serve as a secondary diagnostic tool to assess calf pump function. Valsalva and distal calf maneuvers improve standardization and alleviate the bending/twisting of the sonographer, thereby improving ergonomics.

## Patient Positioning

The deep veins are evaluated initially in a reverse Trendelenburg position with head and torso above the thigh, knee, and feet. The focus is to determine patency more so than unsuspected DVT. The classic recommendation is to evaluate the superficial venous structures CVVI with the patient in a standing position, when appropriate. This is particularly important in those patients with minimal signs of venous disease such as C1 and C2 classifications. A platform facilitates ergonomics and patient stability (Fig. 20-12). Standing allows for optimal dilatation and venous filling. The patient shifts the weight onto the leg not being examined.

Standardization of the study is accomplished with the standing position because the published diagnostic criteria are based on this position. Exceptions to the standing positioning include examination of patients with advanced CVVI with obvious varicose veins and/or severe reflux of the major superficial and/or deep veins. Standing may also be contraindicated in patients who experience pain with standing or those patients who are susceptible to motion sickness because they may become dizzy, lightheaded, or nauseous. The reverse Trendelenburg position is the recommended patient positioning if a standing test cannot be performed. Some centers will choose to examine veins of the calf, knee area, and lower thigh using a less stressful sitting position (Fig. 20-13). If negative reflux results are obtained in positions other than standing, it is imperative to repeat the assessment in a standing position if possible. The goal is of the positioning and is to create a gravitational impact to the venous structures.

The technologist/sonographer position must be addressed. Chapter 3 presented a great deal of information on ergonomics. Ergonometrics are paramount to a technologist's long-term professional health and well-being. The torso should be erect and not forcefully twisted because attention changes between instrument and patient. Elbows should be close to the body. One hand deals with instrument controls, whereas the other handles the transducer. One foot controls compression/decompression maneuvers if using an automated cuff system. Positioning the patient on a platform minimizes arm extension because the veins are examined from the groin to the ankle. Height of the technologist's stool is accommodated to optimize body

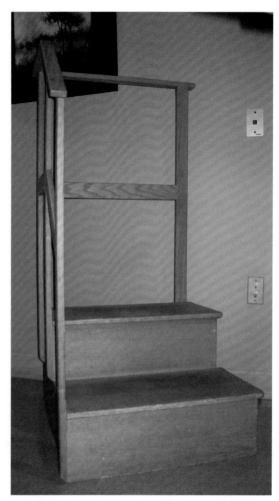

**FIGURE 20-12** A platform device used for evaluation of patients in the standing position.

positioning differences among the groin, thigh, knee, or calf examinations (Fig. 20-14).

## Equipment

High-resolution duplex ultrasound with transducer frequencies ranging from 3.5 to 7.5 MHz and 7.5 to 17.0 MHz is recommended for deep and superficial venous testing, respectively. Linear transducers are ideal for extremity venous applications. Use of proper transducer selection and system optimization is paramount for accurate diagnosis.

## Scanning Technique

The essential protocol includes evaluation of patency and valvular function in the lower extremity deep veins, veins in the saphenous compartments, nonsaphenous superficial veins, and tributaries. Physiologic incompetent perforating veins should be examined in patients presenting with advanced disease. Protocols also include the differential diagnoses of nonvenous pathologies such as arterial and lymphatic abnormalities and masses. Many patients will present with coexisting muscular or bony abnormalities and should be noted within the final report. These findings may compromise the patient's quality of life as well as the venous findings.

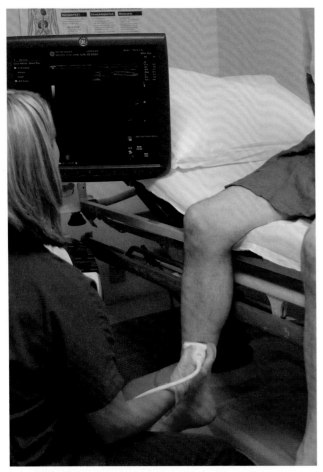

**FIGURE 20-13** Proper patient and technologist position for a sitting CVVI examination.

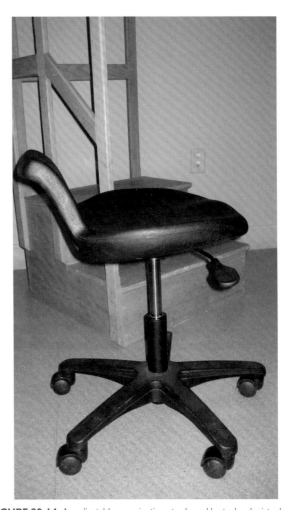

**FIGURE 20-14** An adjustable examination stool used by technologists during venous evaluations.

Evaluation of the deep veins precedes any CVVI testing. Detection of acute DVT is rare; continuation of a CVVI examination becomes secondary and is not recommended. Interpreting and/or referring physicians should be contacted according to preestablished protocols. A preliminary report may be acceptable at certain institutions.

Detection of chronic deep venous obstruction, either total or partial, is part of a CVVI evaluation, and the examination is completed. Chronic venous obstruction is suspected in patients with a history of previous DVT (Fig. 20-15). Patients with chronic DVT may require special hematologic treatment, which is beyond the scope of this chapter. Detection of acute superficial thrombosis or thrombophlebitis (STP) when inflammation is present, does not deter continuation of CVVI examination. Protocol alternatives address location and extension of STP. A recommendation is to treat STP at or near the SFJ or SPJ as potential DVT. Similarly, perforating or muscular vein thrombosis is assessed for potential risk of embolization before completing a CVVI examination.

The examination typically begins at the groin at or just above the level of the SFJ. A focused evaluation of the deep veins documents absence of thrombus. Vein walls are imaged in a transverse plane and compressed with the transducer at the skin surface. Normal veins coapt completely. Chapter 17 described techniques for a DVT examination.

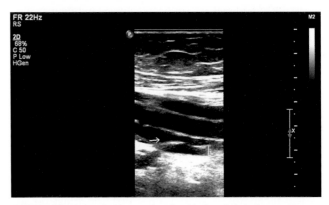

**FIGURE 20-15** A sagittal image of a vein with chronic thrombus present (*arrow*).

## Determination of Venous Flow Patterns

Once venous patency is confirmed, the examination continues with analysis of flow patterns using spectral Doppler. Various maneuvers are employed to stimulate valve closure and to determine whether retrograde flow (i.e., reflux) exists. Color-flow imaging can complement in the determination of flow directions and reflux times. However, the accepted standard for reflux diagnosis is the measurement of reflux time along the axis of the Doppler spectral tracing using the equipment calipers. Flow recordings are localized, and specific patterns of reflux can be inferred from such recordings. A complete evaluation of the GSV, for example, evaluates the terminal valve, preterminal valve, diffuse, proximal, segmental, or distal patterns of reflux, multiple sources of reflux causing multisegmental reflux, or atypical patterns involving multiple veins.[33,34] Reflux patterns may vary when examining a patient with recurrence after treatment.

Classic limb compression techniques using an automatic rapid cuff inflation/deflation system are recommended and may be of use when patients are obese or unable to perform maneuvers on command. A pneumatic cuff is wrapped around the thigh or the calf. Testing is performed in the veins centrally located in relation to the cuff.

A cuff around the upper calf often provides compression sufficient to test the veins from the groin to behind the knee. Even ankle veins can be evaluated with the cuff in this position. Normal flow in a vein proximal to the cuff should increase during compression and stop during decompression. Pathologic flow or reflux occurs during decompression. Flow in a vein distal to the cuff should occur only during decompression. In this case, reflux would occur during compression.

Proper compression techniques using this cuff method require a pressure of 70 to 80 mm Hg to be applied quickly, held for a few seconds, and released quickly. Higher pressures may have to be applied to large extremities. The compressor must be filled with enough air, and the hoses must be large enough, particularly if a large cuff is employed. The applied pressure may vary depending upon the relative size of the cuff to the thigh or the calf. The applied pressure decreases significantly with tissue depth if a small cuff is used. Tissue pressure decreases because the distance between tissue or vein and the skin increases. Large cuffs apply pressure to the deep tissues and veins more uniformly.

Reflux time duration is dependent on the vein filling with blood and the vein emptying with compression. Duration of compression and interval between compressions may affect reflux measurements. Sequential evaluations of reflux at multiple locations are also affected by compression duration and refilling time. As a standard, a minimum of 30 s between testing sites is recommended.

The automatic compression/decompression technique (known as rapid cuff inflation/deflation) is commonly commanded with a foot switch. This relieves the hands of the technologist to concentrate on the transducer and instrument controls. It is also considered a reproducible, standardized technique.

The "parana maneuver" presents physiologic advantages. This method involves a touch provocation to force the patient to shift weight slightly forward and backward while the transducer interrogates the vein in real time. With skill and practice, the parana maneuver is reproducible and may best reflect the patient's own calf pump and valvular function.

Some examiners rely on hand compression, although this technique may introduce testing variability. A major justification is added variety of testing conditions. Unusual venous segments can be specifically tested. Amount and time of compression can be readily adapted to different veins, different anatomies, and different types of patients. Testing alternatives increase at the expense of consistency. Hand compression maneuvers may increase the use of poor

body ergonomics; therefore, proper techniques ensuring correct body positioning is encouraged.

Traditionally, reflux time measurement is performed using the spectral Doppler with the vein in a longitudinal image. Documentation should include this standard method as usual protocol or as validation of other methods used to detect reflux. Many laboratories choose to set the Doppler orientation such that spectral tracings demonstrating normal venous flow are below the baseline and retrograde/abnormal flow demonstrated above the baseline.

A greatly informative way of screening for reflux is with the use of color-flow transverse/oblique images. Multiple veins can be studied simultaneously. This technique is of great value while studying the GSV and one of its superficial tributaries at the lower thigh, for example. Another appropriate double vein evaluation is in the upper calf while observing reflux simultaneously in the GSV proper, or while differentiating the posterior and anterior arches or other tributaries. Recirculating reflux is particularly obvious while studying two veins simultaneously with color flow. Although this technique is adequate for detection of severe reflux, the report must adequately document such findings with spectral Doppler in longitudinal images with caliber measurements of the spectral waveform along the time axis.

## Protocol Requirements

CVVI is concerned primarily with valvular function that permits abnormal reverse flow, or reflux, in superficial (and deep) veins of the lower extremities. Because most types of ultrasound examinations individual laboratory protocols vary, the required documentation also varies. The following are minimal suggestions for images which are needed to document B-mode characteristics, spectral Doppler waveforms, or color flow to demonstrate these findings:

- compressibility or coaptability of the common femoral, femoral, and popliteal veins as well as the GSV and SSV tested by manual compression with the transducer at the skin surface
- patency and flow characteristics of the common femoral vein at one level, with color-flow and spectral Doppler waveforms
- patency and flow characteristics of the femoral vein at one or more levels, with color-flow and spectral Doppler waveforms
- when present, documentation of a dual femoral or dual popliteal vein
- patency and flow characteristics of the popliteal vein at one level, with color-flow and spectral Doppler waveforms
- condition of calf veins in patients with localized signs and symptoms showing risk for DVT or chronic obstruction below the knee (C3 to C6)
- flow characteristics in segmental levels of the saphenous veins, including the GSV, AAGSV, PAGSV, VOG, and SSV
- flow characteristics of nonsaphenous veins potentially associated with varicose veins or pelvic source drainage
- possible involvement of pelvic veins or veins proximal to the groin
- any unusual venous or nonvenous finding.

Documentation may be simplified during screening protocols and may have to be more complex depending on the objectives of pretreatment investigative protocols. Peritreatment protocols are dependent on the type of treatment and specific objectives. Follow-up protocols are also dependent on the objectives of the examination and intended treatment.

### Screening for CVVI with Ultrasonography

The basic protocol includes image documentation of any anomaly of the femoropopliteal veins and a single documentation of saphenous or nonsaphenous abnormality. The scans of the deep and superficial veins follow the pattern described above, but can be interrupted after discovery of a single abnormality. The scan may also focus primarily on the region with the highest suspicion of an abnormality, for example, during the search of the source of obvious varicose veins.

## Definitive Diagnosis for CVVI with Ultrasonography

The protocol may vary, depending on the objective of the test and the potential treatment. There are three common test objectives. The first is the selection of patients for thermal ablation of the GSV in the thigh. The protocol comprises a standard evaluation of the femoropopliteal veins and the GSV in the thigh. Additionally, a limited evaluation of the GSV and SSV in the calf is performed, and the calf deep veins may have to be studied pending signs and symptoms.

The second is the examination of patients of a phlebology clinic with perioperative ultrasound capabilities. A complete examination included the femoropopliteal, the saphenous veins, and nonsaphenous veins related to visible varicose veins. The infrapopliteal deep veins are examined as a function of signs and symptoms. Details of exact location of reflux sources and drainage points are not necessary because the examination is performed at the time of treatment.

The third type of objective is the examination of patients for limited or extensive stripping/ligation/phlebectomy procedures. A complete examination includes a detailed drawing of refluxing and nonrefluxing veins plus segments not visualized. Perforating veins, sources, and drainage points are precisely located. Vertical and circumferential measurements are performed. Distance from the sole of the foot determines the vertical location. Distance from the tibial tuberosity, for example, determines the circumferential position of the venous finding. The physician would then perform treatment based either on a paper drawing or on a mapping on the skin of the patient. Some procedures may require measurements or skin marking very close to treatment day, often with the patient in the standing and operative position.

Saphenous sparing techniques such as a CHIVA (French acronym for Conservative and hemodynamic treatment of venous insufficiency in ambulatory care) procedure may require additional information to determine the new flow pathways through the venous channels left open in the extremity.

### Peritreatment Ultrasound

The role of ultrasonography in the venous treatment room will be discussed fully in Chapter 21. The role of ultrasonography in venous disease has expanded beyond a diagnostic tool and is commonly used during treatments such as thermal and chemical ablation. During thermal ablation. ultrasound is often used to map the course of the vein being treated on the patient's skin. The site of the venous incision is selected with ultrasound, needles, introducers, guidewires, and laser or radiofrequency catheters are inserted under ultrasound guidance. The tip of the thermal ablation catheter is placed at an appropriate distance from the SFJ under direct ultrasound visualization. The introduction of the tumescent anesthesia is performed under ultrasound guidance. At the completion of the ablation procedure, ultrasound confirms obstruction of the treated vein and the lack of DVT. Ultrasound can also demonstrate local recanalization of the treated vein, tributaries approaching the treated vein with potential risk for recanalization, and other superficial veins which may need subsequent, complementary procedures.

Ultrasonography is also used during chemical ablation or foam sclerotherapy. Imaging of the vein is performed during needle insertion. Ultrasound is also used to follow the hyperechoic foam because it flows through the treated vein and can be used to monitor if the foam approaches a perforating vein, the SFJ or SPJ. Transthoracic cardiac ultrasound can be used to observe the foam arrival in the right heart.[35,36] Transthoracic cardiac ultrasound may show bubbles in the left heart, indicating the presence of a right to left shunt or a patent foramen ovale. Transcranial Doppler ultrasonography may demonstrate the presence of high-intensity transient signals in the middle cerebral artery during foam sclerotherapy. Not all laboratories perform these adjunctive ultrasounds.

### Follow-up Ultrasound

Postablation protocols include a limited evaluation of the deep veins to assure patency as well as a complete examination of the treated vein. Ultrasonography can demonstrate whether segments of the treated vein are fully fibrosed or if the vein is recanalized, totally or partially in diameter as well as completely or segmentally in its longitudinal extension.[37,38] Thrombus may be detected immediately after treatment or after months or years because of recanalization and rethrombosis.

Patients are followed serially with ultrasound because of the recurrence of venous disease. As a chronic disease, venous treatments do not offer a "cure" but offer a decrease in the intensity of the disease and a decrease in the patient's symptoms, thus improving quality of life. The opposite leg may develop treatable disease with time, or the treated leg may have new veins requiring treatment. The patient follow-up study is commonly bilateral and follows the same protocols as described for definitive diagnostic ultrasound. A common problem is lack of adequate history on previous procedures. Technologists often discover that veins are absent or that treated veins are present.

### Pitfalls

Equipment settings must be properly adjusted in order to accurately detect venous reflux. Some technical factors affecting reflux measurement are as follows:
- Gain alters the sensitivity of spectral Doppler or color flow
- High persistence may result in false-positive color-flow findings

- Velocity scales (physiologic term) or pulse repetition frequency, PRF (engineering term) also affect the spectral Doppler or color-flow sensitivity to detection of reflux
- Varied instruments have different settings and different characteristics and may affect reflux detection.

There are alternate explanations to retrograde flow, although initially described as "reflux." Flow from a tributary filling in a segment of the vein after a compression/decompression maneuver may produce a reverse flow pattern if this flow enters below a valve sinus. Reverse flow may occur by surgical correction of hemodynamics to preserve drainage. Flush ligation of the SFJ, for example, may create reverse flow through the saphenous vein until the next distal perforating vein. This perforating vein thus becomes a treatment-designed junction where flow is shunted or directed to this new drainage point. CHIVA procedures commonly create reverse flow in successfully treated veins in a similar surgical method as described above.

## DIAGNOSIS

### B-mode Ultrasound Findings

Normal B-mode image findings will reveal smooth, thin-walled veins with no obvious change in venous diameter. The vein is fully compressible, and the lumen is hypoechoic.

B-mode images of an acute DVT show enlarged veins, particularly when compared to a normal, contralateral, equivalent venous segment. Veins are incompressible under transducer pressure, and the lumen may appear hypoechoic or even anechoic. The thrombosed venous lumen becomes more hyperechoic because the DVT progresses to subacute thrombosis and chronic obstruction. Thrombus may be seen filling the vein either partially or completely (Fig. 20-16).

B-mode images of chronic venous obstruction show diameters diminutive in caliber and thickened. The vein may be partially or totally incompressible. The aged thrombus may appear hyperechoic, and fibrous strands may be observed within the lumen (see Fig. 20-15). The veins may display possible tortuosity. Collaterals develop and enlarge with time.

CVVI may present with an increase in the vein's diameter, but the veins are completely compressible. The lumen is hypoechoic. Some of the valve sinuses may appear prominent with thickened valve leaflets. The affected veins may eventually become tortuous, varicose, or even aneurysmal.

Immediately following thermal ablation, the vein is still anesthetized and compressed by tumescence; B-mode imaging may change rapidly or take months to reveal eventual results of treatment. In postprocedural follow-up, typically at 6 to 9 months, the vein may be segmentally sonographically absent, fibrosed, thrombosed, or recanalized simultaneously at different sites along the course of the vein.[37-39]

### Spectral Doppler Waveforms

Normal venous flow waveforms are spontaneous, phasic with respiration, and unidirectional toward the heart. Flow augments with distal compression or release of proximal compression (Fig. 20-17).

In the presence of an acute, fully occlusive DVT, the spectral Doppler waveform shows absence of flow. Partially occlusive DVT, proximal thrombosis, or external compression cause continuous flow. The lack of flow augmentation following distal compression or release of proximal compression is observed in patients with acute DVT. Arterial flow waveforms can be present from within a lysing thrombus.

Flow is also absent with complete chronic venous obstruction. Partial obstruction, proximal obstruction, or external compression cause continuous flow and lack of flow augmentation, similarly to acute DVT. Spectral analysis may also reveal flow through small, tortuous channels within the diseased vein. Arterial, venous, or fistula-like flow may be observed in small vessels near the obstructed vein, and these may be a possible sign of recanalization, neovascularization, or inflammation. Flow via dilated, collateral veins is common.

In patients with CVVI, reverse flow or reflux are noted following proximal compression (includes Valsalva maneuver) or release of distal compression (Fig. 20-18). Turbulent flow may also be present within enlarged valve sinuses.

### Color Flow

Color flow shows the respiratory phasicity and flow augmentation of normal veins, findings better perceived with

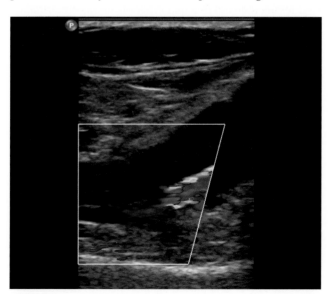

**FIGURE 20-16** A vein with acute thrombus present.

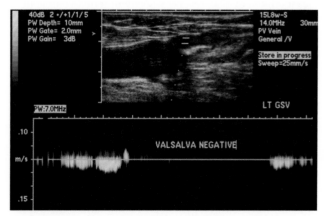

**FIGURE 20-17** A normal venous Doppler signal with no reflux present.

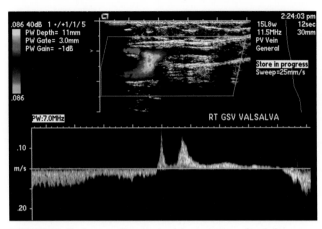

**FIGURE 20-18** A venous Doppler signal demonstrating reflux during a Valsalva maneuver.

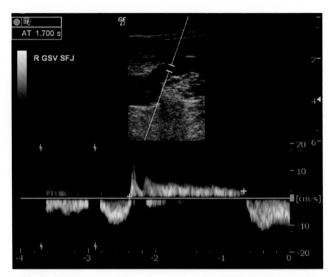

**FIGURE 20-19** A venous Doppler waveform from SFJ illustrating the measurement of 1.7 s of retrograde flow.

Doppler spectral analysis. Colors usually become lighter with increased flow and may alias. Color disparity can often lead to detection of defects missed with grayscale imaging.

Color detects no flow if DVT completely occludes the vessel. If a partial thrombus exists, color flow demonstrated flow around the thrombus. Perception of color-flow augmentation depends on instrument settings and visual acuity.

Color flow has several advantages during the evaluation of chronic venous obstruction. Similar to the findings of spectral Doppler evaluation, color flow through small, tortuous channels inside a chronically obstructed vein may be present. Arterial, venous, or fistula-like flow in small vessels near the obstructed vein may be present and may represent a possible sign of recanalization, neovascularization, or inflammation. Perception of collateral flow is dependent on venous dilation or neoformation, flow patterns, and instrument settings.

CVVI will demonstrate retrograde color flow away from the heart. This may occur spontaneously, under proximal compression, or following the release of distal compression. Turbulent or multiple color-flow patterns may be displayed within enlarged valve sinuses. An advantage of using color flow in transverse and longitudinal planes prior to spectral Doppler is to optimize the location of the sample volume in the region of most perceived flow or reflux.

## Quantification of Reflux

Measurement of reflux duration is commonly preferred to measurement of peak reverse velocity or reflux volume flow rate. A classic, commonly referenced study was originally designed to describe normal values.[40] In the vast majority of *normal* subjects, saphenous vein valves close in less than 500 ms. The valves of the deep femoropopliteal veins close in less than 1 s. Perforating vein valves close in less than 350 ms. Longer durations are commonly considered as abnormal reflux (Fig. 20-19). Another study also suggested there are other factors that may influence reflux time, including study time of day, hydration, patient positioning, and sonographer skill set.[41] Actual duration of reflux may also depend on vein diameter, amount of venous blood volume stored distally, strength and duration of distal compression, and characteristics of the distal venous network. Pathology Box 20-1 summarizes the duplex ultrasound findings of CVVI.

---

**PATHOLOGY BOX 20-1**
*Ultrasound Finding of CVVI*

| B-mode (Grayscale) | Spectral Doppler | Color-flow Imaging |
|---|---|---|
| • Vein diameter enlarged<br>• Valve sinuses enlarged<br>• Tortuosity, varicosities, or venous aneurysms may be present | • Saphenous veins and tributaries retrograde flow >500 ms<br>• Deep veins retrograde flow >1.0 s<br>• Perforating veins retrograde flow >350 ms | • Retrograde color flow<br>• Turbulent or multiple color patterns seen within valve sinuses |

---

# OTHER NONINVASIVE DIAGNOSTIC PROCEDURES

Two classic technologies, PPG and APG, have been used as a screening tool and as a quantifier of venous abnormality, respectively. Recently, another indirect test has been employed in this patient population. This newer test employs a "red" light detector to aid in superficial vein mapping.

## Venous Photoplethysmography

PPG testing should be considered a screening procedure for the detection of reflux.[42] The source of reflux is mostly undetermined. A PPG transducer emits infrared light and detects the signal reflected back from the blood within the cutaneous vessels. Compression/decompression maneuvers alter the quantity of blood under detection by the PPG. The amount of blood detected by the PPG is reduced when blood is pumped back toward the heart. Upon completion of the maneuvers, blood volume returns, and the sensor displays the return.

### Patient Position

The patient is examined in a sitting position with legs dependent. The PPG is placed against the skin in the medial aspect of the calf. A common placement is about 10 to 15 cm above the medial malleolus. Other positions may be used for additional testing. The PPG positioned on the posterior aspect of the lower calf would provide information about SSV reflux.

### Technique and Required Documentation

Once the patient and the PPG transducer are appropriately positioned, the examination begins with recording a baseline tracing while the limb is relaxed and no muscular contractions are occurring. The next step is to produce emptying of the calf venous blood volume. This is done using muscular contractions with flexion/relaxation of the foot. About 5 to 10 foot flexion maneuvers are common practice. The PPG tracing is recorded during these maneuvers. A resting horizontal line is usually placed near the top of a 5-cm wide strip paper. The tracing falls to the bottom of the strip paper during the flexion/relaxation of the foot. The tracing returns to the baseline position during the recovery period with the foot at rest and leg relaxed. The timing of blood return to the region indicates the presence or absence of reflux. Tracings may be observed on a monitor, but paper graphic registration is recommended. A common recording speed is 25 mm/s or about 0.5 to 1 cm/minute.

The test can be repeated with the use of a tourniquet in an attempt to differentiate superficial reflux from deep system reflux. A tourniquet can be placed around the thigh or other location over the GSV. The tourniquet can also be used to occlude the SSV by placing the tourniquet around the upper third of the calf. Changes in the recording both with and without the tourniquets in place may indicate that different portions of the venous system are incompetent.

Paper registry should be filled with information about (a) instrument utilized, (b) time scale, (c) anatomic location of the PPG sensor, (d) resting trace showing arterial pulses and stable baseline, (e) clear tracing during foot flexion, usually toward the bottom of the registry, and (f) enough paper length documenting recovery time.

### Diagnostic Criteria

Venous recovery time or refilling time (VRT) is the parameter measured during PPG. VRT is usually measured from the end of flexion/relation period to about 90% to 95% of the distance between the bottom of the curve and the baseline tracing. Recovery time is usually greater than 20 s.

Venous reflux is suspected if the PPG tracing takes less than 20 s to return to baseline. Severe reflux may be suggested if the recovery time is less than 10 s.

If results are abnormal, the use of a tourniquet proximal to the PPG location may indicate a superficial or deep vein source for reflux. With a tourniquet in place over the GSV in the thigh, if the VRT returns to normal, then GSV incompetence is suspected. If the recovery time remains abnormal with the use of the tourniquet, then deep vein reflux is suspected. Similar principles are applied to the detection of SSV reflux. With a tourniquet placed in the upper third of the calf, if VRT normalizes, then SSV reflux is likely.

## Air Plethysmography

APG is a recommended technique for quantification of CVI.[43] Clinically, APG can be used to detect physiologic abnormalities to clearly differentiate a pathophysiologic condition from an apparent aesthetic problem. Comparison between serial APG testing can demonstrate and quantify disease evolution. Comparison between pre- and posttreatment APG testing can demonstrate immediate quantifiable improvement, particularly in patients in the C4B, C5, and C6 clinical CEAP categories showing skin changes that are not readily modifiable. Immediate- and long-term posttreatment APG testing can be used to demonstrate either improvement because of treatment or disease evolution.

### Patient Position

Patient training and performance is paramount to obtain reliable results. The patient is asked to perform a series of maneuvers requiring the movement from supine to standing positions. The specific positions are described in the following section that discusses these particular techniques.

### Technique and Required Documentation

An APG examination is conducted as follows with particular care in the use of specific patient position sequencing:
- The subject rests supine to relax while receiving instructions and providing information pertinent to the test.
- Sensing cuff is wrapped around the calf; sensing cuff is inflated to 10 mm Hg.
- The leg is elevated to optimize emptying of venous volume (VV).
- The leg is brought back to a horizontal position; pressure in sensing cuff is readjusted to 10 mm Hg; in and out 100 mL calibration is performed with syringe.
- The patient stands over the nontested leg holding onto a support structure, relaxing the leg being tested, a difficult task in this standing position.
- The patient rests the foot of the leg being tested on the floor, performs one toe raise and relaxes; this movement is optional in a short protocol.
- The patient performs 10 toe raises and relaxes.
- The patient returns gently to the horizontal position.

The following simplified APG measurements are recommended:
- blood VV (in mL) accumulated in the veins once the patient moves from supine to standing position
- filling time (FT) demonstrating how long it takes to accumulate blood in the calf to 90% of VV once the patient stands
- volumetric filling rate (FR) indicating blood accumulated per unit time (90% VV/FT in cc/s) as complement to FT
- residual volume (RV) measured as a percentage of VV (100 × RV/VV in %), indicating how much volume is pumped from the calf after 10 toe raises.

An extensive APG testing would also include:
- measurement of the ejection fraction as a complement to a "residual volume" testing following ONE toe raise
- total blood volume accumulated in the calf of a supine patient once a pneumatic cuff placed around the thigh is inflated to 80 mm Hg
- volumetric emptying rate measured after the pneumatic cuff is deflated
- differentiation of data from superficial and deep veins by repeating tests with a tourniquet applied around the knee, for example, to minimize the influence of the superficial veins.

Required documentation for the APG testing includes the tracings obtained during the various maneuvers. The tracing should illustrate the stable baseline at the bottom of the chart, the 100 mL calibration pulse, the exponential filling curve with the estimate of the VV, FT, and FR (90% VV/FT), the one toe raise curve for calculation of the ejection fraction (optional in the limited protocol), the 10 toe raise curve with the estimate of the RV% and return to the baseline showing a posttest baseline curve deviating from pretest baseline curve by no more than 5% to 10% of the VV.

### Diagnostic Criteria

Normal values for VV are variable and will be dependent on gender, age, and other characteristics. Normal FT should be longer than 25 s. The venous FR should be less than 2 mL/s. The RV% is normally less than 20% to 35%.

Abnormal findings include a very-low VV which may indicate calf venous thrombosis or chronic obstruction. A high VV greater than, for example, 100 mL, should indicate abnormally high venous pooling because of large veins or numerous veins. An FT shorter than 10 s indicates severe reflux, whereas an FT shorter than 25 s suggests mild to moderate reflux. An FR greater than 2 mL/s indicates venous insufficiency, and ranges of this variable have been coarsely related to severity of venous diseases. An RV% greater than 20% to 35% has been associated to increased ambulatory venous pressures suggesting severity of disease according to the inability to empty the calf veins. Pathology Box 20-2 summarizes CVVI findings with PPG and APG.

Extensive APG evaluation may give parameters suggesting (a) proximal venous obstruction in the pelvic, abdominal regions, (b) differentiation between superficial and deep

---

**PATHOLOGY BOX 20-2**
**APG and PPG Results with CVVI**

| PPG | VRT <20 s |
|-----|-----------|
| APG | FT <25 s |
|  | FR >2 mL/s |
|  | RV >20%–35% |

---

venous pathologies, (c) nonfunctional calf muscle pump, (d) effectiveness of elastic compression, and (e) venous versus nonvenous edematous changes.[43,44]

## Near-Infrared Imaging

Several imaging technologies are being developed to show superficial veins on the skin.[45,46] These are not commonly employed, but some centers are using this technology to aid venous imaging in this patient population. Imaging in the near-infrared range (880 to 930 nm) demonstrates subcutaneous veins with a diameter of 0.5 to 2 mm at a depth of 1 to 3 mm. This technology may help with guidance of venous access, phlebotomy, injection sclerotherapy, and control of laser interstitial therapy.

A highly processed method detects veins as deep as 8 mm from the skin. The vein is detected with near-infrared technology and is projected on the skin with green light.[46] The green light does not affect the infrared signal. Appropriate projection is the key to localize veins that are going to be treated.

---

### SUMMARY

- CVVIy is one of the most prevalent diseases.
- Proper CEAP description of the patient studied and/or treated is recommended.
- Venous flow patterns are recorded using various maneuvers to determine whether abnormal retrograde flow is present.
- Common diagnostic parameters used to determine abnormal retrograde flow include reflux times in excess of 1.0 s in the deep system, 0.5 s in the superficial system, and 0.35 s in the perforating veins.
- Color-flow duplex ultrasonography has become the most useful technology for definitive diagnosis, pre- and peritreatment imaging, and procedure/patent follow-up.

### CRITICAL THINKING QUESTIONS

1. What is an anatomic feature that differentiates the AAGSV from the GSV?

2. A patient is old and reports episodes of dizziness in the past. Your examination table cannot be put into a reverse Trendelenburg position. What can you do in order to accurately complete your CVVI examination?
3. You are having difficulty demonstrating retrograde flow in a patient with extensive varicose veins. What equipment settings should you check and why?

### MEDIA MENU

Student Resources available on the**Point**® include:
- Audio glossary
- Interactive question bank
- Videos
- Internet resources

---

### REFERENCES

1. Eklöf B, Rutherford RB, Bergan JJ, et al. American Venous Forum International Ad Hoc Committee for Revision of the CEAP Classification. Revision of the CEAP classification for chronic venous disorders: consensus statement. *J Vasc Surg.* 2004;40:1248–1252.
2. Beebe HG, Bergan JJ, Bergqvist D, et al. Classification and grading of chronic venous disease in the lower limbs—a consensus statement. Organized by Straub Foundation with the cooperation of the American Venous Forum at the 6th annual meeting, February 22–25, 1994, Maui, Hawaii. *Vasa.* 1995;24:313–318.
3. Porter JM, Moneta GL. International consensus committee on chronic venous disease. Reporting standards in venous disease: an update. *J Vasc Surg.* 1995;21:625–645.
4. Caggiati A, Bergan, JJ, Gloviczki P, et al. Nomenclature of the veins of the lower limbs: an international interdisciplinary consensus statement. *J Vasc Surg.* 2002;36:416–422.

5. Kachlik D, Pechacek V, Baca V, et al. The superficial venous system of the lower extremity: new nomenclature. *Phlebology*. 2010;25:113–123.

6. Coleridege-Smith P, Labropoulos N, Partsch H, et al. Duplex ultrasound investigation of the veins in chronic venous disease of the lower limbs—UIP consensus document. Part I. Basic principles. *Eur J Vasc Endovasc Surg*. 2006;31:83–92.

7. Cavezzi A, Labropoulos H, Partsch S, et el. Duplex ultrasound investigation of the veins in chronic venous disease of the lower limbs – UIP consensus document. Part II. Anatomy. *Eur J Vasc Endovasc Surg*. 2006;31:288–299.

8. Robertson L, Evans C, Fowkes FG. Epidemiology of chronic venous disease. *Phlebology*. 2008;23:103–111.

9. Cesarone MR, Belcaro G, Nicolaides AN, et al. 'Real' epidemiology of varicose veins and chronic venous diseases: the San Valentino Vascular Screening Project. *Angiology*. 2002;53:119–130.

10. Carpentier PH, Maricq HR, Biro C, et al. Prevalence, risk factors, and clinical patterns of chronic venous disorders of lower limbs: a population-based study in France. *J Vasc Surg*. 2004;40:650–659.

11. Maffei FH, Magaldi C, Pinho SZ, et al. Varicose veins and chronic venous insufficiency in Brazil: prevalence among 1755 inhabitants of a country town. *Int J Epidemiol*. 1986;15:210–217.

12. Evans CJ, Fowkes FG, Ruckley CV, et al. Prevalence of varicose veins and chronic venous insufficiency in men and women in the general population: Edinburgh Vein Study. *J Epidemiol Commun Health*. 1999;53:149–153.

13. McLafferty RB, Lohr JM, Caprini JA, et al. Results of the national pilot screening program for venous disease by the American Venous Forum. *J Vasc Surg*. 2007;45:142–148.

14. McLafferty RB, Passman MA, Caprini JA, et al. Increasing awareness about venous disease: The American Venous Forum expands the National Venous Screening Program. *J Vasc Surg*. 2008;48:394–399.

15. Ruckley CV, Evans CJ, Allan PL, et al. Telangiectasia in the Edinburgh Vein Study: epidemiology and association with trunk varices and symptoms. *Eur J Vasc Endovasc Surg*. 2008;36:719–724.

16. Mäkivaara LA, Ahti TM, Luukkaala T, et al. Persons with varicose veins have a high subsequent incidence of arterial disease: a population-based study in Tampere, Finland. *Angiology*. 2007;58:704–709.

17. Maurins U, Hoffmann BH, Lösch C, et al. Distribution and prevalence of reflux in the superficial and deep venous system in the general population—results from the Bonn Vein Study, Germany. *J Vasc Surg*. 2008;48:680–687.

18. Evans CJ, Allan PL, Lee AJ, et al. Prevalence of venous reflux in the general population on duplex scanning: the Edinburgh vein study. *J Vasc Surg*. 1998;28:767–776.

19. Drinan KJ, Wolfson PM, Steinitz D, et al. Duplex imaging in lymphedema. *J Vasc Technol*. 1993;17:23–26.

20. Rutherford RB, Padberg FT, Comerota AJ, et al. Venous severity scoring: An adjunct to venous outcome assessment. *J Vasc Surg*. 2000;31:1307–1312.

21. Moura RM, Gonçalves GS, Navarro TP, et al. Relationship between quality of life and the CEAP clinical classification in chronic venous disease. *Rev Bras Fisioter*. 2010;14:99–105.

22. Darvall KA, Sam RC, Bate GR, et al. Changes in health-related quality of life after ultrasound-guided foam sclerotherapy for great and small saphenous varicose veins. *J Vasc Surg*. 2010;51:913–920.

23. Shepherd AC, Gohel MS, Brown LC, et al. Randomized clinical trial of VNUS Closure FAST radiofrequency ablation versus laser for varicose veins. *Br J Surg*. 2010;97:810–818.

24. Garratt AM, Macdonald LM, Ruta DA, et al. Towards measurement of outcome for patients with varicose veins. *Qual Health Care*. 1993;2:5–10.

25. Launois R, Reboul-Marty J, Henry B. Construction and validation of a quality of life questionnaire in chronic lower limb venous insufficiency (CIVIQ). *Qual Life Res*. 1996;5:539–554.

26. Engelhorn C, Engelhorn A, Salles-Cunha S,et al. Relationship between reflux and greater saphenous vein diameter. *J Vasc Technol*. 1997;21:167–172.

27. Morrison N, Salles-Cunha SX, Neuhardt DL, et al. Prevalence of reflux in the great saphenous vein as a function of diameter. 21st Annual Congress, American College of Phlebology, Tucson, AZ, November 8–11, 2007 Congress Syllabus, p. 111

28. Morrison N. Saphenous ablation: what are the choices, laser or RF energy. *Semin Vasc Surg*. 2005;18:15–18.

29. Lurie F, Creton D, Eklof B, et al. Prospective randomized study of endovenous radiofrequency obliteration (closure) versus ligation and vein stripping (EVOLVeS): two-year follow-up. *Eur J Vasc Endovasc Surg*. 2005;29:67–73.

30. Tzilinis A, Salles-Cunha SX, Dosick SM, et al. Chronic venous insufficiency due to great saphenous vein incompetence treated with radiofrequency ablation: an effective and safe procedure in the elderly. *Vasc Endovascular Surg*. 2005;39:341–345.

31. Morrison N, Neuhardt DL, Rogers CR, et al. Comparisons of side effects using air and carbon dioxide foam for endovenous chemical ablation. *J Vasc Surg*. 2008;47:830–836.

32. Morrison N, Neuhardt DL, Rogers CR, et al. Incidence of side effects using carbon dioxide-oxygen foam for chemical ablation of superficial veins of the lower extremity. *Eur J Vasc Endovasc Surg*. 2010;40:407–413.

33. Engelhorn CA, Engelhorn AL, Cassou MF, et al. Patterns of saphenous reflux in women with primary varicose veins. *J Vasc Surg*. 2005;41:645–645.

34. Engelhorn CA, Engelhorn AL, Cassou MF, et al. Patterns of saphenous venous reflux in women presenting with lower extremity telangiectasias. *Dermatol Surg*. 2007;33(3):282–288

35. Hansen K, Morrison N, Neuhardt DL, et al. Transthoracic echocardiogram and transcranial doppler detection of emboli after foam sclerotherapy of leg veins. *J Vasc Ultrasound*. 2007;31:213–216.

36. Morrison N, Neuhardt DL. Foam sclerotherapy: cardiac and cerebral monitoring. *Phlebology*. 2009;24:252–259.

37. Salles-Cunha SX, Rajasinghe H, Dosick SM, et al. Fate of the great saphenous vein after radio frequency ablation: detailed ultrasound imaging of the treated segment. *Vasc Endovasc Surg*. 2004;38:339–344.

38. Salles-Cunha SX, Comerota AJ, Tzilinis A, et al. Ultrasound findings after radiofrequency ablation of the great saphenous vein: descriptive analysis. *J Vasc Surg*. 2004;40:1166–1173.

39. Gornik HL, Sharma AM. Duplex ultrasound in the diagnosis of lower extremity deep vein thrombosis. *Circulation*. 2014;129(8):917–921.

40. Labropoulos N, Tiongson J, Pryor L T, et al. Definition of venous reflux in lower-extremity veins. *J Vasc Surg*. 2003;38(4):793–798.

41. Lurie F, Comerota A, Eklof B, et al. Multicenter assessment of venous reflux by duplex ultrasound. *J Vasc Surg*. 2012;55:437–445.

42. Beraldo S, Satpathy A, Dodds SR. A study of the routine use of venous photoplethysmography in a one-stop vascular surgery clinic. *Ann R Coll Surg Engl*. 2007;89:379–383.

43. Christopoulos DG, Nicolaides AN, Szendro G, et al. Air-plethysmography and the effect of elastic compression on venous hemodynamics of the leg. *J Vasc Surg*. 1987;5:148–159.

44. Pizano Ramirez N, director. Guias Colombianas para el Diagnostico y el Manejo de los Desordenes Cronicos de las Venas. Editora Guadalupe S.A, Bogota, D.C., 2009, p. 247

45. Zharov VP, Ferguson S, Eidt JF, et al. Infrared imaging of subcutaneous veins. *Lasers Surg Med*. 2004;34:56–61.

46. Miyake RK, Zeman HD, Duarte FH, et al. Vein imaging: A new method of near infrared imaging, where a processed image is projected onto the skin for the enhancement of vein treatment. *Dermatol Surg*. 2006;32:1031–1038.

# Sonography in the Venous Treatment Room

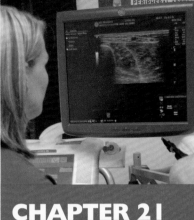

JEAN M. WHITE-MELENDEZ | WILLIAM B. SCHROEDTER

**CHAPTER 21**

## OBJECTIVES

- List the various treatment options for patients suffering from symptomatic chronic venous insufficiency
- Explain the role of imaging in endovenous thermal ablation
- Describe the role of imaging in chemical ablation
- Define the role of the sonographer in the treatment room
- Describe the equipment and room set up for various venous insufficiency treatment options

## KEY TERMS

**ablation**

**chronic venous insufficiency**

**perivenous anesthesia**

**phlebologist**

**reflux**

**sclerosant**

**sclerotherapy**

## GLOSSARY

**chronic venous insufficiency (CVI)** A long-lasting venous valvular or obstructive disorder of the veins

**endovenous ablation** Destruction of the vein by various means (e.g., heat, chemical)

**perivenous (tumescent) anesthesia** Anesthesia that is placed around the vein to be treated with thermal ablation under ultrasound guidance

**phlebologist** Physician who specializes in the diagnosis and treatment of vein disorders

**reflux** Pathologic reflux in a vein is defined as retrograde flow upon release of distal compression in a standing patient[1,2]
- >0.5 seconds in the superficial venous system
- >1.0 second in the deep venous system

**sclerosant** A chemical irritant used in the treatment of varicose veins resulting in inflammation and subsequent fibrosis, thus obliterating the lumen of the vein

**sclerotherapy** A medical procedure involving an injection of a sclerosant into the vein; may be performed visually or under ultrasound guidance

Duplex ultrasound evaluation is the gold standard method for the assessment of the veins of the lower extremity. First used in the detection of venous thrombosis, the technology has been expanded to include evaluation of variable venous anatomy, assessment for valvular incompetence, and documentation of venous stenosis or compression.[3-6] Venous duplex ultrasound is essential in the diagnosis and clinical planning for the patient who suffers from venous disease. Not only does it define the anatomy and particularly the anatomic variants common in venous disease, it also allows for the evaluation of normal and pathologic hemodynamics. Documenting reflux within a given vein segment is used as an indicator of venous system dysfunction. However, the overall goal should be to assess venous system hemodynamics. It is important to understand that the decision to treat a given vein is not based solely on the ultrasound findings but rather on the clinical evaluation of whether the treatment can serve to normalize or improve venous system hemodynamics. Various treatments for venous insufficiency have evolved over the years. Ultrasound guidance is an integral component of modern treatment techniques. This chapter discusses those techniques with an emphasis on the role of ultrasound and the sonographer.

# TREATMENT OPTIONS

Traditionally, chronic venous insufficiency, and specifically superficial venous disease, was treated surgically with what is commonly known as vein stripping and high ligation.[6,7] Vein stripping procedures had their genesis in the 1800s, and many of the techniques were described by Frederick Trendelenburg—a familiar name in vascular surgery. Trendelenburg was a surgeon who first reported many of the venous surgical techniques of the time. Today, vein stripping is rarely performed. It is invasive and painful, requiring general anesthesia and thus involving a hospital stay. Additionally, the recovery is prolonged often requiring weeks to months.

Today, minimally invasive techniques have largely replaced traditional surgical treatment. Treatment options were described in Chapter 20. Many of these techniques require guidance in order to properly place materials such as needles, devices, and drugs. Ultrasound is used for this guidance and is indispensable in the intervention room. Ablation of diseased superficial veins is one of the primary procedures performed. Ablation can include endovenous thermal or chemical ablation of the main superficial veins and chemical ablation of larger bulbous tributaries as well as smaller varicosities, reticular veins, and telangiectasias. Although most of the surface smaller veins can be treated with visual sclerotherapy, patients with clinically significant varicosities and reticular veins often require precise guidance for the delivery of the sclerosants, and this is accomplished with the use of ultrasound. Large superficial varicosities are often addressed using a technique called ambulatory phlebectomy, or microphlebectomy. This is a surgical procedure in which a small incision is created next to the varicosity, a special instrument is employed to hook the vein and extract it.

# TEAMWORK

Minimally invasive venous treatments can involve medical personnel, including a physician, physician's assistant, nurse practitioner, nurse, and sonographer. For the purposes of this chapter, the definition of a sonographer is the person holding the transducer, whether technologist or physician. Some experienced technologists and sonographers have chosen to expand their knowledge base in this discipline to allow them to obtain the credential of Registered Phlebology Sonographer (RPhS) from the organization Cardiovascular Credentialing International (CCI). An individual with the RPhS credential has a thorough knowledge of venous anatomy and hemodynamics.

Venous treatments often include a specialist called a phlebologist. A phlebologist is a physician who specializes in the diagnosis and treatment of vein disorders. This physician may be a vascular surgeon, interventional radiologist, interventional cardiologist, or other physician specialist with the interest, knowledge, and requisite skill set.

Some phlebologists perform the imaging guidance personally without the presence of a sonographer. In some practices, the sonographer works as a first assistant in the interventional room, not only operating the ultrasound instrument imaging but also assisting the phlebologist with adjunctive therapies that are required in the large majority of patients. Experience has shown that the optimal approach is to have the close

| TABLE 21-1 | **Complications of Venous Ablation Procedures** |
|---|---|
| Thermal ablation | Misplaced thermal device into deep venous system |
| | Misplaced thermal device from superficial system through perforating vein into deep system |
| | Acquired arteriovenous fistulae |
| | Endovenous heat-induced thrombosis (EHIT) |
| | Nerve injury |
| | Cutaneous burn |
| | Deep vein thrombosis |
| | Pulmonary embolism |
| Chemical ablation | Misplaced sclerosant into the deep system or unintended location |
| | Sclerosant extravasation |
| | Skin ulceration |
| | Deep vein thrombosis |
| | Pulmonary embolism |
| Perivenous anesthesia administration | Anesthesia misplaced or not completely surrounding the vein |
| | Intravascular injection of anesthesia |
| | Accidental puncture of adjacent artery or vein |
| | Acquired arteriovenous fistula |
| | Anaphylaxis |

teamwork of a phlebologist and sonographer during venous treatments. Minimally invasive endovenous procedures are highly effective and carry a fairly low risk of adverse complications. However, serious complications can occur, and these may be devastating. Table 21-1 lists some of the potential complications encountered. Complications have occurred with the misplacement of the endovenous thermal device, resulting in ablation of the external iliac vein and common femoral vein. Misplacement of chemical sclerosant into the popliteal artery has been reported, resulting in loss of limb. Acquired arterial venous fistulas have resulted from administration of the perivenous anesthesia. The thermal device has been witnessed leaving the great saphenous vein coursing into a perforating vein and then traveling through a segment of the femoral vein before coursing back to the saphenous vein. The phlebologist and phlebology sonographer are a team, working together, providing two set of eyes, ensuring proper placement of any needle or device, or device, and recognizing and minimizing any potential adverse complications.

# SONOGRAPHIC EXAMINATION TECHNIQUES

The primary role of the sonographer within the intervention room is to provide ultrasound guidance but in many vein centers, the sonographer may take on a greatly expanded role. This role may be as expanded or as limited as the center desires. In addition to assisting in the procedure with ultrasound guidance, the sonographer may play a role in the clinical decision-making process as well as the treatment

| TABLE 21-2 | **Sonographer Checklist** |
|---|---|
| Medical record review | Review preprocedure venous ultrasound report |
| | Confirm procedure to be performed |
| | Confirm correct leg and vein to be treated |
| Patient dialogue | Confirm understanding of procedure |
| | Confirm the leg and vein to be treated |
| | Answer patient questions |
| | Provide education |
| Ultrasound | Mark position of vein |
| | Determine area of access and mark |
| Procedure preparation | Set up sterile tray |
| | Prep and drape patient leg |
| Procedure | Provide ultrasound guidance for |
| | • vein access |
| | • device placement |
| | • perivenous (tumescent) anesthesia |
| | • anesthesia for nerve block if performed |
| | Confirm ablation of vein |
| | Confirm proper distribution of sclerosant |
| Postprocedure | Clean up |
| | Apply dressing |
| | Apply compression stocking |
| | Confirm postprocedure ultrasound appointment |
| | Provide postop instructions |

options. Given the variability of the venous system, the sonographer is in an optimal position to aid the physician in the clinical decision making.

Many centers employ a sonographer checklist to aid in the procedure. Table 21-2 presents a concise sonographer checklist for venous procedures. The specific components will vary depending on the practice.

## Patient Preparation

The sonographer must begin with reviewing the patient records to confirm that the procedure scheduled is consistent with the patient's clinical condition as documented in the chart. The correct leg and vein to be treated should be verified. This is a critical step. The diagnostic ultrasound study must be examined again with emphasis on its consistency with the scheduled procedure. If there appears to be any discrepancy, the rest of the team should be notified and the information clarified.

Within the sonographer's Scope of Practice is the provision of patient education. During the procedure room preparations and venous mapping preprocedure, the sonographer spends a considerable amount of time with the patient. This time is ideal for answering any final questions regarding the procedure, reexplaining the venous disease process, long-term consequences of chronic venous insufficiency, and

steps the patient can take to minimize or delay significant recurrence of the disease. Specific clinical questions should be deferred to the physician.

## Patient Positioning

Once the patient arrives, they are typically checked in and prepared by vein center staff. If a patient is also scheduled for microphlebectomy (ambulatory phlebectomy) or vein extraction, he or she should remain standing for a minimum of 5 to 10 minutes to ensure maximum distention of any superficial veins. This period of standing can take place in a secondary examination room or within the procedure room depending on the office configuration. After standing for the appropriate time, the phlebologist often personally marks the veins for extraction (Fig. 21-1). This not only develops rapport with the patient but allows direct visualization of the veins in question. If the sonographer will be assisting in the phlebectomy, they should be present as well in order to similarly view the veins in question. Once the veins are marked, the patient can be taken to the procedure room.

For the ablation procedure, the patient is placed on the procedure table in a position that balances their comfort while optimizing access to the target vein(s). For a great saphenous vein or anterior accessory great saphenous vein, a supine position with the head slightly elevated and the leg externally rotated with the knee slightly bent is used.

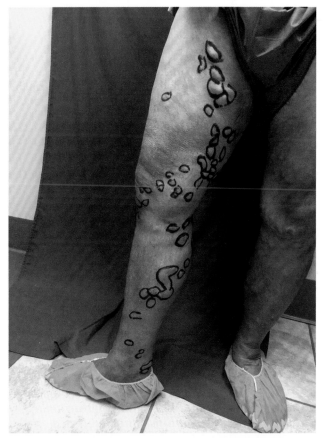

**FIGURE 21-1** A patient marked for an extensive microphlebectomy. Extraction of the large varicosities in the upper thigh may complicate the postprocedure dressing because application of adequate compression can prove difficult at this leg segment.

This can often be facilitated by having the patient turn very slightly on their side or simply just placing most of their weight on the hip of the target leg. A roll or small pillow to support the knee can notably increase patient comfort. For the small saphenous vein, the patient is positioned prone with a pillow placed under the feet for comfort and to prevent popliteal vein compression during the procedure.

## Equipment

Generally, most ultrasound instruments can be successfully used in the intervention room. While Doppler evaluation is occasionally used for confirmation of refluxing segments, ultrasound in the intervention room is primarily an imaging procedure. Therefore, a high-quality image is a prerequisite. Most, but not all, the veins of interest will be superficial, and therefore higher frequencies are optimal to provide the highest-quality image resolution. Ensure proper instrument optimization, including frequency, grayscale settings, frame rate, and proper placement of focal zones to the image of the vein of interest.

## Scanning Technique for Mapping the Vein

Once the patient is positioned, the target vein is identified and reevaluated to confirm the anatomy and pathology described on the diagnostic venous duplex ultrasound report. Once confirmed, the course of the vein is marked on the skin. Drawing a line on the skin through the gel is challenging. An alternate technique involves placing "dots" on the skin with a marker and then connecting the dots once the gel is wiped off the limb. Some sonographers will use a small plastic coffee stirrer. These tiny straws can be pushed into the skin, creating a small ring in the skin surface. It is not uncomfortable for the patient. These small rings on the skin will lasts a remarkably long time. Some centers will use a common purple surgical skin marker, but others have noted the purple marks wipe off with the gel. Permanent magic marker is used by many to draw the line connecting the dots. One must also take care to make the dots on the skin directly over the vein along the likely course of the anesthesia administration. In practice, one can use a more anterior or more posterior scan plane and still see the vein, sometimes with better visualization than directly over it. The sonographer must be cognizant of this fact. The marking procedure is not very precise because if the patient moves or is slightly repositioned, often the vein is no longer under the line. For some, the line can sometimes be a distraction drawing the attention to the line as opposed to what the ultrasound image is actually displaying.

In addition to drawing the line, some centers will also mark 5 and 10 cm intervals along the line. The tumescent anesthesia needle is 10 cm in length. Therefore, if desired, the phlebologist can make a skin wheel of anesthesia with a small gauge needle prior to tumescent administration. The larger gauge tumescent needle is then introduced through the anesthetized skin, resulting in significantly less patient discomfort.

Additionally, the vein can also be evaluated for the presence of any large tributaries or perforating veins. Some believe there is an increased risk of incomplete ablation or subsequent recanalization at the point where these vessels intersect. With the location of large tributaries or perforating

veins marked on the skin, the phlebologist may elect to deliver additional thermal energy in these regions.

The room should be kept warm to prevent vasoconstriction. A heating pad in the intervention room is also helpful. One can also consider the use of a topical application of nitroglycerin paste over the vein. If the vein is not very large or if vasospasmed, the application of heat while the procedure prep is being performed can often relieve this spasm. Vasospasm is not uncommon and has the appearance of a notable thickened vein wall. The patient may be cold, dehydrated, or apprehensive about the procedure, and this can result in the vasospasm. Veins can decrease in size by 300% in minutes. Heat can help alleviate this situation. A blanket can also be used if the patient is feeling chilled.

## Setting up for the Procedure

In some settings, the sonographer sets up the sterile tray, organizing the instruments and devices used in the procedure (Fig. 21-2). It is beyond the scope of this chapter to describe the specific procedures involved with sterile technique, but many treatises on sterile procedures are available. If permitted, one might chose to observe in an operating room or other treatment room. Body position of the sonographer is important and awareness of the surroundings so as not to touch nonsterile items. Should there be a break in sterile technique, a change of gown or gloves will rectify the situation.

Many advocate fairly strict sterile technique for thermal ablation procedures. Although the access is quite limited, a sterile field for the instruments and thermal device (catheter or fiber) is used. Adjunctive procedures such as phlebectomy also necessitate good sterile technique. The patient is optimally positioned, and an iodine-based antiseptic is applied on the leg using either the foam brush included in many surgical packs or with gauze sponges (Fig. 21-3). An iodine-based antiseptic has the advantage of coloring the leg so any areas missed can easily be identified. In the rare instance a patient has an iodine allergy, an alternative such as chlorhexidine or even isopropyl alcohol can be used. The top and sides of the leg are covered with the antiseptic solution. Although it can be done alone, it is very helpful to have a nonsterile assistant hold the leg up in order to access the back of the leg.

Once the entire leg is covered with the antiseptic solution, the sterile split draped is placed on the patient. The split taped

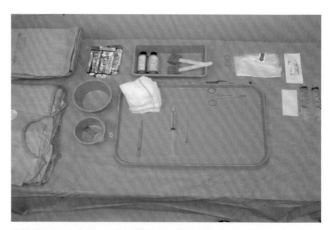

**FIGURE 21-2** Typical setup of the sterile tray. This will vary depending upon the device and interventional techniques used.

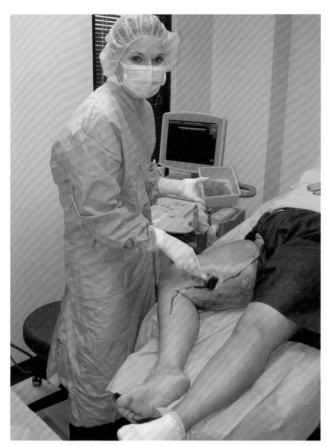

**FIGURE 21-3** An image of a patient being prepped for a procedure and disinfecting the leg with an iodine-based antiseptic scrub prior to draping.

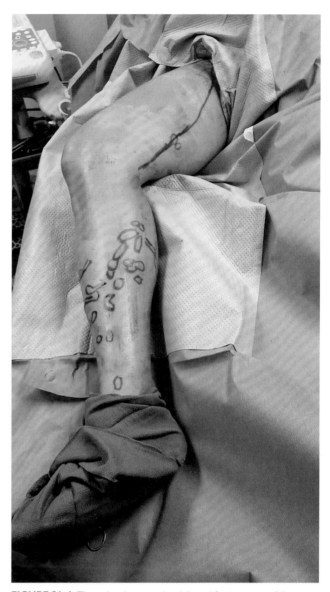

**FIGURE 21-4** The patient is prepped and draped for treatment of the great saphenous vein with concomitant microphlebectomy of bulbous below-knee tributaries.

area is pushed up underneath the leg, and the sides draped around the patient. For a great saphenous, anterior great saphenous, or posterior great saphenous veins, the groin is the most challenging area for an adequate drape. One technique that can be used is to temporarily wrap the drape around the leg and then wrap the foot in a sterile towel. After completing this, reposition the leg using external rotation and then place the roll under the slightly bent knee. Finally, secure the sides of the drape at the groin high enough to allow access several centimeters above the saphenofemoral junction. Often, an additional sponge for extra antiseptic solution at the groin may be necessary. Once the drape is in place, the leg is once again optimally positioned. The transducer is placed within a sterile sleeve, and the location of the vein along with its relationship to the line on the skin is confirmed. Adequate visualization of saphenofemoral junction must also be checked. As mentioned previously, changing the leg position may alter the relationship of the vein to the marking on the skin surface. In the case of small saphenous vein treatment, the patient is placed prone, and the drape is placed higher enough to allow access to the popliteal fossa or higher depending upon the planned length of treatment (Fig. 21-4).

## Imaging Guidance During Venous Treatment Procedures

The exact imaging guidance technique will vary depending upon the preferences of the phlebologist. Some phlebologists prefer to hold the transducer while getting access to the vein. The benefits of the "coupling" of the hands in a coordinated approach can certainly be appreciated. However, many believe the imaging is best accomplished by the sonographer who is a specialist at transducer manipulation and optimizing the image for visualization of the vein, the surrounding structures, the access needle, and guidance of anesthesia. There must be absolute confidence of the location of the different components utilized in an ablation procedure. The experienced sonographer typically sees things in the image possibly missed by less experienced persons. This also allows the phlebologist to concentrate on their role. This team approach has worked successfully for many in a number of varied settings with physicians of many specialties.

If the sonographer is scrubbed in and sterile, operating the instrument may become an issue. In reality, the instrument should be set up to optimize the image for the length of the target vein and in the majority of cases, there are not a large number of adjustments necessary. However, there are clearly instances when the instrument settings may have to be adjusted. Use of a sterile sheet of clear plastic that can be placed over the primary controls will allow the controls to be accessed by the sonographer while maintaining sterility. If a sterile cover is not available for the ultrasound controls, a nonsterile assistant in the room can be instructed to make minor adjustments in the equipment as needed.

## Access

The first step of the ablation procedure is to gain access to the vein. The patient should ideally be in a reverse Trendelenburg position to ensure filling and distention of the vein. The vein is identified, and the sonographer and phlebologist must agree on the exact access site. This is chosen based on the given anatomy. Many times, it is preferable to access below any large tributaries in order to isolate their connection with the truncal vein. However, these are sometimes associated with a valve sinus, remnant valve, or minor tortuosity which can all potentially complicate passage of the device. The size and depth of the vein must also be considered. While deeper vessels are often more challenging to cannulate, superficial vessels come with their own set of challenges. There is less room for manipulation of the needle when attempting to access the vein. Additionally, if the vessel is out of the fascial compartment, it is less supported and tends to move or roll in response to the pressure of the needle.

Once the location is agreed upon, the skin wheel of anesthesia is place subcutaneously, and the access needle is inserted through this anesthetized skin. It typically helps to have the patient in a degree of reverse Trendelenburg position so the veins will distend. Whether to image the vessel in a transverse or longitudinal plane is personal preference. The transverse view has the advantage of being able to determine whether the needle is directed over the middle of the vein or medially or laterally (Fig. 21-5). In a longitudinal view, this is slightly more difficult. The longitudinal view has an advantage in that the needle can be more easily advanced directly under the transducer and can be more easily seen throughout the advancement. If using a transverse view, the phlebologist must have a good awareness of space to determine what angle is needed to advance the needle so the tip will arrive at the chosen

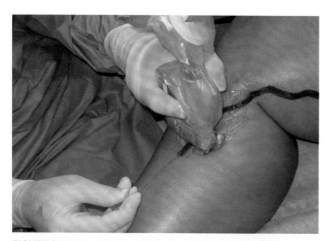

**FIGURE 21-5** The vein is imaged in a transverse plane. The needle is advanced from below the transducer into the field of view where access to the vein can be imaged.

access location under the transducer's field of view. Many times, considerable pressure is necessary to puncture the vein wall with the needle, and it is not uncommon for the needle to perforate not only the anterior or "top" wall but also the posterior wall. This is typically readily obvious on imaging because the needle can be seen perforating both walls which are now held together. With very slow withdrawal of the needle, the back wall of the vein can be seen to "drop off" the needle, and blood return will be noted. The blood return is termed "flash." Many times, the needle will actually core the tissue although within the lumen a "flash" of blood is not appreciated in the needle. Despite of lack of "flash," if the sonographer and phlebologist are confident that the needle is intravascular, the guidewire can be threaded, or a 5 mL syringe can be used to "pull the core of tissue out of the needle" rather than resticking the patient or repositioning the needle.

For those performing these procedures, it is evident that veins do not like to be touched, and if too much contact is made, the vein will vasospasm. This sometimes precludes access at this location. Applying nitropaste and heat to induce vasodilatation can help, but often the solution is to choose another location slightly proximal or distal and reattempt the access.

## Placement of Instrumentation

Once access is obtained, the guidewire is inserted through the needle into the vein. This must be accomplished under ultrasound guidance, and it is imperative to confirm the wire is intraluminal. It has been observed that sometimes wires advance fairly easily but are extravascular. The expertise of the sonographer becomes invaluable in this case. If the wire is in fact outside the vein lumen, the dilator sheath will follow. The patient may tolerate a wire that is extravascular better than one might expect, especially if it is within the saphenous fascia. However, the dilator is not well tolerated if not placed within the vein, and therefore confirmation of intravascular placement is essential. Once the guidewire position is confirmed, the dilator sheath is placed over the wire and into the vein. The wire is removed, and the sheath is left in place. It is through this sheath that the ablation device is introduced into the vessel lumen. The catheter or laser fiber should be imaged with ultrasound and followed up the vein to the saphenofemoral junction (Fig. 21-6). If resistance is encountered, imaging can often demonstrate how the catheter or fiber should be manipulated in order to pass the obstruction. This may occur at a region of a valve or small tortuosity. It is not recommended to simply wait at the saphenofemoral junction for the catheter or fiber to appear into view. As mentioned earlier in this chapter, catheters and fibers have been observed exiting the target vein through large tributaries or going into perforating veins, coursing through the deep system and reemerge into the truncal vein. Constant observation of the catheter or fiber while it is being passed would avoid misplacement of this sort. While this would likely be noted during tumescent administration, the trauma incurred to the vein wall should be avoided.

Position of the device at the truncal junction or terminal point of treatment is clearly the most critical imaging function. Failure to position the device properly can result in endovenous heat-induced thrombosis (EHIT), deep vein

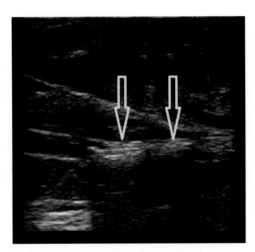

**FIGURE 21-6** Thermal device (at *arrows*) within the vein.

thrombosis, or even worse, thermal ablation of the deep vein itself. In the case of the great saphenous vein, the tip of the device should be positioned distal to the superficial epigastric vein in accordance with the manufacturer's recommendations. This would generally be from 2 to 4 cm distal to this location. In small saphenous vein treatment, it is advised to never advance the device out of the small saphenous compartment. In the case of a saphenopopliteal junction, this is often in proximity to the sciatic nerve and given the dire consequence of nerve injury, it is important to be cautious. The sciatic nerve, and its division into the sural and common peroneal nerves, can be visualized in most patients. Additionally, the sural nerve commonly courses in proximity to the small saphenous vein in the distal calf, and this is also easily visualized. Sonographers should be familiar with the nerve anatomy of the leg and the ultrasound appearance of nerves. Once the device in in place, the patient is positioned in a supine or Trendelenburg position to empty and contract the vein around the device.

### Perivenous Anesthesia

Perivenous administration of anesthesia (tumescent anesthesia) is integral to the provision and success of the treatment. The anesthesia not only anesthetizes the surrounding tissues making the procedure possible but it also serves as a heat sink, insulating the vein from the surrounding tissues, protecting them from thermal damage, and minimizing postoperative patient discomfort. Finally, the anesthesia compresses the vein exsanguinating it and ensuring good contact with the device optimizing thermal delivery. High-quality ultrasound imaging facilitates this process by ensuring precise delivery in the perivenous tissues. Again, this can be accomplished in either a transverse or longitudinal imaging plane, and often both imaging planes are utilized. The use of the longitudinal plane while administering the anesthesia is preferred by this author for the following reasons:

- The needle can be more easily identified in the proper location
- It tends to direct the needle along the course of the vein which upon injection directs the anesthetic along the course of the vein
- The needle can more easily be withdrawn or inserted to place fluid both above and below the vein

- Intraluminal injection can be most readily identified which would be difficult or impossible to detect while imaging transversely

Intravenous injection is not typically associated with dramatic effects, but most anesthetic formulas use epinephrine to induce vasoconstriction and minimize bleeding. This can certainly result in cardiac effects if large volumes are used and therefore should be consciously avoided. Intraluminal injection of anesthesia is more common in large diameter vessels and on imaging typically appears as "snow" or bubbles moving rapidly cephalad within the vein. The goal is to surround the vein with the anesthesia, and this appears as a cocoon of hypoechoic fluid encircling the vein (Fig. 21-7). This fluid compresses the vein, and imaging ensures that the vein walls are compressed and in contact with the device. This is very important at the terminal point of treatment where adequate anesthesia is required in order to completely coapt the vein walls above the tip of the catheter. Additionally, the vein should be adequately separated from the muscular compartment deep to the vein as well separated a minimum of 1 to 2 cm below the skin line. Thermal ablation of vessels superficial to this minimal 1 cm limit may result in superficial skin burns that can be permanent. After the anesthesia has been administered, a transverse sweep along the entire course of the vein is performed to confirm that an adequate "cocoon" of perivenous fluid is visualized. A transverse view may also be utilized when administering perivenous anesthesia of anterior accessory great saphenous vein as to ensure to create enough of a heat sink between the vein and the superficial femoral artery.

### Thermal Treatment

Prior to beginning the actual treatment and delivery of the heat, the exact position of the device should be confirmed. The position of the tip of the ablation device is verified and documented. Many protocols require imaging the vein during the procedure largely to ensure the destruction of the endothelial lining of the vessel. This is seen as a bright hyperechoic echo that actively forms as the device is withdrawn. In some instances, transducer pressure or pressure supplied manually by the sonographer's free hand over the vein ensures that the vessel walls are coapted and in contact with the thermal device. This is most important at

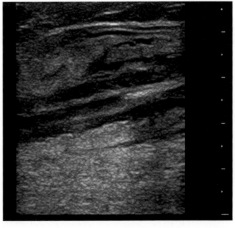

**FIGURE 21-7** Thermal device within the vein with tumescent anesthesia surrounding the vein (hypoechoic areas above and below the vein).

the initial firing of the device to limit any proximal propagation of heat into the junction. Many device manufacturers advocate increased energy delivery to the vein at the junction to ensure ablation and limit potential recanalization. Particularly, large segments or connections with large tributaries or perforating veins as previously marked also warrant additional energy delivery and perhaps increased transducer pressure to ensure wall contact with the device. During thermal ablation, if the patient reports any discomfort, additional perivenous anesthesia will be administered immediately. Once the entire length of vein is treated, the device and sheath are removed, and pressure is maintained over the access site until hemostasis is achieved.

### Posttreatment

Following treatment, a brief imaging of the vein to ensure sclerosis is also warranted, however, complete occlusion of the vein may not be immediately appreciated depending upon the size of the vein, specific anatomy, the device used, and the energy delivered. Follow-up of a patient undergoing venous ablation is routinely conducted with duplex ultrasound 2 to 7 days post-procedure in order to confirm the destruction of the target vein as well as ensure that there has been no EHIT or other deep vein involvement (Fig. 21-8).[8]

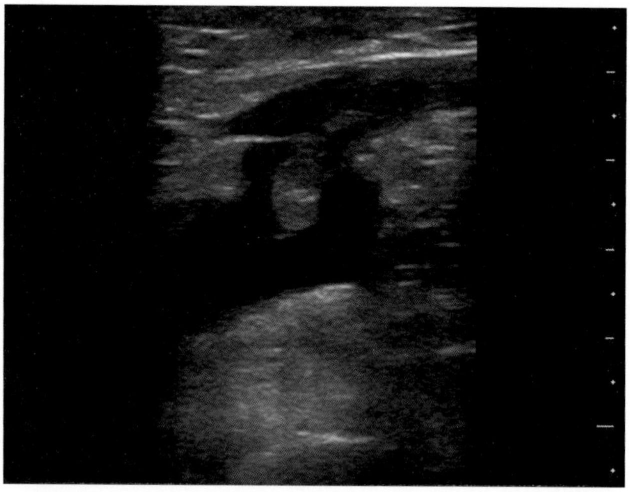

## Ultrasound-Guided Sclerotherapy

The protocol for delivering sclerosants to diseased vein segments is similar to what was described with access for thermal ablation; however, there are some important differences.[9] The goal is to distribute the sclerosant volume to the diseased vein(s). Often, these are associated with clusters of varicosed tributaries, and therefore mapping of the cluster, its extent, and connection is critical to the goal. Optimally, one would desire to identify the primary outflow from these vessels and inject at that segment in order for the sclerosant to fill the varicosities. This can sometimes be accomplished in a reverse Trendelenburg position, but optimal filling of the veins and visualizing the flow abnormalities would be achieved in a standing position. These veins are not traced out on the skin, but the target vein for injection is identified and this is marked on the skin. As these vessels are often tortuous, consideration should be given to the direction the access needle will be inserted

**FIGURE 21-8** Endovenous heat-induced thrombosis (EHIT) 3 days following great saphenous vein thermal ablation with thrombus formation that has propagated into the common femoral vein.

into the field of view as well as the direction the sclerosant will travel. In practice, the sclerosant movement is only somewhat controlled; however, ultrasound can be used to ensure adequate dispersion of the sclerosant throughout the target vessels. This can be accomplished by applying pressure on some vessels or "milking" the tissues, thereby moving the sclerosant in the desired direction.

## Post-Procedure

Once the procedure is completed, the leg is cleaned. The iodine-based antiseptic or prep soap is removed with a towel wetted either with water or hydrogen peroxide and then dried. A small adhesive strip bandage is applied to close the access incision. The leg is then dressed or a stocking applied according to device manufacturer or center protocol. A graduated compression stocking is more than adequate for most patients. Absorbent pads can be applied over the course of the vein because in some instances the anesthesia may leak out of the needle access sites. The room is then thoroughly cleaned and prepared for the next procedure.

---

### SUMMARY

- Understanding the treatment options available for the patient suffering from chronic venous insufficiency, and how the diagnostic ultrasound information will be used to treat the patient optimizes the ability of the sonographer to obtain the necessary data.
- Most modern treatments of chronic venous insufficiency are extremely dependent upon high-quality ultrasound. Active participation of the sonographer within the intervention room can be a great asset to the phlebologist and allow for optimal patient care.
- The phlebology sonographer and the phlebologist working as a team provide valuable interaction and can serve to minimize and avoid potential errors and pitfalls in treatment.

- Both thermal and chemical ablation may be used to treat primary trunks; however, thermal ablation is far more common. Ultrasound guidance for the thermal ablation device involves access to the proper vein, guiding the catheter through the vein segment, and positioning the thermal device tip in the precise location.
- Chemical ablation of larger subcutaneous varicosities is performed under ultrasound guidance. Ultrasound can confirm the presence of the needle within the target vein so there is little or no extravasation of sclerosant outside the vein. As the sclerosant is injected, ultrasound is used to document and even facilitate the distribution of sclerosant through the vein segments.
- Successful treatment of the vein segments can be confirmed immediately upon completion; however, documentation of anatomic success is typically performed 2 to 7 days posttreatment.

## CRITICAL THINKING QUESTIONS

1. While following the catheter up the great saphenous vein, the catheter is lost from view but is subsequently identified in the common femoral vein at the saphenofemoral junction. What is the likely course of the catheter?
2. You are assisting during access of a subcutaneous varicosity for administration of a sclerosant. There is an initial blood return but during injection, the sclerosant does not readily travel through the target vein but is identified surrounding the vein. What is the most likely occurrence?
3. A patient presents for treatment of great saphenous reflux which was noted to be 6 to 8 mm throughout its length on the diagnostic ultrasound. The great saphenous vein was mapped with the patient in a supine position and at the target location just below the knee vein measured 2.2 mm. What would the sonographer do at this point?

## MEDIA MENU

Student Resources available on thePoint* include:
- Audio glossary
- Interactive question bank
- Videos
- Internet resources

## REFERENCES

1. van Bemmelen PS, Bedford G, Beach K, et al. Quantitative segmental evaluation of venous valvular reflux with duplex ultrasound scanning. *J Vasc Surg.* 1989;10:425–431.
2. Labropoulos N, Tiongson J, Pryor L, et al. Definition of venous reflux in lower extremity veins. *J Vasc Surg.* 2003;38:793–798.
3. Caggiati A, Bergan JJ, Gloviczki P, et al. Nomenclature of the veins of the lower limb: extensions, refinements and clinical application. *J Vasc Surg.* 2005;41:719–724.
4. Cavezzi A, Labropoulos N, Partsch H, et al. Duplex ultrasound investigation of the veins in chronic venous disease of the lower limbs—UIP Consensus Document. Part II. Anatomy. *Eur J Vasc Endovasc Surg.* 2006;31:288–299.
5. Coleridge-Smith P, Labropoulos N, Partsch H, et al. Duplex ultrasound investigation of the veins in chronic venous disease of the lower limbs—UIP Consensus Document. Part I. Basic principles. *Eur J Vasc Endovasc Surg.* 2006;31:83–92.
6. Gloviczki P. *Handbook of Venous Disorders: Guidelines of the American Venous Forum.* 3rd ed. New York, NY: Arnold; 2009.
7. Moore W. *Vascular Surgery: A Comprehensive Review.* 4th ed. Philadelphia, PA: W.B. Saunders; 1993.
8. Dexter D, Kabnick L, Berland T, et al. Complications of endovenous lasers. *Phlebology.* 2012;27(Suppl 1):40–45.
9. Goldman M. *Sclerotherapy: Treatment of Varicose and Telangiectatic Leg Veins.* 2nd ed. St. Louis, MO: Mosby Year Book; 1995.

# The Role of Ultrasound in Central Vascular Access Device Placement

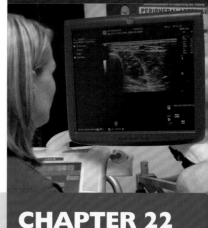

GAIL EGAN | GARY SISKIN

**CHAPTER 22**

## OBJECTIVES

- Describe the different types of vascular access device options
- List the various veins that can be accessed for the placement of a central line
- Describe the ultrasound techniques used to attain venous access
- Define the potential complications of central venous access

## KEY TERMS

**basilic vein**

**jugular vein**

**peripherally inserted central catheter**

**superior vena cava**

**vascular access device**

## GLOSSARY

**air embolism** Inadvertent release of air or gas into the venous system

**collateral veins** Preexisting veins that enlarge to take flow from neighboring but occluded vessels

**fistula** An abnormal connection or passageway between two organs or vessels; may be caused by trauma or intentionally for therapeutic purposes

**gain** The brightness of an ultrasound image, which can be manipulated on most devices

**glidewire** A hydrophilic guidewire

**guidewire** A Nitinol or stainless steel wire used to support sheath or catheter exchanges and to predict vessel patency; measured in diameter and length

**infiltration** Leaking of intravenous fluid from a catheter into the tissue surrounding the vein

**intima** Innermost layer of a vein or artery, composed of one layer of endothelial cells in contact with blood flow; also known as the tunica intima

**microintroducer** Small needles and wires used to make the initial access into a target

**peel away sheath** A sheath that is perforated along the long axis, allowing the device to be split for removal from a catheter

**PICC** A peripherally inserted central catheter; a type of vascular access device that is typically inserted into a vein of the upper extremity and threaded to achieve a tip location in the distal third of the superior vena cava

**pneumothorax** Collection of air in the pleural space (between the lung and chest wall)

**sheath** A thin-walled, hollow plastic tube through which wires and catheters can be advanced; measured in Fr size according to the size of the catheter it can accommodate (e.g., a 5Fr sheath will allow a 5Fr catheter to be passed through it)

**stenosis** Narrowing of a vein or artery because of disease or trauma

Central venous access plays a vital role in the care of critically ill patients as well as patients requiring intravenous antibiotic therapy, central venous pressure monitoring and sampling, hemodialysis, chemotherapy, and total parenteral nutrition. Vascular access devices (VADs) are catheters that allow clinicians to infuse medications and blood components, obtain blood samples, and deliver other exchange therapies. Some patients may require only short-term access, while others are dependent on central vascular access for a lifetime. Central VADs are catheters placed such that the terminal tip of the catheter resides in a central vein, most often the superior vena cava (SVC). There are many different types of central VADs, each with varying characteristics. The goal for device selection is to match the right device to the right patient, with consideration given to therapy duration, number and type of infusions, and patient lifestyle and activity issues. A thorough assessment prior to device placement is critical in selecting the right device and placing it in the right location for the right therapy.

Today, it is virtually the standard of care to use ultrasound guidance to assess potential target sites for VAD placement and to guide the initial venous puncture as the first step in device placement. The Agency for Healthcare Research and Quality has recommended the use of ultrasound as one of their 11 practices to improve patient care in their landmark 2001 publication, "Making Health Care Safer: An Analysis of Patient Safety Practices."[1,2]

In 2011, The American College of Surgeons published a revised statement on recommendations for the use of real-time ultrasound guidance for placement of central venous catheters, recommending ultrasound training for all health professionals placing central venous catheters and that ultrasound be used when placing devices. This chapter will focus on the role ultrasound imaging plays in the placement of central VADs.

## ANATOMY

Central VADs may be placed into a variety of target veins. These most commonly include peripheral, upper extremity veins, such as the basilic, brachial, and cephalic veins, in addition to central veins, such as the subclavian veins (SCVs) and internal jugular veins (IJVs). No matter where the initial puncture site is, the catheter typically passes through the brachiocephalic vein on its way to the SVC (Fig. 22-1). The catheter tip typically resides in the distal third of the SVC (Fig. 22-2). This is also known as the atriocaval junction. This is a desirable location for the tip of a VAD because a flow rate of 2,000 mL/min of venous blood flow is present here. From this location, blood flows directly into the right atrium, then to the right ventricle, and then into the pulmonary circulation. Given the high blood flow in this location, infusates are rapidly dispersed and diluted in this area of high flow. Aspiration for blood return, exchange transfusions, and dialysis or apheresis are also easily accomplished when the VAD tip is accurately located.

## CENTRAL VASCULAR ACCESS DEVICE OPTIONS

There are a variety of VADs available. Each of these devices has different characteristics, which confer different advantages and disadvantages upon them. VADs may be divided into three categories: nontunneled devices, tunneled devices, and implanted ports.

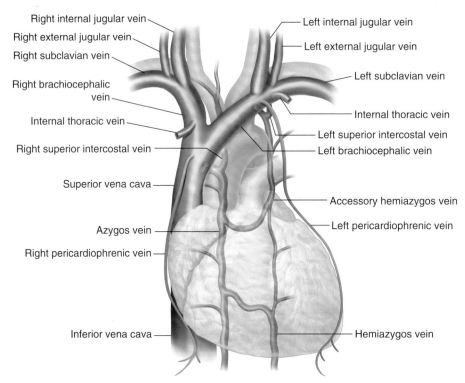

**FIGURE 22-1** An anatomic drawing demonstrating the central veins, including the internal jugular and brachiocephalic veins in addition to the superior vena cava, all of which are important for the placement of vascular access devices. (Image courtesy of Michael Ciarmiello.)

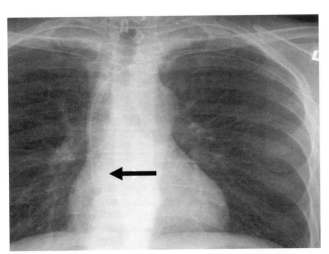

**FIGURE 22-2** A single frontal x-ray of the chest demonstrating a left-sided peripherally inserted central catheter (PICC) placed under ultrasound guidance with the tip of the PICC at the right atrium (RA)–SVC junction (*arrow*).

## Nontunneled Central Vascular Access Devices

Nontunneled central VADs are placed percutaneously into a central or peripheral vein, with the device's tip residing at the atriocaval junction or distal third of the SVC. These devices include critical care catheters, temporary dialysis and apheresis catheters, small bore polyurethane or silicone catheters, and peripherally inserted central catheters (PICCs). They may have one to five lumens, depending on the patient's infusion needs. Nontunneled VADs are secured at the puncture site with sutures, subcutaneous securement devices, or adhesive securement devices. They are typically used for patients requiring access for days to weeks, though they may remain in place longer if needed.

## Tunneled Central Vascular Access Devices

Tunneled VADs are placed via a central vein with their tip residing at the atriocaval junction or in the distal third of the SVC. These devices differ from the devices listed in the previous section because they are tunneled under the skin to an exit site, typically located several centimeters from the puncture site into the vein. The tunnel helps to provide stability for the device and reduces the risk of device-related infection. These devices are often more comfortable for the patient because the exit site is not in the neck or clavicle area and may be hidden for cosmetic reasons. Tunneled VADs may be used for infusions and long-term dialysis or apheresis. They are available in one to three lumen configurations and may remain in place for years.

## Implanted Ports

Implanted ports are VADs with a catheter segment attached to a plastic or titanium reservoir. The entire system is placed under the skin. The reservoir has a silicone septum, which is accessed with a non-coring needle when infusion or sampling is needed. Ports are most often used for patients who require intermittent therapy, such as weekly or monthly treatment. Because the device is under the skin, patients do

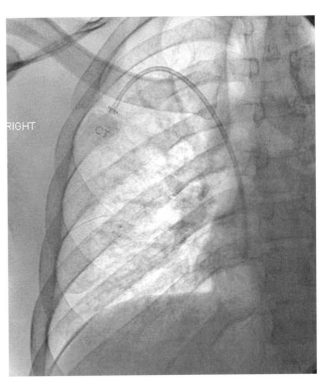

**FIGURE 22-3** A single frontal image obtained during a CT scan showing an implanted port that is compatible with a high-flow contrast injection during that examination. (The letters "CT" seen on the body of the port can confirm this.)

not need to keep a dressing on the site or perform frequent maintenance when not in use. Many implanted ports are now available which will tolerate contrast administration using power injectors. A noncoring needle and extension set which are also approved for power injection must be used in power injectable ports for this purpose (Fig. 22-3).

## PERIPHERAL VAD PLACEMENT

Venous access can be achieved by placing small caliber catheters (also known as peripheral cannulas) via the superficial veins of the upper and lower extremities. Use of the upper extremities is by far more common, with lower extremity access typically limited to use in infants and patients with few access site options. The basilic vein is the dominant superficial vein of the upper extremity and is located on the medial aspect. With a blood flow of approximately 80 mL/min, it is the vein of first choice for placement of PICCs. The basilic vein drains directly into the axillary vein, which becomes the SCV as it enters the chest. The brachial veins are also located medially in the upper extremity and are paired veins in close proximity to the brachial artery. Typically smaller than the basilic vein, they are a good choice for initial access as well. Their location adjacent to the brachial artery imparts a higher risk of inadvertent arterial puncture than other upper extremity veins. The cephalic vein is the smallest of the named upper extremity veins with a blood flow of approximately 30 mL/min and is thus the least preferred choice for VAD placement. It is positioned more laterally on the arm, making it easy to access. It joins the SCV just past the shoulder.

Lower extremity veins such as the saphenous vein or veins of the feet may be used when there are no suitable upper extremity veins for access. This is more common in neonates and children. While many peripheral veins are palpable and visible, ultrasound has been proven useful in achieving initial access and in reducing nontarget puncture-related complications.

Use of peripheral cannulas should be limited to very short-term therapy (less than 1 week). Peripheral cannulas are changed on an as needed basis. Assessment of the site for erythema, edema, and patency are basic tenets of management. Only infusates that are nonirritating and lack vesicant properties should be administered via peripheral cannulas.

## CENTRAL VAD PLACEMENT

The most common sites for central venous access are the IJVs and the SCVs. The IJVs are relatively superficial, facilitating assessment and cannulation. The right IJV approach is preferred over the left because it has a straighter course to the heart, making the procedure technically easier. In close proximity to the IJVs are the smaller external and anterior jugular veins, which drain blood from the face and neck. The external jugular veins are superficial and often tortuous. They join the IJV at the confluence of the SCVs and brachiocephalic veins. Because of their size, they are not preferred for central venous access and are more often used in the setting of IJV occlusion.

## SONOGRAPHIC EXAMINATION TECHNIQUES

Ultrasound allows anatomical assessment of the IJV prior to the procedure as well as dynamic guidance during vein puncture. The IJV can be cannulated blindly using an anatomical landmark approach, formerly a common method for performing this procedure. However, compared with the landmark method, real-time ultrasound guidance has been shown to be both a quicker and safer way to accomplish this goal. Meta-analysis comparing ultrasound to the landmark approach has demonstrated that the overall success rate, procedure time, and a reduced risk of arterial injury are associated with the use of ultrasound guidance.[3] Two-dimensional ultrasound guidance can reduce failure of catheter placement and complication rates related to insertion by 86% and 57%, respectively.[4] When using ultrasound, it is important to assess the depth of the vessel from the skin, vessel patency, vessel diameter, variations in diameter with respiration, and the relationship of the vein to the common carotid artery (CCA). It is important to identify the CCA prior to attempted cannulation of the IJV. Typically, the IJV is located anterior and lateral to the CCA (Fig. 22-4). However, there are several variations of this relationship that can be encountered. In a prospective evaluation of 869 patients who had undergone real-time ultrasound-guided cannulation of the IJV, five anatomical arrangements of the IJV and CCA were found in 659 patients. In 328 cases (49.8%), the IJV was anterolateral to the CCA, whereas in an additional 146 cases (22.2%), it was lateral to the CCA. In 148 cases (22.5%), the vein lies directly anterior to the artery. In the remaining cases, the IJV was anteromedial to the CCA in 30 cases (4.5%) and directly medial to the artery in seven cases (1.0%).[5]

The SCVs are commonly used to attain central venous access. The SCVs are located in the chest, adjacent to the subclavian arteries. They usually lie directly under the

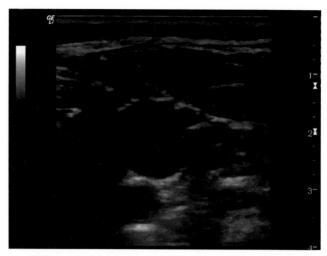

**FIGURE 22-4** The transverse image of the left side of the neck showing both the larger internal jugular vein anterior and slightly lateral to the smaller common carotid artery.

clavicle. Because of this location, they are more difficult to visualize with ultrasound than other target veins. The SCVs are typically large and have historically been used for the placement of nontunneled VADs in critical care medicine. They terminate in the brachiocephalic veins, at the confluence with the IJVs. Ultimately, the right and left brachiocephalic veins join to form the SVC. Neither the SCVs nor the upper extremity veins should be utilized for cannulation in patients with chronic renal insufficiency or chronic kidney disease. Because use of these veins for VAD placement may be associated with thrombus and stenosis, avoidance of these veins preserves them for use for permanent access for hemodialysis (arteriovenous fistula or graft formation) in the future.[6]

The common femoral veins (CFVs) are located in the groin, medial to the common femoral artery. The CFVs drain blood from the lower extremities into the external iliac veins. These ultimately become the common iliac veins, which join to form the inferior vena cava. The CFVs are most often used for central venous access in emergent situations and in patients in whom other potential access veins are occluded. VAD placement via the CFV is associated with a higher rate of mechanical and infectious complications and therefore should be avoided unless other access sites are not available or the patient's clinical condition precludes placement elsewhere.

### Scanning Technique

Ultrasound imaging is used to both assess potential access sites for VAD placement and guide the initial needle puncture into the access site. Initial assessment includes evaluation of available patent vessels, their location in relation to other structures (arteries, other implanted devices, etc.), and the ability to access the target. The specific target vein is assessed for size and patency. A stenotic (or scarred) vein will appear smaller than expected. Patency is determined by a test of vessel compressibility, similar to that used in the assessment of a patient for deep venous thrombosis. Gentle pressure is applied on the skin overlying the vein using the transducer. A patent vein should compress easily

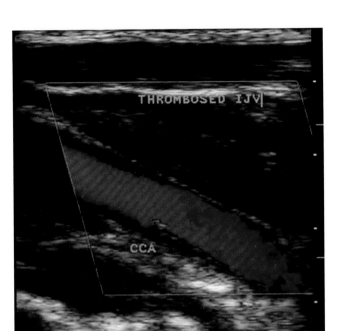

**FIGURE 22-5** The longitudinal image of the neck showing a noncompressible, thrombosed internal jugular vein and its relationship to the common carotid artery.

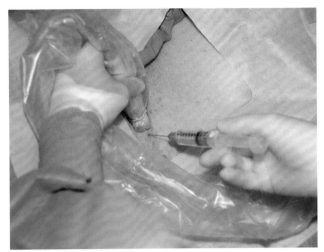

**FIGURE 22-6** A single image during VAD placement showing the longitudinal approach to venous access.

under pressure and re-expand once pressure is released. A thrombosed vein will not compress using this technique; and in addition, its lumen will appear more echogenic than that of a patent vein (Fig. 22-5). In comparison, compression of an artery will result in less reduction of vessel diameter, and pulsation will be visible. Clearly differentiating venous from arterial vessels is a key factor in reducing the risk of inadvertent arterial puncture. Vessel caliber should also be assessed using ultrasound. The target vein must be of adequate diameter to accommodate the selected VAD, so that complete occlusion of the vein can be avoided.

Ultrasound guidance is used to guide the initial needle puncture into the target vessel. Once the patient is positioned, the skin is prepped with antiseptic solution, and sterile barrier drapes are applied. The skin is anesthetized with a local anesthetic. Additionally, systemic sedation or anesthesia may be used depending on the type of device placed and the patient's overall clinical condition. Sterile ultrasound gel is then applied to the skin overlying the target vessel. A sterile sheath is used to cover the transducer. The ultrasound probe is positioned on the patient's skin in either a longitudinal or transverse position, depending on the preference of the clinician (Fig. 22-6). A needle guide may be attached to the probe depending on clinician preference as well. The depth of the ultrasound image is adjusted to accommodate for the size of the target vessel and its depth below the skin. Typically, a small (21 g) hyperechoic needle is used to attain access. The needle should be visualized once it enters the skin, as it approaches the target vessel, and as a successful puncture has been attained. Confirmation of successful access is noted by flashback of blood in the needle hub or by aspiration for blood return with an attached syringe. Upon confirmation of accurate access, a small guidewire is advanced into the target vessel. A small skin incision is typically performed to allow the VAD to

pass through the skin with minimal resistance. The needle is exchanged for a small venous sheath. Smaller VADs may be advanced into position directly through this sheath. Larger, guiding wires are often inserted for placement of larger VADs. Some VADs may be advanced directly over these wires, while others are advanced through a larger sheath following a series of exchange maneuvers. Once the VAD is in place, confirmation of appropriate tip placement is made with fluoroscopy or chest x-ray. On ultrasound, the VAD is easily observed within the vein producing a parallel hyperechoic linear structure (Fig. 22-7).

## Technical Considerations

Complications associated with central venous access device placement include vein damage, nontarget puncture, bleeding, air embolism, and cardiac arrhythmias (Pathology Box 22-1). Each can be minimized with careful assessment of the target vein coupled with ultrasound guidance to attain access. Expert placement of VADs, along with minimizing additional venous interventions, serves to reduce and

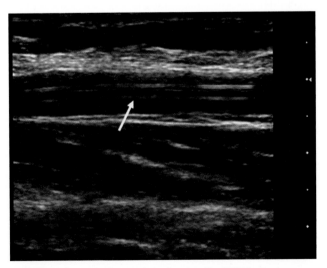

**FIGURE 22-7** A sagittal image of a basilic vein with a PICC line in place (*arrow*).

**PATHOLOGY BOX 22-1**
*Complications Associated with VAD Placement*

| Complication | Ultrasound Appearance |
|---|---|
| Vein damage | Irregular intimal surface<br>Anechoic to hypoechoic area indicating extravascular accumulation of blood<br>Arteriovenous fistula with flow evident between vein and companion artery on color or spectral Doppler |
| Nontarget puncture | Anechoic to hypoechoic area indicating extravascular accumulation of blood<br>Expanding hematoma indicated by enlarging extravascular mass |
| Bleeding | Anechoic to hypoechoic area indicating extravascular accumulation of blood; may be diffuse within tissue |
| Air embolism | Rounded hyperechoic structure in blood stream producing an acoustic shadow |
| Cardiac arrhythmia | Uneven, irregularly spaced cardiac cycles displayed on arterial spectral analysis |

preserve access sites for future use. Consideration should be given to assessment of a patient's access needs early in the patient's entry into the health care system. If the correct vascular access is placed in the right location early in the patient's therapy, other potential access sites are preserved. It should be noted that the presence of collateral veins does not constitute a neovascularization process. Rather, collateral veins are small veins that have enlarged to divert venous flow in the presence of a stenosis or thrombosis. Their presence on physical exam or ultrasound assessment should alert the clinician to potential difficulties in successfully placing a VAD.

### Vein Damage

Vein damage occurs each time a vein is accessed, whether for sampling purposes or for placement of a VAD. Veins are composed of three layers—the intima, the media, and the adventitia. The innermost lining of the vein is the intima, composed of a single layer of endothelial cells. Each time a vein is accessed, this layer is disrupted. This disrupted surface allows platelets to adhere to its surface, beginning the clotting cascade. An arterial venous fistula is another form of vein damage that can occur with device placement. This is most likely to occur when the initial needle is placed through both walls of the vein into a neighboring artery. When recognized, the device should be removed and pressure applied to the site. An arteriovenous fistula may close on its own or may require intervention to close.

### Nontarget Puncture

Nontarget puncture occurs when the access needle is directed to a neighboring structure such as an artery or lung. Careful identification and differentiation of arteries from veins prior to and during initial puncture will minimize the likelihood of inadvertent arterial puncture. Use of a small

access needle will minimize the risk of bleeding, should non-target puncture occur. In the event of arterial puncture, the needle should be immediately removed and gentle pressure should be applied to achieve hemostasis. A sterile occlusive dressing should be applied once hemostasis is achieved, and the patient's vital signs should be monitored. The site should be assessed frequently for an expanding hematoma, which could compromise venous blood flow or respiratory status, particularly with carotid artery puncture. Inadvertent puncture of the lung may result in pneumothorax or a collapsed lung. Pneumothorax is one of the most serious and potentially life-threatening complications of central venous catheterization. The complication rate varies from 0% to 6% but has been reported as high as 12.4% with inexperienced practitioners.[7] Pneumothorax accounts for 25% to 30% of all reported complications of central vein catheter insertion.[8,9] The IJV approach has been shown to have a lower risk of pneumothorax compared to SCV cannulation.[10-12] The failure of the first attempt at catheter insertion is also associated with a significant increase in pneumothorax risk. A small pneumothorax can be treated conservatively with observation. If the patient is symptomatic or the pneumothorax enlarges, placement of a pleural drainage catheter may be required.

### Bleeding

Bleeding with or following VAD placement may occur because of traumatic or difficult VAD insertion, comorbid conditions such as a coagulopathy or other hematologic disorder, and concurrent treatment with certain medications. Medications that increase the likelihood of bleeding include clopidrogel, warfarin, aspirin, other nonsteroidal anti-inflammatory drugs, and heparin. When possible, these medications may be discontinued prior to device placement. If discontinuation is not clinically feasible, other measures can be taken to reduce bleeding risk. These include the use of hemostatic dressing materials, change in VAD selection to a less invasive device, and administration of blood components or reversal agents.

### Air Embolism

Air embolism during central VAD placement occurs when air enters the venous system via the needle, sheath, or device. Although unusual, it is a serious complication that can result in respiratory compromise and even death. The risk of air embolism can be minimized by utilizing valved sheaths; performing exchange maneuvers efficiently; and assuring that catheter lumens are flushed, secured, and locked. If the patient is symptomatic, the patient should be treated symptomatically with oxygen and supportive care. Air emboli are not often seen within the target vessel because these emboli move quickly within the blood stream.

### Cardiac Arrhythmias

Cardiac arrhythmias during VAD placement typically occur when guidewires are advanced into the heart, triggering the heart's conduction system. This is often transient, and patients are often asymptomatic. In the absence of symptoms, arrhythmias are detected using intraprocedure cardiac monitoring.

## SUMMARY

- Ultrasound imaging has allowed clinicians to improve assessment and decision making prior to device placement by helping identify target vessels and determining their suitability for use.
- Coupled with optimal device selection and development of an infusion plan, ultrasound imaging is an integral component of access planning and placement.
- Real-time ultrasound imaging helps minimize placement complications by allowing the clinician to visualize venous access, avoid neighboring structures, and guide devices into position.
- Once thought to be a useful tool for access limited or challenging patients, ultrasound imaging is now the standard of practice for central VAD placement.

## CRITICAL THINKING QUESTIONS

1. While examining the subclavian vein of a patient with a peripherally inserted central vein access device, you notice the bright acoustic reflections of the catheter within the vein. A colleague who is observing the ultrasound asks whether that is the catheter tip. What is your answer?
2. You are assisting during the placement of a central venous line via the IJV. Following the procedure, a hematoma is observed in the area of the puncture. Is this a normal occurrence and what could be done next?

## MEDIA MENU

Student Resources available on the**Point**® include:
- Audio glossary
- Interactive question bank
- Videos
- Internet resource

## REFERENCES

1. Rothschild JM. Ultrasound Guidance of Central Vein Catheterization. 2001. Available at: http://www.ahrq.gov/clinic/ptsafety/chap21.htm. Accessed June 4, 2007.
2. Making Health Care Safer: A Critical Analysis of Patient Safety Practices. 2001. Available at: https://archive.ahrq.gov/clinic/ptsafety/. Accessed June 4, 2007.
3. Bowdle A. Vascular complications of central venous catheter placement: evidence-based methods for prevention and treatment. *J Cardiothorac Vasc Anesth*. 2014;28:358–368.
4. Lameris JS, Post PJ, Zonderland HM. Percutaneous placement of Hickman catheters: comparison of sonographically guided and blind techniques. *AJR Am J Roentgenol*. 1990;155(5):1097–1099.
5. Gordon AC, Saliken JC, Johns D, et al. US-guided puncture of the internal jugular vein: complications and anatomic considerations. *J Vasc Interv Radiol*. 1998;9:333–338.
6. National Kidney Foundation Kidney Disease Outcomes Quality Initiative. Clinical Practice Guidelines and Recommendations: Vascular Access. 2006. Available at: http://www.kidney.org/professionals/kdoqi/guideline_uphd_pd_va/index.htm. Accessed May 5, 2017.
7. Seneff MG. Central venous catheters. In: Rippe JM, Irwin RS, Alpert JS, et al, eds. *Intensive Care Medicine*. 2nd ed. Boston, MA: Little Brown and Co; 1991:17–37.
8. Sofocleous CT, Schur I, Cooper SG, et al. Sonographically guided placement of peripherally inserted central venous catheters: review of 355 procedures. *AJR Am J Roentgenol*. 1998;170:1613–1616.
9. Funaki B. Central venous access: a primer for the diagnostic radiologist. *AJR Am J Roentgenol*. 2002;179:309–318.
10. Lefrant JY, Muller L, De La Coussaye JE. Risk factors of failure and immediate complication of subclavian vein catheterization in critically ill patients. *Intensive Care Med*. 2002;28:1036–1041.
11. Chimochowski GE, Worley E, Rutherford WE, et al. Superiority of the internal jugular over the subclavian access for temporary dialysis. *Nephron*. 1990;54:154–161.
12. McGee DC, Gould MK. Preventing complications of central venous catheterization. *N Engl J Med*. 2003;348:1123–1133.

# PART SIX

# ABDOMINAL

# Aorta and Iliac Arteries

KATHLEEN A. CARTER  |  JENIFER F. KIDD

## CHAPTER 23

## OBJECTIVES

- Identify the characteristics of a complete aortoiliac duplex imaging examination
- Define aortic and iliac aneurysms
- Describe the importance of orthogonal orientation in the measurement of aneurysms
- Identify three key characteristics that should be evaluated when assessing iliac stents
- List three frequent complications associated with aortic endograft repair (EVAR)
- List four types of endoleaks and their frequency

## GLOSSARY

**aneurysm**  A localized dilatation of the wall of an artery

**endoleak**  The continued blood flow into an excluded aneurysm after endovascular placement of a stent graft

**endovascular aneurysm repair**  A form of minimally invasive surgery in which a stent graft is placed inside an aneurysm, providing a new channel for blood flow and excluding flow from the dilated walls of an artery

**fusiform**  Elongated, spindle-shaped

**saccular**  A sac-like or pouch-like bulging

**stent**  A tube-like structure placed inside a blood vessel to provide patency and support

## KEY TERMS

**aneurysm**

**aortoiliac**

**aortoiliac disease**

**atherosclerosis**

**endoleak**

**endovascular aneurysm repair (EVAR)**

**fusiform**

**iliac stent**

**long-term surveillance**

**saccular**

Color duplex ultrasonography (CDU) can be an important modality for the diagnosis and postintervention follow-up of pathology in the aorta and iliac arteries. Ultrasound has been used for many years to detect and follow the presence of abdominal aortic aneurysm (AAA).[1] The first use of ultrasound to demonstrate the size of an AAA was reported in 1961 by Donald and Brown.[2] Studies have also shown excellent correlation of ultrasound with arteriography in the detection of aortoiliac atherosclerotic disease.[3,4] CDU provides both anatomic and physiologic information, is noninvasive, nontoxic, and well tolerated by patients. It allows the examiner to make both qualitative and quantitative assessment of blood flow using a combination of pulsed wave and color Doppler.

Ultrasound can rapidly differentiate aortic aneurysmal disease from tortuosity, adjacent visceral aneurysms, or retroperitoneal lymphadenopathy.[5] The incidence of AAA in the United States population is 60/1,000.[6] It is the 13th leading cause of death with approximately 15,000 deaths from ruptured aortic aneurysms in the United States annually.[7] AAA occurs with more frequency in older men and is found most often inferior to the renal arteries. Aortic aneurysms are commonly associated with iliac, femoral, and popliteal aneurysms, with some reports of almost a 20% incidence of associated popliteal aneurysms.[8] The most common abnormality of the iliac arteries noted on ultrasound is aneurysmal dilatation with an incidence one-tenth as common as aneurysms of the aorta.[9,10]

# SONOGRAPHIC EXAMINATION TECHNIQUES

A complete aortoiliac duplex ultrasound or a limited aortoiliac duplex ultrasound is performed based on the indication for the study and whether the examination is conducted pre- or postintervention. Indications for aortoiliac duplex ultrasound include pulsatile abdominal mass, suspected or known aortic or iliac aneurysm disease, claudication (usually of the hip or buttock areas) that interferes with the patient's occupation or lifestyle, ischemic rest pain, decreased femoral pulses, abdominal bruit, and emboli in ischemic digits (also known as blue toe syndrome). Additionally, duplex may be performed following lower extremity physiologic studies indicating inflow disease, after intervention (postangioplasty or poststent evaluation) or as follow-up to iliac revascularization.

## Patient Preparation

Patients should fast overnight (8 to 12 hours) to minimize the amount of scatter and attenuation from bowel gas. Medication or bowel prep is usually not necessary. Patients can take morning medications with water. Gum chewing or smoking in the morning of the examination is discouraged because this may increase the swallowing of air that could further obscure the field of view. The procedure and its length should be explained to the patient.

## Patient Positioning

The patient should be supine in a comfortable position with the head elevated. The examiner should be seated comfortably slightly higher than the patient with the scanning arm supported. In patients with large abdominal girth, it may sometimes be necessary for the sonographer to push on the abdomen to bring the aorta and iliac arteries into better view. Considerable transducer pressure on the abdomen can help displace abdominal contents and bowel gas without too much discomfort to the patient. When using this technique, inform the patient and request that they report if there is any discomfort. In addition, it is ergonomically important that the examiner's shoulder be positioned over the transducer to allow the examiner's body weight to help push, rather than to put strain on the arm or elbow. It is often helpful to place the patient in a lateral decubitus view when an anterioposterior approach is obscured by abdominal contents, bowel gas, or scar tissue.

## Equipment

High-resolution ultrasound equipment utilizing robust color flow and spectral Doppler capability is necessary for good assessment of the aortoiliac segments deep in the abdomen. The system must have the penetration ability to clearly image deep vessels and structures with good tissue differentiation as well as adequate color Doppler sensitivity. Low-frequency transducers with imaging and Doppler carrier frequencies ranging from 1 to 5 MHz are utilized most often. Curved linear transducers are best for optimum resolution. However, based on patient girth and condition, the sector transducers with frequencies of 1 to 4 MHz can be used. Additionally, gel, wipes, and hardcopy worksheet documentation supplies are needed. Images obtained throughout the study are stored on the hard drive and transferred to appropriate digital format at completion of examination.

## Scanning Technique

### AAA Protocol

When an ultrasound study is performed for assessment of AAA, subdiaphragmatic aorta and the common iliac arteries (CIAs) are evaluated. Beginning at the level of the celiac axis and extending to the femoral bifurcation, examine the aorta and iliac arteries with B-mode in both transverse and sagittal planes. The iliac arteries are usually easier to follow in a longitudinal plane. The normal aorta lies immediately adjacent to the spine, has smooth margins, has no focal dilatation, and tapers toward the terminal aorta at the level of the umbilicus (Fig. 23-1). Transverse images with diameter measurements are documented from the proximal aorta (near the diaphragm), mid aorta (near the renal arteries), and distal aorta above the bifurcation of the iliac arteries. The diameter measurements may include both anterior to posterior (AP) wall measurement and left to right lateral wall measurements; however, it is the AP measurement that is most reliable. The lateral wall edges are subject to acoustic dropout and thus less accurate (Fig. 23-2). Measurements of

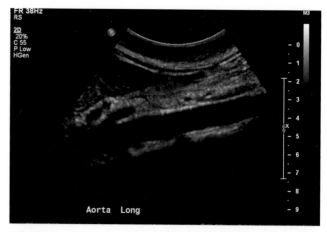

**FIGURE 23-1**  Longitudinal view of normal tapering aorta.

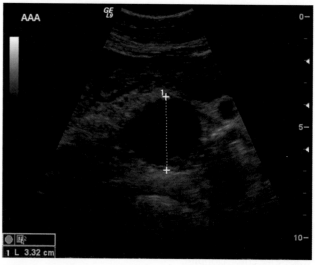

**FIGURE 23-2**  Transverse view of the aorta with an AP diameter measurement.

the proximal CIA are also documented. Longitudinal images with AP diameter measurements are taken from the outer wall to outer wall of the aorta, taking care that the measurements are perpendicular to the long axis of the aorta (Fig. 23-3).[11] This is particularly important in those patients with angulation of the aortic neck. Angulation can occur because the aorta enlarges in diameter, when it often elongates. This elongation results in angulation of the proximal neck, with larger diameter aneurysms having more angulated necks.[12] Studies comparing three-dimensional (3-D) computed tomography (CT) reconstruction with ultrasound have shown that both allow for the assessment of the aorta in the orthogonal plane and avoid oblique cuts caused by aortic neck angulation that would overestimate the diameter.[13] Because the decisions for management of AAAs depend on precise determination of aneurysm size, it is critically important that the sonographer makes sure that the transducer is orthogonal or perpendicular to the aorta itself, not necessarily transverse or parallel to the long axis of the body. In addition to aortic measurements, in the presence of a focal aneurysm, it is important to note its length, its proximity to the renal arteries, and the presence and extent of any intraluminal thrombus. The presence of thrombus, residual lumen, dissection, flaps, pseudoaneurysms, wall defects, stenoses, and/or occlusion is documented. When plaque is encountered, characterize the plaque as to its echogenicity and presence of calcification.

Additional segmental Doppler sampling of velocities along the course of the aorta and iliac arteries will reveal any concurrent atherosclerotic disease of hemodynamic significance. All spectral Doppler waveforms are collected maintaining an angle of 60° or less, parallel to the wall and with the sample volume placed in the center stream of the vessel. This often requires manipulation of the transducer to avoid angles greater than 60°. The peak systolic velocity (PSV) should be recorded from the proximal, mid, and distal aorta as well as from each CIA.

### Preintervention Aortoiliac Protocol

The increasing use of endovascular therapy has changed the role of the vascular laboratory in many centers. In addition to having a diagnostic role, the vascular laboratory is often used today to assist in determining what type of treatment the patient may undergo. The scope of the stenoses and disease identified should be noted. This careful duplex assessment can determine whether the disease is focal or diffuse; determine the location, length, and severity of lesions; and, with good visualization, can assist in determining residual diameters. Whether the disease is present proximal or distal to the inguinal ligament is an important differentiation in the management of patients with lower extremity ischemia. In addition, duplex ultrasound can determine the important distinction between severely stenotic iliac lesions from occlusion. This data will aid the physician in planning potential angioplasty/stent procedures and help determine what type of intervention will be appropriate for the patient.

When the duplex ultrasound is performed preintervention for atherosclerotic disease, symptoms of claudication, follow-up to known stenosis, or based on a positive physiologic exam, a comprehensive study is done. The general techniques described for AAA evaluation are utilized for the preintervention evaluation. A combination of transverse and longitudinal views should be employed. The study should include the entire aorta (proximal, mid, and distal); visceral vessel origins (celiac, superior mesenteric artery, inferior mesenteric artery [IMA], and renal artery origins); proximal, mid, and distal CIAs; proximal, mid, and distal external iliac arteries (EIAs); internal iliac (hypogastric) arteries; common femoral arteries (CFAs); and the superficial femoral artery (SFA) and profunda femoral artery (PFA) origins. The origin of the internal iliac artery is important to identify as a landmark ending the CIA segment and beginning as the EIA. The internal iliac artery is not always seen in the same plane as the EIA. Diameter measurements and velocities are recorded from each of these segments.

### Postintervention Aortoiliac Protocol

The rationale of following patients after intervention is based on several indications. First, identification and treatment of restenosis prior to complete occlusion may improve patency rates. Second, it is thought that stenoses are technically easier to manage compared to occlusion. Finally, percutaneous angioplasty (PTA) and stent procedures are associated with a significant restenosis rate. The follow-up of aortic and iliac arteries following endovascular intervention requires knowledge of the location and extent of angioplasty treatment area and/or stent placement. The stent structure within the arteries is not always easily visible by B-mode evaluation. Therefore, it is important to know where the stents have been placed to ensure the Doppler cursor is carefully walked throughout the entire length of the stent. The stent should be evaluated for alignment, full deployment, and relationship to the vessel wall (Fig. 23-4). Images of the stent and adjacent vessels should be recorded. As mentioned in the preceding sections, the Doppler angles ideally should be 45° to 60° and always be parallel to the vessel wall in the longitudinal plane when collecting peak systolic and end diastolic waveforms. A limited duplex exam for postintervention patients typically may include assessment of the terminal aorta, CIAs, EIAs, and internal iliac arteries. The assessment can also include the CFA, SFA, and PFA origins, depending on what type of intervention has been done. A general rule of thumb is to image several centimeters above and below any area treated by PTA and/ or stenting as well as a thorough assessment of the treated

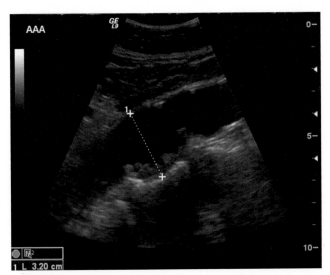

**FIGURE 23-3** Longitudinal view of the aorta with calipers placed perpendicular to the long axis or the aorta.

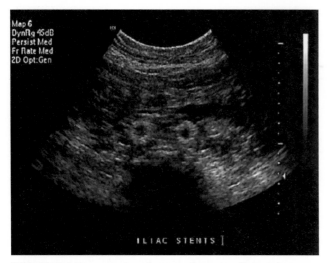

**FIGURE 23-4** Transverse view of common iliac stents with normal stent deployment.

segment(s). The PSV should be documented in the terminal aorta; the proximal, mid, and distal CIAs; proximal internal iliac artery; and proximal, mid, and distal EIAs.

## Technical Considerations

Color-flow imaging is a useful component of aortoiliac ultra-sounds because it assists with vessel localization and aids in following these vessels. Color-flow imaging is especially helpful in assessing the iliac arteries. They are often deep and tortu-ous as they travel within the pelvis. It may be helpful to place patients in a lateral decubitus position in order to evaluate the length of the iliac arteries. Using color-flow imaging in a sagittal view can help obtain properly aligned spectral Doppler waveforms. Care should be taken to adjust the color scale or pulse repetition frequency (PRF) appropriate to the segment being assessed in order to identify areas of increased velocity.

## Pitfalls

Although all abdominal duplex ultrasound examinations have challenges (bowel gas, obesity, and tortuosity of vessels), in most instances the aortoiliac segments can

be adequately assessed using thorough protocols, proper technique, and adequate time allowance. There are certain limitations that may prevent complete evaluation of the aortoiliac segments, such as recent abdominal surgery, open wounds, indwelling abdominal catheters, or pregnancy in the second or third trimester.

## DIAGNOSIS

Normal aortic diameter is usually less than 2 cm and tapers as it courses distally. Aneurysms are usually defined as a focal dilation of the aorta involving all three layers of the aortic wall that exceeds the normal diameter by more than 50%, usually 3 cm or larger. The larger the dilation, the more the risk is for potential rupture. Focal diameter measurements greater than 3 cm are considered to be consistent with AAA. Ectasia is present when there are areas of dilation less than 3 cm or irregular margins and a nontapering profile. Most aortic aneurysms are fusiform (Fig. 23-5A,B) which involve the entire circumference of the affected portions of the aorta, whereas fewer aneurysms are saccular (Fig. 23-6). Saccular aneurysms are asymmetric outpouching dilations and are often caused by trauma or penetrating aortic ulcers.

The iliac artery is also considered to be aneurysmal when the diameter increases by 50% as compared to the adjacent segment. Generally, when the iliac arteries exceeded a diameter of 1.5 cm, they are considered aneurysmal. Iliac aneurysms are usually associated with atherosclerotic disease and are often bilateral. Complications of iliac aneurysms can include rupture, hydronephrosis secondary to compression of the ureter, or even bladder compression in the presence of large bilateral iliac aneurysms.[14]

Thrombus, plaque, and calcification can also be identified within the aortoiliac system and will have the same ultra-sound appearance as observed elsewhere within the vascular system. Plaque may appear heterogeneous or homogeneous with either smooth or irregular borders. Calcification will appear as bright hyperechoic areas that produce an acoustic shadowing. Thrombus is often homogeneous with smooth borders and is found within the sac of the aneurysm.

Wall defects can be encountered within the aorta and iliac arteries. Intimal tears may appear as small isolated defects on the vessel wall where a short piece of the vessel wall is

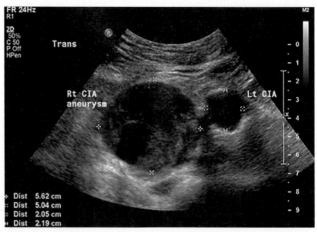

**A**

**B**

**FIGURE 23-5 A:** Transverse image of fusiform aneurysm. **B:** Transverse image of right CIA aneurysm.

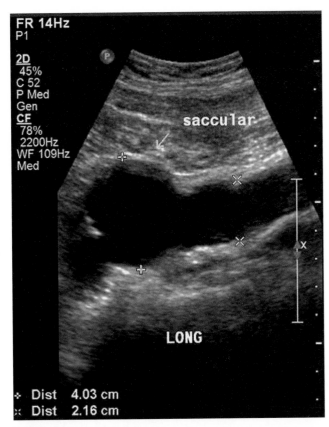

FIGURE 23-6 Longitudinal view of a saccular aneurysm.

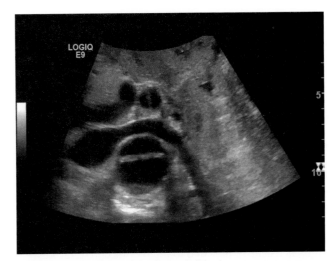

FIGURE 23-7 Transverse view of an aortic dissection.

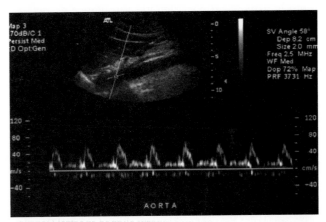

FIGURE 23-8 Lower resistance aortic spectral waveform superior to visceral vessel origins.

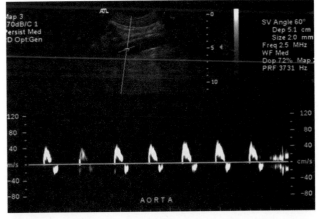

FIGURE 23-9 Spectral waveform of normally high-resistance distal aortic signal.

separated from the remaining wall. This small piece of the wall will protrude into the vessel lumen. Dissections occur when a tear forms between the layers of the wall, usually at the intimal–medial interface and then extends for several centimeters (Fig. 23-7). The initial tear weakens the wall of the aorta, which may enlarge. Existing aneurysms can also dissect. Acute dissections are readily identified by two channels of flow. Chronic dissection may be more challenging to identify when the false lumen has thrombosed and can be confused with stenosis or atherosclerotic disease.

In postinterventional patients, stents should be observed completely expanded to fill the vessel lumen. The walls of the stent should be opposed to the walls of the vessel. The stents should be closely examined to document any irregularities or changes in the shape. The stents should appear circular in transverse view. Elliptical shaped stents may indicate partial stent compression. A kink within a stent may appear as a sharp angulation of the stent walls in an otherwise straight vessel segment.

Hemodynamics in the proximal aorta will have different waveform characteristics than the distal aorta. This is because the proximal aorta supplies the visceral arteries which supply lower resistant vascular beds such as the liver and kidneys. This is reflected in the waveform as shown in Figure 23-8. The distal aorta should be reflective of the higher resistant peripheral vascular bed, which normally has a reverse flow component in early diastole (Fig. 23-9). The hemodynamics in normal iliac segments should also be multiphasic with reversal of flow below the baseline in early diastole, reflective of the normally high-resistant peripheral vascular system.

If a stenosis is identified, it is important to carefully assess throughout the lesion with spectral Doppler and document poststenotic turbulence. When a stent is in place, the spectral Doppler is "walked" through the proximal, mid, and distal ends of the stent. The sonographer should be aware of the location of all the stents to ensure a complete assessment.

The examination is completed with evaluation of the CFA, SFA, and PFA origins. Their accompanying hemodynamics should validate the more proximal findings. For example, severe proximal disease will often result in turbulent or multiphasic to monophasic distal signals (Fig. 23-10A). Be sure to clearly denote any areas not well visualized. This is important because iliac arteries can have focal severe stenoses or occlusions with multiphasic flow distally including the reverse flow component below the baseline if good collateralization is present. If a stenosis is encountered, the PSV of the prestenotic signal prior to the stenosis, the maximum PSV within the stenosis (Fig. 23-10B), and the poststenotic signal should be documented. When a ratio of 2:1 (or 100% increase in velocity) with poststenotic turbulence is documented, there is at least a 50% stenosis present. Care should be taken to remain in the artery of interest because elevated velocities in collateral vessels could be mistaken for stenosis. Tortuosity can also cause elevated velocities. In the absence of a stenosis, however, there is usually no post-stenotic turbulence associated with the elevated velocity. Chronic iliac occlusions can be difficult to identify. The artery can become contracted and echogenic, and differentiation with the surrounding tissue may be challenging. It is helpful to identify and follow the companion vein when chronic occlusion is suspected (Fig. 23-11A,B).

## AORTOILIAC DUPLEX ULTRASOUND FOLLOWING ENDOVASCULAR AORTIC STENT GRAFT REPAIR

The endovascular stent graft repair method of treating AAA has proven to be a much less invasive alternative procedure with lower perioperative mortality compared with conventional open surgical repair.[15] The recovery from this procedure is considerably shorter than with the traditional method, and there is no abdominal incision.

The endovascular aneurysm method of repair (EVAR) involves the placement of a stent graft device within the aortic aneurysm sac via a catheter-based delivery system through small groin incisions into the CFA, and deployment is under angiographic or ultrasound imaging guidance. The goal of this minimally invasive treatment is to achieve

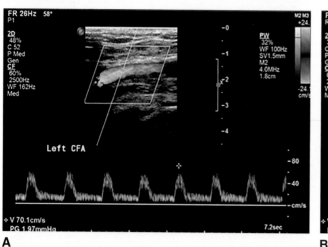

A

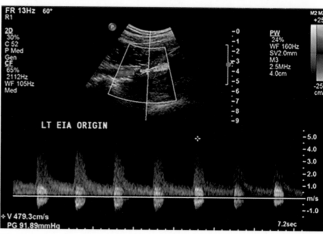

B

**FIGURE 23-10 A:** Abnormal spectral waveform in left CFA distal to the proximal hemodynamically significant stenosis in left EIA. **B:** Left EIA spectral waveform within stenosis with a PSV 479 cm/s.

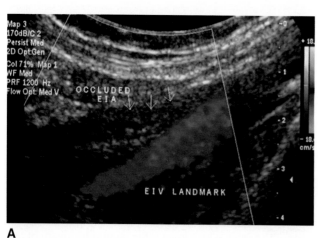

A

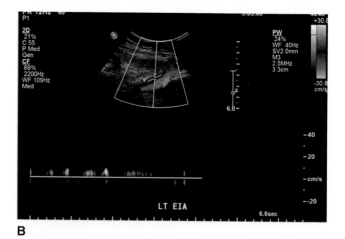

B

**FIGURE 23-11 A:** Identification of iliac vein in the presence of iliac artery occlusion. **B:** Spectral analysis documents iliac artery occlusion.

exclusion of the aneurysm sac from the general circulation, thereby reducing its risk of rupture.[16,17] Failure to isolate the aneurysm from the circulation where persistent blood flow is demonstrated outside the graft lumen but within the aneurysm sac has been defined as "endoleak" and is a common complication associated with many of the commercially available aortic stent graft devices.[18–20] Close surveillance, therefore, is mandatory after EVAR because rupture is still possible if an endoleak is present since the aneurysm continues to be perfused at near systemic arterial pressure. This has been shown to be true even with very small endoleaks. It is long-term surveillance and patient compliance that have become the key issues following the repair of AAAs by the endovascular method. CT angiography and CDU imaging have been the imaging modalities of choice postoperatively to evaluate and monitor stent grafts, either alone or in combination. Studies that have compared CT with CDU in the diagnosis of endoleaks have shown conflicting results. Certain studies suggested that the predictive value of CDU is equal to or higher in detecting and identifying the source of endoleaks,[21–30] whereas others estimated that the sensitivity of CDU is less than that of CT.[31–35] CDU has an important advantage over CTA for the identification of endoleak flow direction because this parameter is difficult to assess by CTA. The disadvantage of the CDU is that the results are influenced by the equipment, examiner, bowel gas, and obesity.

CDU has emerged as a low-cost and low-risk alternative imaging modality that is widely available without the exposure to ionizing radiation as well as the risk of nephrotoxicity in patients with marginal renal function. In many institutions, CDU is now used as a primary method of surveillance post-EVAR, thus allowing CT scanning and aortography to be used more selectively to plan secondary intervention. CDU can accurately monitor the residual aneurysm sac size, demonstrate graft and limb patency,[36] has the ability to identify endoleak and determine the leak source, detect graft limb dysfunction and kinking, and in some cases, migration of the stent graft device. It can provide the examiner with hemodynamic information that is not available with other imaging modalities.[24,25,37–39] Other complications associated with the procedural graft deployment that can cause iatrogenic injury because of the use of large bore catheters in the groin include arteriovenous fistula, hematoma, intimal flaps, dissection, or pseudoaneurysm.

## EVAR Devices

Prior to commencing the examination, it is important for the examiner to have a good working knowledge and understanding of the endovascular technique as well as the aortic stent graft designs and configurations that are currently available. The examiner should have the relevant patient information about what type of endograft device has been deployed and details of the operative procedure performed.

There are three basic types of aortic stent grafts currently used: bifurcated, straight tube, and uni-iliac grafts. These may be used in conjunction with side branch occluding devices, coil embolization of branch vessels, extension grafts, and femorofemoral crossover grafting. It is, however, the bifurcated modular stent graft that is most frequently

deployed. The examiner should also be aware of the recent development and implantation of fenestrated grafts where there is transrenal or suprarenal aortic endograft fixation with renal artery stenting and or superior mesenteric artery stenting. The examiner will observe the graft material and metal struts extending above the usual position (below the renal arteries), and it is essential to identify renal artery patency after graft deployment to evaluate the technical success of the proximal fixation which could adversely affect renal perfusion. The superior mesenteric and celiac arteries should also be examined to document patency.

## Scanning Technique

The examination is performed with the patient lying in the supine position, and the examiner commences the study using B-mode imaging in the transverse plane identifying the aorta at the level of the celiac axis and superior mesenteric arteries. The reflective metal struts of the aortic stent graft should be identified; and as previously discussed in some grafts, these struts can be visualized above the level of the renal arteries. The proximal extent of the graft fabric is seen as a hyperechoic signal along the anterior and posterior walls of the aortic lumen (Fig. 23-12); it can be visualized just below the level of the renal arteries. This is the proximal attachment or fixation site. If the stent graft is bifurcated or uni-iliac, then the distal attachment or fixation site(s) would be the native CIA or EIA. Often the reflective struts or dilatation of the distal end of the graft limb to the native vessel can be readily observed (Fig. 23-13A,B).

The examiner then uses the caliper measurement on the ultrasound machine to measure the aorta at the level of the renal arteries in the both the anteroposterior and transverse diameters as a baseline for comparison on follow-up studies to assess for possible dilatation of the aneurysm neck. The distance should be measured from landmarks such as the superior mesenteric or renal arteries in the longitudinal plane to the proximal attachment site for detection of possible graft device migration. The assessment should be repeated along the entire length of the aorta, taking maximum orthogonal diameter measurements of the residual aneurysm sac. The

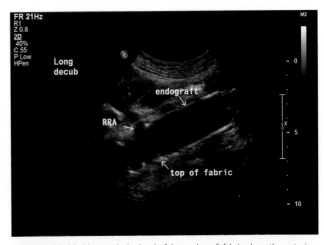

**FIGURE 23-12** Hyperechoic signal of the endograft fabric along the anterior and posterior walls of the aortic lumen.

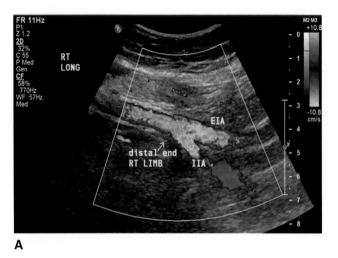

**A**

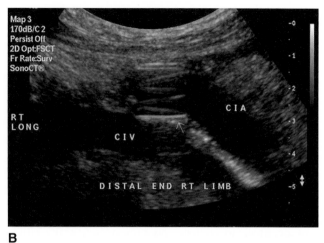

**B**

**FIGURE 23-13  A:** CDI demonstrates distal end of right limb aortic endograft; the graft limb ends just proximal to the internal iliac and external iliac bifurcation. **B:** B-mode image illustrating the reflective struts at the distal end of the right graft limb to the CIA.

vessel axis should be followed with measurements made perpendicular to the aorta accommodating for vessel tortuosity to accurately obtain baseline transverse measurements that will be used for ongoing serial follow-up of the residual sac (Fig. 23-14). The B-mode characteristics of the excluded sac should be noted, paying particular attention to any areas of hypoechogenecity or heterogeneity because these may be associated with an endoleak. Transverse and sagittal views of the distal attachment/fixation site(s) are obtained to identify any evidence of graft kinking or graft limbs that appear crossed because of device rotation during deployment. The additional use of harmonic imaging by the examiner will assist in facilitating the accurate identification of the attachment sites and characterize the thrombus within the sac by improving the overall quality and contrast resolution of the image.

With spectral Doppler, record a PSV measurement in the suprarenal aorta and confirm patency of the renal arteries. For all velocity measurements, the Doppler angle is maintained at 60° or less and the angle cursor is aligned parallel to the vessel wall in the longitudinal approach. Using color and spectral Doppler, the stent graft is assessed from the proximal attachment site throughout the body of the graft and the graft limbs to the distal attachment site(s) looking for any perigraft flow, graft stenosis, thrombosis, or kinking recording waveforms and velocities throughout. It is important to have a small color box to incorporate the entire residual aneurysm sac and to fill the lumen of the graft and graft limbs, thus avoiding excessive artifact (Fig. 23-15). If flow is identified within the sac, it is easier to differentiate between a true endoleak and color artifact from bowel gas or excessive color gain. Any suspected color endoleak should be confirmed with spectral Doppler.

The examination continues distally beyond the distal attachment/fixation site(s) with color and spectral Doppler to assess the patency of the native iliac and femoral arteries. Any complications following endograft placement (i.e., stenosis, occlusion, hematoma, or pseudoaneurysm at access site) should be thoroughly documented.

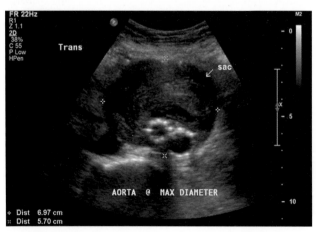

**FIGURE 23-14** Transverse and AP measurements of the residual AAA sac.

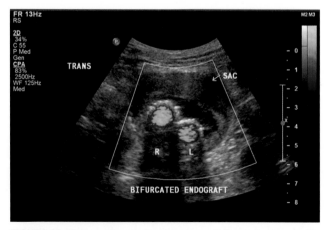

**FIGURE 23-15** Power Doppler imaging of normal bifurcated endograft with color box appropriately placed to include the excluded AAA sac.

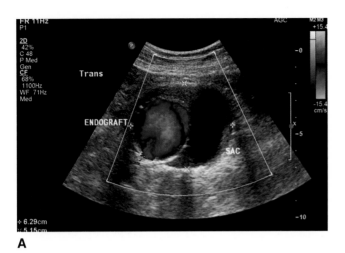

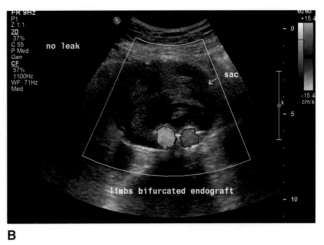

**A**          **B**

**FIGURE 23-16** **A:** Residual AAA sac that appears very heterogeneous in texture ("spongy") with hypoechoic areas. **B:** Unstable sac—hypoechoic areas above bifurcated limbs.

## Diagnosis

Over time, there should be a decrease in the size of the aneurysm sac. However, any increase in the sac size, pulsatility of the sac or areas of echolucency within the sac on B-mode should alert the examiner to probable sac instability (Fig. 23-16A,B). A residual sac that appears very heterogeneous in texture ("spongy") with hypoechoic areas combined with an increase in size or a sac size that has not decreased since the last assessment would suggest impending endograft complication and a possible endoleak.[40]

Flow patterns will normally be multiphasic in the aortic stent graft and outflow vessels of the iliofemoral segment arteries. This is caused by the normally high-resistance lower extremity arterial bed.

It is essential for the examiner to recognize flow patterns associated with perigraft leak and their potential sites (Fig. 23-17). A real leak will have reproducible arterial waveforms with different spectral Doppler characteristics compared to flow within the aortic endograft. The examiner should try to determine the source(s) of the leak and identify the flow direction (i.e., a leak arising from a lumbar artery and exiting via the IMA). Endoleaks may result from an inadequate or ineffective seal at the proximal or distal attachment site (Type I) or an endoleak originating from a branch vessel (Fig. 23-18A-F) resulting in retrograde flow may include the inferior mesenteric, lumbar, accessory renal, or internal iliac arteries (Type II). Both the Type I and II endoleaks are the most common endoleaks observed with implanted EVAR devices now in current use. Less common causes of endoleak are flow from modular disconnection, an inadequate seal at the modular junction or through a defect in the graft fabric (Type III), or flow in the sac caused by graft porosity or microleak (Type IV). Another form of unstable AAA sac where the aneurysm continues to expand because of persistent or recurrent pressurization in the absence of an endoleak has been termed endotension[41] or Type V.[42] Endotension may be from missed low flow in the sac or stagnant endoleak.[43–45] Other theories include intrasac hygroma causing increased pressure and sac enlargement or transudation of fluid through the graft fabric.

The ability for the examiner to recognize B-mode characteristics of an unstable AAA sac and then identify any endoleak may depend on using other diagnostic maneuvers to determine if there is perigraft flow. In some instances, an endoleak may be very subtle or intermittent, and these maneuvers can include changing the position of the patient from supine to left and right decubitus positions, optimizing the color settings by decreasing the color PRF and increasing persistence and gain to assure there is no flow in the residual sac.[46] The additional use of power Doppler can facilitate the detection of low-flow amplitude endoleaks that may course off-axis to the sound beam. This may be seen as an atypical signal on the stent graft wall in the presence of a Type IV endoleak. Pathology Box 23-1 summarizes the various findings with endoleaks.

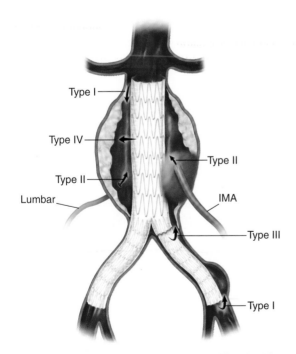

**FIGURE 23-17** Potential sites of perigraft leak diagram (Types I to IV).

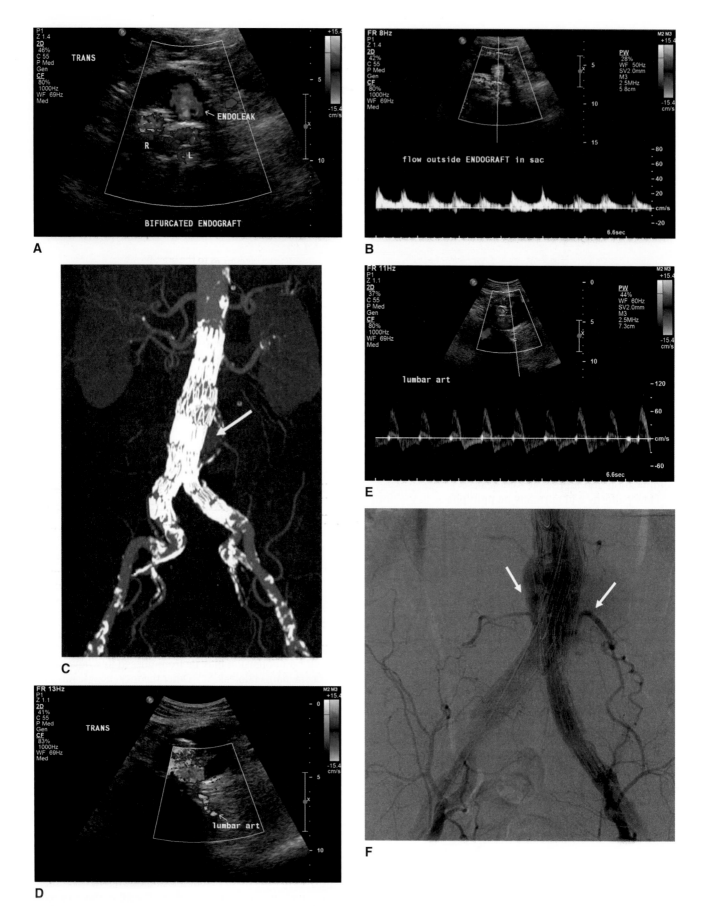

**FIGURE 23-18** **A:** B-mode and color appearance of Type II endoleak. **B:** Spectral waveforms from a Type II endoleak. **C:** Type II endoleak (*arrow*) demonstrated on CT. **D:** Type II endoleak from posterior lumbar artery. **E:** Spectral waveform of Type II endoleak from posterior lumbar artery. **F:** Type II endoleak (*arrows*) from posterior lumbar artery demonstrated on CT.

**PATHOLOGY BOX 23-1**
*Classification of Endoleaks*

| Type | Cause of Perigraft Flow | Usual Hemodynamics |
|------|-------------------------|--------------------|
| I | Inadequate seal at endograft attachment or fixation site(s) | Because the endoleak originates from the graft, the Doppler waveform morphology should be the same as that within the graft. Usually high-flow rates |
| II | Branch vessel flow without communication with attachment site (lumbar, IMA, occasionally accessory renal artery, internal iliac artery) | Can be monophasic or multiphasic but most often is bidirectional. Can be very slow flow or higher flow rates<br>Doppler waveform morphology reflects the end source—for example, a single branch vessel entering the sac will be bidirectional or "to-and-fro"<br>If the flow is entering IMA and exiting lumbar, the waveform morphology would likely be multiphasic reflective of the peripheral vascular bed |
| III | Flow from modular disconnect[a] between segments of the endograft[b]<br>Flow from fabric disruption | Similar waveform morphology as to the graft flow because that is the source<br>Usually high flow |
| IV | Flow from fabric porosity (more than 30 days after placement) | Similar waveform morphology as to the graft flow because that is the source. Can be very subtle and difficult to define |
| **Undefined source** | Flow identified but source undetermined | Varies |
| V | No flow detected continued sac expansion | |

[a]Would only be seen in devices with modular configuration.
[b]These can occur in isolation or in combination with Type II branch vessels.

## SUMMARY

- The long-term outcome of the endovascular method of AAA repair and the durability of the prosthesis is unknown; structural device failure and complications have been reported in the literature.
- Duplex ultrasound imaging with color and power Doppler is an accurate modality to detect early and late endoleak and device complications following endoluminal aortic surgery.
- Duplex ultrasound has emerged as a reliable tool for follow-up surveillance and the diagnostic test of first choice that is cost-effective, noninvasive, and can be repeated without exposure to ionizing radiation.
- Duplex ultrasound, however, is a very operator-dependent and operator-driven modality that requires experience and a sound knowledge of the endovascular technique with standard laboratory imaging protocol and good quality equipment to achieve a thorough and optimal examination.

## CRITICAL THINKING QUESTION

1. You are examining a patient for a follow-up examination of an infrarenal AAA. As you are scanning in transverse,
the AAA appears to be fusiform but is not round but rather ovoid. What can you do to ensure that you are measuring this AAA transverse measurement most accurately?
2. When an increase in velocity is encountered when performing an aortoiliac duplex ultrasound, what are the three most important pieces of information to collect in order to determine whether this is a hemodynamically significant stenosis versus some other reason for increased velocity?
3. "Endoleak" is the term used to describe what complication following endograft implantation in the treatment of AAA?
4. Draw a diagram of an aortic endograft and discuss the potential sites of endoleak the examiner should be aware of.
5. What are the ultrasound features suggestive of graft or sac instability?

## MEDIA MENU

Student Resources available on thePoint® include:
- Audio glossary
- Interactive question bank
- Videos
- Internet resources

# REFERENCES

1. Kohler TR, Nance DR, Cramer MM, et al. Duplex scanning for diagnosis of aortoiliac and femoropopliteal disease: a prospective study. *Circulation.* 1987;5:1074–1080.

2. Donald I, Brown TG. Demonstration of tissue interfaces within the body by ultrasonic echo sounding. *Br J Radiol.* 1961;34:539–546.

3. Yehuda GW, Otis SM, Bernstein EF. Screening for abdominal aortic aneurysm in the vascular laboratory. In: Bernstein EF, ed. *Vascular Diagnosis.* 4th ed. St. Louis, MO: Mosby; 1993:645–651.

4. Currie JC, Jones AJ, Wakeley CJ, et al. Non-invasive aortoiliac assessment. *Eur J Vasc Endovasc Surg.* 1995;9:24–28.

5. Rizzo RJ, Vogelzang RL, Bergan JJ, et al. Use of imaging techniques for aortic evaluation. In: Bergan JJ, Yao JS, eds. *Aortic Surgery.* Philadelphia, PA: W. B. Saunders Company; 1989:48.

6. Melton LK, Bickerstaff LK, Hollier LH, et al. Changing incidence of abdominal aortic aneurysms: a population based study. *Am J Epidemiol.* 1984;120(3):379–386.

7. Kuivaniemi H, Platsoucas CD, Tilson MD. Aortic aneurysms: an immune disease with a strong genetic component. *Circulation.* 2008;117:242–252.

8. Grimm JJ, Wise MM, Meissner MH, et al. The incidence of popliteal artery aneurysms in patients with abdominal aortic aneurysms. *J Vasc Ultrasound.* 2007;31(2):71–73.

9. Gooding GAW. Aneurysms of the abdominal aorta, iliac and femoral arteries. *Semin Ultrasound.* 1982;3(2):170–179.

10. Marcus Redell SL. Sonographic evaluation of iliac artery aneurysms. *Am J Surg.* 1980;140:666–670.

11. American College of Radiology(ACR) Practice Guideline for the Performance of Diagnostic and Screening Ultrasound of the Abdominal Aorta—collaborative with AIUM. 2005 (Resolution 32), Amended 2006 (Resolution 35). Available at: www.acr.org.

12. Veith FJ, Hobson RW, Williams RA, et al, eds. *Vascular Surgery, Principles and Practice.* New York, NY: McGraw Hill Publishers, Inc.; 1994:1250, 372.

13. Sprouse LR, Meier GH III, Parent FN, et al. Is ultrasound more accurate than axial computed tomography for maximal abdominal aortic aneurysm? *Eur J Vasc Endovasc Surg.* 2004;28(1):28–35.

14. Gooding GAW. B mode and duplex examination of the aorta, iliac arteries and portal vein. In: Zweibel WJ, ed. *Introduction to Vascular Ultrasonography.* 2nd ed. San Diego, CA: Harcourt Brace Jovanovich; 1986:433.

15. May J, White GH, Yu W, et al. Concurrent comparison of endoluminal versus open repair in the treatment of abdominal aortic aneurysms: analysis of 303 patients by life table method. *J Vasc Surg.* 1998;27:231–222.

16. Parodi J, Palmaz JC, Barone HD. Transfemoral intraluminal graft implantation for abdominal aortic aneurysms. *Ann Vasc Surg.* 1991;5:491–499.

17. May J, White GH, Harris JP. Endoluminal repair of abdominal aortic aneurysms—state of the art. *Eur J Radiol.* 2001;39:16–21.

18. White GH, Yu W, May J, et al. Endoleak as a complication of endoluminal grafting of AAA: classification, incidence, diagnosis and management. *J Endovasc Surg.* 1997;4:152–168.

19. White GH, May J, Petrasek P, et al. Type III and type IV endoleak: Toward a complete definition of blood flow in the sac after endoluminal repair of AAA. *J Endovasc Surg.* 1998;5:305–309.

20. Buth J, Laheij RFJ, on behalf of EUROSTAR Collaborators. Early complications and endoleaks after endovascular abdominal aortic aneurysm repair: report of a multi-centre study. *J Vasc Surg.* 2001;34:98–105.

21. Heilberger P, Schunn C, Ritter W, et al. Postoperative color flow duplex scanning in aortic endografting. *J Endovasc Surg.* 1997;4(3):262–271.

22. Sato DT, Goff CD, Gregory RT, et al. Endoleak after aortic stent graft repair: diagnosis by color duplex ultrasound scan versus computed tomography scan. *J Vasc Surg.* 1998;28(4):657–663.

23. Thompson MM, Boyle JR, Hartshorn T, et al. Comparison of computed tomography and duplex imaging in assessing aortic morphology following endovascular aneurysm repair. *Br J Surg.* 1998;85(3):346–350.

24. Zannetti S, De Rango P, Parente B. et al. Role of duplex scan in endoleak detection after endoluminal abdominal aortic aneurysm repair. *Eur J Vasc Endovasc Surg.* 2000;19(5):531–535.

25. Wolf YG, Johnson BL, Hill BB, et al. Duplex ultrasound scanning versus computed tomographic angiography for postoperative evaluation of endovascular abdominal aortic aneurysm repair. *J Vasc Surg.* 2000;32(6):1142–1148.

26. Fletcher J, Saker K, Batiste P, et al. Colour Doppler diagnosis of perigraft flow following endovascular repair of abdominal aortic aneurysm. *Int Angiol.* 2000;19(4):326–330.

27. d'Audiffret A, Desgranges P, Kobeiter DH, et al. Follow-up evaluation of endoluminally treated abdominal aortic aneurysms with duplex ultrasonography: validation with computed tomography. *J Vasc Surg.* 2001;33(1):42–50.

28. McLafferty RB, McCrary BS, Mattos MA, et al. The use of color-flow duplex scan for the detection of endoleaks. *J Vasc Surg.* 2002;36(1):100–104.

29. Collins JT, Boros MJ, Combs K. Ultrasound surveillance of endovascular aneurysm repair: a safe modality versus computed tomography. *Ann Vasc Surg.* 2007;21(6):671–675.

30. Schmieder GC, Stout CL, Stokes GK, et al. Endoleak after endovascular aneurysm repair: duplex ultrasound imaging is better than computed tomography at determining the need for intervention. *J Vasc Surg.* 2009;50(5):1012–1017.

31. McWilliams RG, Martin J, White D, et al. Detection of endoleak with enhanced ultrasound imaging: comparison with biphasic computed tomography. *J Endovasc Ther.* 2002;9(2):170–179.

32. Sandford RM, Brown MJ, Fishwick G, et al. Duplex scanning is reliable in the detection of endoleak following endovascular aneurysm repair. *Eur J Vasc Endovasc Surg.* 2006;32:537–531.

33. Raman KG, Missig-Carroll N, Richardson T, et al. Color-flow duplex ultrasound scan versus computed tomographic scan in the surveillance of endovascular aneurysm repair. *J Vasc Surg.* 2003;38(4):645–651.

34. Elkouri S, Panneton JM, Andrews JC, et al. Computed tomography and ultrasound in follow-up of patients after endovascular repair of abdominal aortic aneurysm. *Ann Vasc Surg.* 2004;18(3):271–279.

35. AbuRahma AF, Welch CA, Mullins BB, et al. Computed tomography versus color duplex ultrasound for surveillance of abdominal aortic stent-grafts. *J Endovasc Ther.* 2005;12(5):568–573.

36. Blom AS, Troutman D, Beeman B, et al. Duplex ultrasound imaging to detect limb stenosis or kinking of endovascular device. *J Vasc Surg.* 2012;55(6):1577–1580.

37. Carter KA, Gayle RG, DeMasi RJ, et al. The incidence and natural history of Type 1 and 11 endoleak: a 5 year follow-up assessment with color duplex ultrasound scan. *J Vasc Surg.* 2003;35:595–597.

38. May J, Harris JP, Kidd JF, et al. Imaging modalities for the diagnosis of endoleak. In: Mansour M, Labropoulos N, eds. *Vascular Diagnosis.* Philadelphia, PA: Elsevier Saunders; 2005:407–419.

39. Berdejo GL, Lipsitz E. Ultrasound imaging assessment following endovascular aortic aneurysm repair. In: Zweibel W, Pellerito J, eds. *Introduction to Vascular Ultrasonography.* 5th ed. Philadelphia, PA: Elsevier Saunders; 2005:553–570.

40. Nelms C, Carter K, DeMasi R, et al. Color duplex ultrasound characteristics: Can we predict aortic aneurysm expansion following endovascular repair? *J Vasc Ultrasound.* 2005;29(3):143–146.

41. White GH, May J, Petrasek P, et al. Endotension: an explanation for continued AAA growth after successful endoluminal repair. *J Endovasc Surg.* 1999;(6):308–315.

42. Belchos J, Wheatcroft M, Prabhudesai V, et al. Development of endotension after multiple rounds of thrombolysis after endovascular aneurysm repair. *J Vasc Surg Cases.* 2015;1:24–27.

43. Meier GH, Parker FM, Godziachvili V, et al. Endotension after endovascular aneurysm repair: the Ancure experience. *J Vasc Surg.* 2001;34:421–427.

44. Blackwood S, Mix D, Wingate M, et al. Endotension: net flow through an endoleak determines its visibility. *J Vasc Surg.* 2013;57(5):84S–85S.

45. Yoshitake A, Hachiya T, Itoh T, et al. Nonvisualized type III endoleak masquerading as endotension: a case report. *Ann Vasc Surg.* 2015;29(3):595.

46. Busch K, Kidd JF, White GH, et al. What are the duplex ultrasound signs that characterize an "unstable abdominal aortic aneurysm sac" after endograft implantation? *J Vasc Ultrasound.* 2007;31(3):143–146.

# The Mesenteric Arteries

ANNE M. MUSSON | ROBERT M. ZWOLAK

**CHAPTER 24**

## OBJECTIVES

- Describe typical symptoms of chronic mesenteric ischemia
- List the vessels for which the Intersocietal Accreditation Commission for Vascular Testing requires documentation
- Describe a collateral pathway of blood flow to the hepatic and splenic arteries when the celiac artery is occluded
- Describe the differences in Doppler waveform characteristics between the celiac and superior mesenteric arteries
- Define compensatory flow
- List indications other than chronic mesenteric ischemia for which mesenteric artery duplex ultrasound scanning has clinical utility
- Define median arcuate ligament compression syndrome

## GLOSSARY

**collateral flow** Relating to additional blood vessels that aid or add to circulation

**postprandial** Occurring after a meal

**splanchnic** Relating to or affecting the viscera

**visceral** Relating to internal organs or blood vessels in the abdominal cavity

---

The first case report describing the use of ultrasound in the diagnosis of mesenteric artery disease was published by Jager and associates from the University of Washington in 1984.[1] Subsequently, many researchers reported the use of ultrasound to describe normal splanchnic blood flow and the physiologic response to eating.[2-4] In 1991, two retrospective studies identified duplex ultrasound flow velocities that allowed accurate identification of mesenteric artery stenosis.[5,6] Since then, the mesenteric duplex ultrasound examination has been adopted by many laboratories, and prospective studies as well as additional larger retrospective studies have established the accuracy of the velocity thresholds.[7-10]

Today, the mesenteric duplex ultrasound examination is a widely accepted and accurate test to identify stenosis or occlusion of the mesenteric arteries. This duplex ultrasound scan examines the celiac artery, superior mesenteric artery (SMA), and inferior mesenteric artery (IMA). The typical indications for this examination include patients with suspected chronic mesenteric ischemia (CMI), median arcuate ligament syndrome (MALS), and patients who have undergone prior mesenteric intervention, either stent placement or bypass graft. Less common indications include assessment of visceral artery dissection and aneurysm. The value of the mesenteric duplex ultrasound lies in the ability to help identify those patients who may go on to require initial or repeat percutaneous endovascular intervention or open surgical repair. Duplex ultrasound examination holds an advantage over computed tomographic angiography (CTA) as an early examination in patient evaluation because it is noninvasive, does not involve contrast administration, does not expose the patient to radiation, and is less expensive. Additionally, the duplex ultrasound provides physiologic information about collateral development.

CMI occurs more frequently in women than men (3:1) with a typical age range of 40 to 70 years. Almost all CMI patients are active smokers or have a history of tobacco abuse. The clinical diagnosis of CMI is challenging because the disorder is rare and the most common symptom, abdominal pain, may be due to a vast number of more common abdominal disorders. Thus, CMI is often overlooked for prolonged periods of time because the patient is worked up for malignancy, ulcer, gallbladder disease, and/or psychologic etiologies. One of the challenges of diagnosing CMI is that atherosclerotic stenosis or occlusion of the visceral arteries is not uncommon. In one study, 27% of patients undergoing aortic angiography for evaluation of aortic aneurysm or lower extremity arterial occlusive disease were found to have ≥50% stenosis of either the celiac artery or the SMA.[11] Only a small fraction of patients with mesenteric arterial stenosis, however, develop chronic intestinal ischemia because these arteries are interconnected by a rich collateral network. It is in patients with extensive disease involving two or all three of these vessels that symptoms generally develop and can become life threatening. The importance of evaluating the IMA increases if disease is identified in the celiac artery or SMA. An exception to this multivessel standard is the patient in whom previous abdominal surgery has interrupted the collateral network.

## HISTORY AND PHYSICAL

Obtaining a focused history is especially important in patients with possible mesenteric vascular disease because the examination performed may be modified based on patient history and indication. The most common indication in most laboratories will be assessment of patients for possible CMI. In this setting, the typical patient has postprandial abdominal pain, weight loss, and almost always, a history of smoking. The pain is often referred to as intestinal angina. In effect, eating is the "stress test" for the mesenteric circulation. Similar to the cramping pain in the leg that occurs with exercise, postprandial abdominal pain occurs when there is insufficient visceral blood flow to support the increased oxygen demand required by intestinal motility, secretion, and absorption. Typically, epigastric or periumbilical pain starts approximately 30 minutes after eating and lasts for 1 to 2 hours. Because of the intense severity of the pain, patients often develop sitophobia or "food fear," and limit the size of meals. It is primarily decreased nutritional intake that leads to weight loss rather than malabsorption. Malabsorption causing diarrhea may occur, but is not a consistent feature. Constipation or normal bowel habits may also be present in patients with chronic intestinal ischemia.

Some patients will be sent for this examination with a possible diagnosis of MALS. These patients are younger, and again more likely to be female. The history provided by MALS patients includes months or years of diffuse upper abdominal pain. MALS patients are not necessarily smokers. They are almost all very thin.

Patients may be referred for the mesenteric duplex ultrasound examination as surveillance following mesenteric stenting or bypass surgery. Knowledge of the patient history is important because different diagnostic velocity criteria may be used in patients who have previously undergone mesenteric stent placement or bypass surgery. Finally, obtaining a history of small mesenteric aneurysms or dissections will be extremely important in terms of directing which segments of vessels are evaluated and what measurements are recorded.

There are only a few relevant physical findings for the vascular technologist to look for in patients sent for a mesenteric duplex ultrasound examination. Surgical scars may indicate prior open mesenteric bypass surgery. Patients with an obese abdomen are less likely to have CMI or MALS than those with thin or cachectic body habitus.

## ANATOMY

As with every duplex ultrasound examination, it is important to know the expected anatomy of these arteries (Fig. 24-1) as well as the common variants. The celiac artery is the first abdominal branch arising from the abdominal aorta, and its origin from the anterior aspect of the aorta usually lies 1 to 2 cm below the diaphragm. The celiac artery is short, 2 to 4 cm, branching into the common hepatic and splenic arteries. The SMA typically originates from the anterior surface of the aorta 1 to 2 cm below the celiac. The IMA arises from the distal aorta just proximal to the aortic bifurcation.

The extensive collaterals that enable many patients to remain asymptomatic despite harboring significant occlusive disease are primarily the superior and inferior pancreaticoduodenal arteries (pancreaticoduodenal arcade) that bridge the celiac and SMA. Likewise, the arc of Riolan, or meandering mesenteric artery, provides communication between the inferior artery and SMA. There are additional collaterals between the internal iliac arteries and the IMA.

### Anatomic Variants

Anomalous mesenteric artery anatomy has been reported in approximately 20% of the general population, and this can substantially increase the complexity of a mesenteric duplex ultrasound examination (Table 24-1). Awareness of the possible anomalies facilitates recognition of unusual ultrasound findings. A right hepatic artery originating from an artery other than the celiac is described as a replaced right hepatic artery. This is the most common anomaly, with a prevalence of approximately 17%. Most often, a replaced right hepatic originates from the SMA (approximately 10% to 12%), with the remainder originating from a variety of alternative sites.[12] This finding should be suspected when a low-resistance flow pattern (flow throughout diastole) is found in an otherwise normal appearing proximal SMA. Occasionally, a replaced right hepatic artery may actually be visualized arising from the SMA and arching back toward the liver. The SMA Doppler waveform morphology distal to the take-off of the hepatic artery will revert to the normal high-resistance pattern. Other important mesenteric artery anomalies include the common hepatic artery originating from the SMA, the common hepatic artery originating from the aorta, and a common origin of the celiac artery and SMA (celiacomesenteric artery) from the aorta.

## SONOGRAPHIC EXAMINATION TECHNIQUES

### Patient Preparation

An important difference in this scan from all others performed in the vascular laboratory is that it is essential for the patient to fast for at least 6 hours. The fasting patient typically demonstrates a low-flow, high-resistance SMA Doppler waveform,

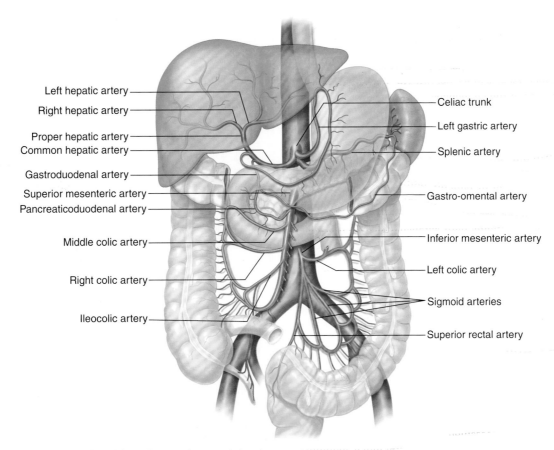

Left hepatic artery

Right hepatic artery

Proper hepatic artery

Common hepatic artery

Gastroduodenal artery

Superior mesenteric artery

Pancreaticoduodenal artery

Middle colic artery

Right colic artery

Ileocolic artery

Celiac trunk

Left gastric artery

Splenic artery

Gastro-omental artery

Inferior mesenteric artery

Left colic artery

Sigmoid arteries

Superior rectal artery

**FIGURE 24-1** The anatomy of the abdominal aorta and mesenteric branches.

| TABLE 24-1 | **Anatomic Variants of the Mesenteric Arteries** |
|---|---|
| **Four Most Common Celiac and Mesenteric Variants** | |
| **Variant** | **% Incidence** |
| Replaced right hepatic originating from the SMA | 10–12 |
| Replaced common hepatic originating from the SMA | 2.5 |
| Common hepatic originating from the aorta | 2 |
| Common origin of the celiac and SMA—celiacomesenteric | <1 |

but this changes to a high-flow, low-resistance pattern after eating. Velocity thresholds for identifying stenosis of the celiac artery and SMA have been established for patients in the fasting state. Typically, the patient is asked not to eat or drink anything starting at midnight and is then scheduled for their duplex ultrasound scan in the early morning to minimize abdominal gas and disruption of the patient's meal and medication cycles. Regular medications can be taken with sips of water. Diabetic patients may need to consult with their primary care provider to alter insulin or other medications appropriately. All patients are asked to refrain from smoking or chewing gum in the morning of the examination. If scanning a nonfasting patient, it is important to state in the report that the standard criteria for determining stenosis do not apply and report only on the patency of the vessels. The results should include an explanation that criteria for stenosis identification in the celiac and SMA are based on data obtained from patients in a fasting state.

## Patient Position

The examination is typically performed with the patient supine. A slight reverse Trendelenburg position or head elevation may be helpful. As with the renal duplex ultrasound scan, low-frequency transducers (2 to 5 MHz) are required, with the frequency range determined by the body habitus of the patient.

## Required Documentation

While details of scanning technique follow, it is important to know exactly what documentation should be collected from each major artery. Current minimum standards established by the Intersocietal Accreditation Commission (IAC) for visceral vascular documentation of the mesenteric arterial system include images and Doppler waveforms of the following vessels:
- Aorta adjacent to visceral vessel origins
- Celiac artery origin
- Common hepatic artery
- SMA origin
- Proximal SMA
- IMA

The Society for Vascular Ultrasound publishes recommended Performance Guidelines. The current document lists the same minimum requirements as the IAC and also suggests including Doppler waveforms from the splenic artery and the mid and distal SMA, in addition to documenting patency of the superior mesenteric vein and inferior vena cava.

## Scanning Technique

The transducer is initially placed just below the xyphoid process for identification of the proximal abdominal aorta (Fig. 24-2). The aorta, celiac, proximal common hepatic, splenic, SMA, and IMA should all be interrogated thoroughly by pulsed Doppler. Spectral waveforms should be recorded. This will require a combination of sagittal and transverse scanning. The Doppler sample volume should be "walked" from the aorta through the origins and into the proximal segments of the major arteries to identify the highest peak systolic velocity (PSV) and end-diastolic velocity (EDV). In the case of a suspected stenosis, care should be taken to document the presence of poststenotic turbulence which serves to confirm a flow-limiting stenosis.

### Celiac, Hepatic, and Splenic Arteries

The celiac artery, from its origin to the bifurcation into common hepatic and splenic arteries, is usually best viewed in a transverse plane. This image of the celiac bifurcation is often referred to as the "seagull sign" (Fig. 24-3). The "wings" of the seagull are formed from the common hepatic artery (coursing toward the liver) and the splenic artery (coursing toward the spleen). The normal celiac artery Doppler waveform has a sharp systolic upstroke and a low-resistance flow pattern characterized by forward flow throughout the cardiac cycle. This Doppler waveform morphology occurs because the celiac artery supplies low-resistance solid organs, the liver and spleen (Fig. 24-4). Careful attention to Doppler angle correction for velocity determination is necessary because these vessels may be very tortuous. It is not unusual for the celiac to have a sharp anterior and superior angulation as it exits from under the crus of the diaphragm. The splenic and common hepatic arteries should also display low-resistance signals with flow throughout the cardiac cycle.

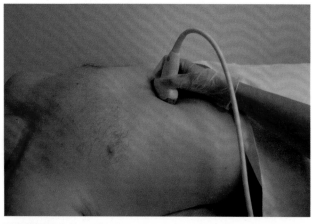

FIGURE 24-2 Photo showing patient, technologist, and transducer position.

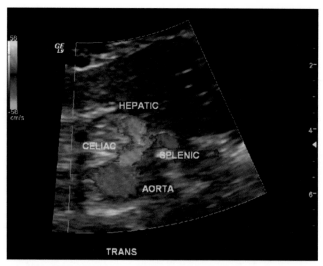

FIGURE 24-3 Color-flow image in transverse showing the origin of the celiac artery and the aorta. The "seagull sign" is formed by the celiac artery bifurcation into the common hepatic and splenic arteries.

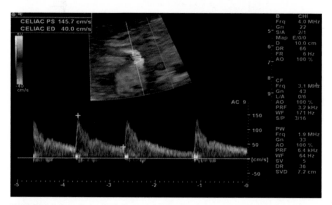

FIGURE 24-4 Color-flow image and Doppler spectral waveform from a normal celiac artery. The flow pattern is typical of a low-resistance vascular bed, with forward flow throughout the cardiac cycle.

### Superior Mesenteric Artery

The SMA is best visualized in a sagittal plane as it courses parallel to the aorta. The normal fasting Doppler waveform has a high-resistance flow pattern (biphasic or triphasic) and little or no flow in the second half of the cardiac cycle. This is similar to the pattern found in the major upper and lower extremity arteries (Fig. 24-5). It is recommended that the SMA be scanned as far distally as possible, obtaining Doppler waveforms from the proximal, middle, and distal segments.

### Inferior Mesenteric Artery

The IMA is most easily identified in a transverse view by locating the aortic bifurcation and then scanning proximally up the distal abdominal aorta for 1 to 3 cm. The IMA usually originates from the anterior aorta slightly to the left of the midline (Fig. 24-6). Normal Doppler waveforms from the IMA resemble those from the fasting SMA, with a high-resistance waveform pattern.

## Test Meal

Researchers have studied the dynamic effects of mesenteric blood flow in normal subjects following a test meal,

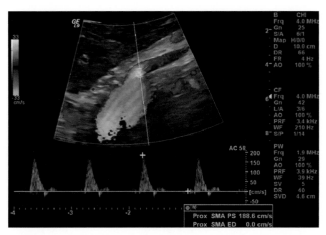

**FIGURE 24-5** Normal high-resistance, triphasic SMA spectral waveform flow pattern in a fasting patient. The color-flow image shows the origin of the SMA in sagittal view. Note the placement of the angle cursor for Doppler angle correction along the curve near the vessel origin.

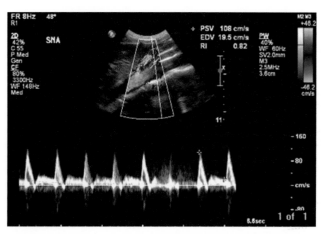

**FIGURE 24-7** Duplex ultrasound image showing the origins of both the celiac artery and SMA in a sagittal view. The pulsed Doppler sample volume is positioned in the SMA, just distal to the origin of the celiac artery. The corresponding SMA spectral waveform shows a normal high-resistance flow pattern.

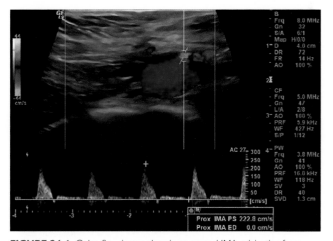

**FIGURE 24-6** Color-flow image showing a normal IMA originating from the anterior distal aorta slightly to the left of midline (usually seen at "1 to 2 o'clock" from the aorta on a transverse image). The spectral waveform shows a high-resistance flow pattern. The angle correction is aligned to the vessel origin.

demonstrating substantial changes in normal SMA flow, with the PSV nearly doubling and the EDV nearly tripling compared to the baseline velocities.[2–4] Gentile et al.[13] studied 80 patients with vascular disease and concluded that adding postprandial duplex ultrasound scanning increased specificity and positive predictive value slightly but did not improve overall accuracy for identification of >70% stenosis. Thus, a test meal may be included on a selective basis but generally is not needed because the elevated fasting velocities provide excellent diagnostic discrimination.

## Technical Considerations

### Positive Vessel Identification/Accurate Angle Determination

Attempts should be made to visualize the origins of both the celiac artery and SMA in the same duplex ultrasound image to confirm the presence of separate origins (Fig. 24-7). This is particularly important when both arteries have elevated

velocities and abnormal Doppler waveforms. This may require rotating the transducer slightly or moving laterally and angling the transducer back toward the midline. Asking the patient to suspend breathing momentarily increases one's ability to capture the Doppler waveform and determine the correct angle. The angulation of the proximal SMA is acute and changes quickly over a short distance. As with other types of arterial spectral Doppler evaluation, waveforms should be collected at angles of ≤60°.

### Use of Color Features: Aliasing, Turbulence, and Flow Direction

A color bruit frequently offers an instant clue to the presence of a significant stenosis. Once observed, inspect thoroughly with spectral Doppler to find the maximum velocity (Fig. 24-8). Close attention should also be given to the Doppler pulse repetition frequency (PRF) and the orientation of the color-scale bar. The PRF scale should be adjusted (usually increasing the frequency range to limit aliasing of the color scale) to more reliably determine flow direction. The color on the top half of the color bar scale is assigned to flow coming

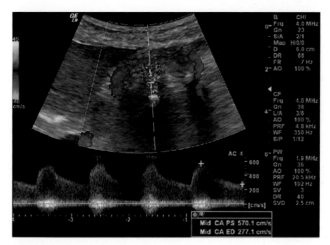

**FIGURE 24-8** Color bruit in a celiac artery. Doppler velocities indicate significant stenosis, with PSV = 570 cm/s and EDV = 277 cm/s.

toward the transducer, whereas the colors on the bottom half represent flow away from the transducer. This feature allows the technologist to identify and track antegrade flow in tortuous vessels and more readily identify retrograde flow. Flow direction becomes particularly important when the celiac artery is occluded or severely stenotic. In this situation, low pressure in the celiac artery induces SMA collaterals to divert blood toward the liver and spleen through the gastroduodenal artery (GDA). The GDA backfills the common hepatic artery such that retrograde flow in the common hepatic crosses the celiac artery origin to perfuse the splenic artery (Figs. 24-9 and 24-10). The finding of retrograde flow direction in the common hepatic artery is always associated with severe celiac artery stenosis or occlusion.[14] Thus, even when the celiac artery cannot be well visualized, the finding of retrograde flow in the common hepatic is significant.

## Turn Color Off: Inspect with B-Mode

Color can mask important features that are well visualized in grayscale. For example, although there are distinct color cues seen in arterial dissections, the thin echogenic line identified by grayscale is a very important piece of the puzzle in diagnosis of dissection (Fig. 24-11). Grayscale imaging is also useful in locating stents, with their brightly echogenic walls (Fig. 24-12). Additionally, we find that observing tortuous vessels in grayscale can assist accurate angle determination.

## Tips for Scanning Patients with Bypass Grafts

Mesenteric bypass grafting remains a durable option for selected patients, including those who have failed stenting or have anatomy unsuitable for stenting. Having access to the operative note may be extremely helpful in guiding the duplex ultrasound scan because there are several different graft configurations. The inflow artery may be the supraceliac aorta, the infrarenal aorta, or the common iliac artery. Likewise, mesenteric bypass grafts can have a single or dual outflow, commonly with distal anastomosis with the

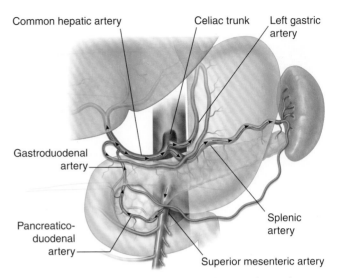

**FIGURE 24-9** When the celiac artery is occluded or severely stenotic, collaterals from the SMA divert blood through the GDA toward the liver and spleen. Retrograde flow in the common hepatic artery fills the splenic artery.

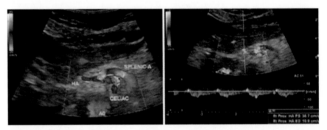

**FIGURE 24-10** Color-flow image (left) and Doppler spectral waveform (right) illustrating the importance of color scale and PRF. The pulsed Doppler sample volume is positioned in the common hepatic artery, and both the spectral waveform and color-flow (*blue*) image indicate flow away from the transducer. This represents retrograde collateral flow in the common hepatic artery and antegrade flow (*red*) into the splenic artery.

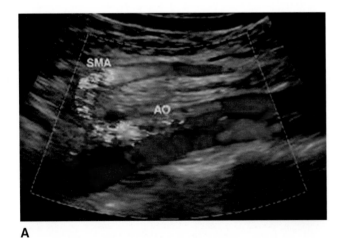

**A**

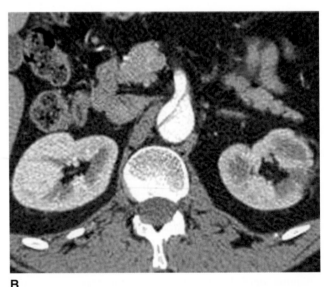

**B**

**FIGURE 24-11** Color flow abnormalities with definite separation of *red* and *blue* channels is classic for dissection. Dissections of the visceral arteries frequently start in the aorta. **A:** Color image of an aortic dissection extending into the SMA with associated turbulence. **B:** CT image showing the echogenic line produced by the dissection, a feature that can also be seen in a grayscale image of the aorta.

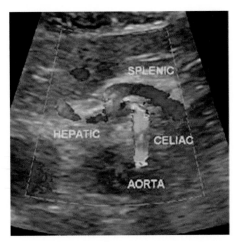
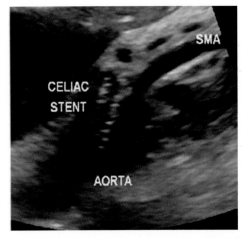

**FIGURE 24-12** Turning color off aids in identifying the location of a stent. On the left, the color flow image demonstrates adequate filling of the celiac artery but masks the stent which is more clearly visualized in the grayscale image on the right.

SMA, or the celiac, or both. If one knows where to look for inflow and outflow in advance, it can save much time and frustration. The inflow artery supplying the bypass graft should be evaluated, and the Doppler sample volume walked through the proximal anastomosis, body of the graft, the distal anastomosis, and into the outflow artery (Figs. 24-13 and 24-14). It is difficult, if not impossible, depending on the length of the bypass, to show the entire graft in one image (e.g., Ilio-SMA bypass graft), and it is often necessary to

concentrate on one segment at a time. Particular attention should be directed to the proximal and distal anastomoses because those are the most common locations for stenosis.

Liem et al.[15] reviewed 167 duplex ultrasound scans from 38 patients to characterize duplex ultrasound findings in mesenteric bypass grafts with respect to type of revascularization, graft caliber, and changes over time. They found that midgraft mean PSV, typically 140 to 200 cm/s, may be affected by graft diameter, but not significantly by the choice

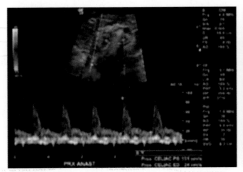
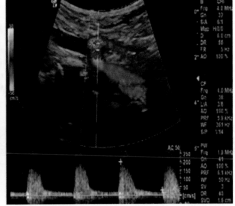

**FIGURE 24-13** Duplex ultrasound images of an external iliac artery to SMA bypass graft. The distal anastomosis to the SMA is shown on the left. The image on the right shows a high-resistance spectral waveform. This bypass was too long to visualize in one image.

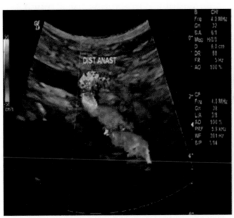
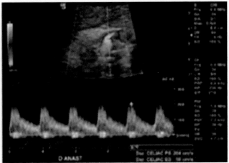

**FIGURE 24-14** Duplex ultrasound images of an aortoceliac bypass graft with Doppler spectrum of the proximal (left image) and distal (right image) anastomoses. This bypass graft was visualized in one image.

of inflow artery. If the PSV is ≥300 cm/s or <50 cm/s in the bypass, the recommendation is to decrease the time between surveillance scans to less than 6 months or to use secondary imaging (CTA or angiography). Velocity trending is also important. The likelihood to recommend confirmatory diagnostic imaging is greater if a high PSV has been trending upward over sequential studies, or a low PSV is trending downward.

### Compensatory Flow

Elevated velocities may be noted in a normal mesenteric artery (celiac or SMA) when compensatory flow occurs because of critical stenosis or occlusion of the companion visceral vessel. For example, when the celiac artery has a critical stenosis or occlusion, SMA flow and velocity will often increase. A prominent IMA may suggest occlusion or stenosis of the SMA with collateralization through a meandering mesenteric artery. However, in this setting, it may be difficult to distinguish compensatory flow in a widely patent artery from increased velocities because of a pathologic stenosis. Doppler waveform analysis may be helpful in this situation. A stenosis usually elicits a flow disturbance with high-velocities and poststenotic spectral broadening. With compensatory flow, there is little spectral broadening, no prestenotic, stenotic, poststenotic velocity profile, and velocities may be uniformly elevated throughout.

### Pitfalls

Abdominal gas can be the source of particular frustration during mesenteric duplex ultrasound examinations. If there is air in the epigastrium, light massage with the transducer will sometimes move it out of the way. If midline scars from abdominal surgery cause shadowing, sliding the transducer to the right or left and angling toward midline may help visualization. Having the patient turn into a slight left lateral decubitus position (left side down) occasionally provides an adequate acoustic window through the liver. Doing so, however, requires that one reconfirm identification of the celiac and SMA.

## DIAGNOSIS

Diagnostic velocity criteria for stenosis of the celiac and SMA have been reported by multiple authors. The initial report was a retrospective analysis that determined PSV criteria for a >70% angiographic stenosis. This was published in 1991 by Moneta et al.[5] at Oregon Health Sciences University. In 1993, this group reported the accuracy of these thresholds when tested prospectively. They found excellent accuracy by using a threshold PSV >275 cm/s for the SMA with 92% sensitivity and 96% specificity and a threshold PSV >200 cm/s for the celiac artery with 87% sensitivity and 90% specificity.[7] In similar studies, also in 1991, Bowersox et al.[6] at Dartmouth-Hitchcock Medical Center evaluated criteria for a >50% angiographic stenosis retrospectively and subsequently published a prospective analysis of their criteria in 1998.[9] In their retrospective study, the Dartmouth group found better sensitivity and specificity using EDV criteria. In their prospective study, EDV criteria again proved more accurate. They found an EDV > 45 cm/s in the SMA resulted in a sensitivity of 90% and a specificity of 91% and an EDV > 55 cm/s in the celiac artery provided 93% sensitivity and 100% specificity. PSV analysis demonstrated SMA PSV >300 cm/s was not as accurate (81%) as EDV criteria (91%), but celiac PSV >200 cm/s had excellent accuracy (93%). Perko et al.[8] in their 1997 report also found increased diastolic velocities to be the most accurate predictors of stenosis (EDV >70 cm/s for the SMA and EDV >100 cm/s for the celiac artery to identify >50% stenosis).

In 2012, AbuRahma et al.[10] published mesenteric duplex/angiography correlations for a much larger cohort of 153 patients and analyzed PSV and EDV data retrospectively for both the 50% and 70% angiographic stenosis breakpoints. Overall, they found PSV values to be better than EDV values for detecting stenosis. The velocity threshold criteria reported in these studies for the celiac artery and SMA are summarized in Tables 24-2 and 24-3. In 2013, van Petersen et al.[16] published another large retrospective analysis correlating

---

**TABLE 24-2　Summary of Velocity Thresholds for Diagnosis of Celiac Artery Stenosis by Duplex Scanning**

| Author | Stenosis (%) | PSV (cm/s) | Sensitivity (%) | Specificity (%) | EDV (cm/s) | Sensitivity (%) | Specificity (%) |
|---|---|---|---|---|---|---|---|
| Moneta[5,6] | ≥70 | ≥200 | 87 | 80 | | | |
| Zwolak[6,9] | ≥50 | ≥200 | 93 | 94 | ≥55 | 93 | 100 |
| AbuRahma[10] | ≥70 | ≥320 | 80 | 89 | ≥100 | 58 | 91 |
| AbuRahma[10] | ≥50 | ≥240 | 87 | 83 | ≥40 | 84 | 48 |

---

**TABLE 24-3　Summary of Velocity Thresholds for Diagnosis of SMA Stenosis by Duplex Scanning**

| Author | Stenosis (%) | PSV (cm/s) | Sensitivity (%) | Specificity (%) | EDV (cm/) | Sensitivity (%) | Specificity (%) |
|---|---|---|---|---|---|---|---|
| Moneta[5,6] | ≥70 | ≥275 | 92 | 96 | | | |
| Zwolak[6,9] | ≥50 | ≥300 | 60 | 100 | ≥45 | 90 | 91 |
| AbuRahma[10] | ≥70 | ≥400 | 72 | 93 | ≥70 | 65 | 95 |
| AbuRahma[10] | ≥50 | ≥295 | 87 | 89 | ≥45 | 79 | 79 |

duplex ultrasound velocities with angiographic stenosis in the SMA and celiac. They identified duplex ultrasound velocity thresholds for 50% and 70% stenosis that were similar to prior authors. Interestingly, they found velocity differences occurred with respiration in the SMA as well as in the celiac artery.

Because the diagnosis of CMI generally relies on the identification of significant disease in at least two of the three mesenteric arteries, inclusion of data from the IMA is important. Several investigators have reported successful visualization of the IMA, ranging from 86% to 92% of mesenteric scans. Although the patient group with significant IMA stenosis was small in the following two studies, they recommend similar guidelines for identifying IMA stenosis. For the identification of >50% angiographic stenosis, Pellerito et al.[17] found that PSV was the best criterion and that a threshold >200 cm/s provided 90% sensitivity and 97% specificity. AbuRahma et al.[18] determined the most accurate PSV for detecting >50% stenosis to be a PSV >250 cm/s, with 90% sensitivity and 96% specificity. In this study, they found that PSV, EDV and IMA/aortic systolic ratios all provided reasonable accuracy. The IMA PSV criteria are summarized in Table 24-4.

In summary, although there are multiple recommendations for 50% and 70% stenosis identification, they don't vary that much. One should choose a set of the published criteria and thereafter employ quality assurance data to confirm accuracy of the choice.

## Stented Visceral Arteries

Stenting has surpassed open bypass as the most frequently utilized method of visceral artery revascularization.[19] Indes et al.[20] reported a steady increase in the proportion of stenting compared to open surgical repair, from 28% in 2000 to 75% in 2006. It is generally accepted that percutaneous visceral artery intervention has a lower morbidity/mortality rate and shorter or no hospital stay while providing high technical and early clinical success rates. However, percutaneous intervention is associated with substantial rates of restenosis, recurrent symptoms, and the requirement for re-do intervention. Based on propensity for restenosis, duplex ultrasound scanning is an ideal monitoring method. In contrast, open surgical repair has a lower restenosis rate but carries a higher likelihood of perioperative complications as well as a longer hospital stay. With less chance for postoperative restenosis, the evidence to surveil mesenteric bypass grafts is less compelling.

As reported for stented internal carotid and renal arteries, several studies provide evidence that the duplex ultrasound velocity criteria for native SMA and celiac artery may overestimate the severity of stenosis if applied to stented vessels.[21-24] In 2009, Mitchell and coworkers from the Oregon Health & Science University reported velocity data on patients who underwent SMA stent placement. Despite proven resolution of stenosis, early poststent duplex ultrasound scanning revealed SMA velocities ranging from 279 to 416 cm/s, with a mean PSV of 336 cm/s.[22] Thus, successfully stented SMA or celiac artery may harbor elevated velocities in the absence of restenosis.

In 2012, AbuRahma et al.[23] reported duplex ultrasound velocity data following SMA and celiac artery stent placement. As in previous reports, they found higher velocities in stented mesenteric arteries in comparison with native arteries. These velocity data are summarized in Table 24-5. Also in 2012, Baker and coworkers[24] reviewed duplex ultrasound data for detection of in-stent stenosis of the SMA. They found a significant decrease between the prestent and first poststent mean SMA PSV. However, in successfully stented SMAs, the PSV often remained higher than the threshold criteria for significant stenosis in a native SMA. They concluded that obtaining an early baseline study was important, and that a progressive increase above this baseline, or an in-stent SMA PSV approaching 500 cm/s, should be considered suspicious for in-stent restenosis.[24]

Although further prospective validation studies are needed, this is an important step toward revised duplex ultrasound criteria for evaluation after mesenteric stenting.

| TABLE 24-4 | Summary of Velocity Thresholds for Diagnosis of IMA Stenosis by Duplex Scanning | | | | | | |
|---|---|---|---|---|---|---|---|
| Author | Stenosis (%) | PSV (cm/s) | Sensitivity (%) | Specificity (%) | EDV (cm/s) | Sensitivity (%) | Specificity (%) |
| Pellerito[17] | ≥50 | ≥200 | 90 | 97 | ≥25 | 40 | 91 |
| AbuRahma[18] | ≥50 | ≥250 | 90 | 96 | ≥80 | 60 | 100 |

| TABLE 24-5 | Summary of Velocity Thresholds to Identify In-Stent Stenosis[23] | | | | |
|---|---|---|---|---|---|
| | Stenosis (%) | PSV (cm/s) | Sensitivity (%) | Specificity (%) | Overall Accuracy (%) |
| Celiac artery | >70 | >363 | 88 | 92 | 90 |
| Celiac artery | >50 | >274 | 96 | 86 | 93 |
| SMA | >70 | >412 | 100 | 95 | 97 |
| SMA | >50 | >325 | 89 | 100 | 91 |

## OTHER DISORDERS

Several other visceral vascular disorders can be assessed with mesenteric duplex ultrasound scanning. Several publications indicate that median arcuate ligament compression syndrome can be diagnosed by duplex. In addition, visceral artery aneurysms and dissections may be identified on duplex ultrasound. Rarely, an ultrasound is performed to detect thromboembolic disease.

### Median Arcuate Ligament Compression Syndrome

Individuals with median arcuate ligament compression syndrome (MALS) have transient compression of the celiac artery origin by the median arcuate ligament of the diaphragm during exhalation which is relieved or lessened by descent of the diaphragm with inhalation. Thus, the PSV of the celiac artery is increased during exhalation and decreased during inhalation. Duplex ultrasound interrogation can readily identify these velocity changes. The image of the proximal celiac artery in MALS patients demonstrates a characteristic hooked appearance (Fig. 24-15). When scanning patients with possible MALS, representative Doppler waveforms should be obtained from the celiac artery during deep inhalation and compared with waveforms obtained during complete exhalation (Fig. 24-16A,B). Typically, these respiratory maneuvers are enough to establish the diagnosis. However, several investigators have recently identified a subset of

MALS patients whose celiac artery velocity will normalize only when standing.[25–27] Consider standing a suspected MALS patient when the velocities fail to normalize with inspiration.

### Aneurysm

Visceral artery aneurysms are rare, occurring in 0.1% to 0.2% of routine autopsies.[28] Most are identified incidentally during CT and magnetic resonance imaging studies, although there are several case studies reporting identification by duplex ultrasound. Among visceral artery aneurysms, the greatest incidence occurs in the splenic artery at 60%, with

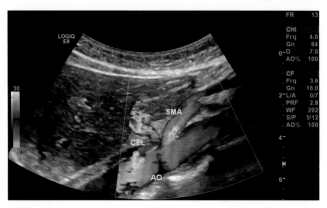

**FIGURE 24-15** Image of the proximal celiac artery in an MALS patient demonstrating a characteristic hooked appearance.

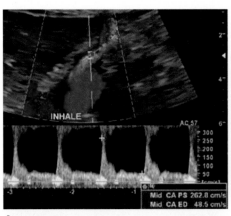

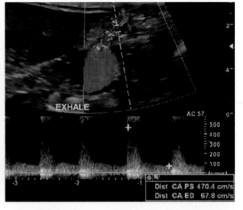

**A**

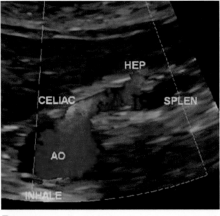

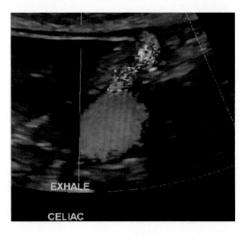

**B**

**FIGURE 24-16** **A:** Doppler spectral waveforms from a celiac artery during inhalation (left) and exhalation (right) illustrating the findings in median arcuate ligament compression syndrome. Note the change in PSV from 263 (inhalation) to 470 cm/s (exhalation) and EDV from 49 (inhalation) to 68 cm/s (exhalation). These changes are because of transient compression of the celiac artery by the median arcuate ligament during exhalation. **B:** Visual color changes were apparent before interrogation with Doppler: These images demonstrate the color increase in velocity and turbulence associated with compression of the celiac artery with exhalation (on the right).

female patients affected four times more often than male patients. Medial degeneration of the splenic artery most often occurs as a result of arterial fibrodysplasia, portal hypertension with splenomegaly, and repeated pregnancies. Although the incidence of splenic artery aneurysm is very rare, rupture can be catastrophic. A 95% rupture rate has been reported in the splenic aneurysm recognized during pregnancy, with an associated 70% maternal mortality rate and 95% fetal mortality rate.[29] Other locations of visceral artery aneurysms include the hepatic (men affected twice as often as women), SMA, or celiac artery (men and women affected equally) (Table 24-6, Figs. 24-17 and 24-18). Treatment options for visceral artery aneurysms include open surgery and endovascular repair, with the goal of preventing aneurysm expansion and/or rupture. Duplex ultrasound imaging can be used for follow-up scans after treatment.

## Dissection

Causes of celiac artery, SMA, and IMA dissections include atherosclerosis, fibromuscular dysplasia, trauma, connective tissue disorders, vasculitis, and iatrogenic events. Some dissections occur without any identifiable etiology. Dissections occur most frequently in the SMA, and many are extensions of an aortic dissection. Treatment of SMA dissection may include conservative management with anticoagulation, endovascular stent placement, or surgical procedures.

Dissections provide a unique pattern of color separation with antegrade flow along one wall of the artery and retrograde flow along the other wall (Figs. 24-11A,B and 24-19). Duplex ultrasound can be used to monitor dissections and posttreatment.

Pathology Box 24-1 summarizes the common pathology observed during a mesenteric duplex ultrasound examination.

## Acute Mesenteric Ischemia

Acute mesenteric ischemia can result from embolus to the mesenteric arteries or thrombosis of an artery with existing chronic disease. Approximately two-thirds of these patients are women, with a median age of 70 years. The nature of the pain varies, but generally is described as pain out of proportion to physical findings. Time spent in the vascular laboratory is generally not useful and should be discouraged. If the diagnosis is not made quickly, bowel necrosis rapidly ensues, with a high mortality rate. In an analysis of 103 cases of acute occlusion of the SMA at Massachusetts General Hospital, the mortality rate was 85%.[30] In addition to the critical time factor, there is a possibility that a distal embolus in the

### TABLE 24-6 Relative Incidence of Visceral Artery Aneurysm

| Visceral Artery | % Incidence |
|---|---|
| Splenic | 60 |
| Hepatic | 20 |
| Superior mesenteric | 5 |
| Celiac | 4 |
| Gastric and gastroepiploic | 4 |
| Jejunal ileal colic | 3 |
| Pancreaticoduodenal | 2 |
| Gastroduodenal | 1.5 |
| Inferior mesenteric | Rare |

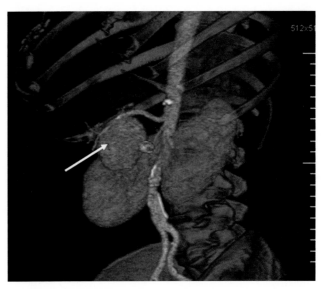

**FIGURE 24-17** CT scan of 5.5 cm SMA aneurysm (*arrow*).

SMA may go undetected by ultrasound. It is important for the requesting provider to understand that although patency of the proximal SMA may be verified, embolus to the more distal branches cannot be excluded and to consider alternative imaging, such as CTA. The majority of visceral emboli lodge in the SMA, often 3 to 8 cm beyond the SMA origin and first several branches, at the origin of the middle colic artery.

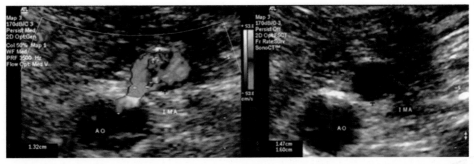

**FIGURE 24-18** IMA aneurysm as seen on duplex ultrasound examination: the typical color pattern of an aneurysm is demonstrated on the left. Measurements, obtained in grayscale on the right, were 1.5 × 1.6 cm.

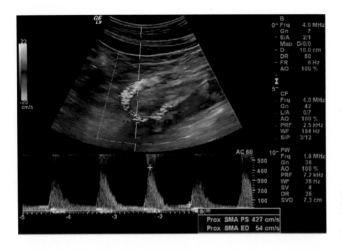

**FIGURE 24-19** Taken from the same patient as in Fig. 24-11A,B; high velocities consistent with stenosis were documented in the proximal SMA. The stenosis was likely the result of thrombosis of the false lumen of this portion of the dissection extending into the SMA from the aorta.

### PATHOLOGY BOX 24-1
#### Celiac and Mesenteric Artery Pathology

| Pathology | Sonographic Appearance | |
| --- | --- | --- |
| | **Color** | **Doppler** |
| Stenosis >50% | High-velocity flow with aliasing, color bruit | High-velocity flow with poststenotic turbulence |
| Celiac artery occlusion | No color filling at the origin, retrograde hepatic artery flow | Absent Doppler flow signal at the origin, retrograde Doppler flow in the hepatic artery |
| Celiac artery compression syndrome | Increase in color velocity with exhalation | Increase in velocity with exhalation and decrease with inhalation |
| Superior mesenteric artery occlusion | No color filling at the origin, reconstitutes distally | Absent Doppler flow signal in proximal artery |
| Aneurysm | Focal dilation with mixed color filling observed in dilated region | Disturbed flow usually present in dilated regions |
| Dissection | Color separation with separate flow channels of antegrade and retrograde flow | Disturbed or stenotic signals may be present, sometimes with separate flow channels of antegrade and retrograde flow |

## SUMMARY

- The mesenteric arteries can be successfully interrogated by duplex ultrasound.
- In an era where CT and CTA are used frequently, many appropriate clinical situations remain wherein duplex ultrasound scanning is a valuable and appropriate test.
- Screening patients for suspected CMI and MALS are two such clinical situations.
- Likewise, surveillance following stent placement is an excellent indication for duplex ultrasound because patients may require multiple and relatively frequent exams.
- This test also provides a reasonable noninvasive method for monitoring open surgical revascularization procedures.
- Duplex ultrasound remains a cost-effective alternative to CTA and avoids the small but real incidence of complications related to CT contrast injection.

## CRITICAL THINKING QUESTIONS

1. A nonfasting patient arrives for a mesenteric duplex ultrasound examination. The patient lives 2 hours away, is unhappy she was not told to be (nothing by mouth) NPO, and wants to get the test done. Do you proceed with the duplex ultrasound examination?

2. During a mesenteric duplex ultrasound scan, you are only able to identify one artery originating from the aorta, and it appears to be the SMA because it parallels the aorta. Scanning more proximally, you identify the splenic and hepatic arteries "seagull" sign, but you cannot demonstrate flow in the celiac artery by color or Doppler. Blood flow in the common hepatic artery is retrograde in direction, headed toward the splenic artery. How do you interpret these findings?

3. You find a celiac artery stenosis with PSV of 435 cm/s and EDV of 70 cm/s with poststenotic turbulence. The SMA PSV is 325 cm/s and EDV is 50 cm/s. The SMA waveform demonstrates a normal systolic window, and there is no poststenotic turbulence. Do you conclude that the patient has significant stenosis in both the celiac artery and SMA? Why or why not?

4. A patient in whom you found a significant stenosis of the celiac artery returns to the lab for follow-up scan status post stenting. On your examination, you find the celiac PSV = 250 cm/s and EDV = 65 cm/s, which are above your lab's standard criteria for celiac stenosis. The

prestent velocities were PSV=450 cm/s and EDV=75 cm/s. Do you conclude that there is a residual stenosis? How might you write an interpretation?

5. A young woman is referred to your lab for a mesenteric duplex ultrasound study with a question of MALS. Do you alter your standard protocol for identifying significant mesenteric artery stenosis? Why or why not?

## REFERENCES

1. Jager KA, Fortner GS, Thiele BL, et al. Noninvasive diagnosis of intestinal angina. *J Clin Ultrasound*. 1984;12:588–591.
2. Jager K, Bollinger A, Valli C, et al. Measurement of mesenteric blood flow by duplex scanning. *J Vasc Surg*. 1986;3:462–469.
3. Moneta GL, Taylor DC, Helton WS, et al. Duplex ultrasound measurement of postprandial intestinal blood flow: effect of meal composition. *Gastroenterology*. 1988;95:1294–1301.
4. Flinn WR, Rizzo RJ, Park JS, et al. Duplex scanning for assessment of mesenteric ischemia. *Surg Clin North Am*. 1990;70:99–107.
5. Moneta GL, Yeager RA, Dalman R, et al. Duplex ultrasound criteria for diagnosis of splanchnic artery stenosis or occlusion. *J Vasc Surg*. 1991;14:511–518; discussion 8–20.
6. Bowersox JC, Zwolak RM, Walsh DB, et al. Duplex ultrasonography in the diagnosis of celiac and mesenteric artery occlusive disease. *J Vasc Surg*. 1991;14:780–786; discussion 6–8.
7. Moneta GL, Lee RW, Yeager RA, et al. Mesenteric duplex scanning: a blinded prospective study. *J Vasc Surg*. 1993;17:79–84; discussion 5–6.
8. Perko MJ, Just S, Schroeder TV. Importance of diastolic velocities in the detection of celiac and mesenteric artery disease by duplex ultrasound. *J Vasc Surg*. 1997;26:288–293.
9. Zwolak RM, Fillinger MF, Walsh DB, et al. Mesenteric and celiac duplex scanning: a validation study. *J Vasc Surg*. 1998;27:1078–1087; discussion 88.
10. AbuRahma AF, Stone PA, Srivastava M, et al. Mesenteric/celiac duplex ultrasound interpretation criteria revisited. *J Vasc Surg*. 2012;55:428–436.
11. Valentine RJ, Martin JD, Myers SI, et al. Asymptomatic celiac and superior mesenteric artery stenoses are more prevalent among patients with unsuspected renal artery stenoses. *J Vasc Surg*. 1991;14:195–199.
12. Kadir S. Atlas of normal and variant angiographic anatomy. Philadelphia, PA: W. B. Saunders Company; 1991.
13. Gentile AT, Moneta GL, Lee RW, et al. Usefulness of fasting and postprandial duplex ultrasound examinations for predicting high-grade superior mesenteric artery stenosis. *Am J Surg*. 1995;169:476–479.
14. LaBombard FE, Musson A, Bowersox JC, et al. Hepatic artery duplex as an adjunct in the evaluation of chronic mesenteric ischemia. *J Vasc Technol*. 1992;16:7–11.
15. Liem TK, Segall JA, Wei W, et al. Duplex scan characteristics of bypass grafts to mesenteric arteries. *J Vasc Surg*. 2007;45:922–927; discussion 7–8.
16. van Petersen AS, Meerwaldt R, Kolkman JJ, et al. The influence of respiration on criteria for transabdominal duplex examination of the splanchnic arteries in patients with suspected chronic splanchnic ischemia. *J Vasc Surg*. 2013;57:1603–1611.
17. Pellerito JS, Revzin MV, Tsang JC, et al. Doppler sonographic criteria for the diagnosis of inferior mesenteric artery stenosis. *J Ultrasound Med*. 2009;28:641–650.
18. AbuRahma AF, Dean LS. Duplex ultrasound interpretation criteria for inferior mesenteric arteries. *Vascular*. 2012;20:145–149.
19. Schermerhorn ML, Giles KA, Hamdan AD, et al. Mesenteric revascularization: management and outcomes in the United States 1988–2006. *J Vasc Surg*. 2009;50:341–348.
20. Indes, JE, Giacovelli JK, Muhs BE, et al. Outcomes of endovascular and open treatment for chronic mesenteric ischemia. *J Endovasc Ther*. 2009;16:624–630.
21. Armstrong PA. Visceral duplex scanning: evaluation before and after artery intervention for chronic mesenteric ischemia. *Perspect Vasc Surg Endovasc Ther*. 2007;19:386–392.
22. Mitchell EL, Chang EY, Landry GJ, et al. Duplex criteria for native superior mesenteric artery stenosis overestimate stenosis in stented superior mesenteric arteries. *J Vasc Surg*. 2009;50:335–340.
23. AbuRahma AF, Mousa AY, Stone PA, et al. Duplex velocity criteria for native celiac/superior mesenteric artery stenosis vs in-stent stenosis. *J Vasc Surg*. 2012;55:730–738.
24. Baker AC, Chew V, Chin-Shang Li, et al. Application of duplex ultrasound imaging in determining in-stent stenosis during surveillance after mesenteric artery revascularization. *J Vasc Surg*. 2012;56:1364–1371.
25. Wolfman D, Bluth EI, Sossaman J. Median arcuate ligament syndrome. *J Ultrasound Med*. 2003;22:1377–1380.
26. Downing MC, AyoubK, Sakarwala A, et al. Utility of standing maneuvers during abdominal duplex ultrasound examination to diagnose median arcuate ligament compression. *JVU*. 2009;33:69–74.
27. Ozel A, Toksoy G, Ozdogan O, et al. Ultrasonographic diagnosis of median arcuate ligament syndrome: a report of two cases. *Med Ultrason*. 2012;14:154–157.
28. Grotemeyer D, Duran M, Park EJ, et al. Visceral artery aneurysms-follow-up of 23 patients with 31 aneurysms after surgical or interventional therapy. *Langenbecks Arch Surg*. 2009;394:1093.
29. Stanley JC, Wakefield TW, Graham LM, et al. Clinical importance and management of splanchnic artery aneurysms. *J Vasc Surg*. 1986;3:836–840.
30. Ottinger LW. The surgical management of acute occlusion of the superior mesenteric artery. *Ann Surg*. 1978;188:721–731.

# The Renal Vasculature

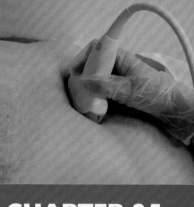

MARSHA M. NEUMYER

## CHAPTER 25

## OBJECTIVES

- Describe the anatomy of the renal vasculature
- Relate the most common pathologies found during a sonographic examination of the renal circulatory system
- Describe patient preparation and positioning used for sonographic evaluation of the renal arteries, renal veins, and kidneys
- Define the technical applications of the B-mode, spectral, color, and power Doppler evaluations of the renal vasculature
- List the validated diagnostic criteria used for defining renal artery stenosis, occlusion, and renal parenchymal dysfunction

## GLOSSARY

**poststenotic signal** A Doppler spectral waveform recorded immediately distal to a flow-reducing stenosis. The waveform exhibits decreased peak systolic velocity and disordered flow during systolic deceleration and diastole as a result of the pressure-flow gradient associated with the lesion

**renal–aortic velocity ratio** The peak systolic renal artery velocity divided by the peak systolic aortic velocity recorded at the level of the celiac and/or superior mesenteric arteries. The ratio is used to identify flow-limiting renal artery stenosis

**renal artery stenosis** Narrowing of the renal artery most commonly as a result of atherosclerotic disease or medial fibromuscular dysplasia

**renal artery stent** A tiny tube inserted into a stenotic renal artery at the time of arterial dilation (angioplasty). The stent, usually a metallic mesh structure, helps to hold the artery open.

**renal cortex** The outermost area of the kidney tissue lying just beneath the renal capsule, the fibrous covering of the kidney

**renal hilum** The area through which the renal artery, vein, and ureter enter the kidney

**renal medulla** The middle area of the kidney lying between the sinus and the cortex. The medullary tissue contains the renal pyramids.

**renal ostium** The opening of the renal artery from the aortic wall

**renal parenchymal disease** A medical disorder affecting the tissue function of the kidneys

**renal sinus** The central echogenic cavity of the kidney. It contains the renal artery, renal vein, collecting and lymphatic systems

**suprasternal notch** The visible indentation at the base of the neck where the neck joins the sternum

**symphysis pubis/pubic bones** The prominence of the pelvic bones noted in the lower abdomen

## KEY TERMS

renal–aortic velocity ratio

renal artery stenosis

renal artery stent

renal cortex

renal hilum

renal medulla

renal ostium

renal parenchymal disease

renal sinus

The true prevalence of renovascular hypertension is unknown but is estimated to affect approximately 50 million people in the United States alone.[1,2] As many as 6% of hypertensive patients have underlying renal disease as the cause of their elevated blood pressure.[2,3] In patients with severe diastolic hypertension, the prevalence of renal artery stenosis approaches 40%. Progression of stenosis occurs in 31% to 49% of patients depending on the initial severity of narrowing of the renal artery.[3-5] Given these facts, it is understandable that renal artery stenosis is a significant cause of incident end-stage renal disease in many patients.[6,7]

Renal artery stenosis should be suspected in adults with an abdominal bruit, sudden onset or worsening of chronic hypertension, azotemia which is induced by angiotensin-converting enzyme inhibitor, decreased serum potassium, unexplained renal insufficiency, recurrent congestive heart failure, or pulmonary edema, and in hypertensive children.[8] In the majority of patients, renal artery disease is correctable with treatment providing control or cure for renovascular hypertension, retention of renal mass, and stabilization of renal function in patients with chronic renal failure.[9]

For identification of renovascular disease, contrast arteriography has historically been the procedure of choice. Although providing anatomic information, this diagnostic test does not identify the functional significance of renal artery disease in hypertensive patients nor does it provide hemodynamic information. Because of its associated, albeit low, morbidity, this invasive test is most often reserved for defining therapeutic intervention. Magnetic resonance angiography (MRA) and computed tomography angiography (CTA) offer less invasive diagnostic testing and excellent sensitivity and specificity, but are relatively expensive and require injection of intravenous contrast.[10] It should be noted that in the case of CTA, the contrast agent may be nephrotoxic and is, therefore, unsuitable for use in patients with renal insufficiency. Given these deficiencies, many clinicians reserve MRA and CTA for use as secondary confirmatory studies and have focused their attention on duplex sonography as a primary diagnostic tool. Sonographic imaging can be performed on an outpatient basis at low cost without risk of ionizing radiation or use of nephrotoxic contrast agents. This modality has the additional advantages of being noninvasive and painless and has demonstrated an overall accuracy of 80% to 90% for identification of renal artery stenosis and definition of its hemodynamic significance.[11]

## ANATOMY

The kidneys are located retroperitoneally in the dorsal abdominal cavity between the 12th thoracic and third lumbar vertebrae with the right kidney usually lying more inferior to the left (Fig. 25-1). The normal organ length is 8 to 13 cm with a width of 5 to 7 cm. The kidneys decrease in size with increasing age. An uncommon finding is a horseshoe kidney which occurs in less than 1% of the population. In excess of 90% of cases of horseshoe kidney, the organs are joined at their lower poles by an isthmus of tissue which lies anterior to the aorta at the level of the fourth or fifth lumbar vertebrae.

For the purpose of sonographic interrogation, the kidneys are segmented into four main areas (Fig. 25-2). The *renal hilum* is the area through which the renal artery, vein, and ureter enter the kidney. The hilum forms a cavity, *the renal sinus*, which contains the renal artery and vein, the collecting and lymphatic systems. The sinus is in large part made up of fat and fibrous tissue. For this reason, it is normally brightly echogenic on sonographic imaging (Fig. 25-3). The tissue of the kidney is referred to as the renal parenchyma. The parenchyma is divided into two parts: *the medulla* and *cortex*. The renal pyramids, which appear triangular shaped when the kidney is imaged longitudinally, carry

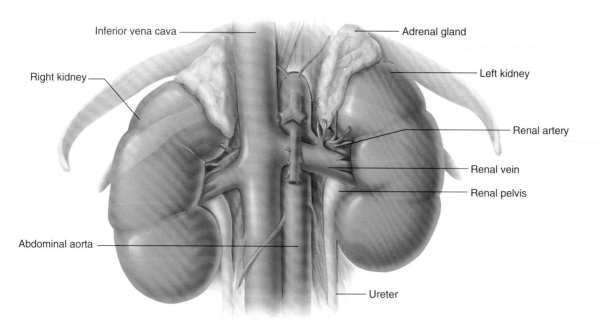

**FIGURE 25-1** Diagram illustrating anatomic location of the kidneys.

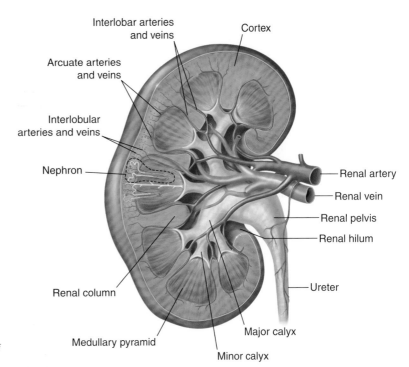

**FIGURE 25-2** Diagram illustrating the vasculature of the kidneys.

urine from the cortex to the renal pelvis. The cortex is the outermost area of the kidney and lies just beneath the renal capsule. This is the area where urine is produced. Cortical tissue, called columns of Bertin, lies between the medullary pyramids. The 12 to 18 pyramids generally have lower echogenicity than the cortex and are usually seen well in the normal adult patient.

The transpyloric plane serves as an important surface anatomic landmark for sonographic localization of the renal arteries (Fig. 25-4). This transverse plane is located halfway between the suprasternal notch and the symphysis pubis cutting through the lower border of the first lumbar vertebrae, the ninth costal cartilages, and the pylorus. The renal arteries can be identified approximately 2 cm below the transpyloric plane arising from the anterior, lateral, or posterolateral wall of the abdominal aorta. The left renal artery usually originates slightly more cephalad than the right. The right renal artery initially courses anterolaterally

and then moves posterior to the inferior vena cava (IVC) and the right renal vein (Fig. 25-5A). In a small number of cases, the right renal artery will originate from the aortic wall anteriorly and course superior to the IVC (Fig. 25-5B) The left renal artery courses on a slightly inferior path from the posterolateral aortic wall, passes posterior to the left renal vein, and is crossed by the inferior mesenteric vein. Between 12% and 22% of patients have duplicate main renal arteries that enter the kidney through the renal hilum or accessory polar arteries, a feature found more often on the left than on the right[12] (Fig. 25-6). Most often, the accessory renal arteries arise from the aortic wall below the main renal artery and course to the polar surfaces of the kidney instead of entering the renal hilum. Occasionally, accessory renal arteries originate from the common or internal iliac arteries.

Along its course, the renal artery normally gives rise to two to five branches that supply blood to segments of the kidney. At the level of the renal hilum, the renal artery divides into a large anterior and a smaller posterior branch which give rise to interlobar, arcuate, and interlobular arteries within the renal parenchyma (refer to Fig. 25-2).

On each side, the renal vein courses anteriorly from the renal hilum with the ureter arising posteriorly. The renal artery normally lies between the vein and the ureter. The right renal vein has a short course from the hilum of the kidney to the IVC, whereas the left renal vein courses anterior to the aorta just below the origin of the superior mesenteric artery (SMA) (refer to Fig. 25-1). In 2% to 5% of patients, the left renal vein takes a retroaortic path. Approximately 9% of patients will demonstrate a bifid left renal vein with both a retroaortic branch and another branch coursing anterior to the aorta. It is important to be aware of these anatomic anomalies because the left renal vein is used as a major anatomic landmark for locating the renal arteries during the sonographic examination.

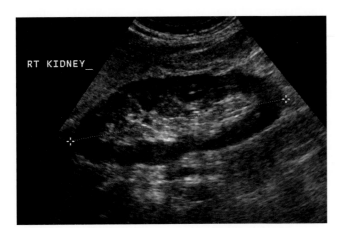

**FIGURE 25-3** B-mode longitudinal image of a kidney illustrating the echogenic sinus, the medulla, cortex, and renal pyramids.

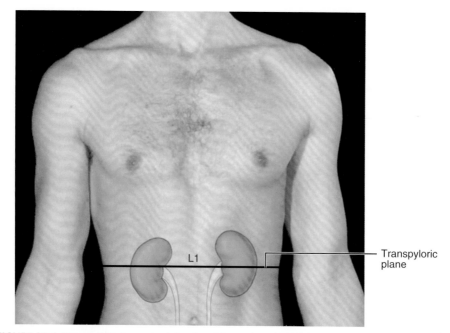

**FIGURE 25-4**  Diagram illustrating anatomic location of the renal arteries and the transpyloric plane.

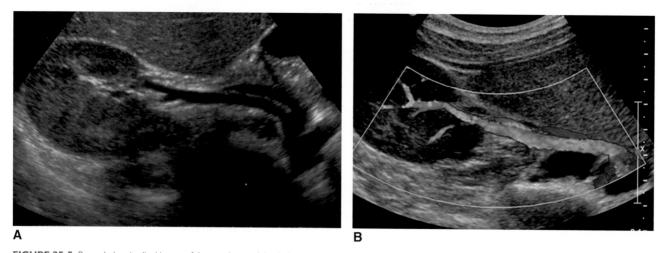

**FIGURE 25-5**  B-mode longitudinal image of the renal artery lying in its normal anatomic position posterior to the IVC (**A**). Color-flow image demonstrating the right renal artery lying anterior to the IVC (**B**).

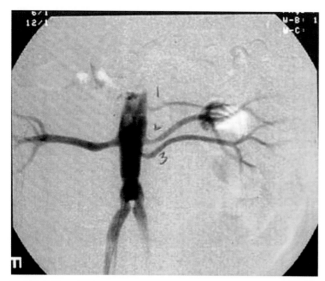

**FIGURE 25-6**  Arteriogram demonstrating multiple renal arteries on the left side.

## ETIOLOGY OF RENAL ARTERY DISEASE

The majority of renovascular disease is caused by atherosclerotic renal artery stenosis.[9,13] As noted in Pathology Box 25-1, these lesions primarily affect the ostium and proximal third of the renal artery but may be found in any segment of the vessel, including the interlobar and smaller branches within the renal medulla and cortex.[14] For reasons that are not well understood, renal artery stenosis is found more often in men than in women with lesions occurring bilaterally in more than 30% of patients.[15] Those most at risk for atherosclerotic renal artery stenosis include elderly, hypertensive patients; smokers; and patients with coronary and/or peripheral arterial disease, hyperlipidemia, or diabetes.

Medial fibromuscular dysplasia is the second most common curable cause of renovascular disease. This nonatherosclerotic disease entity commonly affects the mid-to-distal segments of the renal artery in females aged 25 to 50 years. Although most often the disease is found bilaterally, it may

**PATHOLOGY BOX 25-1**
*Characterization of the Most Common Types of Renal Artery Pathology Encountered During Sonographic Evaluation of the Renal Arteries*

| Pathology | Location | Sonographic Appearance | Spectral Doppler |
|---|---|---|---|
| Atherosclerosis | Usually ostial or proximal Any segment of main renal Parenchymal arteries | Acoustically homogeneous or heterogeneous Smooth or irregular surfaced | High velocity with poststenotic turbulence if >60% diameter-reducing stenosis Low velocity if stenosis is preocclusive |
| Medial fibromuscular dysplasia | Mid-to-distal renal artery Parenchymal arteries | Segmental narrowing and dilation of the renal artery Alternating regions of forward and reversed flow | High velocity compared to proximal arterial segment |
| Occlusion | Focal or entire length | Intraluminal echoes of varying echogenicity dependent on chronicity Kidney length <8–9 cm | Absent Doppler signal in imaged artery Low-velocity, low-amplitude signals in the renal parenchyma |

involve one side only with the right side being affected more frequently than the left.[16] As noted sonographically and angiographically, the lesions produce segmental concentric narrowing and dilation, resulting in a "string of beads" appearance (Fig. 25-7A,B).[17,18] An intimal form of this disease, found more commonly in males, produces focal narrowing of the mid or distal segment of the renal artery. Whereas intimal fibromuscular dysplasia has been associated with progressive dissection and thrombosis of the renal artery, the medial expression of the disorder progresses in fewer than 30% of patients and rarely leads to arterial dissection and thrombosis.

Although atherosclerotic stenosis and fibromuscular dysplasia are the most commonly observed renal artery pathology, other complications must be considered during the sonographic examination. These include aortic dissection extending into the renal arteries, aneurysms of the main or segmental renal arteries, aortic coarctation proximal to the renal artery origins, arteriovenous fistulae, arteritis, and extrinsic compression of the renal artery and/or vein by tumors or other masses.[14,19]

## SONOGRAPHIC EXAMINATION TECHNIQUES

### Patient Preparation and Positioning

To reduce excessive abdominal gas that may obviate adequate visualization of the renal arteries and veins, patients are asked to fast for 8 to 10 hours prior to their examination. Elective studies are scheduled in the morning; diabetic patients are prioritized according to their insulin schedules. To prevent development of hypoglycemia while awaiting their renal duplex examination, diabetic patients are permitted to have dry

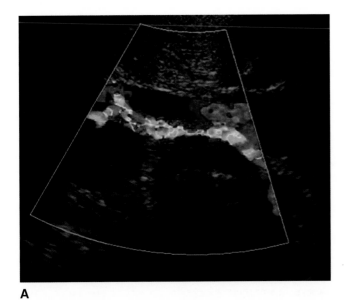

**A**

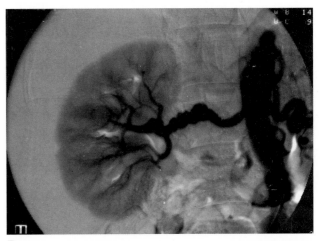

**B**

**FIGURE 25-7** Color-flow image of a renal artery with fibromuscular dysplasia (FMD). Note the regions of forward and reversed flow associated with the segmental concentric narrowing and dilation (**A**). Arteriogram illustrating FMD in the mid-to-distal renal artery segments on the right (**B**).

toast and clear liquids. Patients are permitted to take morning medications with sips of water and are asked to refrain from smoking or chewing gum to reduce the amount of swallowed air.

## Patient Positioning

Prior to initiating the examination, patients are asked to lie supine on the examination table with their head slightly elevated. The examination table is placed in the reverse Trendelenburg position with the patient's feet 15° to 20° lower than their heart. This allows the visceral contents to descend into the lower abdomen and pelvis enhancing the acoustic windows used for access to the renal arteries and kidneys. From the supine position, the sonographer is able to examine the aorta, celiac trunk, proximal SMA, the renal ostia, and the proximal-to-mid segments of the renal arteries. To facilitate visualization of the mid-to-distal segments of the renal arteries and the kidneys, the patient may be moved to the right or left lateral decubitus position with their arm placed over their head and their legs extended to elongate the body. In some cases, the patients may be asked to lie prone with their midsection flexed over a pillow or foam wedge. This position allows access to the kidneys and distal renal arteries through an intercostal image plane.

The sonographer should be positioned on either side of the examination table which is elevated to a height that allows scanning without overextension of their arm. It is also important to ensure that the patient is lying close to the sonographer's side of the table. This facilitates ease of movement of the transducer from the midline of the patient's abdomen to the flank while allowing the sonographer to maintain correct ergonomic positioning. If at all possible, sonographers should learn to scan with both hands, moving the ultrasound system to the opposite side of the bed as appropriate to the study.

## Equipment

Examination of the abdominal vasculature is performed using a high-resolution ultrasound system with phased or curved array transducers ranging in frequency from 2.0 to 5.0 MHz. The grayscale image is used to localize vessels and organs, and to identify atherosclerotic plaque, aneurysmal dilation, and dissections. Color and power Doppler imaging facilitate visualization of arteries and veins, identification of anatomic landmarks, detection of regions of disordered flow, and confirmation of vessel occlusion. Differentiation of normal and abnormal flow patterns is based on Doppler velocity spectral waveform parameters. A diagnosis of renal artery stenosis or occlusion requires accurate interpretation of Doppler spectral waveform data and integration of all accompanying sonographic information. Throughout the study, careful attention must be given to optimization of spectral and color Doppler pulse repetition frequency (velocity scale), gain, wall filters, and most importantly, angle of insonation.

## Scanning Technique[20]

### Interrogation of the Aorta, Mesenteric, and Renal Arteries

With the patient lying supine, a sagittal image of the aorta is obtained from the left paramedian scan plane beginning at the level of the xyphoid process and continuing through the aortic bifurcation to include the common iliac arteries. Care is taken to identify atherosclerotic plaque, duplicate main and accessory renal arteries, aneurysmal dilation, dissection, and regions of flow disturbance using B-mode, color, and power Doppler imaging. Using a small Doppler sample volume size and an appropriate angle of insonation less than or equal to 60°, spectral waveforms are recorded from the abdominal aorta at the level of the celiac artery and SMA. The peak systolic velocity (PSV) from the aorta is retained for calculation of the renal–aortic velocity ratio.

Because the branches of the celiac artery and SMA may course in close proximity to the main or accessory renal arteries, it is important to recognize the mesenteric arterial flow patterns. To achieve this goal, representative Doppler spectral waveforms should be obtained from the proximal celiac artery and SMA. A secondary benefit may be identification of flow-limiting mesenteric artery stenosis. This is most likely to occur in patients where atherosclerotic plaque is noted along the aortic walls in the region of the mesenteric artery origins.

A cross-sectional image of the aorta is obtained at the level of the SMA. Just inferior to the SMA, the left renal vein is identified as it crosses either anterior to the aorta or in a retroaortic position (Fig. 25-8). Optimized B-mode and color-flow imaging should be used to determine the presence of renal vein thrombosis or entrapment of the renal vein by small bowel or the SMA. Extrinsic compression of the vein may result in "nutcracker" or mesenteric compression syndrome.

The renal arteries normally lie immediately inferior to the left renal vein. Visualization of the proximal segments of these vessels may be facilitated by moving the transducer upright so that it is perpendicular to the patient's abdominal wall (Fig. 25-9). This position allows compression of the left renal vein. While remaining upright, the transducer is then angled slightly to the right or left to create a sagittal image of the renal artery (Fig. 25-10). Color-flow imaging may facilitate identification of the vessels and optimal visualization of the renal artery origins and accessory renal arteries. From this scan plane, the renal arteries can most often be visualized from the ostium to the midsegment. To rule out orificial renal artery stenosis, the Doppler sample volume is swept slowly from the aortic lumen through the renal ostium. Demonstration of the change in spectral waveform pattern from the high-resistance, low-diastolic aortic flow

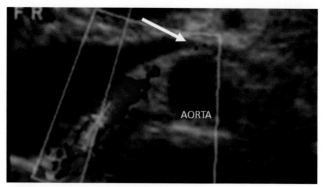

**FIGURE 25-8** Transverse color-flow image of the aorta demonstrating the left renal vein (*arrow*) crossing over the anterior aortic wall.

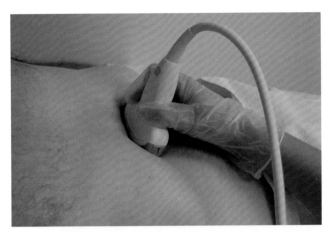

**FIGURE 25-9** An image demonstrating appropriate positioning of the ultrasound transducer for acquisition of images and Doppler spectral waveforms from the ostium and proximal renal arteries.

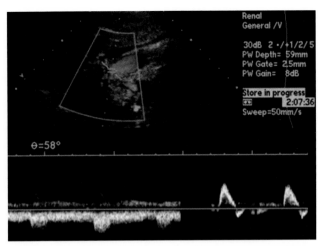

**FIGURE 25-11** Doppler spectral waveforms demonstrating the transition from the high-resistance (low-diastolic flow) aortic signal to the low-resistance (high-diastolic flow) signal obtained as the sample volume is slowly swept from the aortic lumen into the renal artery ostium.

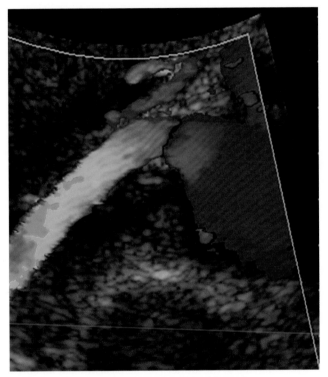

**FIGURE 25-10** Sagittal color-flow image of the right renal artery.

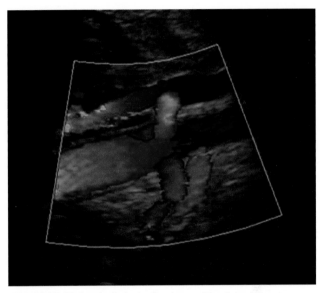

**FIGURE 25-12** Longitudinal color-flow image of the abdominal aorta illustrating the "banana peel" approach used for identifying the renal ostia and proximal renal artery segments.

to the low-resistance, high-diastolic renal artery flow allows recognition of abnormal flow patterns and ostial lesions (Fig. 25-11). Thereafter, Doppler spectral waveforms are obtained continuously throughout all visualized segments, and representative signals are then recorded taking care to ensure that all waveforms are obtained at appropriate angles of insonation.

Another imaging technique that has proven to be quite useful for identifying the ostia and proximal segments of the renal arteries is termed the "banana peel" approach. To achieve the best views, the patient is moved to the decubitus position opposite the side of interest. The aorta is imaged with the transducer oriented longitudinally. Using a "heel-toe" maneuver to achieve a near-zero Doppler angle of insonation, the renal arteries are identified as they arise from the lateral aortic walls (Fig. 25-12).

To interrogate the mid-to-distal segments of the renal arteries and parenchymal flow, the patient is moved to the lateral decubitus or prone position. With the patient lying in the decubitus position, a transverse image of the kidney can be obtained through an intercostal window using a coronal plane from the patient's flank. The right renal artery is relatively easy to follow from the renal hilum to its origin at the aortic wall. The left renal artery may be more difficult to visualize. It is helpful to image from a posterolateral plane, using the left kidney as an acoustic window. Assuming the positions of the hands on a clock, an image of the left kidney is obtained so that the renal pelvis is positioned at either 5, 6, or 7 o'clock. From the 5 o'clock position, the left renal artery will be noted to course slightly to the right before entering the kidney. At the 6 o'clock position, the renal artery will enter the hilum on a straight course. When imaged from the 7 o'clock position, the artery will

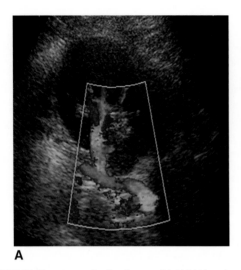 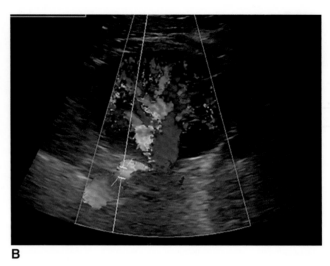

A                                                        B

**FIGURE 25-13** Transverse color-flow images of the left kidney demonstrating the renal artery entering the renal hilum at the 5 o'clock position (**A**) and the 7 o'clock position (**B**).

course slightly to the left just before entering the pelvis of the kidney (Fig. 25-13A,B).

Access to the distal segment of the renal artery can also be obtained by having the patient lie prone, flexed in the midsection over a pillow or foam wedge. Using an intercostal window, excellent images of the kidney and distal-to-mid segments of the renal artery are readily obtained. With both approaches, attention must be given to appropriate angle correction taking care to use a range of angles similar to those used for Doppler spectral interrogation of the proximal-to-mid segments of the artery.

### Identification of Accessory Renal Arteries

Several imaging approaches may be used to facilitate identification of accessory or multiple renal arteries. Duplicate renal arteries may be detected on a longitudinal, oblique image of the aorta or from a transverse view of the kidney where the arteries can be noted coursing to the polar surfaces rather than to the renal hilum (Fig. 25-14).

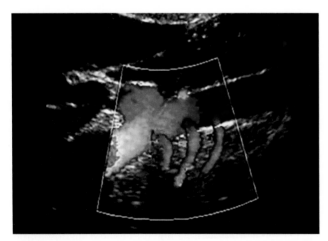

**FIGURE 25-14** Longitudinal color-flow image of the abdominal aorta demonstrating multiple renal arteries. (Image courtesy of Patricia A. (Tish) Poe, BA, RVT, FSVU.)

Whereas color-flow imaging is helpful in highlighting these small vessels, power Doppler imaging has shown value because of the lower angle dependence of this modality compared to color-flow imaging. Clues to the presence of additional renal arteries can also be obtained by increasing the sample volume size and scanning in the para-aortic region from the level of the SMA through the aortic bifurcation. Because the renal arteries are the only low-resistance vessels distal to the SMA, detection of multiple low-resistance Doppler signals should encourage the examiner to pursue one or more of the previously mentioned acoustic planes.

### Evaluation of Blood Flow within the Kidney

Blood flow patterns are recorded at a 0° angle of insonation throughout the upper, mid, and lower poles of the renal sinus, medulla, and cortex. Color and/or power Doppler imaging may facilitate detection of regions of absent or disturbed flow or increased signal amplitude. The Doppler spectral waveforms with the highest PSV and end-diastolic velocity (EDV) from each segment of the organ should be retained. In addition to evaluation of the renal vasculature, the parenchyma of the kidney should be examined for cortical thinning, renal calculi, masses, cysts, or hydronephrosis. The presence of perinephric fluid collections should also be noted.

### Determination of Renal Size

Because renal atrophy could preclude successful revascularization in patients with flow-limiting renal artery lesions, it is important to document kidney size during every examination. The normal renal length is between 9 and 13 cm. Comparing side to side, a difference in renal length greater than 1 cm suggests compromised flow on the side with the smaller kidney. With the patient lying in the lateral decubitus position and the transducer angled anterolaterally just below the costal border, a coronal or lateral flank approach can be used to obtain a long-axis view of the kidney. The pole-to-pole length of the kidney is measured during deep inspiration. Accuracy is enhanced by averaging three separate measurements.

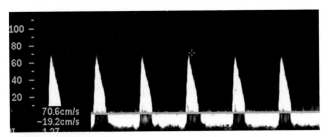

**FIGURE 25-15** Doppler spectral waveforms recorded within the renal parenchyma in a patient with renal vein thrombosis. Note the reversed, blunted diastolic flow component.

### Evaluation for Renal Vein Thrombosis

Patients may be referred to the vascular laboratory to rule out renal vein thrombosis. Patients with acute renal failure may present with pain and hematuria. Other patients may be suspected of renal cell carcinoma with extension of the tumor into the renal veins or IVC. The renal veins and IVC should always be examined in patients with an IVC filter or thrombosed IVC because retrograde thrombosis may extend into the renal veins.

Confirmation of renal vein thrombosis can be technically challenging. It is important to optimize the grayscale image because acute thrombus may have acoustic properties similar to flowing blood. Whereas venous dilation suggests acute thrombosis, the renal vein may be contracted when the condition is chronic. The absence of an optimized spectral, color, or power Doppler signal suggests thrombosis of the renal vein. In this setting, Doppler spectral waveforms with retrograde, blunted diastolic flow components are usually recorded throughout the arteries of the renal parenchyma (Fig. 25-15).

### Use of Contrast-Enhanced Imaging

There are many factors that may influence the ability to visualize the entire length of the renal artery, including excessive bowel gas, patient body habitus, and inability to adequately position the patient to gain optimal acoustic windows.[11] Quite often, imaging can be improved and diagnostic accuracy increased by employing intravenous ultrasound contrast agents to enhance visualization of the renal arteries. Although not yet approved by the Food and Drug Administration for clinical vascular evaluations, investigators have shown improved diagnostic accuracy when these agents are used in the liver, mesenteric, and peripheral vessels.[19,21]

A study from 2003 demonstrated improved ability to identify the renal ostium, the length of the renal artery, accessory renal arteries, and flow-limiting renal artery stenoses in select cases following intravenous injection of contrast (Fig. 25-16A,B).[22] Further discussion of ultrasound contrast agents will be found in Chapter 32 of this text.

## DIAGNOSIS

### The Abdominal Aorta and Common Iliac Arteries

The B-mode images of the normal abdominal aorta and common iliac arteries should demonstrate anechoic lumens with smooth arterial walls. Care should be taken to identify aneurysmal dilation, dissection, and/or atherosclerotic plaque with particular attention to the regions surrounding the aortic branch vessels. Recognition of narrowed or tortuous arterial segments may be facilitated by using color-flow or power Doppler imaging.

The proximal abdominal aorta carries blood to the low-resistance vascular beds of the liver, spleen, and kidneys. This flow demand is reflected in the Doppler spectral waveform morphology. At this level, the Doppler spectral waveform is characterized by rapid systolic upstroke, sharp systolic peak, and forward diastolic flow. The PSV ranges from 60 to 100 cm/s. Distal to the renal arteries, the aortic waveform exhibits slightly lower velocity and a triphasic flow pattern. This waveform pattern reflects the elevated vascular resistance of the lumbar arteries and lower extremity circulation.

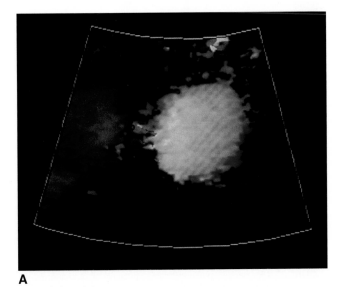

**A**

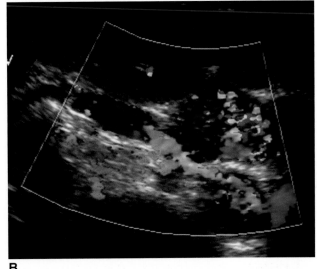

**B**

**FIGURE 25-16** Color-flow images of a renal artery prior to (**A**) and following (**B**) intravenous injection of an ultrasound contrast agent. (Image courtesy of John Pellerito, MD, North Shore University Medical Center, Long Island, NY.)

Flow should be laminar throughout the normal proximal abdominal aorta with the exception of slight flow disturbance, which may be evident at the ostia of the renal and mesenteric arteries. Increased velocity may be noted in tortuous vessels in the absence of disease, but high-velocity, turbulent signals suggest significant arterial narrowing.

## The Normal Renal Artery

The lumen of the normal renal artery should be anechoic, and the vessel should have smooth walls throughout its length. Color-flow and/or power Doppler imaging may demonstrate regions of narrowing caused by tortuosity, kinking, or extrinsic compression.

The Doppler spectral waveform from the normal renal artery is characterized by rapid systolic upstroke, a sharp systolic peak, and forward diastolic flow. An early systolic peak (ESP) or compliance peak may be seen on the upstroke to systole (Fig. 25-17). It is thought that the ESP or compliance peak is a reflection of the elasticity of the arterial wall and, therefore, its presence is usually variable throughout the renal artery and smaller vessels within the kidney.

The PSV of the adult renal artery ranges from 90 to 120 cm/s with EDV exceeding one-third the systolic value. Normally, PSV and EDV decrease proportionately from the main renal artery to the level of the renal cortex. The PSV in the distal renal artery ranges from 70 to 90 cm/s, decreasing to 30 to 50 cm/s in the renal sinus, and 10 to 20 cm/s at the level of the renal cortex.

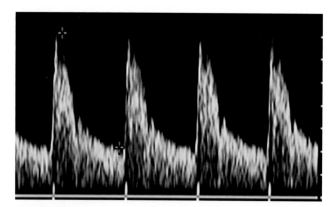

**FIGURE 25-17** Doppler spectral waveforms illustrating normal renal arterial waveform morphology.

## Renal Artery Stenosis of Less Than Hemodynamic Significance (<60%)

B-mode imaging may demonstrate atherosclerotic plaque extending from the aortic wall into the orifice or proximal segment of the renal artery. Color-flow imaging is helpful in identifying regions of disordered flow and narrowing of the arterial lumen.

As the diameter of the renal artery decreases, the flow demands of the kidney increase. Narrowing of the renal artery diameter by 30% to 60% results in an increase in renal artery PSV in excess of 180 cm/s. The degree of narrowing is not yet severe enough to cause a decrease in pressure or flow distal to the lesion. Therefore, poststenotic turbulence is not present with this degree of luminal compromise.

## Flow-reducing Renal Artery Stenosis (>60%)

When the diameter of the renal artery is reduced by more than 60%, the PSV increases significantly above 180 cm/s, and poststenotic turbulence develops immediately downstream (Fig. 25-18A–D). Beyond this region, in the absence

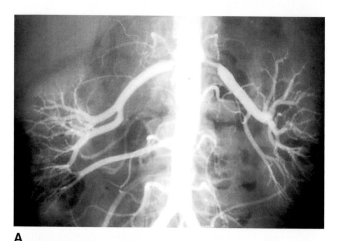

**A**

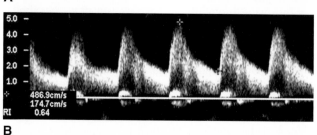

**B**

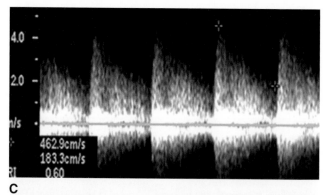

**C**

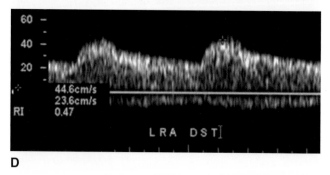

**D**

**FIGURE 25-18** Arteriogram demonstrating a proximal left renal artery stenosis (**A**) and the associated Doppler spectral waveforms demonstrating high velocity at the site of stenosis (**B**), poststenotic turbulence (**C**), and dampening (parvus tardus signal) distally (**D**).

of tandem or critical lesions, flow will gradually return to a normal laminar profile. It is important to confirm the poststenotic signal that differentiates a flow-reducing stenosis from one that is of less than hemodynamic significance (<60%). When the degree of arterial narrowing exceeds 80%, systolic upstroke will be delayed, the compliance peak will be lost, and the PSV will decrease distally (parvus tardus signal). In the absence of elevated renovascular resistance, diastolic forward flow will be maintained.

## Renal Artery Occlusion

Occlusion of the renal artery is confirmed by using optimized spectral, color, and power Doppler to demonstrate the absence of flow in the main renal artery. Multiple image planes may be required to ensure complete visualization of the full length of the vessel. Because the kidney is supplied by adrenal and ureteral collaterals, low-amplitude, low-velocity Doppler signals are usually noted throughout the renal medulla and cortex. With chronic renal artery occlusion, the PSV in the cortex will be less than 10 cm/s, and pole-to-pole length of the kidney will be less than 9 cm.

## Intrinsic Parenchymal Dysfunction

Using a 0° angle of insonation, Doppler spectral waveforms should be recorded throughout the parenchymal vessels in the medulla and cortex of the kidney. The spectral pattern differentiates normal renovascular resistance from intrinsic parenchymal dysfunction (medical renal disease). In the normal kidney, the Doppler spectral pattern demonstrates continuous high-diastolic flow throughout all segments of the kidney. In the absence of parenchymal disease, diastolic flow normally approximates 40% to 50% of the systolic velocity. Surprisingly, elevated diastolic flow is sustained even in normal kidneys with flow-limiting renal artery stenosis. It is most likely that the reduction in flow triggers compensatory vasodilation and renovascular resistance remains low.

Parenchymal disease most often results in accumulation of interstitial cellular infiltrates and edema, resulting in impedance to arterial inflow to the kidney and increased renovascular resistance. This finding is associated with a broad spectrum of renal disorders, including glomerulonephritis, polycystic disease, acute tubular necrosis, obstructive hydronephrosis, and diabetic nephropathy. In 1979, Arima et al.[23] and Norris and his colleagues[24] demonstrated that increased renovascular resistance is associated with decreased diastolic flow in native and transplanted kidneys. The amount of arterial impedance is dependent on age and the region of the renal arterial system that is sampled. The degree of renovascular resistance can be determined using a calculated resistive index (RI). Investigators have shown that the RI is normally highest in the renal hilum (0.65 ± 0.17) and lowest in the interlobar arteries (0.54 ± 0.20).[25-27] A diastolic to systolic velocity ratio less than 0.3 (RI greater than 0.8) is also predictive of medical renal disease; further decline in diastolic flow is associated with elevated blood urea nitrogen and serum creatinine levels.[28] Most modern ultrasound systems include the calculation of end diastolic to peak systolic ratio (EDR) or RI. The EDR is the EDV/PSV whereas the RI is the (PSV − EDV)/PSV.

## Indirect Renal Hilar Evaluations

Based on the knowledge that in peripheral arteries pulsatility decreases and systolic upstroke is delayed as a consequence of more proximal significant disease, several investigators have advocated use of a limited, indirect assessment of the arteries within the renal hilum. This approach is attractive because it overcomes the technical challenges associated with interrogation of the entire length of the renal artery and decreases the time required to perform the study. Handa et al.[29] demonstrated an accuracy of 95%, sensitivity of 100%, and specificity of 93% for identification of proximal flow-reducing renal artery stenosis using an *acceleration index (AI)* of less than 3.78. The *AI* is defined as the slope of the systolic upstroke (kHz/s) divided by the transmitted frequency. When translated into velocity units, an AI equal to or less than 291 cm/s$^2$ is suggestive of proximal flow-reducing renal artery stenosis. Martin and his colleagues found an *acceleration time* (AT), defined as the time interval between the onset of systole and the initial compliance peak, greater than 100 ms to be more predictive of significant proximal renal artery disease in their patient population than an AI.[30] The AT can be calculated automatically on most high-end ultrasound systems by indicating with calipers the onset of systole and the early systolic (compliance) peak. The value can also be determined by manual calculation by using hand-held calipers to measure the distance between these two points. Because the smallest time interval measured on most state-of-the art ultrasound systems is 40 ms, 2.5 time intervals demonstrated on the spectral display is equal to 100 ms. Stavros et al.[31] combined the AI and AT with loss of the compliance peak to identify proximal flow-limiting renal artery lesions and to differentiate 60% to 79% stenosis from more critical lesions as detailed in Figure 25-19. Other investigators have found low diagnostic sensitivity using hilar waveform evaluation for detection of significant renal artery disease.[32,33]

As noted previously, the main renal artery divides into several segmental branches proximal to the renal hilum. Because each of these branches originates from the main renal artery, in theory, it should not matter which branch is used for Doppler signal analysis. Inaccurate information could be obtained if Doppler waveforms were recorded in accessory, polar renal arteries because each of these could give rise to segmental branches with varying Doppler spectral waveform contours.

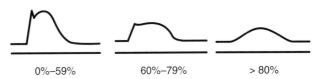

0%-59%          60%-79%          > 80%

**FIGURE 25-19** Diagram illustrating comparison of Doppler waveform morphology recorded in the distal main renal artery and segmental renal artery branches in normal and stenotic renal arteries. Note that rapid systolic upstroke and the compliance peak or ESP are commonly found in arteries with less than hemodynamically significant stenosis (0% to 59%). Some investigators have noted the loss of the compliance peak or ESP with renal artery stenosis in the range of 60% to 79%. The most validated observation is the dampened waveform found with renal artery stenosis exceeding 80%. (Modified from Stavros et al.[31])

The indirect renal hilar examination is performed with the patient lying in the lateral decubitus or prone position. Using an intercostal approach, a transverse image of the kidney is obtained at a depth between 4 and 8 cm in most patients. From this plane of view, the renal hilum and distal segmental branches of the main renal artery can be interrogated using a 0 degree angle of insonation. It is important to record a strong Doppler signal in order to optimize waveform clarity. This is accomplished by using the highest possible transducer frequency to improve Doppler sensitivity,[31] a large (3 to 5 mm) Doppler sample volume, and a sweep speed of 100 ms.

It has been estimated that hypertension affects 10% of the population of the United States, and that less than 6% of this group has renal artery disease. In order to detect disease that has such a low prevalence, a diagnostic test procedure must have high sensitivity. Unfortunately, although indirect hilar assessment is an attractive option, investigators report varying results ranging from high sensitivity to lack of correlation between the duplex sonographic findings and angiography.[12,31,34–40] There are multiple reasons for this variation in accuracy. Doppler waveform contour is affected by arterial compliance, obstruction to arterial inflow, and the degree of resistance in the microcirculation.[41,42] The AT and AI may remain normal in patients with elevated renovascular resistance (parenchymal dysfunction, medical renal disease) or systemic arterial stiffness. While delayed systolic upstroke and loss of a compliance peak are common findings in cases of renal artery stenosis exceeding 80% diameter reduction, the Doppler spectral waveform may remain normal when there is stenosis in the range of 60% to 79%. To complicate matters further, low-velocity, dampened intrarenal spectral waveforms have been noted in patients with aortic coarctation or aortic occlusion in the absence of significant renal artery stenosis. As a consequence of these and other issues, indirect renal hilar assessment is not recommended as the sole diagnostic tool for detection of renal artery disease. As long as the deficiencies of this approach are recognized, it does serve as a valuable tool to complement direct renal artery interrogation, particularly in cases where the direct examination is technically limited. It is important to keep in mind that hilar studies do not define the anatomic location of proximal renal artery lesions nor can they differentiate a well-collateralized renal artery occlusion from a high-grade stenosis.[30] Care must be taken to ensure that spectral waveforms are recorded in the distal main renal artery and its hilar branches and not in segmental branches of accessory renal arteries.

## Renal–Aortic Ratio and Current Criteria

Current diagnostic criteria for identification of renal artery stenosis are based on the renal–aortic ratio (RAR) which is the ratio of the renal artery PSV to the aortic PSV recorded at the level of the mesenteric arteries. Narrowing of the renal artery diameter by more than 60% to 70% results in significant increase in PSV while the velocity in the aorta remains relatively unchanged. Kohler and his colleagues[43] demonstrated excellent sensitivity for confirming the absence of flow-limiting (>60% diameter reduction)

renal artery stenosis using an RAR <3.5. Similarly, an RAR >3.5 has shown excellent value for identification of significant renal artery stenosis. As such, the RAR may be used as a primary diagnostic criterion as long as caveats are recognized. In patients with increased cardiac output or significant abdominal aortic stenosis, the aortic PSV may exceed 100 cm/s. In such cases, the calculated renal–aortic velocity ratio will be too low, and the severity of renal artery stenosis will be underestimated. For example, if the aortic velocity is 140 cm/s and the renal artery velocity is 320 cm/s, the renal–aortic velocity ratio is 2.3, mistakenly suggesting the absence of significant renal artery stenosis. Similarly, in cases with low cardiac output, aortic occlusion, coarctation, or aortic aneurysm, the aortic PSV will be lower than normal (<40 cm/s). Use of the calculated RAR could result in overestimation of the severity of renal artery stenosis.

Recently, investigators have compared the use of the conventional renal–aortic ratio (RAR) to use of a renal–renal ratio (RRR) for identification of >50% diameter-reducing renal artery stenosis.[44] The RRR is defined as the ratio between the PSV recorded in the proximal or midsegment of the renal artery compared to the PSV recorded in the distal segment of the renal artery. An RRR of 2.7 demonstrated a 97% sensitivity, 96% specificity, and 97% positive and negative predictive values.

Elevated renal artery velocity accompanied by poststenotic turbulence has been shown to be a sensitive predictor of flow-limiting renal artery stenosis.[45–47] Hoffman et al.[48] used a renal artery PSV greater than 180 cm/s as an indicator of stenotic renal artery disease. A pressure-flow gradient results when the diameter of the artery is reduced by more than 60% and poststenotic turbulence is apparent immediately distal to the site of narrowing. Renal artery stenosis of less than hemodynamic significance is identified by an elevated PSV (>180 cm/s), an RAR <3.5 and, most notably, the absence of a poststenotic signal. Inclusion of these criteria should be used in addition to, or in place of, the RAR to increase diagnostic accuracy. Table 25-1 summarizes the commonly utilized diagnostic criteria for renal artery stenosis.

## Evaluation of the Renal Veins

Duplex sonography should demonstrate an anechoic lumen and respirophasicity throughout all visualized segments of the normal renal vein. Intraluminal echoes will be apparent when the vein is obstructed. Care must be taken to optimize B-mode, spectral, and color Doppler parameters to ensure identification of acute thrombus, partial venous obstruction, recanalization, collateralization, and/or extrinsic compression. Continuous, nonphasic, low-velocity flow will be noted proximal to thrombosed venous segments. Minimally, phasic flow is often recorded distally if the thrombosed segment has recanalized or if venous collaterals have developed. If the kidney has been severely damaged by the thrombotic process, renal atrophy may be apparent, and the kidney may demonstrate increased echogenicity compared to the acoustic pattern of the normal contralateral organ. If the left renal vein is compressed by the mesentery artery or SMA,

| Stenosis (%) | RAR | PSV (cm/s) | PST | Kidney Length (cm) |
|---|---|---|---|---|
| Normal | <3.5 | <180 | Absent | 9–13 |
| <60 | <3.5 | >180 | Absent | 9–13 |
| >60 | >3.5 | >180 | Present | Variable |
| Occluded | N/A | N/A | N/A | <8 |

**TABLE 25-1  Classification of Renal Artery Stenosis Based on the Renal–Aortic Velocity Ratio, Peak Systolic Renal Artery Velocity, and Kidney Length**

PST, poststenotic turbulence.

a high-velocity signal associated with a color bruit may be noted in the vein as it crosses anterior to the aorta.

## SONOGRAPHIC EXAMINATION OF RENAL STENTS

It has been estimated that the restenosis rate following renal artery stenting ranges between 10% and 20%. Several technical and interpretive considerations must be applied to evaluation of renal arteries with stents.[49] While the majority of stents will be placed in the ostium or proximal renal artery, the number and location of stents may be variable. Proximal renal artery stents are most readily visualized from a cross-sectional image of the aorta at the level of the renal artery origins (Fig. 25-20). Harmonic and/or real-time compound imaging is used to improve resolution and conspicuity of lesions and to decrease artifacts. A slight velocity increase is to be expected in stented arterial segments because of the reduction in arterial compliance. Increased velocity may also be noted at the distal end of the stent when the diameter of the stented segment exceeds the diameter of the native renal artery. This most often occurs when the stent is placed in the smaller diameter distal renal artery.

It is important to note whether elevated velocity is focal or associated with downstream propagation of flow disturbance. Diameter mismatches are more likely to produce focal elevation in velocity without associated turbulence, whereas the flow profile of a flow-reducing stenosis exhibits high-velocity, poststenotic turbulence, and dampening of the distal waveform. Additionally, temporal changes in velocity will likely be noted when stenotic disease is present, but velocity elevations should remain stable if related to a diameter mismatch.

In 1999, Bakker et al.[50] reported 100% sensitivity and 90% specificity using a PSV threshold value of 226 cm/s and an RAR of 2.7 for recognition of in-stent restenosis. In 2007, using a PSV of 180 cm/s, Girndt et al[51] maintained the excellent sensitivity (100%), but noted that the sensitivity and specificity decreased to 50% and 89%, respectively, if an RAR of 3.5 was used. A few years later, Mohabbat et al.[52] reported a sensitivity of 93% and a specificity of 99% when using a PSV >280 cm/s and an RAR >4.5 to determine a significant in-stent stenosis. Most recently, Pellerito and his colleagues revealed unpublished retrospective data obtained from 98 renal stent evaluations. They documented 93% sensitivity and 92% specificity for recognition of flow-reducing in-stent renal artery stenosis using a peak systolic renal artery velocity equal to or greater than 240 cm/s. Excellent sensitivity and specificity (93% and 94%, respectively) were also obtained by applying a stent–aortic ratio equal to or greater than 3.2 to their studies. To date, diagnostic criteria have not been well validated for classification of renal artery stent stenosis and, in general, native renal artery criteria are being applied with special consideration to the issues of compliance, diameter mismatch, and stent location.[53,54]

## PREDICTION OF SUCCESSFUL RENAL REVASCULARIZATION

Although duplex sonography has been accepted as a valued noninvasive tool for identification of renal artery stenosis and renal parenchymal dysfunction, it has been difficult to define parameters that can be used to successfully select patients whose blood pressure or renal function will improve following renal revascularization. In 2001, Radermacher and his colleagues investigated the use of an RI = [1 − (EDV ÷ highest PSV)] × 100 in 138 patients with unilateral or bilateral significant renal artery stenosis to predict successful revascularization.[55] They also documented creatinine clearance and ambulatory blood pressure prior to the procedure and at three-monthly intervals

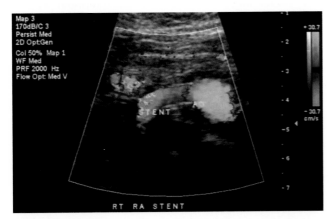

**FIGURE 25-20** Transverse aortic color-flow image illustrating a proximal right renal artery stent.

throughout the first year and yearly thereafter with a mean follow-up of 32 months. They found that an RI of 0.80 or greater could be used to predict which patients would be unlikely to benefit from either renal artery angioplasty or surgical bypass.

Numerous studies have shown that severe renal artery stenosis is associated with renal atrophy.[56–61] Caps et al.[62] demonstrated a high risk for progression to renal atrophy in patients with a renal artery PSV greater than 400 cm/s and a cortical EDV equal to or less than 5 cm/s. If renal artery stenosis is recognized before it critically affects blood flow to the kidney, it is likely that intervention may salvage or improve renal function.[61,63] Conversely, revascularization is most often unsuccessful in kidneys with a pole-to-pole length less than 8 cm.[64] As such, the measurement of kidney length should be a component of the scanning protocol whenever renal artery stenosis is suspected.

## DIAGNOSIS OF PEDIATRIC RENAL ARTERY STENOSIS

Approximately 85% of pediatric hypertension cases occur secondary to another abnormality; renovascular disease accounts for 10% to 25% of these cases. The secondary causes of pediatric hypertension include umbilical artery thrombosis with subsequent thromboembolism in the newborn, idiopathic hypercalcemia in infancy (Williams–Bueren's syndrome), renal parenchymal disease, obstructive uropathies, aortic coarctation, drug-induced hypertension, renin-producing tumors, and pheochromocytomas. In up to 70% of cases, renal artery stenosis is caused by fibromuscular dysplasia with medial hyperplasia being the predominant subtype. Multicystic renal dysplasia is the second most common type of childhood renal disorder.

When compared to adult kidneys, a number of distinct anatomic differences in size, location, and appearance will be noted. In a neonate, the pole-to-pole kidney length is usually less than 4 cm and increases only slightly (to less than 6 cm) throughout the first year. In children, the kidney is positioned lower in the abdomen than an adult kidney and is most often fully ascended when the child is around 6 years old. Newborn kidneys are lobulated with fetal lobulations remaining apparent in the renal cortex for the first 5 years. In infants, the renal parenchyma is more echogenic than in an adult kidney, and the renal pyramids are quite prominent. The renal sinus is less echogenic in a child because it is not infiltrated with fat as it is in an adult kidney (Fig. 25-21).

For evaluation of pediatric renal vascular cases, patients are fasted for approximately 3 hours prior to the examination. Low-frequency curved array or linear transducers are employed for the study. The scanning technique does not differ significantly from that used for adult patients. While most children can be positioned as previously described, the examination of an infant's renal vessels and kidneys may be facilitated by placing the child prone with the abdomen flexed over a pillow and using an intercostal scan plane. As necessary, the mother is permitted to lie near the child,

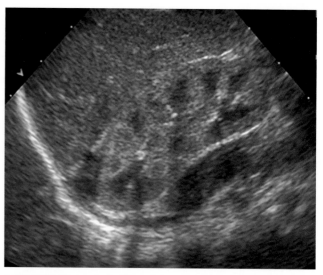

**FIGURE 25-21** Longitudinal B-mode image of an infant's kidney. Note the prominent pyramids, indistinct renal sinus, and increased echogenicity compared to that seen in the normal adult kidney.

and the study is performed when the child is calm and breathing quietly.

Given that the diagnosis of renal artery stenosis is based on velocity parameters and Doppler waveform morphology, it is important to remember that velocity within the renal artery and parenchymal vessels is dependent on age and location of Doppler sampling. The highest velocity is commonly found in the main renal artery, whereas the lowest velocity is in the interlobar arteries. Deeg et al.[65] reported a PSV of 51.5 ± 13.4 cm/s in the main renal artery and 19.5 ± 5 cm/s in the interlobar arteries of children less than 1 year of age. In contrast, in children between 6 and 12 years of age, the PSV in the main renal artery was 80 ± 18 and 27.9 ± 5.3 cm/s in the interlobar arteries. The values did not change significantly in children between 12 and 18 years of age. These investigators also noted that the RI decreased with age. The RI in the main renal artery of infants was 0.82 ± 0.11 and 0.73 ± 0.17 in the interlobar arteries. In children between 6 and 12 years of age, the RI values were 0.71 ± 0.09 and 0.58 ± 0.10 for the main renal artery and the interlobar arteries, respectively. No significant change in these values was noted for children between 12 and 18 years of age. Several investigators have noted that the RI is normally higher in children than in adults and following cardiac bypass, the RI in children is normally elevated (>1.0) for at least the first 3 days.[66–69]

In infants, the RI is most often less than 0.85 in the absence of flow-reducing renal artery stenosis but will exceed that value when flow-limiting renal artery disease is present. At present, well-validated diagnostic criteria for identification of renal artery stenosis in pediatric patients have not been reported in the literature. In general, diagnosis is based on elevated PSV, poststenotic turbulence, and delayed systolic upstroke and run-off distal to the stenotic site.

## SUMMARY

- Duplex sonography of the renal vasculature and kidneys has become the initial primary diagnostic procedure for evaluation of renovascular hypertension and suspected renal artery pathology in both adult and pediatric patients.
- Although technically challenging, renal vascular sonography provides noninvasive, cost-effective, accurate diagnostic information.
- Duplex ultrasound technology allows definition of vessel and tissue pathology, detection of altered blood flow patterns, and quantitation of hemodynamic disturbances.
- The length of the abdominal aorta, renal arteries, and kidneys can be evaluated with B-mode imaging to localize atherosclerotic disease, fibromuscular dysplasia, aneurysms, dissections, cysts, and masses and to demonstrate extrinsic compression of the renal vessels because of masses or entrapment.
- This modality has also shown value as a tool for confirming progression of renal artery stenosis and defining therapeutic options based on kidney size and cortical flow patterns.
- Color-flow and power Doppler imaging facilitate recognition of regions of flow disturbance, stenosis, occlusion, and anatomic anomalies.
- Visualization of the blood flow vectors eases placement of the Doppler sample volume for waveform analysis and measurement of velocities.
- The determination of disease severity is based on the PSV and the presence or absence of a poststenotic signal in the main renal artery.
- Assessment of velocity waveform parameters recorded within the renal parenchyma yields clues to the presence of intrinsic renal disease and the likelihood of successful revascularization.
- The role of indirect, renal hilar duplex sonography for identification of flow-limiting renal artery disease remains controversial. At present, studies have shown that it is best used to complement direct, complete examination of the renal arteries and kidneys.
- Given the broad scope of diagnostic information that can be obtained using ultrasound to interrogate the renal vasculature, it is not surprising that duplex sonography is recognized as the ideal technology for identification of renal vascular disease in children and adults and for follow-up after endovascular or surgical intervention.

- The technical success of each study is influenced by the experience of the examiner and physician interpreter. Complete, accurate examinations of the renal vasculature are possible in more than 90% of patients when the study is performed in high-volume laboratories by experienced, credentialed sonographers and interpreted by qualified physicians both of whom have a knowledge of renal vascular disease, the validated techniques used for assessment of the renal vasculature, and the current diagnostic criteria used for classification of renal artery stenosis.

## CRITICAL THINKING QUESTIONS

1. A patient presents for a renal duplex scan. Prior to initiating the examination, you can determine the approximate location of this patient's renal arteries by noting several body surface landmarks. What are the most important landmarks to use to accomplish this goal?
2. During the renal sonographic examination, there are other important anatomic landmarks to use for locating the renal arteries. Which of the landmarks are most commonly used?
3. It is always important to consider the patient's clinical presentation. For example, if you had a 40-year-old hypertensive female present for renal duplex sonography, what would be the most likely pathology responsible for her renovascular hypertension?
4. A patient of large body habitus presents for a renal duplex ultrasound examination. With the patient lying supine, you are able to image the abdominal aorta in both sagittal and cross-sectional planes, but you cannot visualize the right renal artery. What steps can you take to determine whether the renal artery is patent or occluded?
5. A PSV of 220 cm/s is recorded in the proximal segment of a tortuous right renal artery. How would you determine whether the elevated velocity is the result of flow-limiting stenosis or vessel angulation?

## MEDIA MENU

Student Resources available on thePoint® include:
- Audio glossary
- Interactive question bank
- Videos
- Internet resources

## REFERENCES

1. Berglund G, Anderson O, Wilhelmensen L. Prevalence of primary and secondary hypertension: studies in a random population sample. *BMJ.* 1976;2:554–556.
2. Dunnick NR, Sfakianakis GN. Screening for renovascular hypertension. *Radiol Clin North Am.* 1991;29:497–510.
3. Holley KE, Hunt JC, Brown AL, et al. Renal artery stenosis: a clinical-pathologic study in normotensive and hypertensive patients. *Am J Med.* 1964;37:14–18.
4. Eyler WR, Clark MD, Garman JE, et al. Angiography of the renal arteries including a comparative study of renal arterial stenoses in patients with and without hypertension. *Radiology.* 1962;78:879–882.

5. Caps MT, Perissinotto C, Zierler RE, et al. A prospective study of atherosclerotic disease progression in the renal artery. *Circulation.* 1998;98:2866–2872.
6. Plouin PF, Rossignol P, Brobie G. Atherosclerotic renal artery stenosis: to treat conservatively, to dilate, to stent, or o operate? *J Am Soc Nephrol.* 2001;12:2190–2196.
7. Mailloux LU, Husain A. Atherosclerotic ischemic nephropathy as a cause of chronic kidney disease; what can be done to prevent end-stage renal disease? *Saudi J Kidney Dis Transpl.* 2002;13(3):311–319.
8. Chobanian AV, Bakris GL, Black HR, et al. The Seventh Report of the Joint National Committee on Prevention, Detection, Evaluation, and Treatment of High Blood Pressure. *JAMA.* 2003;289:2560–2572.

9. Safian RD, Textor SC. Renal artery stenosis. *N Engl J Med.* 2001;344(6):431–442.
10. Johnson PT, Halpern EJ, Kuszyk BS, et al. Renal artery stenosis: CT angiography: comparison of real-time volume rendering and maximum intensity projection algorithms. *Radiology.* 1999;211(2):337–343.
11. Hansen KJ, Tribble RW, Reavis SW, et al. Renal duplex sonography: evaluation of clinical utility. *J Vasc Surg.* 1990;12:227–236.
12. Kliewer MA, Tupler RH, Hertzberg BS, et al. Doppler evaluation of renal artery stenosis: interobserver agreement in the interpretation of waveform morphology. *Am J Roentgenol.* 1994;162:1371–1376.
13. Stanley JC. Natural history of renal artery stenosis and aneurysms. In: Calligaro KD, Dougherty MJ, Dean RH, eds. *Modern Management of Renovascular Hypertension and Renal Salvage.* Baltimore, MD: Williams & Wilkins; 1996:14–45.
14. Working Group on Renovascular Hypertension. Detection, evaluation, and treatment of renovascular hypertension. *Arch Intern Med.* 1987;147:820–829.
15. Bookstein JJ, Maxwell MH, Abrams HL, et al. Cooperative study of radiologic aspects of renovascular hypertension. *JAMA.* 1977;237:1706–1709.
16. Stanley JC, Gewertz BL, Bove BL, et al. Arterial fibrodysplasia: histopathologic character and current etiologic concepts. *Arch Surg.* 1975;110:561–566.
17. Treadway KK, Slater EE. Renovascular hypertension. *Annu Rev Med.* 1984;35:665–692.
18. Harrison EG, McCormack U. Pathological classification of renal artery disease in renovascular hypertension. *Mayo Clin Proc.* 1971;46:161–167.
19. Cotter B, Mahmud E, Kwan OL, DeMaria AN. New ultrasound agents: expanding upon existing clinical applications. In: Goldberg BB, ed. *Ultrasound Contrast Agents.* St. Louis, MO: Mosby; 1997:31–42.
20. Neumyer MM, Thiele BL, Strandness DE Jr. *Techniques of Abdominal Vascular Sonography. A Videotape Production.* Pasadena, CA: Davies Publishing, Inc.; 1996.
21. Goldberg BB, Liu JB, Forsberg F. Ultrasound contrast agents: a review. *Ultrasound Med Biol.* 1994;20(4):319–333.
22. Blebea J, Zickler R, Volteas N, et al. Duplex imaging of the renal arteries with contrast enhancement. *Vasc Endovascular Surg.* 2003;37:429–436.
23. Arima M, Ishibashi M, Usami M, et al. Analysis of the arterial blood flow patterns of normal and allografted kidneys by the directional ultrasonic Doppler technique. *J Urol.* 1979;122:587–591.
24. Norris CS, Pfeiffer JS, Rittgers SE, et al. Noninvasive evaluation of renal artery stenosis and renovascular resistance. *J Vasc Surg.* 1984;1:192–201.
25. Zubarev AV. Ultrasound of renal vessels. *Eur Radiol.* 2001;11:1902–1915.
26. Korst MB, Joosten FB, Postma CT, et al. Accuracy of normal-dose contrast-enhanced MR angiography in assessing renal artery stenosis and accessory renal artery stenosis and accessory renal arteries. *Am J Roentgenol.* 2000;174:629–634.
27. Krumme B. Renal Doppler sonography-Update in clinical nephrology. *Nephron Clin Pract.* 2006;103:c24–c28.
28. Neumyer MM, Wengrovitz M, Ward T, et al. Differentiation of renal artery stenosis from renal parenchymal disease using duplex ultrasonography. *J Vasc Technol.*
29. Handa N, Fukunaga R, Etani H, et al. Efficacy of echo-Doppler examination for the evaluation of renovascular disease. *Ultrasound Med Biol.* 1988;14:1–5.
30. Martin RL, Nanra RS, Wlodarczyk J. Renal hilar Doppler analysis in the detection of renal artery stenosis. *J Vasc Technol.* 1991;15(4):173–180.
31. Stavros TA, Parker SH, Yakes YF, et al. Segmental stenosis of the renal artery: pattern recognition of the tardus and parvus abnormalities with duplex sonography. *Radiology.* 1992;184:487–492.
32. Isaacson JA, Neumyer MM. Direct and indirect renal arterial duplex and Doppler color flow evaluations. *J Vasc Technol.* 1995;19:309–316.
33. Isaacson JA, Zierler RE, Spittell PC, et al. Noninvasive screening for renal artery stenosis: comparison of renal artery and renal hilar duplex scanning. *J Vasc Technol.* 1995;19:105–110.
34. Baxter GM, Aitchison F, Sheppard D, et al. Colour Doppler ultrasound in renal artery stenosis: intrarenal waveform analysis. *Br J Radiol.* 1996;69:810–815.
35. Kliewer MA, Hertzberg BS, Keogan MT, et al. Early systole in the healthy kidney: variability of Doppler US waveform parameters. *Radiology.* 1997;205:109–113.
36. Helenon O, Rody FE, Correas JM, et al. Color Doppler US of renovascular disease in native kidneys. *Radiographics.* 1995;15:833–854.
37. Postma CT, Bijlstra PJ, Rosenbusch G, et al. Pattern recognition of loss of early systolic peak by Doppler ultrasound has a low sensitivity for the detection of renal artery stenosis. *J Hum Hypertens.* 1996;10:181–184.
38. Nazal MM, Hoballah JJ, Miller EV, et al. Renal hilar Doppler analysis is of value in the management of patients with renovascular disease. *Am J Surg.* 1997;174:164–168.
39. Kliewer MA, Tupler RH, Carroll BA, et al. Renal artery stenosis: analysis of Doppler waveform parameters and tardus-parvus pattern. *Radiology.* 1993;189:779–787.
40. Patriquin HB, LaFortune M, Jequier J-C, et al. Stenosis of the renal artery: assessment of slowed systole in the downstream circulation with Doppler sonography. *Radiology.* 1992;184:470–485.
41. van der Hulst VPM, van Baalen J, Kool LS, et al. Renal artery stenosis: endovascular flow wire study for validation of Doppler US. *Radiology.* 1996;100:165–168.
42. Bude RO, Rubin JM, Platt JF, et al. Pulsus tardus: its cause and potential limitations in detection of arterial stenosis. *Radiology.* 1994;190:779–784.
43. Kohler TR, Zierler RE, Martin RL, et al. Noninvasive diagnosis of renal artery stenosis by ultrasonic duplex scanning. *J Vasc Surg.* 1986;4:450–456.
44. Chain S, Luciardi H, Feldman G, et al. Diagnostic role of new Doppler index in assessment of renal artery stenosis. *Cardiovasc Ultrasound,* 2006;4:4.
45. Taylor DC, Kettler MD, Moneta GL, et al. Duplex ultrasound scanning in the diagnosis of renal artery stenosis: a prospective evaluation. *J Vasc Surg.* 1988;7:363–369.
46. Taylor DC, Moneta GL, Strandness DE Jr. Follow-up renal artery stenosis by duplex ultrasound. *J Vasc Surg.* 1989;9:410–415.
47. Neumyer MM, Wengrovitz M, Ward T, et al. The differentiation of renal artery stenosis from renal parenchymal disease by duplex ultrasonography. *J Vasc Technol.* 1989;13:205–216.
48. Hoffman U, Edwards JM, Carter S, et al. Role of duplex scanning for the detection of atherosclerotic renal artery disease. *Kidney Int.* 1991;39:1232–1239.
49. Neumyer MM. Duplex scanning after renal artery stenting. *J Vasc Technol.* 2003;27(3):177–183.
50. Bakker J, Beutler JJ, Elgersma OE, et al. Duplex ultrasonography in assessing restenosis of renal artery stents. *Cardiovasc Interv Radiol.* 1999;22:475–480.
51. Girndt M, Kaul H, Maute C, et al. Enhanced flow velocity after stenting of renal arteries is associated with decreased renal function. *Nephron Clin Pract.* 2007;105:c84–c89.
52. Mohabbat W, Greenberg RK, Mastracci TM, et al. Revised duplex criteria and outcomes for renal stents and stent grafts following endovascular repair of juxtarenal and thoracoabdominal aneurysms. *J Vasc Surg.* 2009;49(4):827–837.
53. Rocha-Singh K, Jaff MR, Kelley Lynne E. Renal artery stenting with noninvasive duplex ultrasound follow-up: 3-year results from the RENAISSANCE renal stent trial. *Catheter Cardiovasc Interv.* 2008;72(6):853–862.
54. Chi YW, White CJ, Thomton S, et al. Ultrasound velocity criteria for renal in-stent restenosis. *J Vasc Surg.* 2009;50(1):119–123.
55. Radermacher J, Chavan A, Bleck J, et al. Use of Doppler ultrasonography to predict the outcome of therapy for renal artery stenosis. *N Engl J Med,* 2001;344(6):410–417.
56. Moran K, Muihall J, Kelly D, et al. Morphological changes and alterations in regional intrarenal blood flow induced by graded renal ischemia. *J Urol.* 1992;148:1463–1466.
57. Truong LD, Farhood A, Tasby J, et al. Experimental chronic renal ischemia: morphologic and immunologic studies. *Kidney Int.* 1992;41:1676–1689.
58. Gob'e GC, Axelsen RA, Searle JW. Cellular events in experimental unilateral ischemic renal atrophy and regeneration after contralateral nephrectomy. *Lab Invest.* 1990;63:770–779.
59. Sabbatini M, Sansone G, Uccello F, et al. Functional versus structural changes in the pathophysiology of acute ischemic renal failure in aging rats. *Kidney Int.* 1994;45:1355–1361.
60. Shanley PF. The pathology of chronic renal ischemia. *Semin Nephrol.* 1996;16:21–32.
61. Guzman RP, Zierler RE, Isaacson JA, et al. Renal atrophy and renal artery stenosis: a prospective study with duplex ultrasound. *Hypertension.* 1994;23:346–350.

62. Caps MT, Zierler RE, Polissar NL, et al. The risk of atrophy in kidneys with atherosclerotic renal artery stenosis. *Kidney Int.* 1998;53:735–742.

63. Cambria RP, Brewster DC, L'Italien GJ, et al. Renal artery reconstruction for the preservation of renal function. *J Vasc Surg.* 1996;24:371–380.

64. Hallett JW Jr, Fowl R, O'Brien PC, et al. Renovascular operations in patients with chronic renal insufficiency: do the benefits justify the risks? *J Vasc Surg.* 1987;5:622–627.

65. Deeg KH, Worle K, Wolf A. Doppler sonographic estimation of normal values for flow velocity and resistance indices in renal arteries of healthy infants. *Ultraschall Med.* 2003;24(5):312–322.

66. Wong SN, Lo RN, Yu EC. Renal blood flow pattern by noninvasive Doppler ultrasound in normal children and acute renal failure patients. *J Ultrasound Med.* 1989;8:135–141.

67. Keller MS. Renal Doppler sonography in infants and children. *Radiology.* 1989;172:603–604.

68. Grunert D, Schoning M, Rosendahl W. Renal blood flow and flow velocity in children and adolescents; duplex Doppler evaluation. *Eur J Pediatr.* 1990;149:287–292.

69. Patriquin H. Doppler examination of the kidney in infants and children. *Urol Radiol.* 1991;12:220–227.

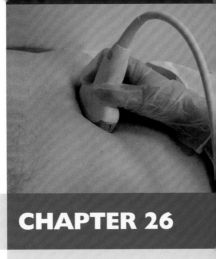

# The Inferior Vena Cava and Iliac Veins

MICHAEL J. COSTANZA

**CHAPTER 26**

## OBJECTIVES

- Describe the anatomy and physiology of the inferior vena cava and iliac veins

- Identify the most useful positions for the patient and sonographer for conducting an ultrasound examination of the inferior vena cava and iliac veins

- Recognize useful maneuvers to improve the ergonomics and imaging quality of an ultrasound examination of the inferior vena cava and iliac veins

- List the required images for an ultrasound examination of the inferior vena cava and iliac veins

- Understand the most common pathologic conditions and anatomic variants of the inferior vena cava and iliac veins

- Describe how color, spectral, and power Doppler evaluations are complementary to each other and grayscale images

- List the grayscale, color, and spectral Doppler characteristics of the most common pathologic conditions and anatomic variants of the inferior vena cava and iliac veins

## GLOSSARY

**confluence** The union of two or more veins to form a larger vein; the equivalent of a bifurcation in the arterial system

**inferior vena cava filter** A typically cone-shaped medical device designed to prevent pulmonary embolism; an IVC filter is placed into the inferior vena cava so that it can trap venous thromboemboli from the lower extremities before they travel to the heart and lungs

**pulmonary embolus** The obstruction of the pulmonary arteries usually from detached fragments of a blood clot that travels from the lower extremity veins

**retroperitoneum** The space between the abdominal cavity and the muscles and bones of the posterior abdominal wall; vascular structures in the retroperitoneum include the inferior vena cava, the iliac veins, and the abdominal aorta

**thrombosis** Partial or complete occlusion of a blood vessel as a result of clot

The retroperitoneal location of the inferior vena cava (IVC) and iliac veins makes them challenging to examine sonographically. Successful imaging of the IVC and iliac veins requires knowledge of their anatomy and physiology as well as appropriate preparation and patient positioning. Because these vessels can be the source of a pulmonary embolus, careful evaluation is essential. In addition to detecting thrombus, ultrasound has proven to be a useful tool to aid in the placement of IVC filters and their follow-up.

## ANATOMY

The external iliac veins drain the lower extremities as a continuation of the common femoral veins. They begin at the inguinal ligament and course cephalad as they dive deep into the pelvis. The internal iliac veins drain the pelvic viscera and musculature and join the external iliac veins at the level of the sacroiliac joints to form the common iliac veins. The IVC begins at the junction of the right and left common iliac veins at the level of the fifth lumbar vertebra. It ascends in the retroperitoneum to the right of the abdominal aorta and courses through the deep fossa on the posterior surface of the liver between the caudate lobe and bare area. After passing through the diaphragm at the level of the eighth thoracic vertebra, the IVC terminates in the right atrium. The venous tributaries of the IVC are listed in Table 26-1.

The IVC receives blood from all organs and tissues inferior to the diaphragm. It returns the deoxygenated blood to the heart for oxygenation and recirculation. The diameter of the IVC depends on the hydration status of the patient. In well-hydrated patients, the IVC appears distended, and the mean diameter at the level of the renal veins is 17 to 20 mm.[1] Mega cava (excessively large IVC diameter) is a rare condition that tends to occur only in patients of very large stature or in patients with congestive heart failure. Most large series reported less than 3% of examined patients had an IVC larger than 28 mm in diameter.[2] Dehydration causes collapse of the IVC, making it narrow and difficult to detect and evaluate with ultrasound. In these situations, having an assistant elevate the patient's legs often increases the caliber of the vein, making it easier to visualize.[3]

### Anatomic Variants

Because several precursor veins contribute to its formation during embryogenesis, the IVC can display a wide spectrum of anatomic variation. Persistence of the left precursor of the IVC can result in paired vena cavae or a left-sided IVC. In the case of paired vena cavae, the duplication typically terminates at the level of the renal veins when the left IVC drains into the left renal vein. A completely left-sided IVC can either terminate in the left renal vein or extend cranially to drain into the azygos vein in the chest.[4]

Anomalies of the IVC may also involve its intrahepatic portion. When the intrahepatic portion of the IVC is congenitally absent, blood is returned to the heart via the azygos or hemiazygos veins. Although ultrasound may not detect this anomalous collateral venous pathway, the diagnosis can be made by demonstrating direct drainage of the hepatic veins into the right atrium as well as absence of the intrahepatic IVC. In membranous obstruction of the intrahepatic IVC, ultrasound demonstrates a fibrous septum in the IVC just cephalad to the insertion of the right hepatic vein. Flow may be reversed in the IVC, and flow in the distal hepatic veins is sluggish and continuous.

## SONOGRAPHIC EXAMINATION TECHNIQUES

### Patient Preparation

Extensive bowel gas represents the most common impediment to a successful sonographic examination of the IVC and iliac veins. The bowel gas prevents transmission of the ultrasound signal and precludes accurate identification of any deep abdominal structures. Having the patient fast for 8 hours prior to the examination can decrease the likelihood of bowel gas; however, the examination should still be attempted even if the patient has eaten. Although morbid obesity can make abdominal imaging difficult because of the depth of penetration necessary, it rarely precludes adequate IVC visualization. In surgical patients, open abdominal wounds can encroach on the areas of the abdomen typically used to place the ultrasound probe. These patients may require alternative probe placement and the assistance of the nursing staff to achieve a complete ultrasound examination.

### History and Physical

The history and physical should focus on detecting signs and symptoms of deep venous thrombosis (DVT) and venous insufficiency. Patients should be questioned about lower extremity edema, including the duration of symptoms, location (unilateral vs. bilateral), associated skin changes, and recent injury, illness, or surgery. Recent onset of unilateral lower extremity edema following a recent illness or surgery could indicate an acute ileofemoral DVT. Long-term, bilateral lower extremity edema associated with skin hyperpigmentation or lower leg ulcers could indicate chronic venous insufficiency. Patients with a previous history of DVT or pulmonary embolism may have an IVC filter in place which should be evaluated during the sonographic exam.

### Patient Positioning

The examination begins with the patient in supine position and the sonographer standing to the patient's right side. The height of the bed or stretcher should be adjusted

| TABLE 26-1 | **IVC Venous Tributaries** |
|---|---|
| Hepatic veins | |
| Renal veins | |
| Common iliac veins | |
| Right adrenal vein | |
| Right ovarian vein or testicular vein | |
| Inferior phrenic vein | |
| Four lumbar veins | |
| Medial sacral vein | |

so that the level of the patient's abdomen is slightly lower than the sonographer's waist. In this configuration, the sonographer can extend his or her scanning arm downward and ergonomically apply pressure to the patient's abdomen. The ability to easily and comfortably apply pressure with the probe often allows the sonographer to disperse bowel gas and obtain better images of deep abdominal structures. The amount of force exerted on the transducer must be regulated because excessive pressure will also compress the IVC, making it difficult to visualize.

## Scanning Technique

Achieving adequate penetration usually requires a 1 to 4 MHz probe; however, a 5 MHz probe may be more appropriate for thin patients. A complete examination requires a longitudinal and transverse survey of the IVC from the diaphragm to the confluence of the common iliac veins.

The examination begins with the probe perpendicular, at the midline of the body, just distal to the xyphoid process of the sternum. Angling the transducer to the patient's left allows visualization of the proximal abdominal aorta posterior to the liver. After identifying this landmark, the transducer can be angled to the patient's right side to obtain a longitudinal image of the IVC posterior to the liver (Fig. 26-1). The hepatic veins which are anterior tributaries of the proximal IVC should be recognized and evaluated. The transducer can then be slowly moved inferiorly using a rock and slide motion. By slightly rocking to the right and then to the left, each side of the IVC is scanned while sliding the probe inferiorly.[5] Rotating the transducer may be required to keep the IVC in view. This technique uses the sagittal plane to obtain longitudinal images of the proximal, mid, and distal IVC to the common iliac vein confluence (usually at the level of the umbilicus).

To scan in the transverse plane, the transducer is returned to the anterior, subxyphoid location and angled superiorly. Once the heart is visualized, the transducer should be slowly straightened to look for the IVC just to the right of the midline. In the transverse plane, the IVC will appear oval (Fig. 26-2). While keeping the IVC in view, the transducer is moved inferiorly with the rock and slide motion as previously described. The renal veins which are lateral

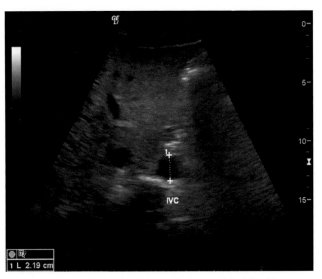

**FIGURE 26-2** Grayscale image of a transverse view of the IVC with a diameter measurement.

tributaries of the IVC should be noted and evaluated. The examination continues inferiorly through the level of the common iliac veins until they can no longer be visualized.

The coronal plane may offer better imaging of the distal IVC and the confluence of the common iliac veins. With the patient in the left lateral decubitus position, the probe is placed superior to the right iliac crest in the mid-coronal plane. The inferior pole of the right kidney provides a landmark, and the IVC bifurcation is usually medial and inferior to it. Although scanning in the coronal plane is possible with the patient in supine position, the left lateral decubitus position offers an ergonomic advantage and may produce superior images in patients who have bowel gas that obscures an anterior acoustic window.

A portion of the common iliac veins will most likely be identified and evaluated during the IVC survey. For the rest of the iliac venous examination, the patient should be supine with the bed or stretcher in reverse Trendelenburg position. The same 1 to 4 MHz probe can be used or a 5 MHz probe may be more appropriate for thin patients. Starting at the groin, the common femoral vein can be followed proximally to identify and examine the distal external iliac vein. When the external iliac begins to dive deep into the pelvis, the examination continues using an anterolateral approach with the transducer placed lateral to the rectus muscle.[6] The external and common iliac veins are then followed proximally to their confluence. Imaging the entire iliac venous system can be challenging. The confluence of the external and common iliac veins often cannot be definitively identified, and the deep location of the iliac veins can compromise image quality.

The efficiency of the examination can be improved by minimizing the number of times the patient changes position. With the patient supine, the IVC survey to obtain longitudinal and transverse images should be performed, followed by the iliac vein evaluation. The patient can then be turned to the left lateral decubitus position for scanning in the coronal plane to obtain images of the distal IVC and the common iliac confluence. The required images for the IVC and iliac venous examination are listed in Table 26-2.

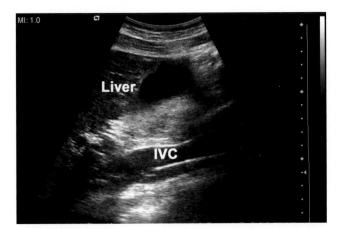

**FIGURE 26-1** Grayscale image of a longitudinal view of the IVC.

**TABLE 26-2　Required Images for IVC and Iliac Veins**

| Image Plane | Anatomic Level | Landmarks |
|---|---|---|
| Longitudinal | Proximal IVC | Diaphragm and hepatic vein(s) |
| | Middle IVC | Head of the pancreas |
| | Distal IVC | |
| | Common iliac vein confluence | Common iliac veins |
| | External iliac veins | |
| Transverse | Proximal IVC | Hepatic veins |
| | Middle IVC | Renal veins |
| | Distal IVC | |
| | Common iliac vein confluence | Common iliac veins |
| | External iliac veins | |

## DIAGNOSIS

The normal IVC and iliac veins have echogenic, muscular walls. The lumen of these vessels should appear anechoic. With quiet respiration, the diameter of the IVC may appear to change with the phasic changes in abdominal pressure produced during respiration. The grayscale image can be evaluated for various pathologies, including thrombosis, intraluminal tumor, and extrinsic compression (Pathology Box 26-1).

### Thrombosis

Thrombosis that results from propagation of a lower extremity venous thromboembolism represents the most common pathologic finding. Grayscale imaging may reveal a distended

IVC or iliac vein with echogenic material within the lumen. Recently formed thrombus can be virtually anechoic and undetectable by grayscale imaging. This situation highlights the importance of color-flow and Doppler examination to evaluate IVC and iliac vein patency (Fig. 26-3). The echogenicity of a thrombus increases as it ages over the course of several days and weeks. Thrombus that does not obstruct flow may only be detected by grayscale imaging demonstrating free-floating echogenic material within the IVC or iliac vein lumen.

### Neoplastic Obstruction

Compared to thrombotic occlusion, neoplastic obstruction of the IVC and iliac veins is rare. Grayscale imaging reveals an intraluminal tumor or an extrinsic mass. Intraluminal

**PATHOLOGY BOX 26-1**
*Common Pathology of the Inferior Vena Cava and the Iliac Veins*

| Condition | Sonographic Findings | | |
|---|---|---|---|
| | **Grayscale** | **Color** | **Doppler** |
| Thrombus (occlusive) | Distended vein with echogenic material within lumen | Absent flow | No signal |
| Thrombus (partially occlusive) | Echogenic material that appears partially free floating and partially attached to the vessel wall | Present or diminished flow | Continuous signal; loss of respiratory and cardiac variation |
| Neoplastic obstruction | Intraluminal tumor originating from renal or hepatic veins or extrinsic mass | Absent flow; collateral veins may be detected | No signal or continuous signal in partial obstruction; look for arterial flow with tumor |
| IVC filter with thrombus | Echogenic metal struts of filter; echogenic material within lumen | Absent flow | No signal or continuous signal with partial obstruction |
| Left-sided IVC | Paired IVC or IVC on left side only | Anomalous IVC drains into left renal vein or azygous vein | Normal |
| Absent intrahepatic IVC | Intrahepatic IVC not visualized | Hepatic veins drain directly into right atrium | Normal |
| Caval fistulas | Dilated vein | Tissue bruit | Pulsatile flow cephalad to fistula |
| Iliac vein compression syndrome (May–Thurner's) | Left iliac vein compressed by right common iliac artery | Increased velocity and possible turbulent flow at compression point | Monophasic waveform distal to compression point |

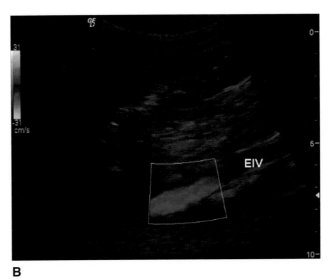

**A**                                    **B**

FIGURE 26-3 **A:** The external iliac vein (EIV) has a homogenous, hypoechoic appearance, and no color flow is detected. These findings are consistent with acute DVT of the EIV. **B:** A normal EIV with an anechoic lumen on grayscale imaging and complete filling to the vessel walls on color-flow imaging.

tumors typically arise from hepatic or renal veins and may secondarily obstruct or thrombose the IVC.[7] Extrinsic tumors may completely or partially obstruct the IVC or iliac veins, resulting in dilated collateral veins and distention of the distal IVC and iliac veins. Intraluminal tumor is typically moderately echogenic and will demonstrate flow within the mass on color-flow imaging. Small vessels can be seen within the tumor itself.

## Inferior Vena Caval Interruption

Sonography of the IVC may demonstrate the presence of an IVC filter, a device used to protect patients from pulmonary emboli. IVC filters are typically placed just distal to the renal veins in order to trap lower extremity venous thromboemboli before they can travel to the heart and lungs. Most IVC filters consist of thin metal struts joined at one end to form the shape of a cone (Fig. 26-4). In longitudinal views of the IVC, a filter's metal struts appear as echogenic lines that converge to a point near the level of the renal veins (Fig. 26-5). In transverse view, the filter appears as a central echogenic dot with lines radiating to the IVC wall. The patency of the IVC proximal and distal to the filter should be evaluated. Echogenic material within and around the filter represents trapped thrombus and should be considered an abnormal finding.[8] Rarely, an IVC filter strut may perforate the IVC causing a hematoma. In most cases, ultrasound can only visualize the hematoma, not the penetrating strut.[9] Computerized tomography scans usually prove to be more useful for diagnosing this condition.

## Color and Power Doppler

Color Doppler provides a useful method for evaluating the patency of the IVC. Although a complete IVC survey requires imaging in the longitudinal and transverse planes, longitudinal images prove to be more informative in the assessment of color flow. Color flow may be difficult to demonstrate in the transverse plane because blood flow is perpendicular to

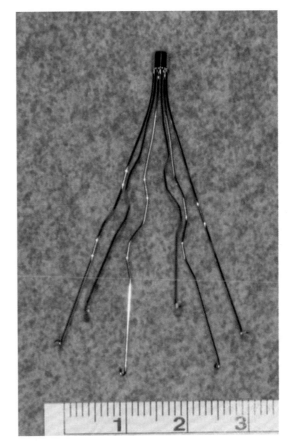

FIGURE 26-4 Greenfield IVC filter.

the ultrasound beam. The entire IVC should be evaluated with color flow, including the suprahepatic, intrahepatic, and infrahepatic IVC as well as the IVC proximal and distal to an IVC filter, if present.

Color Doppler can also detect caval fistulas which are abnormal connections between the IVC and surrounding

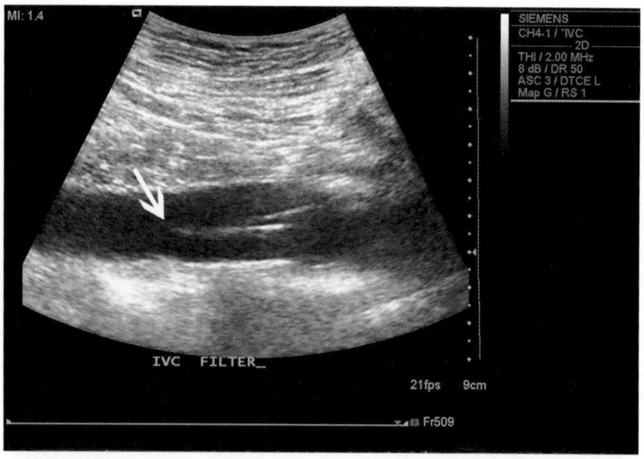

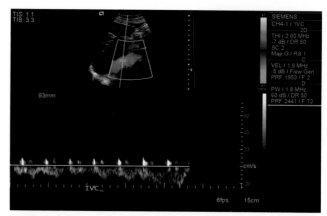

**FIGURE 26-5** Longitudinal grayscale image of the IVC with a filter in place. The *arrow* points to the superior tip of the filter.

**FIGURE 26-6** Color-flow and spectral waveform analysis of the proximal IVC showing cardiac pulsatility superimposed on respiratory phasicity.

vessels. Caval fistulas may occur spontaneously or they may be surgically created. Spontaneous aortocaval fistulas represent a rare complication of large abdominal aortic aneurysms. Color flow demonstrates visible tissue bruit and pulsatile flow in the IVC above the fistula. Directly imaging the connection between the aorta and the IVC may be difficult. Surgically created portacaval fistulas usually involve a side to side connection between the portal vein and the IVC. The fistula creates a tissue bruit, and optimal visualization often requires using the liver as an acoustical window with the patient turned onto his or her left side.

The deep location and relatively low-flow state of the IVC and iliac veins stress the limits of the color Doppler examination. Power Doppler offers a complementary assessment that can overcome these imaging challenges. Because power Doppler functions independent of the ultrasound angle of incidence, it can evaluate patency even when the only images obtainable are in the transverse plane. Power Doppler can also detect slow flow better than color Doppler. This increased sensitivity allows power Doppler to detect extremely low flow in the IVC or iliac veins that could otherwise result in a false-positive diagnosis of venous thrombosis based on the color Doppler findings alone. The use of power Doppler to detect and define low-flow conditions such as intrahepatic portacaval shunts has also been reported.[10]

## Spectral Doppler Characteristics

Blood flows slowly through the IVC, and the caval waveform varies with respiration and the cardiac cycle. During quiet respiration, the diaphragm descends creating positive pressure in the abdomen and negative pressure in the chest. Blood, therefore, flows from the abdomen to the chest during inspiration, and the reverse occurs during expiration. Superimposed on this respiratory variation are the rapidly cycling pressure waves transmitted from the heart, specifically the right atrium (Fig. 26-6). The prominence of cardiac pulsatility in the IVC depends on the fluid status of the patient. Normally, the proximal IVC near the heart has a pulsatile waveform pattern, whereas flow in the distal IVC and iliac veins remains phasic, resembling the pattern seen in the lower extremity veins. Severe fluid overload may allow cardiac pulsations to be detected as far distally

as the iliac veins. Partial obstruction of the IVC eliminates the normal respiratory and cardiac variation in the IVC and iliac veins. In this case, spectral analysis demonstrates continuous Doppler signals with a uniform flow velocity.

Spectral Doppler analysis plays an important role in detecting iliac vein thrombosis. Unlike the lower extremity veins, the patency of iliac veins cannot be evaluated with compression maneuvers, and direct grayscale imaging may not be possible deep in the pelvis. In these circumstances, the diagnosis of an iliac vein thrombosis relies on indirect evidence from the spectral Doppler analysis (Fig. 26-7). Loss of respiratory phasicity and inability to augment the signal with distal thigh compression indicate a proximal obstruction consistent with iliac veins thrombosis. These findings are usually absent in the setting of nonocclusive thrombosis, and duplex ultrasound cannot detect obstruction or thrombosis of the internal iliac veins.

### Iliac Vein Compression Syndrome

Iliac vein compression syndrome (IVCS) occurs when the left common iliac vein is compressed between the overlying right common iliac artery and the underlying vertebral body.

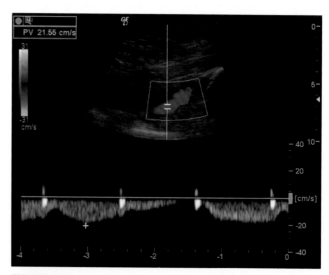

**FIGURE 26-7** Color-flow and spectral waveform analysis of the external iliac vein showing respiratory phasicity.

Also known as May–Thurner's syndrome, this condition most commonly presents as a left iliofemoral DVT; however, it may also cause chronic left lower extremity pain and edema secondary to venous insufficiency. Grayscale imaging can localize the point at which the right common iliac artery crosses the left common iliac vein. Doppler examination can then determine whether this crossing point causes significant compression. Monophasic flow without respiratory variation caudad to the compression and increased flow velocity at the point of compression are signs of a localized iliac vein stenosis consistent with IVCS.[11] Definitive imaging studies, including venography with intraluminal pressures, intravascular ultrasonography, computed tomography, or magnetic resonance imaging, may be required to confirm the diagnosis.

## DUPLEX ULTRASOUND GUIDANCE FOR IVC FILTER PLACEMENT

The utility of duplex ultrasound has expanded beyond the diagnosis of thrombus to now include guidance during IVC filter placement. Percutaneous IVC filter placement has traditionally been performed with contrast venography in an operating room or interventional radiology suite. Duplex ultrasound guidance can transform IVC filter placement into a bedside procedure that does not require exposure to radiation or intravenous contrast.[12]

### Patient Preparation and Positioning

Imaging the IVC for filter placement follows the same basic preparation and techniques outlined in the previous sections. The sonographer stands on the patient's right side, and the ultrasound machine is positioned on the same side toward the head of the bed so that it can be viewed by the sonographer and the physician performing the procedure. Ideally, the filter should be placed just distal to the level of the renal veins. In some patients, the right renal vein can be visualized during grayscale imaging of the IVC. More commonly, the right renal artery is easier to locate and provides a dependable and consistent marker for the level of the renal veins. With the IVC in a longitudinal projection, the right renal artery is easily identified in cross section as it passes posterior to the IVC (Fig. 26-8). Doppler interrogation can confirm the identity of the right renal artery by demonstrating the characteristic spectral waveform tracing of a renal artery.

### Scanning Technique

While the physician gains percutaneous access to the right or left common femoral vein, the sonographer maintains a longitudinal image of IVC with the right renal artery in cross section. Maintaining this grayscale image allows real-time visualization of the wire and delivery sheath as the physician advances them into the IVC. The sheath should then be identified and advanced with ultrasound guidance so that its tip is just below the level of the right renal artery. Flushing saline through the sheath creates echogenic turbulence at the tip that can often aid in its identification.

Once the sheath tip is in a satisfactory infrarenal location, the IVC filter is advanced through the sheath and into

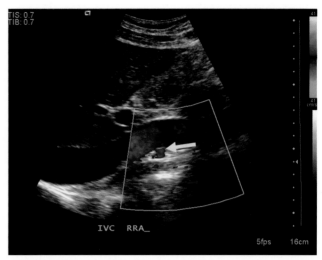

**FIGURE 26-8** In a longitudinal view, the right renal artery (*arrow*) is identified posterior to the IVC.

the IVC. Once the filter tip is at the level of the right renal artery, the physician deploys it under real-time sonographic visualization (Fig. 26-9). The grayscale image will show the filter quickly expanding and engaging the IVC sidewalls. A transverse image should then be obtained and recorded to confirm that the filter is completely expanded with its struts apposed to the sidewalls of the IVC.

## INTRAVASCULAR ULTRASOUND

Intravascular ultrasound can function as a valuable imaging tool during endovascular procedures on the iliac veins. Balloon angioplasty and stenting of stenotic and obstructed iliac veins have shown promise as a means of improving chronic edema and accelerating ulcer healing. Traditional venous sonography during these procedures is often impractical

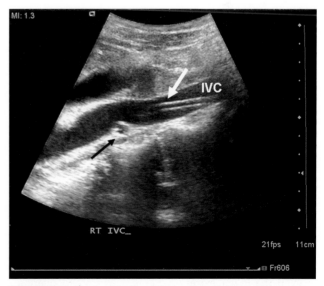

**FIGURE 26-9** The tip of the filter delivery catheter (*white arrow*) is advanced in the IVC to the level of the right renal artery (*black arrow*).

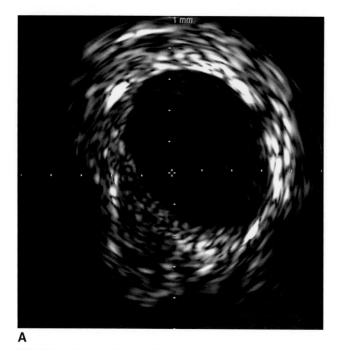

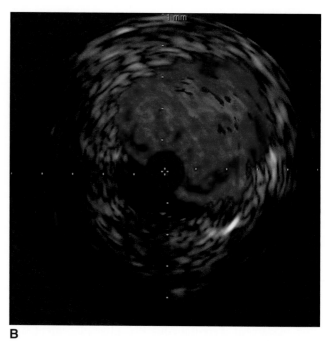

**A**　　　　　　　　　　　　　　　　　　　　　**B**

**FIGURE 26-10 A:** IVUS image of the right common iliac vein. The small gray circle in the middle of the image represents the location of the IVUS catheter. The dark, circular area around the catheter is the patent lumen of the common iliac vein. The walls of the vein are echogenic and appear lighter gray and white on the image. **B:** IVUS image of the right common iliac vein demonstrating color flow within the vessel lumen.

and limited because of the depth of the iliac veins as they traverse the pelvis. Contrast venography produces planar images that tend to underestimate the true severity of iliac vein stenosis.[13] IVUS provides real-time images of the vein lumen with more detail and accuracy than duplex sonography or contrast venography. As an intraoperative imaging technique, IVUS can diagnose iliac vein stenosis and evaluate the effect of endovascular intervention.

Flexible IVUS catheters have ultrasound crystals embedded at their tip to provide imaging of the vessel lumen and wall structure. After obtaining percutaneous venous access, the physician uses fluoroscopic guidance to advance the IVUS catheter over a wire to the area of interest. The ultrasound crystals in the IVUS catheter emit sound waves covering 360 degrees of the vessel and insonate the vessel at right angles to the axis of the catheter. The catheter is connected to a console in which the screen displays a grayscale, transectional image of the lumen and vessel wall in a plane perpendicular to the long axis of the catheter. Many IVUS catheters can display color flow by sampling up to 30 frames of IVUS images per second and recording any difference in position of the echogenic blood particles between images (Fig. 26-10). Although it cannot quantify blood flow velocity, color imaging with IVUS can help differentiate the flow lumen from the vessel wall.

During iliac vein interventions, IVUS has excellent sensitivity in detecting stenotic and obstructed vein segments. In patients with May–Thurner's syndrome, external compression usually flattens the vein in the anteriorposterior dimension. Contrast venography may not detect this compressed area because the flattened vein will not appear stenotic in the standard anteriorposterior planar projection. IVUS imaging easily demonstrates the compressed area by showing a change in the shape of the vessel (circular to elliptical) and quantifying the decreased vessel diameter and area.[14] Other

subtle vessel changes that the IVUS can detect include wall thickening, webs, trabeculations, and nonocclusive thrombus (Fig. 26-11). After balloon angioplasty and stenting, IVUS can evaluate the flow lumen and ensure that the stent has been completely expanded and apposed to the vessel wall (Fig. 26-12). IVUS can also guide IVC filter placement at the bedside potentially obviating the need for patient transport, fluoroscopy, and intravascular contrast.[15]

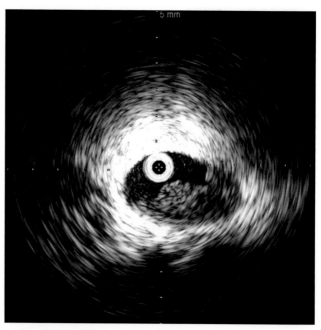

**FIGURE 26-11** IVUS image of the left common iliac vein. The vein is compressed and elliptical in shape. There is also nonocclusive, echogenic thrombus within the vessel lumen.

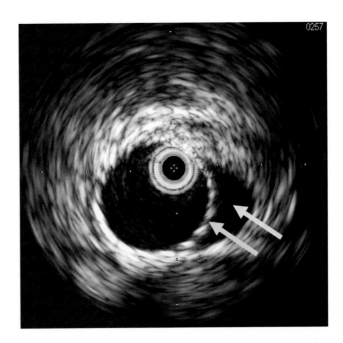

**FIGURE 26-12** IVUS image of a stent (echogenic circular structure pointed to by *yellow arrow*) within the larger diameter common iliac vein (*white arrow*).

## SUMMARY

- Ultrasonography of the IVC and iliac veins offers several advantages over other imaging modalities.
- It is a noninvasive examination that does not require radiation exposure or contrast administration.
- As a diagnostic tool, ultrasonography provides an accurate anatomic and physiologic assessment of the IVC and iliac veins.
- Optimizing the sonographic examination requires adequate patient preparation and positioning as well as knowledge of the pathophysiology of the IVC and iliac veins.

## CRITICAL THINKING QUESTIONS

1. You receive a request for an ultrasound examination of the inferior cava and iliac veins in an obese patient who ate breakfast 2 hours ago. How should you proceed? What, if anything, can be done to optimize the quality of the exam?
2. During an ultrasound of the IVC, you note that the IVC appears distended; however, the lumen appears to be anechoic. You cannot detect a color Doppler signal in the IVC, and the spectral Doppler signal in the common iliac veins is continuous without respiratory variation. What is the likely clinical scenario to explain these findings?
3. You are performing an ultrasound of the IVC on a patient who has had an IVC filter and now presents with bilateral lower extremity edema. You note that the echogenic struts of the filter extend to the vena caval wall. The filter appears to be located above the level of the renal veins, and there is echogenic material within and cephalad to the filter. Which of these findings are abnormal and why?

## MEDIA MENU

Student Resources available on thePoint® include:
- Audio glossary
- Interactive question bank
- Videos
- Internet resources

## REFERENCES

1. Mintz GS, Kotler MN, Parry WR, et al. Real-time inferior vena caval ultrasonography: normal and abnormal findings and its use in assessing right-heart function. *Circulation.* 1981;64:1018–1025.
2. Skyes AM, McLoughlin RF, So CB, et al. Sonographic assessment of infrarenal vena caval dimensions. *J Ultrasound Med.* 1995;14:665–668.
3. Allan PL. The aorta and inferior vena cava. In: Allan PL, Dubbins PA, Pozniak MA, McDicken WN, eds. *Clinical Doppler Ultrasound.* 2nd ed. Philadelphia, PA: Churchill Livingstone Elsevier; 2006:127–140.
4. Moore KL. *Clinically Oriented Anatomy.* 3rd ed. Baltimore, MD: Williams & Wilkins; 1992.
5. Tempkin BB. Inferior vena cava scanning protocol. In: Tempkin BB, ed. *Ultrasound Scanning Principles and Protocols.* 2nd ed. Philadelphia, PA: W.B. Saunders Company; 1999:41–52.
6. Zwiebel WJ. Extremity venous examination: technical considerations. In: Zwiebel WJ, ed. *Introduction to Vascular Ultrasonography.* 4th ed. Philadelphia, PA: W.B. Saunders Company; 2000:311–328.
7. Pussell SJ, Cosgrove DO. Ultrasound features of tumor thrombus in the IVC in retroperitoneal tumours. *Br J Radiol.* 1981;54:866–869.
8. Asward MA, Sandager GP, Pais SO, et al. Early duplex scan evaluation of four vena caval interruption devices. *J Vasc Surg.* 1996;24:809–818.
9. Mohan CR, Hoballah JJ, Sharp WJ, et al. Comparative efficacy and complications of vena caval filters. *J Vasc Surg.* 1995;21:235–246.
10. Oquz B, Akata D, Balkanci F, et al. Intrahepatic portosystemic venous shunt: diagnosis by colour/power Doppler imaging and three dimensional ultrasound. *Br J Radiol.* 2003;76:487–490.
11. Oguzkurt L, Ozkan U, Tercan F, et al. Ultrasonographic diagnosis of iliac vein compression (May-Thruner) syndrome. *Diag Interv Radiol.* 2007;13:152–155.
12. Connors MS, Becker S, Guzman RJ, et al. Duplex scan-directed placement of inferior vena cava filters: a five year institutional experience. *J Vasc Surg.* 2002;35:286–291.
13. Neglen P, Raju S. Intravascular ultrasound scan evaluation of the obstructed vein. *J Vasc Surg.* 2002;35:694–700.
14. Forauer AR, Gemmete JJ, Dasika NL, et al. Intravascular ultrasound in the diagnosis and treatment of iliac vein compression (May-Thurner) syndrome. *J Vasc Interv Radiol.* 2002;13:523–527.
15. Jacobs DL, Motahanhalli RL, Peterson BG. Bedside vena cava filter placement with intravascular ultrasound: a simple accurate, single venous access method. *J Vasc Surg.* 2007;46:1284–1286.

# The Hepatoportal System

WAYNE C. LEONHARDT | ANN MARIE KUPINSKI

## CHAPTER 27

## OBJECTIVES

- Identify normal hepatoportal anatomy
- Describe normal hepatoportal Doppler waveforms
- List acoustic scanning planes and windows when evaluating hepatoportal vasculature
- List the causes and anatomic levels of obstruction resulting in portal hypertension
- Describe portosystemic collateral pathways associated with portal hypertension
- List sonographic findings associated with portal hypertension

## GLOSSARY

**ascites** An abnormal accumulation of fluid within the peritoneal cavity. It is the most common complication of cirrhosis

**Budd-Chiari's syndrome** Hepatic venous outflow obstruction at any level from the small hepatic veins to the junction of the inferior vena cava and the right atrium, regardless of the cause of obstruction

**hepatopetal** Refers to antegrade flow, toward the liver (physiologically normal direction of flow within the portal–splenic venous system)

**hepatofugal** Refers to retrograde flow, away from the liver (physiologically abnormal direction of flow within the portal–splenic venous system)

**helical portal vein flow** Spiraling, swirling, "Helix" flow pattern demonstrating hepatopetal, hepatofugal, or simultaneous bidirectional flow; uncommon flow pattern seen in 2% of normal patients

**hepatic arterial buffer response** Compensatory mechanism to maintain perfusion to the liver by arterial vasodilation when portal vein flow is obstructed in patients with advanced cirrhosis

**hepatic hydrothorax** Hepatic hydrothorax is defined as a pleural effusion in patients with liver cirrhosis in the absence of cardiopulmonary disease. The pathophysiology involves the passage of ascitic fluid from the peritoneal cavity to the pleural space through diaphragmatic defects

**portal hypertension** Elevated pressure gradient between the portal vein and IVC or hepatic veins of 10 to 12 mm Hg or greater

**portosystemic collaterals** Formation of abnormal blood vessels that shunt portal blood flow bypassing the liver to the systemic circulation, decompressing increased portal venous pressure

**sinusoidal obstruction syndrome (SOS)** Formerly known as hepatic veno-occlusive disease, is a syndrome of tender hepatomegaly, right upper quadrant pain, jaundice,

## KEY TERMS

**helical flow**

**hepatic artery**

**hepatic arterial buffer response**

**hepatic veins**

**hepatofugal**

**hepatopetal**

**portal hypertension**

**portal vein**

**portosystemic collaterals**

**TIPS**

and ascites; most often occurring in patients undergoing hematopoietic cell transplantation, and less commonly following radiation therapy to the liver, liver transplantation, and ingestion of alkaloid toxins. High doses of radiation and toxins damage hepatic sinusoidal endothelial cells and hepatocytes, leading to hepatocellular necrosis

**TIPS** Transjugular intrahepatic portosystemic shunt is a percutaneously created connection within the liver between the hepatic vein and portal vein that allow blood flow to bypass the liver as a means to reduce portal pressure in patients with complications related to portal hypertension

Duplex sonography is the most common imaging technique used to evaluate the liver and its vasculature. This important noninvasive imaging technique is paramount in evaluating the liver parenchyma, determining the presence of flow, direction, and velocity within the hepatoportal vascular system and in transjugular intrahepatic portosystemic shunts (TIPS). A variety of vascular disorders alter blood flow into, within, and out of the liver. Duplex ultrasound with color Doppler is particularly useful in the detection of intraluminal thrombus, tumor infiltration, hepatofugal flow, portosystemic collaterals, and arterioportal fistulae. This chapter reviews sonographic and hemodynamic characteristics of the normal hepatoportal vascular system, as well as TIPS and other various pathologic conditions, including portal hypertension, cirrhosis, portal and splenic vein (SV) thrombosis, tumor thrombus, hepatic vein obstruction (Budd-Chiari's syndrome), and congestive heart failure.

## ANATOMY

The liver receives a dual blood supply from the hepatic artery and portal vein. These two vessels constitute the hepatic inflow. The hepatic artery supplies approximately 30% of the total blood flow into the liver. It carries oxygenated blood through branches in the portal triad and enters the sinusoids (capillaries) to reach the central veins within the liver. The portal vein supplies approximately 70% of hepatic blood flow.[1] It carries nutrient-rich blood from the gastrointestinal tract to the portal triad, where it enters the sinusoids to reach the central veins. Central veins are the actual beginnings of the hepatic venous system. They enter sublobular veins, which unite and converge to form three hepatic veins that drain into the inferior vena cava (IVC). The hepatic veins comprise the primary hepatic outflow vessels. Figure 27-1 illustrates the microscopic anatomy of a liver lobule constructed around a central vein. The corners of the lobule each contain a branch of the hepatic artery, a branch of the portal vein, and a bile duct (portal triad). Figure 27-2 illustrates the intrahepatic distribution of hepatic arteries, hepatic veins, portal veins, and biliary ducts in the upper abdomen.

## PORTAL VENOUS SYSTEM

Just slightly to the right of midline, the main portal vein (MPV) begins the junction of the SV, and superior mesenteric vein (SMV). The inferior mesenteric vein drains into the SV to the left of the portal/splenic confluence. The left gastric or coronary vein usually joins the SV superiorly

near its junction with the SMV. The MPV courses cephalad approaching the porta hepatis and lies anterior to the IVC. The porta hepatis is the transverse fissure on the visceral surface of the liver between the caudate and quadrate lobes where the portal vein and hepatic artery enter the liver and the hepatic duct leaves the liver.[2] Figure 27-3 illustrates the normal portal venous anatomy and flow direction. Entering the portal hepatis, the MPV divides into a smaller, more anterior, and cranial left portal vein (LPV) and a larger, more posterior, and caudal right portal vein (RPV).[3] The portal veins then branch into medial and lateral divisions on the left, and anterior and posterior divisions on the right. The right branch of the portal vein receives the cystic vein. Portal veins have no valves. Their walls are composed mostly of loosely arrayed, nonparallel connective tissue fibers, and only a minor amount of collagen. The composition of the portal vein results in a hyperechoic wall over a wide range of beam-vessel angles.[4] Portal veins course within the liver segments (intrasegmental) and emanate from the porta hepatis.

### Hepatic Veins

Hepatic veins are anatomically separate from the portal venous system. Unlike the portal veins, hepatic vein walls are composed mostly of tightly packed collagen fibers. The distinct composition of the hepatic vein wall renders it a specular reflector, which is hyperechoic only when the incident beam and the vessel wall are perpendicular.[4] Hepatic veins run between the lobes of the liver (intersegmental) and increase in caliber as they approach the diaphragm. Three main hepatic veins (right, middle, and left) provide the primary outflow route of blood from the liver. They drain into the IVC close to the right atrium. Hepatic veins have no valves.[2] The right hepatic vein (RHV) is usually the largest. In 96% of individuals, the middle hepatic vein (MHV) and left hepatic vein (LHV) join to form a common trunk before entering the IVC (Fig. 27-4). Accessory hepatic veins are common, but are seldom identified sonographically. Of note, the caudate lobe of the liver drains directly into the IVC with the caudate vein being the largest draining vein of this lobe.[5] This is important in the presence of venous outflow diseases, which will be discussed later in the chapter.

### Hepatic Artery

The hepatic artery branches off the celiac trunk to the right. At this level, the hepatic artery is known as the common hepatic artery. It continues over the anterior superior edge

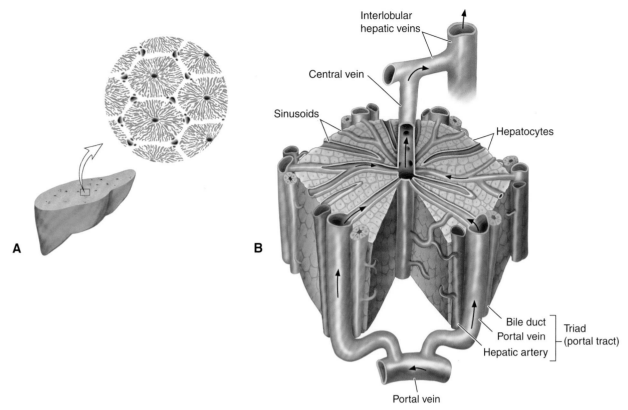

**FIGURE 27-1** Anatomic diagram illustrating the microscopic anatomy of a liver lobule constructed around a central vein. **A:** An enlarged cross-sectional view illustrating the shape of the liver lobules. **B:** The corners of the lobule each contain a branch of the hepatic artery, a branch of the portal vein, and a bile duct (portal triad). The arrows indicate the direction of blood flow. (From Kawamura D, Lunsford B. *Diagnostic Medical Sonography: Abdomen and Superficial Structures*, 3rd ed. Philadelphia, PA: Wolters Kluwer; 2012: Figure 5-13.)

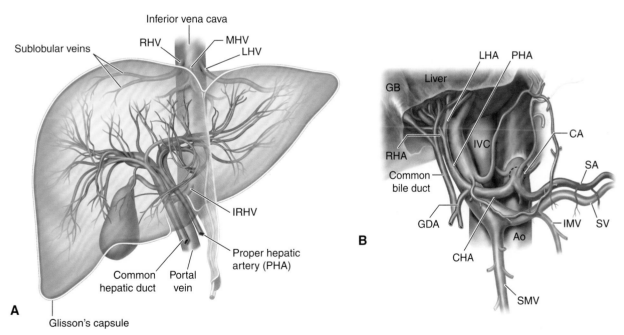

**FIGURE 27-2** Anatomic diagram of the liver illustrating **(A)** the intrahepatic distribution of hepatic arteries, hepatic veins, portal veins, and biliary ducts and; **(B)** the vessels and ducts of the upper abdomen. AO, aorta; CA, celiac artery; CHA, common hepatic artery; GB, gallbladder; GDA, gastroduodenal artery; IRHV, inferior right hepatic vein; LHA, left hepatic artery; PHA, proper hepatic artery; RHA, right hepatic artery; SA, splenic artery. (From Kawamura D, Lunsford B. *Diagnostic Medical Sonography: Abdomen and Superficial Structures*, 3rd ed. Philadelphia, PA: Wolters Kluwer; 2012: Figure 5-11.)

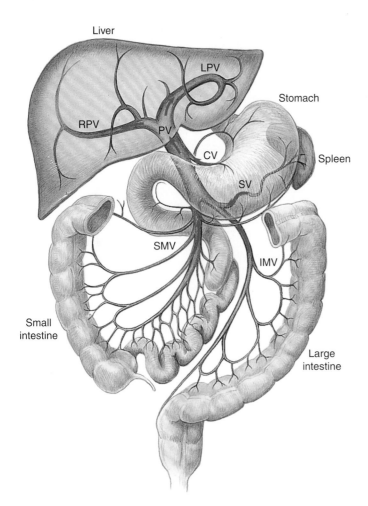

Liver

LPV

Stomach

RPV

PV

CV

Spleen

SV

SMV

IMV

Small intestine

Large intestine

**FIGURE 27-3** A diagram illustrating the normal portal vascular anatomy. The red arrows depict normal direction of blood flow. PV, portal vein; CV, coronary vein.

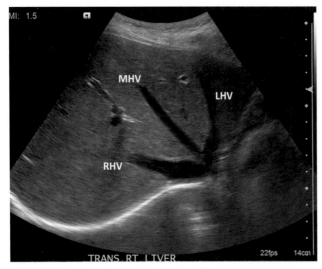

**FIGURE 27-4** Normal grayscale appearance of the three hepatic veins converging toward the inferior vena cava.

# SONOGRAPHIC EXAMINATION TECHNIQUES

There are various indications for hepatoportal duplex ultrasound. Table 27-1 lists several indications for hepatoportal scanning. Any of these conditions can alter the blood flow patterns within the inflow and outflow vessels in the liver.

## Patient Preparation

Patients should fast for 8 to 12 hours. Patients are instructed to abstain from smoking and chewing gum because these activities introduce air into the stomach.

## Patient Positioning

Patient positions while scanning the hepatoportal system include supine, left posterior oblique (LPO), left lateral decubitus (LLD), and right posterior oblique (RPO). A combination of sagittal, transverse, and oblique scanning planes and various acoustic windows is necessary to assess the portal and hepatic vessels. Primary scanning planes include right coronal oblique, transverse epigastric, transverse right costal margin, left coronal oblique, and sagittal left lobes.

### Right Coronal Oblique

The right coronal oblique scanning plane using an intercostal approach provides excellent visualization of the porta

of the pancreas where it gives rise to the gastroduodenal artery. At this point, the common hepatic artery becomes the proper hepatic artery, terminating at the porta hepatis giving off right and left branches. In the majority of patients, the hepatic artery lies anteromedial to the portal vein. Hepatic artery branches accompany portal veins.

| TABLE 27-1 | Indications for Hepatoportal Duplex Ultrasound |
|---|---|
| Liver cirrhosis caused by alcoholic/nonalcoholic steatohepatitis, viral, Hepatitis B and C ||
| Portal hypertension, ascites of unknown etiology or esophageal varices ||
| Thrombosis of the portal, splenic, and superior mesenteric veins ||
| Budd-Chiari's syndrome (hepatic vein thrombosis) ||
| Pre/postinterventional procedures and monitoring of portosystemic shunts ||
| Abdominal trauma ||
| Sudden onset of ascites, acute abdominal pain, elevated D-dimer ||
| Patients with a history of abdominal malignancy ||

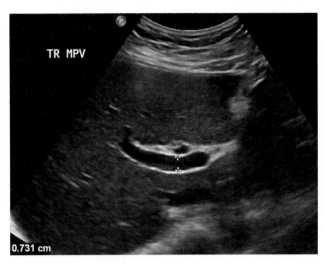

**FIGURE 27-5** Portal vein diameter measured near where the main portal vein (MPV) crosses the inferior vena cava.

hepatis. When patients present with large amounts of ascites and bowel gas, this increases abdominal girth, making it very difficult to image the liver and portal–hepatic venous anatomy. The intercostal approach results in the following: Doppler angles varying from 0 degrees to about 60 degrees, decreases the anterioposterior distance, uses the liver as an acoustic window, and facilitates diagnostic imaging when patients are not compliant holding their breath. To obtain this scanning plane, position the patient in the LPO or LLD positions. Place the transducer in the interspace parallel to the rib margins, aimed at the hepatic hilum.

**Transverse Epigastric**

With the patient supine or in the LPO position, place the transducer over the left lobe of the liver. Angle the transducer cephalad at the level of the diaphragm. This will provide visualization of the hepatic venous confluence. Next, angle the transducer caudad at the level of the left lobe of the liver. Here, the ascending branch of the LPV and accompanying hepatic artery are visualized. Finally, angle the transducer caudad to detect the SV and portal confluence.

**Right Transverse Costal Margin**

Position the patient supine and with the transducer in the transverse plane, place it over the right costal margin at the midclavicular line. The transducer is then angled superior to inferior until a transverse view of the porta hepatis is obtained. Here, the main portal and right anterior and posterior branches are seen together with accompanying hepatic artery.

**Left Coronal Oblique**

Place the patient in the RPO position with the transducer between the left lateral intercostal spaces. Aim the transducer toward the splenic hilum. This window provides optimal visualization of the SV and artery.

**Sagittal Left Lobe**

Position the patient supine and place the transducer in longitudinal plane midline over the left lobe of the liver. This scanning approach demonstrates the LHV, ascending branch of the LPV and accompanying artery. The LHV is seen in the long axis draining into the IVC.

## Scanning Technique

The ultrasound examination begins with the patient in the supine position. As the examination progresses, multiple views and patient positions are used to obtain the various required images.

Duplex ultrasound imaging of the liver includes a complete abdominal examination as well as Doppler assessment of the portal–hepatic vasculature. During the abdominal examination, the liver is evaluated for anatomic features, including size, texture, and surface contour. The presence of hepatic masses, portosystemic collaterals, hepatofugal flow, ascites, and splenomegaly is noted. The portal vein, SV, and SMV are examined for thrombus. Grayscale and color ultrasound images are obtained of the extrahepatic portal vein, intrahepatic portal veins, SV, SMV, proper hepatic artery, hepatic veins, and IVC. These images should include clear views of the adjacent liver parenchyma. The MPV diameter is measured during quiet respiration where it crosses anterior to the IVC (Fig. 27-5).

Perform spectral Doppler and color imaging to evaluate patency and direction of flow from the following hepatoportal vasculature:
- MPV (angle corrected)
- RPV (anterior/posterior branches) nonangle corrected
- LPV (nonangle corrected)
- Proper hepatic artery (angle corrected)
- RHV, MHV, and LHVs (nonangle corrected)
- SV hilum/pancreas (nonangle corrected)
- SMV (nonangle corrected)
- IVC (nonangle corrected)

## Technical Considerations

When scanning the abdominal vasculature, imaging parameters such as depth, field of view, frame rate, and flow sensitivity are very important. While imaging depths vary based on patient body habitus, transducer frequencies between 2.5 and 4.5 MHz may be required to penetrate depths of up to 20 cm. Higher transducer frequencies between 4 and 6 MHz are used in thin adults and children. Selection of the transducer should be made such that adequate depth penetration is achieved while selecting the highest transducer frequency because the higher frequencies provide better resolution. Most often a 3 to 6 MHz pulsed Doppler is required for spectral analysis of abdominal vessels. Electronic-phased sector transducers with 13 to 20 mm scan heads are more effective in obtaining acoustic windows using the intercostal approach. High-resolution convex (4 to 6 MHz) and linear (7 to 9 MHz) transducers are useful when imaging anterior abdominal wall varices and assessing the liver surface for nodularity.

## Pitfalls

The ability to complete a hepatoportal examination depends in part on the experience of the technologist or sonographer as well as the patient. Major limitations affecting the success of the examination include patient obesity, diffuse liver disease, ascites, and bowel gas. Patients with severe abdominal pain, those unable to remain still, those unable to breathe quietly or vary their depth of respiration, and combative patients also present limitations to the examination.

## DIAGNOSIS

There are multiple criteria to assess when evaluating the hepatoportal system. Major diagnostic characteristics are summarized as follows.

## Portal Vein

Respiration and ingestion of food affect portal vein diameter and velocity flow. In normal patients, the portal vein diameter is ≤13 mm in quiet respiration and may increase to 16 mm with deep inspiration.[6] Portal vein diameter is increased in patients with portal hypertension, congestive heart failure, constrictive pericarditis, and portal vein thrombosis (PVT).

Normal portal venous flow is laminar, directed toward the liver with constant antegrade flow throughout the cardiac cycle. This is referred to as "hepatopetal" flow. Helical flow in the portal vein is unusual in normal individuals (2%) and seen in 20% of patients with severe liver disease. When helical flow is present, the monochromatic color Doppler appearance is replaced by alternating red and blue bands. Duplex ultrasound will show hepatopetal, hepatofugal, or simultaneous bidirectional flow depending on the placement of the cursor within the helix (Fig. 27-6). Portal vein velocity varies with cardiac activity and respiration. During inspiration it decreases, and increases during expiration. This is because of the diaphragm descending during inspiration, resulting in an increase in intra-abdominal pressure. This also impedes venous return to the right atrium, thus decreasing flow in the IVC and its tributaries, including the hepatic veins. Portal venous flow and velocity also decrease during exercise (related to the significant reduction in mesenteric arterial blood flow that occurs with exercise) and changes in posture (from supine to sitting or standing) attributed to venous pooling in the legs. It increases with expiration and ingestion of food as a result of splanchnic vasodilatation and hyperemia. Postprandially, flow velocity increases 50% to 100%. There is considerable variation in the reported value for normal portal vein velocity. This variation is dependent

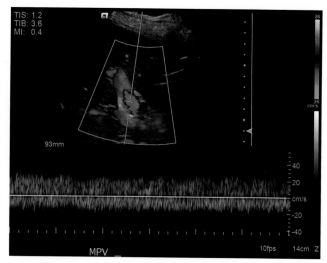

**FIGURE 27-6** Helical flow in the main portal vein (MPV). Spectral Doppler shows both antegrade and retrograde flows because of the wide sample gate within the helix.

on whether the maximum velocity or the time-averaged mean velocity is being reported. Resting peak systolic velocities range from 16 to 31 cm/s.[7] Mean flow velocity has been reported as 19.6+2.6 cm/s by Zironi and 22.9+2.8 cm/s by Cioni.[8,9] The normal spectral Doppler waveform in the portal vein is hepatopetal, monophasic, slightly pulsatile, or undulating (Fig. 27-7). Increased pulsatility has been described particularly in thin patients. Reversed pulsatile flow is seen in patients with tricuspid regurgitation, right-sided congestive heart failure, cirrhosis with vascular arterioportal shunting, and arteriovenous fistulas. Principle determinants attributing to portal vein pulsatility may include trans-sinusoidal transmission of atrial pulsations, the respiratory cycle and the transmission of vena cava, hepatic arterial, or splanchnic pulsations.

## Splenic Vein

In normal patients, the diameter of the SV (in the transverse view at the level of the superior mesenteric artery, SMA) measures up to 10 mm (inner wall to inner wall) and increases by

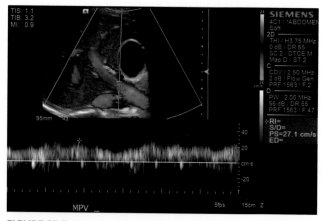

**FIGURE 27-7** Normal spectral waveform in the main portal vein (MPV). Flow direction is toward the liver.

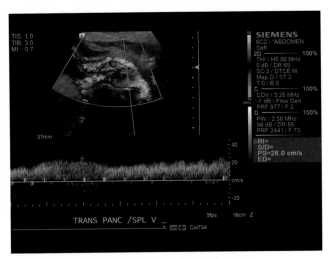

**FIGURE 27-8** Normal splenic vein Doppler waveform.

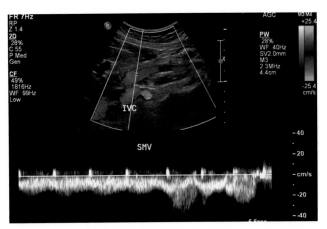

**FIGURE 27-9** Normal superior mesenteric vein waveform (SMV). The inferior vena cava (IVC) is seen deep to the SMV in this image.

20% to 100% from quiet respiration to deep inspiration. An SV diameter of >10 mm and an increase in caliber of less than 20% from quiet respiration to deep inspiration suggests portal hypertension with an 80% sensitivity and a 100% specificity.[10]

Normal SV flow direction is hepatopetal (toward the liver). As seen in the portal vein, respiration and cardiac activity can also affect SV velocity. Flow velocity decreases during inspiration and increases during expiration. Peak systolic velocity in the SV normally ranges from 9 to 30 cm/s. The mean velocity ranges from 5 to 12 cm/s. The normal spectral Doppler waveform in the SV is monophasic with slight pulsatility (Fig. 27-8).

## Superior Mesenteric Vein

In normal patients, the diameter of the SMV can measure up to 10 mm at the trunk (inner wall to inner wall) and increases by 20% to 100% from quiet respiration to deep inspiration. As with the SV, an SMV diameter of >10 mm and an increase in caliber of less than 20% from quiet respiration to deep inspiration suggests portal hypertension.[10]

Normal SMV flow is hepatopetal (toward the liver). Peak systolic velocity in the SMV normally ranges between 8 and 40 cm/s. The mean velocity range is 9 to 18 cm/s. Doppler spectral analysis of the SMV shows a monophasic waveform with slight pulsatility (Fig. 27-9). Flow in the portal confluence is turbulent because the SV joins the SMV to form the portal vein. Respiratory maneuvers and ingestion of food affect flow velocity. Flow velocity decreases during inspiration and increases with expiration, similar to that of the portal vein and SV. Postprandially, SMV velocity increases 50% to 100%.

## Hepatic Veins

The normal diameter of the RHV is less than 6 mm. In patients with congestive heart failure, the RHV diameter increases to a mean diameter of 9 mm or greater.[11]

The hepatic veins normally exhibit a pulsatile triphasic waveform with both antegrade and retrograde flows (Fig. 27-10). This waveform corresponds to cyclic pressure changes within the heart. The initial wave is termed the S wave

(ventricular systole) and is directed toward the heart. During ventricular systole, the tricuspid annulus moves toward the cardiac apex, causing suction of blood into the right atrium from the liver. The result is a dominant antegrade S wave. The next component of the waveform is referred to as the D wave (ventricular diastole). During diastole, with the heart relaxed and the tricuspid valve open, blood flows passively from the liver into the heart, yielding an antegrade D wave. The last feature of the waveform is the A wave (atrial contraction). During atrial contraction, blood flow is toward the liver, yielding retrograde flow. The color-flow imaging will display both red and blue fillings, representing the multiphasic flow within the vessels. Hepatic vein PSV ranges between 22 and 39 cm/s. Normal respiratory variations can augment waveforms with inspiration, causing a slight decrease in the systolic wave and expiration increasing the systolic wave. The Valsalva maneuver diminishes waveform pulsatility.

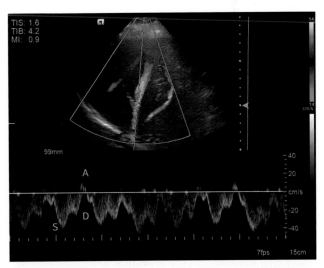

**FIGURE 27-10** Normal hepatic vein waveform. Triphasic, consisting of two periods of antegrade flow below the baseline, corresponding to ventricular systole (S) wave and ventricular diastole (D) wave. Brief transient flow reversal corresponding to atrial contraction (A) wave.

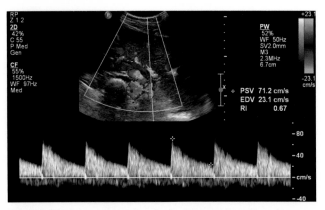

**FIGURE 27-11** Normal hepatic artery Doppler waveforms illustrating a low-resistance pattern with forward flow throughout diastole.

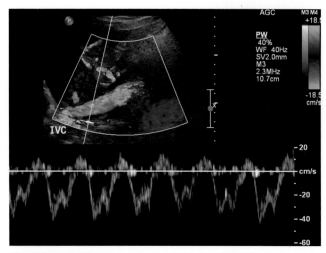

**FIGURE 27-12** Normal Doppler waveforms from the inferior vena cava (IVC). At this level, the flow within the IVC demonstrates slight pulsatility caused by the proximity of the heart.

## Hepatic Artery

The hepatic artery can be readily distinguished from the adjacent portal vein because the hepatic artery demonstrates a higher velocity and is smaller in diameter. Both the hepatic artery and portal vein exhibit flow in the same direction, hepatopetal. Doppler spectral waveforms exhibit a low-resistance flow pattern with antegrade flow throughout the cardiac cycle (Fig. 27-11). This is similar to the pattern observed within the internal carotid artery or renal arteries. Hepatic circulation differs from that of other arterial beds. When portal venous perfusion decreases, hepatic arterial flow increases. This phenomenon has been described as the "hepatic arterial buffer response." Hepatic arterial buffer response is an important compensatory mechanism to maintain perfusion to the liver by hepatic artery vasodilation (enlargement) and increased flow when portal venous flow is reduced as a result of advanced cirrhosis and PVT. With the ingestion of food, portal vein velocity increases and hepatic arterial diastolic flow diminishes, exhibiting increased pulsatility in healthy individuals with a normal liver. The peak systolic velocity in the hepatic artery ranges from 70 to 120 cm/s. The normal resistance index is between 0.5 and 0.7.[12]

## Inferior Vena Cava

Normal blood flow within the IVC is toward the right atrium. The Doppler waveform of the IVC near the heart is pulsatile and triphasic because of reflected right atrial pulsations (Fig. 27-12). The flow pattern becomes more phasic with respiration when sampling velocity flow in the lower abdomen. Peak systolic velocities range from 44 to 118 cm/s.

The size of the IVC varies markedly with respiration and the cardiac cycle. It ranges from 15 to 25 mm in diameter. Deep inspiration limits venous return to the chest, increasing the IVC diameter. Expiration improves venous return, decreasing its diameter. The Valsalva maneuver blocks venous return and flow is temporarily reversed in the IVC, causing it to dilate to its maximum diameter. When the IVC is obstructed, it tends to dilate below the level of obstruction. Respiratory changes are decreased or absent below the obstructed segment. The IVC diameter is also dependent on patient size, right atrial pressure, and fluid overload or heart failure.

## DISORDERS

As with any organ system, there are a multitude of pathologic conditions which can occur. Diseases of the hepatoportal system often produce significant changes, which are evident on ultrasound examination. Some of the more commonly encountered disorders are described in the following sections.

## Portal Hypertension

Portal hypertension is defined as an abnormal increase in portal venous pressure as a result of obstruction of blood flow through the liver. In portal hypertension, hepatopetal flow is rerouted away from the liver through collateral channels to low-pressure systemic vessels. Portal hypertension is defined as an increase in the gradient between the portal vein and IVC or hepatic veins. Normal pressure is between 5 and 10 mm Hg. When the pressure gradient exceeds 10 to 12 mm Hg, the condition becomes clinically significant.[2] Life-threatening complications of variceal hemorrhage associated with portal hypertension account for more than 15,000 hospital admissions per year in the United States.

### Etiology

Portal hypertension results when venous blood flow is obstructed within the liver or in the extrahepatic portal–hepatic venous system. The most common etiology for portal hypertension in North America is sinusoidal obstruction due to cirrhosis. Until recently, the most common cause of cirrhosis was alcohol abuse. Because of the rapid increase of Hepatitis C virus infection, Hepatitis C is now the leader (26%) with alcohol abuse falling second (21%).[13] Other causes include Hepatitis B, primary biliary cirrhosis, nonalcoholic steatohepatitis, primary sclerosing cholangitis, Wilson's disease, cardiac cirrhosis, sinusoidal obstruction syndrome (SOS), sarcoidosis, schistosomiasis, autoimmune hepatitis, and hereditary hemochromatosis. Seventy five percent of deaths attributable to alcoholism are caused by cirrhosis. In cirrhosis, most of the normal liver architecture is replaced by fibrotic scar tissue, steatosis, and regenerating nodules.

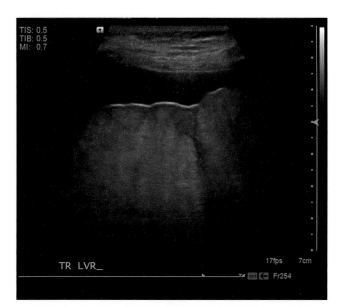

**FIGURE 27-13** A grayscale image of a cirrhotic liver with scalloped contour.

Three stages of cirrhosis include infiltration, inflammation, and scarring. Initially, the liver is enlarged with an echogenic and attenuative echo patterns. With advanced cirrhosis, the liver atrophies and becomes nodular. The contour of the liver is nodular (Fig. 27-13), and the caudate lobe becomes hypertrophied. Distorted liver parenchyma alters biliary and hepatoportal vascular channels that provide increased resistance to portal venous blood flow and obstruction to hepatic venous outflow. The primary complication of portal hypertension is gastrointestinal bleeding from ruptured esophageal and gastric varices. Etiologies of hypertension are divided into three levels: prehepatic (inflow), intrahepatic (liver, sinusoids, and hepatocytes), and posthepatic (outflow). Disease processes associated with each level are listed in Table 27-2.

## TABLE 27-2   Causes of Portal Hypertension

**Prehepatic:**
- Portal/splenic vein thrombosis
- Splanchnic arteriovenous fistula
- Malignancy
- Trauma
- Sepsis
- Pancreatitis
- Hypercoagulable states

**Intrahepatic:**
- Cirrhosis
- Malignancy
- Lymphoma
- Schistosomiasis
- Sinusoidal obstruction syndrome (SOS)
- Sarcoidosis

**Posthepatic:**
- Budd-Chiari's syndrome (hepatic vein/IVC obstruction)
- Congestive heart failure/constrictive pericarditis
- IVC obstruction

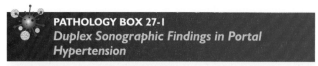

**PATHOLOGY BOX 27-1**
*Duplex Sonographic Findings in Portal Hypertension*

- Increased portal vein diameter (>13–15 mm)
- Increased splenic vein and SMV diameters (>10 mm)
- <20% increase in SMV or splenic vein diameter quiet respiration to deep inspiration
- Decreased or absent respiratory variation (portal/splenic veins)
- Diminished, static, altered pulsatility of portal and hepatic venous flow
- Hepatofugal flow (portal/splenic veins)
- Portosystemic collaterals (varices)
- Ascites and splenomegaly
- Liver parenchyma pathology (cirrhosis, tumor infiltration, Budd-Chiari's syndrome)
- Portal vein obstruction (thrombus, tumor invasion)
- Increased hepatic artery flow (arterialization)

### Duplex Sonographic Findings in Portal Hypertension

Several sonographic findings are associated with portal hypertension. Pathology Box 27-1 lists the duplex sonographic findings.[14]

With the development of portal hypertension, the MPV diameter initially increases because of increasing portal venous pressure (Fig. 27-14). In cases of severe portal hypertension, the diameter of the portal vein may decrease because of (decompression) portosystemic collaterals. An increased portal vein diameter greater than 13 mm indicates portal hypertension with a high degree of specificity 100% but with low sensitivity 40%.[15] Reversed or hepatofugal portal flow is generally associated with a significant reduction in the diameter of the portal vein because more blood is diverted to portosystemic collaterals. Hepatofugal flow in the MPV has been reported in the literature with an overall prevalence of 8.3% in patients.[10] Other studies have reported hepatofugal flow in the portal venous system (portal vein, SV, and SMV) of patients with cirrhosis between 3% and 23%.[16] In some patients with cirrhosis, hepatofugal flow is identified in isolated intrahepatic portal vein branches

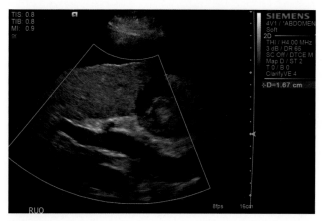

**FIGURE 27-14** A portal vein with an increased diameter (1.67 cm) associated with portal hypertension.

only. Hepatofugal flow can change to hepatopetal flow after ingestion of a meal, because of a postprandial increase in splanchnic venous flow. This phenomenon may be blunted in cirrhotic patients. In addition, hepatofugal flow can revert to hepatopetal flow if the patient's condition improves after medication.

With severe portal hypertension, flow velocity within the portal vein generally decreases because of increased resistance. Spectral Doppler demonstrates continuous (losing normal fluctuations), biphasic (to and fro in some patients), and eventually reverse flow (hepatofugal) in patients with advanced disease (Fig. 27-15).

While several studies advocate decreased portal vein flow as an indicator of portal hypertension, collateral pathways can augment portal vein hemodynamics. For example, a recanalized paraumbilical vein can increase portal vein velocity, whereas splenorenal collaterals can reduce and reverse flow.

An increased SV diameter greater than 10 mm with reduced flow or retrograde hepatofugal flow and no detectable thrombus is an indicator for portal hypertension. In this situation, the mesenteric venous blood is transported to the vena cava through portosystemic collaterals. In the splenic hilum, dilated veins sometimes show anastomoses to veins of the stomach or esophagus.

### Portosystemic Collateral Anatomy

Detection of portosystemic collateral veins (varices) is the most specific finding of portal hypertension (Fig. 27-16). Varices are reported to occur in approximately 39% of patients with biopsy proven cirrhosis and are more common in patients with advanced disease.[17] Color duplex sonography visualizes approximately 65% to 90% of collateral shunts.[18] Commonly seen collaterals include splenorenal varices which are the most common (seen in 21% of patients with spontaneous shunts), the paraumbilical vein (next most common seen in 14% of patients with spontaneous shunts), and gastroesophageal veins (Figs. 27-17 to 27-20).

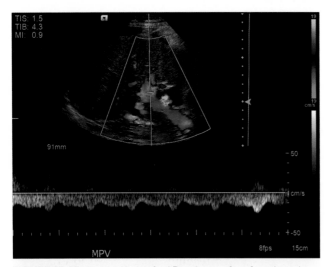

**FIGURE 27-15** Abnormal hepatofugal Doppler waveform from the main portal vein (MPV) in a patient with portal hypertension. The abnormal portal venous flow is displayed below the baseline and is color coded in blue within the image. Normal antegrade hepatic artery flow is displayed above the baseline.

The most prevalent collateral pathway is the coronary vein or left gastric vein. It is identified angiographically in 80% to 90% of patients with portal hypertension. The coronary vein is infrequently seen by ultrasound in normal patients (Fig. 27-21) when dilated, enhancing sonographic visualization. Pathology Box 27-2 describes various portosystemic collateral pathways.[2,14]

### Arterialization (Increased Hepatic Artery Flow)

When portal venous pressure increases as a result of portal vein obstruction, such as advanced cirrhosis and PVT, hepatic arterial flow increases as a homeostatic mechanism to maintain hepatic perfusion. Enlargement, increased flow, and a tortuous "corkscrew" appearance are commonly seen in patients with cirrhosis, portal hypertension, PVT, and inflammation related to chronic active hepatitis. Color duplex imaging demonstrates an enlarged hepatic artery with high-velocity turbulent flow (mixed color flow) referred to as "arterializations."

### Arteriovenous Fistulae

Hepatic arterioportal fistula may cause life-threatening portal hypertension. Causes of arterioportal fistulae include penetrating trauma, iatrogenic trauma secondary to liver biopsies, transhepatic cholangiography, and transhepatic catheterization of the bile ducts or portal veins. Profuse collateral flow typically accompanies severe portal hypertension in patients with hepatic artery to portal vein communications. With an arterioportal fistula, the resulting pressure gradient causes blood to flow from the artery to the vein. Duplex sonography demonstrates arterialized hepatofugal flow in the portal vein. Large anechoic spaces are seen within the liver in the area of the communication. Color Doppler shows turbulent high-velocity flow "color bruit" detected between the communication of the artery and vein.

Another type of fistula can arise between the portal vein and a hepatic vein. The causes responsible for venovenous fistulae are trauma, surgery, organ punctures, perforated aneurysms, and idiopathic causes. The pressure gradients associated with venovenous fistulae cause blood to flow from the portal vein to the hepatic vein. In cases of hepatic vein to portal vein fistulae, the triphasic spectral pattern of the hepatic veins is reflected back to the portal system, producing increased pulsatility in the portal vein waveform.

### Transjugular Intrahepatic Portosystemic Shunt (TIPS)

TIPS is a nonsurgical procedure performed to decompress the portal venous system, for the management of uncontrollable variceal bleeding and refractory ascites. Other indications for TIPS include patients with hepatic venous outflow obstruction (Budd-Chiari's syndrome), hepatic hydrothorax, or hepatorenal syndrome. Before placement of TIPS, a pre-TIPS sonographic evaluation of the abdomen, hepatoportal vasculature, and right jugular vein (patency and flow direction) is paramount to assess for contraindications. Contraindications include hepatoma, PVT, congestive heart failure, unrelieved biliary obstruction, multiple hepatic cysts, severe pulmonary hypertension, and uncontrollable systemic infection or sepsis.

The technique for constructing a TIPS involves passing a catheter under fluoroscopic guidance via the right jugular

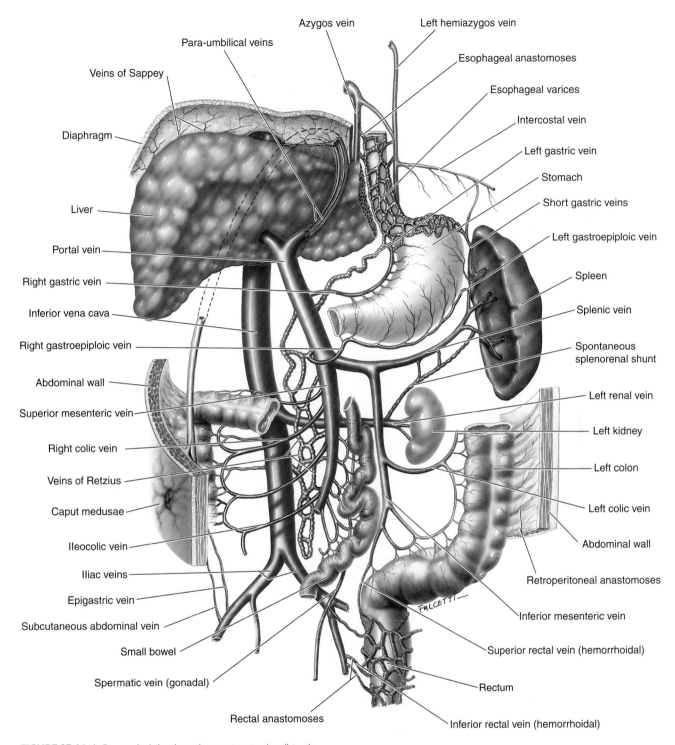

**FIGURE 27-16** A diagram depicting the various portosystemic collaterals.

vein to the level of the hepatic veins. A percutaneous intraparenchymal tract is created by passing a needle through the wall of the hepatic vein (preferably the right, because of its angle and diameter) through the liver parenchyma to a branch of the portal vein (usually the right) adjacent to its junction with the MPV. An angioplasty balloon dilates the track, and an expandable polytetrafluoroethylene (PTFE) covered metallic stent is deployed rerouting blood away

from the liver, out through the stent, into the hepatic vein, and back to the heart. A portion of the stent near the portal vein end is often uncovered.

The ultrasound techniques employed to evaluate a patient with a TIPS are much the same as a conventional evaluation of the native portal system. These include the same transducers and scanning approaches as well as the same patient preparation of having the patient fast prior

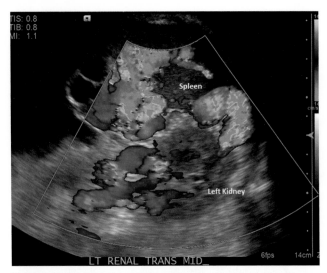

**FIGURE 27-17** Color Doppler image demonstrating varices within the splenic hilum and medial and lateral to the left kidney.

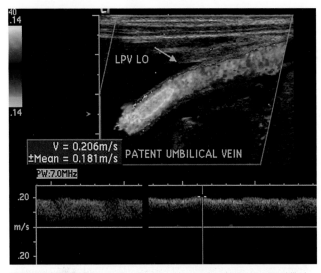

**FIGURE 27-18** Color duplex ultrasound image showing a patent umbilical vein. The velocity is 0.206 m/s.

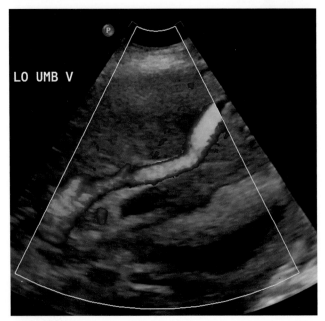

**FIGURE 27-19** Power Doppler image showing a patent umbilical vein.

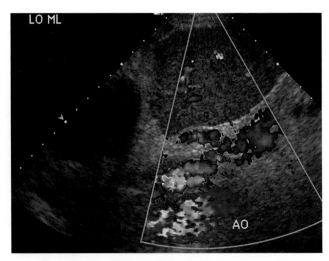

**FIGURE 27-20** Color Doppler image longitudinal midline showing esophageal varices anterior to the abdominal aorta.

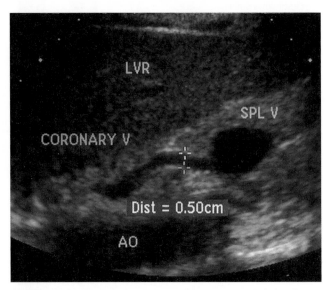

**FIGURE 27-21** Normal grayscale image of the coronary vein (calipers) measuring 5 mm. The coronary vein is running cephalad from the splenic vein (SPL V). AO, aorta; LVR, liver.

to the ultrasound. Technical considerations while imaging TIPS include appropriate color gain, filter, and scale tailored for stent velocities and portal vein branches. Color flow throughout the stent is uniform and enhances areas of focal aliasing. Portal vein branches require a lower color scale to enhance flow direction. Lastly, flow velocity is measured during quiet respiration because intra-TIPS velocity decreases by approximately 22 cm/s during deep inspiration.[19]

Angle-corrected velocities are recorded from the MPV, the portal vein end of the stent, midstent, the hepatic vein end of the stent and the IVC, or outflow hepatic vein. Direction of flow should be noted within these vessels in addition to adjacent intrahepatic portal vein branches, hepatic veins, and SV. The presence of ascites, varices, and stent complications should be noted. Post-TIPS complications include intraperitoneal bleeding, acute stent thrombosis and hepatic artery biliary duct, gallbladder or transcpsular punctures.

| Collateral | Features |
|---|---|
| Coronary vein (left gastric vein) | • Most often joins the portal system at the splenoportal confluence<br>• With portal hypertension, diameter >7 mm<br>• Can demonstrate hepatofugal flow that often leads to esophageal varices |
| Gastroesophageal veins | • Located posterior to left lobe of liver<br>• Can be large and tortuous |
| Recanalized paraumbilical vein | • Located in the fissure for the ligamentum teres<br>• Diameter >3 mm is diagnostic for portal hypertension |
| Splenorenal | • Prominent varices at splenic hilum<br>• Enlarged left renal vein |
| Gallbladder varices | • Portosystemic shunts between the cystic vein branch of the portal vein and either anterior abdominal wall veins or portal vein branches within the liver<br>• Found in 30% of patients with portal vein thrombosis<br>• 3–8 mm in diameter<br>• Tortuous vessels along gallbladder wall |

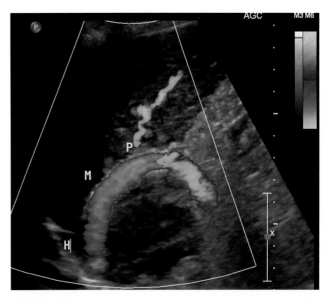

**FIGURE 27-22** Color image of a normal TIPS. H, hepatic vein end; M, mid stent; P, portal vein end.

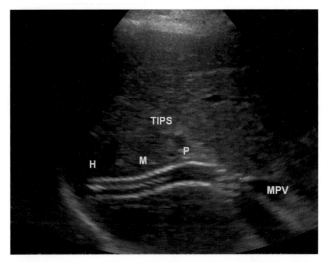

**FIGURE 27-23** Grayscale image of a TIPS stent. The main portal vein (MPV) is also seen.

In a well-functioning TIPS, hepatofugal flow is present within the intrahepatic portal vein branches beyond the site of the stent connection with the portal vein. Color-flow imaging should reveal hepatopetal flow in the MPV with flow directed into the stent. The flow should continue in the direction of the hepatic vein and then out via the IVC. Color should be observed completely filling the stent (Fig. 27-22). It should be noted that color Doppler performed in patients less than 48 to 72 hours after TIPS placement, may produce shadowing along the stent resulting in false-positive results. This is a result of air being trapped within the layers of the PTFE material used to cover the stent. After a brief period of time (usually 2 to 3 days), the air dissipates and the stent will be able to be completely insonated. The frequency of follow-up studies varies among imaging centers. In general, follow-up studies are performed within 24 to 48 hours, at 3 and 6 months, and then yearly. The sonographic appearance of a TIPS stent is a curvilinear echogenic structure with corrugated borders that course through the hepatic parenchyma and extends squarely into both inflowing portal vein and outflowing RHV (Fig. 27-23).

TIPS velocities vary somewhat in different studies. Normal-accepted published velocities within the stent range from 90 to 190 cm/s.[20] Velocities tend to increase from the portal end to the hepatic end of the stent, with the mean velocity of 95 cm/s at the portal venous end and 120 cm/s at the mid portion of the stent. The normal waveform within the TIPS is high velocity, hepatopetal, monophasic, turbulent, with slight pulsatility (Fig. 27-24). A baseline study of each patient is important to gauge further follow-up examinations.

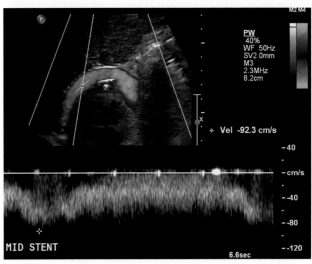

**FIGURE 27-24** Normal Doppler waveforms from a TIPS.

**PATHOLOGY BOX 27-3**
*Duplex Ultrasound Criteria for TIPS Stenosis*

Hepatopetal flow in the left and right portal vein branches as compared to baseline studies

Retrograde flow within the hepatic vein serving as the outflow for the shunt

A velocity of less than 50 cm/s within the stent

A velocity less than 30 cm/s within the main portal vein

A focal region of increased velocity within the stent or hepatic vein

An increase or a decrease in velocity of greater than 50 cm/s within the same portion of the stent as compared to previous studies

Hepatofugal flow in the main portal vein

Recurrent ascites, varices, or splenomegaly

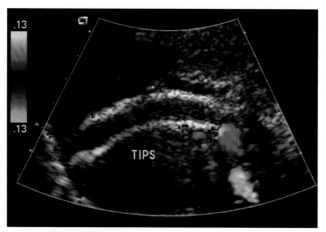

**FIGURE 27-26** An occluded TIPS with no filling on color-flow imaging and echogenic material within the shunt itself.

Within the MPV and hepatic artery, flow velocities are increased. Portal vein velocities may increase to 37 to 47 cm/s greater than the pre-TIPS velocities. Hepatic artery peak systolic velocity may exceed 130 cm/s$^2$. SV velocities are also observed to increase post-TIPS placement.

Multiple duplex ultrasound changes have been associated with TIPS stenosis.[18] Pathology Box 27-3 lists criteria commonly employed in cases of suspected stenosis. Figure 27-25 illustrates a TIPS stenosis.

No single ultrasound criterion has yielded a strong predictive value or sensitivity in detecting stenosis. When multiple criteria are used, sensitivity in identifying TIPS stenosis improves.

TIPS occlusion should be suspected if echogenic material is observed within the stent and no flow is detected on spectral Doppler or color-flow imaging techniques (Fig. 27-26). Care should be taken to optimize Doppler and color imaging techniques to avoid a false-positive finding of thrombosis. Multiple scanning planes as well as appropriate Doppler and color frequencies, color priority settings and Doppler, and color scale or pulse repetition frequencies should be used.

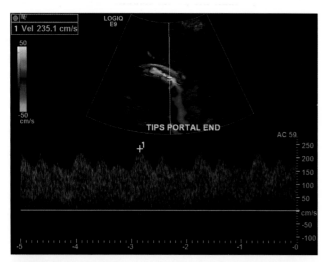

**FIGURE 27-25** An image from a TIPS with a stenosis. Note the elevated velocity of 235 cm/s.

## Portal Venous Thrombosis

PVT results from flow stasis secondary to cirrhosis and portal hypertension. Approximately 20% of all cases of PVT are due to cirrhosis. Malignancies (hepatic and pancreatic) are also responsible for approximately 20% of PVT caused by direct invasion and extrinsic compression. PVT may also involve the splenic and/or mesenteric veins. Other etiologies of PVT include inflammatory processes (such as pancreatitis, appendicitis, and diverticulitis), various hypercoagulable states (including protein C or S deficiencies, antithrombin deficiency, and polycythemia vera), surgical intervention, abdominal malignancy (hepatocellular or pancreatic carcinomas), sepsis, and trauma.[1] Patients with hepatocellular carcinoma are at greater risk of developing malignant thrombus (intravascular tumor) because of direct invasion of the portal vein. Pancreatitis and pancreatic carcinoma are frequent causes of thrombosis and tumor infiltration in the portal vein, SV, and SMV. A sudden onset of ascites, acute abdominal pain, and elevated D-dimer in patients, may indicate the presence of PVT.

Because the MPV is easily visualized in most patients, when a normal appearing portal vein is not readily seen, portal vein occlusion should be suspected. Diagnostic sonographic findings supporting the diagnosis of acute occlusive PVT are the absence of flow by spectral, color, or power Doppler (Figs. 27-27 and 27-28). The portal vein diameter of the thrombosed segment is enlarged in 38% of cases. Acute portal vein thrombus may appear anechoic to hypoechoic and go undetected when performing grayscale imaging. Tumor in the portal vein may present identical to that of thrombosis. Tumor thrombus may be partial or complete and be mixed with benign thrombus. Color Doppler imaging can aid in differentiating benign thrombus from tumor infiltration by identifying small vascular channels that exhibit low-resistance pulsatile arterial signals within a soft tissue mass in the portal veins.[21] (Fig. 27-29). Color imaging and Doppler waveforms help to distinguish complete versus partial PVT.

The sonographic appearance of SMV and SV thrombosis is similar to PVT (Fig. 27-30).

If PVT persists (up to 12 months) without substantial lysis, this leads to the development of periportal collateral

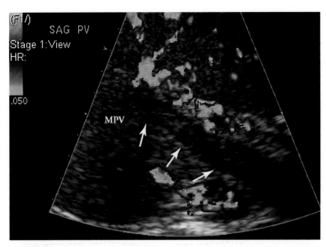

**FIGURE 27-27** A thrombosed main portal vein (MPV) with no flow present using color Doppler techniques. Flow is seen in the adjacent hepatic artery.

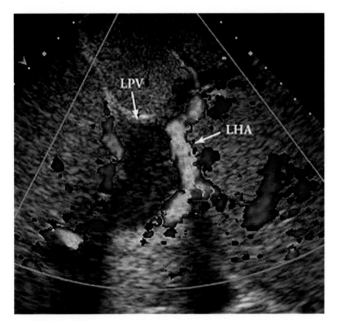

**FIGURE 27-28** Color Doppler image of an acute thrombosed left portal vein (LPV). Note arterialization of the left hepatic artery (LHA) to maintain perfusion to the liver.

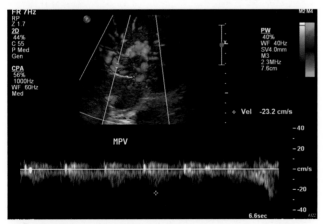

**FIGURE 27-29** Color duplex ultrasound image of tumor thrombus within the main portal vein (MPV). Note the low-resistance arterial flow, below the baseline representing tumor infiltration.

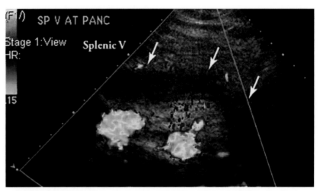

**FIGURE 27-30** Color Doppler image of an acute thrombosed splenic vein in a patient with portal hypertension.

veins known as "cavernous transformation".[2] With cavernous transformation, multiple serpiginous vessels are seen in and around the occluded portal vein. They can appear within 6 to 20 days after acute occlusion to reestablish portal flow. The thrombosed portal vein has a sponge-like mass appearance on grayscale, representing numerous venous recanalizing channels. Color duplex ultrasound imaging demonstrates absent flow in the MPV and recanalizing hepatopetal portal venous flow (2 to 7 cm/s) within periportal collateral veins (Fig. 27-31). Because cavernous transformation results from long-standing portal vein occlusion, it is more likely to be caused by benign processes. The sonographic findings for PVT are listed in Pathology Box 27-4.

## Cardiac Cirrhosis (Congestive Hepatopathy) and Congestive Heart Failure

Cardiac cirrhosis (congestive hepatopathy) includes a spectrum of hepatic disorders that occur in the setting of right-sided heart failure. Edema of the liver secondary to vascular congestion is a complication related to congestive heart failure. Impedance of flow into the right side of the heart due to cardiac or pulmonary disorders causes secondary dilatation and absence of vein wall motion with respiratory maneuvers, within the portal–hepatic venous system and IVC (Fig. 27-32). Increased right heart pressure will impact the portal and hepatic waveforms. Portal vein flow becomes markedly pulsatile, corresponding to pressure transmitted from the right atrium (Fig. 27-33). Hepatic vein waveforms demonstrate a highly pulsatile inverted "W"-type pattern, showing flow reversal during systole, secondary to severe

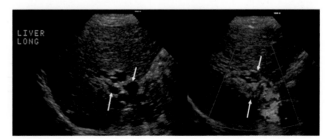

**FIGURE 27-31** A thrombosed portal vein with cavernous transformation (arrows indicate the periportal collateral veins).

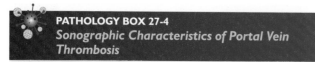

**PATHOLOGY BOX 27-4**
*Sonographic Characteristics of Portal Vein Thrombosis*

- Increased portal vein caliber (>15 mm), intraluminal echoes with variable echogenicity (anechoic, hypoechoic, hyperechoic)
- Massive portal vein caliber (>23 mm) with intraluminal echoes suggests tumor thrombus not specific
- Failure to visualize the portal vein (acute)
- Absent flow by color and power Doppler within a completely obstructed portal vein (occlusive)
- Hepatofugal pulsatile arterial waveform within a soft tissue mass in the main portal vein (tumor thrombus)
- Small vascular arterial channels within a soft tissue mass in the main portal vein (tumor thrombus)
- Increased hepatic arterial flow (arterialization)
- Small echogenic/fibrotic portal channel with intraluminal echoes (chronic)
- Cavernous transformation; periportal collaterals (chronic)
- Gallbladder varices

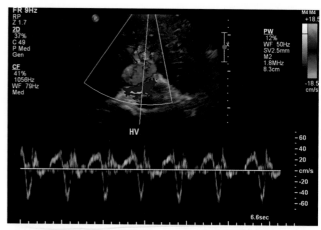

**FIGURE 27-34** Hepatic vein duplex ultrasound image demonstrating marked pulsatility from a patient with severe tricuspid regurgitation.

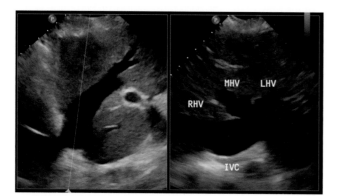

**FIGURE 27-32** Grayscale image in both longitudinal and transverse showing marked dilatation of the hepatic veins and inferior vena cava (IVC) due to congestive heart failure.

tricuspid regurgitation (Fig. 27-34). Hepatomegaly is associated with hepatic congestion. Congestive hepatopathy results from chronically increased pressure and sinusoidal stasis, which causes an accumulation of deoxygenated blood, parenchymal atrophy, necrosis, collagen deposition, and ultimately fibrosis.

## Budd-Chiari's Syndrome

Obstruction of the hepatic venous outflow tract at any level from the small to large hepatic veins, to the junction of the IVC and right atrium as well as concomitant clinical features include acute right upper quadrant pain, jaundice, ascites, hepatomegaly, and liver function abnormalities, suggesting hepatocellular dysfunctions are collectively known as Budd-Chiari's syndrome.[1] There are many causes of Budd-Chiari's syndrome, and these are related to the primary site of obstruction. Primary hepatic vein obstruction results from thrombus or webs (Fig. 27-35). Secondary hepatic venous outflow obstruction results from malignant tumor infiltration, parasitic mass, or from extrinsic compression by a neighboring mass

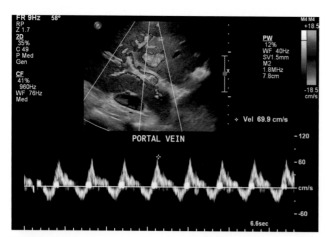

**FIGURE 27-33** A portal vein duplex ultrasound image demonstrating markedly pulsatile flow from a patient with severe tricuspid regurgitation.

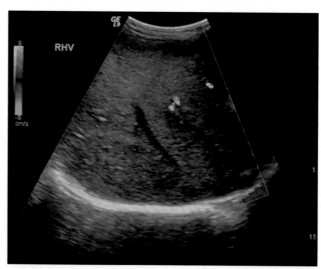

**FIGURE 27-35** Color Doppler image of thrombosed hepatic veins in a patient with Budd-Chiari's syndrome.

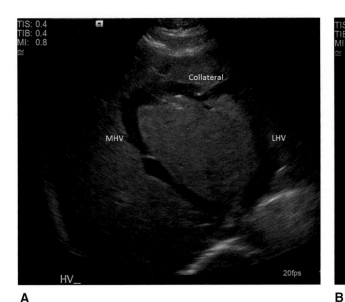
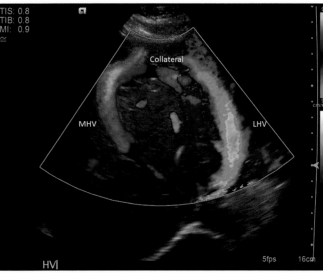

A                                    B

**FIGURE 27-36** **A:** Grayscale image of a patient with chronic Budd-Chiari's syndrome. Absent right hepatic vein. A collateral vessel is seen from middle hepatic vein (MHV) feeding the left hepatic vein (LHV). **B:** Color Doppler image from the same patient. Note the narrowing at the proximal portion of the MHV and reverse flow in the distal portion. Color imaging illustrating the direction of flow from the MHV through the large collateral vessel into the left hepatic vein.

(abscess, cysts, and benign/malignant tumors). Thrombus can occur with cirrhosis, hypercoagulable disorders, the use of oral contraceptives, and abdominal trauma.[14] Approximately 25% of patients with Budd-Chiari's syndrome also have PVT.[22]Tumor invasion is most often associated with hepatocellular carcinoma. IVC occlusion or stenosis cephalad to the hepatic veins can cause Budd-Chiari's syndrome by creating hepatic vein congestion. Obstruction of the IVC may be caused by congenital stenosis or occlusion, thrombosis from hypercoagulable states, or tumor invasion.

Hepatic venous obstruction is often accompanied by stenosis or obstruction of the IVC. When the IVC is involved, lower

extremity edema may be present. With severe obstruction, collateral channels are formed. The collaterals that are most frequently seen that drain into unobstructed hepatic veins include accessory hepatic veins, caudate lobe veins, subcapsular veins, or portal veins (Fig. 27-36). Flow in the portal vein maybe slow or reversed. The caudate lobe enlarges because of blood volume overload because the other lobes of the liver will try to drain out via the caudate veins which empty directly into the IVC[4] (Fig. 27-37). The sonographic findings of Budd-Chiari's syndrome are listed in Pathology Box 27-5.

## Sinusoidal Obstruction Syndrome (SOS)

SOS, formerly known as hepatic veno-occlusive disease, is a condition resulting from toxic injury to hepatic sinusoidal epithelial cells, which then undergo necrosis and sloughing, occluding the hepatic sinusoids and terminal hepatic

**FIGURE 27-37** Color Doppler image of an enlarged caudate lobe compressing the inferior vena cava (IVC) in a patient with Budd-Chiari's syndrome.

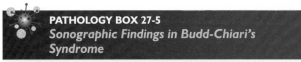

**PATHOLOGY BOX 27-5**
*Sonographic Findings in Budd-Chiari's Syndrome*

- Dilatation of the IVC with intraluminal echoes
- Dilatation of the hepatic veins with intraluminal echoes
- Stenosis or occlusion of the hepatic veins and IVC
- Absence of hepatic vein and IVC flow
- Continuous, turbulent, and reversed flow in the nonoccluded portions of hepatic veins and IVC
- Enlarged caudate lobe (greater than 3.5 cm in anteroposterior diameter)
- Enlarged caudate vein >3 mm in diameter
- Slow or reversed flow in the portal vein
- Portal vein thrombus (25%)
- Ascites/hepatomegaly
- Splenomegaly (25%)
- Portosystemic collaterals

venules. It most commonly occurs after hematopoietic stem cell transplantation. Cases have been reported following radiation to the liver, liver transplantation, and ingestion of traditional herbal remedies or dietary supplements, particularly those containing pyrrolizidine alkaloids.

Clinical features of acute (presents 1 to 3 weeks after initial sinusoidal insult) SOS include a sudden onset of hepatomegaly, abdominal pain, fluid retention, jaundice, and ascites. The subacute and chronic forms (several weeks, months, years after initial sinusoidal insult) of SOS typically present with fatigue, abdominal swelling, with signs and symptoms of portal hypertension. The disease resembles the Budd-Chiari's syndrome clinically; however, the obstruction is because of narrowing and occlusion of sinusoids and terminal hepatic venules (central and interlobular veins) rather than thrombosis of the larger hepatic veins and IVC. Ultrasound can help to exclude acute Budd-Chiari's syndrome and PVT by demonstrating patency of large hepatic veins and portal veins.

## SUMMARY

- Duplex sonography provides important quantitative and qualitative information about the liver and portal–hepatic vascular hemodynamics.
- A thorough working knowledge of the anatomy, hemodynamics, instrumentation, scanning windows, and patience are essential to best utilize this medical imaging tool.
- Furthermore, knowledge about abnormal vascular disorders and altered hemodynamics increases examination efficacy, sonographer knowledge, and contributes to quality patient care.

## CRITICAL THINKING QUESTION

1. A patient presents for an add-on portal system ultrasound examination. The patient is not fasted, obese, and known to have ascites. What scanning plane might you use to begin the scan and why?

2. Why is the breathing pattern of a patient important during a hepatoportal ultrasound examination?
3. You are asked to examine a patient who is 1-day post-procedure from a TIPS shunt being placed. You begin your ultrasound examination and observe a brightly reflective structure within the right lobe of the liver. However, a strong acoustic shadow is present. What is a likely explanation of this finding and what can be done?

## MEDIA MENU

Student Resources available on thePoint° include:
- Audio glossary
- Interactive question bank
- Videos
- Internet resources

## REFERENCES

1. Leonhardt WC. Duplex sonography of the hepatoportal vascular system. *Vasc US Today*. 2012;17:105–172.
2. Wilson SR, Withers CE. The liver. In: Rumack CM, Wilson SR, Charboneau JW, Levine D, eds. *Diagnostic Ultrasound*. 4th ed. Philadelphia, PA: Elsevier Mosby Company; 2011:78–145.
3. Marks WM, Filly RA, Callen PW. Ultrasonic anatomy of the liver: a review with new applications. *J Clin Ultrasound*. 1979;7:137–146.
4. Wachsberg RH, Angyal EA, Klein KM, et al. Echogenicity of hepatic versus portal vein walls revisited with histologic correlation. *J Ultrasound Med*. 1997;16(12):807–810.
5. Bargallo X, Gilbert R, Nicolau C, et al. Sonography of the caudate vein: value in diagnosing Budd-Chiari Syndrome. *Am J Roentgenol*. 2003;181:1641–1645.
6. Weinreb J, Kumari S, Phillips G, et al. Portal vein measurements by real-time sonography. *Am J Roentgenol*. 1982;139:497–499.
7. Abu-Yousef MM, Milam SG, Farner RM. Pulsatile portal vein flow: a sign of tricuspid regurgitation on duplex Doppler. *Am J Roentgenol*. 1990;155:785–788.
8. Zironi G, Garani S, Fenyves D, et al. Value of measurement of mean portal flow velocity by Doppler flowmetry in the diagnosis of portal hypertension. *J Hepatol* 1992;16:298–303.
9. Cioni G, D'Alimonte PI, Cristani A, et al. Duplex-Doppler assessment of cirrhosis in patients with chronic compensated liver disease. *J Gastroenterol Hepatl*. 1992;7:382–384.
10. Bolondi L, Galani S, Gebel M. Portohepatic vascular pathology and liver disease: diagnosis and monitoring. *Eur J Ultrasound*. 1998;7:S41–S52.
11. Henriksson L, Hedman A, Johansson R, et al. Ultrasound assessment of liver veins in congestive heart failure. *Acta Radiol*. 1982;23:361–363.
12. Al-Nakahabandi NA. The role of ultrasonography in portal hypertension. *Saudi J Gastroentero*. 2006;12:111–117.
13. NIDDK. *Cirrhosis of the Liver, NIH Publ No 00-1134*. Bethesda, MD: National Institute of Diabetes and Digestive and Kidney Diseases, 2000.
14. Zwiebel WJ. Vascular conditions. In: Ahuja AT, ed. *Diagnostic Imaging: Ultrasound*. Philadelphia, PA: Elsevier Saunders Company; 2007:1–110.
15. Bolondi L, Gandolfi L, Arienti V, et al. Ultrasonography in the diagnosis of portal hypertension: diminished response of portal vessels to respiration. *Radiology*. 1982;142:167–172.
16. Wachsberg RH, Bahramipour P, Sofocleous CT, Barone A. Hepatofugal flow in the portal venous system: pathophysiology, imaging findings, and diagnostic pitfalls. *Radiographics*. 2002;22:123–140.
17. Andrew A. Portal hypertension: a review. *JDMS*. 2001;17:193–200.
18. Zwiebel WJ. Ultrasound assessment of the hepatic vasculature. In: Zwiebel WJ, Pellerito JS, eds. *Introduction to Vascular Ultrasonography*. 5th ed. Philadelphia, PA: Elsevier Saunders Company; 2005:585–609.
19. Vignali C, Bargellini I, Grosso M, et al. TIPS with expanded polytetrafluoroethylene-covered stent : result of an Italian multicenter study. *Am J Roentgenol*. 2005;185:472–480.
20. Kanterman RY, Darcy MD, Middleton WD, et al. Doppler sonography findings associated with transjugular intrahepatic portosystemic shunt malfunction. *AJR Am J Roentgenol*. 1997;168:467–472.
21. Dodd GD, Memel DS, Baron RL, et al. Portal vein thrombosis in patients with cirrhosis: does sonographic detection of intrathrombus flow allow differentiation of benign and malignant thrombus? *AJR Am J Roentgenol*. 1995;165:573–577.
22. McNaughton DA, Abu-Yousef MM. Doppler US of the liver made simple. *Radiographics*. 2011;31:161–188.

# Evaluation of Kidney and Liver Transplants

M. ROBERT DEJONG | LESLIE M. SCOUTT | MONICA FULLER

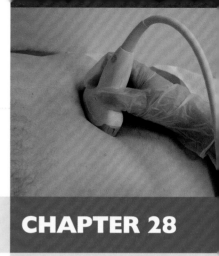

**CHAPTER 28**

## OBJECTIVES

- Describe the types of transplant procedures and vascular anastomoses
- Define the essential components of transplant ultrasound examinations
- Define the vascular complications associated with transplants

## GLOSSARY

**allograft** Any tissue transplanted from one human to another human

**arteriovenous fistula** A connection between an artery and a vein, usually posttraumatic in origin

**immunosuppression drugs** Drugs used to inhibit the body's formation of antibodies to the allograft

**orthotopic transplant** A transplant that is placed in the same anatomic location as the native organ. A whole liver transplant is an orthotopic transplant. Renal transplants are not orthotopic in location

**pseudoaneurysm** Develops secondary to a tear in the arterial wall, allowing extravasation of blood from the arterial lumen that is contained by a compacted rim of surrounding soft tissue

**transplant rejection** The failure of a transplant occurring secondary to the formation of antidonor antibodies by the recipient, thereby leading to loss of the transplant

## KEY TERMS

**arteriovenous fistula**

**liver transplant**

**pseudoaneurysm**

**rejection**

**renal transplant**

**vascular stenosis**

**vascular thrombosis**

Ultrasound (US) evaluation of transplanted organs has become an established and important routine component of posttransplant patient follow-up. Modern advances in surgical techniques and in immunosuppression regimens have resulted in increased long-term survival of both allografts and transplant recipients. Renal and hepatic transplantations are the preferred treatment for patients with renal and hepatic failure, respectively. Pancreatic, small bowel, lung, and cardiac transplants are also increasingly performed. Currently, arm transplants have become possible. This program was started to help veterans who lost their arm or arms while being deployed and suffered the loss in battle. In most series, vascular complications are the second most common cause of graft loss, and US is considered the initial screening modality of choice for the evaluation of a suspected vascular complication in a renal or hepatic transplant recipient. This chapter reviews the US techniques and criteria for US examination of kidney and liver transplants.

## KIDNEY TRANSPLANTATION

The first successful kidney transplant was performed in 1954 at the Peter Bent Brigham Hospital in Boston, MA, between identical twin brothers, which eliminated the potential for any adverse immune reaction.[1,2] However, kidney transplants continued to be very limited because of incompatibility issues until the early 1960s when significant advances occurred in tissue typing, allowing for better matching of donor and recipients. In addition, immunosuppression therapy was introduced in 1961 which dramatically improved graft survival, because these drugs helped the recipient accept the foreign tissue in the allograft. With immunosuppression therapy, transplantation of a deceased donor (DD) allograft became a realistic possibility, and in 1962, the first DD kidney transplant was performed, again at the Peter Bent Brigham Hospital. In 1983, cyclosporine, a highly effective relatively nontoxic immunosuppressant agent, was introduced and resulted in a significant improvement in patient outcomes by reducing the risk of rejection. Since then, continued evolution and refinement of immunosuppression protocols have decreased even further the rate of graft loss caused by rejection in renal transplant recipients.

Currently, renal transplantation is considered the treatment of choice for the majority of patients with end-stage renal disease, providing better quality of life and long-term survival when compared to either peritoneal dialysis or hemodialysis.[3-5] Common causes of end-stage renal disease include diabetes mellitus, autosomal-dominant polycystic kidney disease, glomerulonephritis, hypertension, atherosclerosis, and systemic lupus erythematosus, with diabetes being the most common cause of kidney transplantation.

According to the United Network for Organ Sharing 19,061 kidney transplants, including 13,431 DD and 5,630 living donors (LD), were performed in the United States in 2016.[6] However, there were over 101,000 people on the waiting list for a kidney transplant in 2016. In fact, it is estimated that a new name is added to the waiting list approximately every 14 minutes, and that 13 people will die every day waiting for a kidney transplant.[6] Thus, organ shortage is the major rate-limiting factor for patients awaiting renal transplantation. The current organ shortage has resulted in loosening of the criteria for DD, an increase in the use of LD as well as other creative means of increasing organ availability. One program is called "the Paired Kidney Exchange Program" where finding compatible matches is facilitated and patients are helped to arrange kidney swaps.[7] For example, the wife of patient A gives her kidney to the son of patient B, and the mother of patient B gives her kidney to patient C, whereas the friend of patient C gives his kidney to patient A. The paired kidney exchange program allows for a patient to receive a better matched kidney, as well as help to significantly decrease the wait time for other patients to receive a matched donor. At the time of writing, the largest paired kidney exchange involved 35 donors and 35 recipients, involving multiple hospitals across the United States.

There has been a steady increase in graft survival since the first kidney was transplanted in the 1950s because of significant advances in immunosuppression protocols, surgical techniques, and the improvement in rapid, efficient organ distribution of human leukocyte antigen (HLA)-matched DD grafts by the United Network of Organ Sharing. In 2016, the Organ Procurement and Transplantation Network (OPTN) reported an 80% 5-year graft survival rate for living HLA-matched donors and a 67% 5-year graft survival rate for DD grafts.[8] Risk factors for graft loss include the number of HLA mismatches, increased age of donor or recipient, African-American race, cold ischemic time greater than 24 hours, and diabetic nephropathy as the cause of the recipient's renal failure.[8]

Once a person has received a transplant, they are closely monitored for any signs of graft failure or complication. Patients with graft failure most commonly present with anuria or a rising serum creatinine level. Pain, tenderness, fever, chills, or elevated white blood cell count may also indicate graft dysfunction. However, these are all quite nonspecific signs and symptoms. Hence, imaging, particularly Doppler US, plays a vital role in the clinical assessment of graft dysfunction following renal transplantation by helping to differentiate anatomic and/or vascular problems that may require surgical intervention from functional abnormalities such as acute tubular necrosis (ATN), drug toxicity, and rejection, which are treated medically.

## The Operation

In adults, renal transplants are most commonly placed extraperitoneally in the right iliac fossa. The right iliac fossa is preferred over the left simply because the sigmoid colon usually occupies more space than the right colon, thereby making the vascular anastomoses technically slightly more difficult on the left. In children, the transplanted kidney may be placed intraperitoneally. For DD transplants, the donor's main renal artery is harvested along with a surrounding cuff or patch of the aortic wall called the "Carrel Patch." This oval piece of the donor's aortic wall typically is anastomosed in an end-to-side fashion with the recipient external iliac artery (EIA) (Fig. 28-1). If the donor kidney has multiple renal arteries, either a larger "Carrel Patch" surrounding the ostia of all the main renal arteries is harvested or multiple separate patches are obtained. Alternatively, the donor renal arteries may be grafted together in a "Y" graft with only a single anastomosis to the recipient EIA. For a LD graft, the donor main renal artery is directly anastomosed either in an end-to-side fashion with the recipient EIA or in an end-to-end fashion with the recipient internal iliac artery. Because the harvesting and use of a "Carrel Patch" results in a larger anastomosis without direct suturing into the renal artery ostium, the incidence of renal artery stenosis (RAS) is believed to be reduced in DD transplants in comparison to LD renal transplants. The donor main renal vein is typically anastomosed to the recipient external iliac vein (EIV) in an end-to-side approach. The ureteral anastomosis is most commonly made by creating an ureteroneocystostomy, implanting the donor ureter into the dome of the bladder above the native ureteral orifice.

One special type of kidney transplant is called an en bloc transplant.[9,10] This type of transplant is obtained from cadavers of small pediatric patients aged less than 5 years. Because one kidney would not be able to function adequately in an adult, both kidneys are removed and placed into the recipient. In these patients, the recipient will receive both

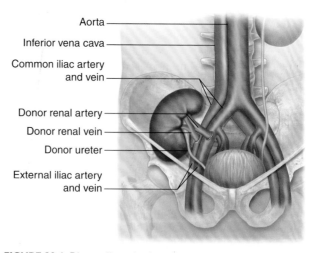

**FIGURE 28-1** Diagram illustrating the most common surgical anatomy for renal transplantation.

kidneys, two ureters, the main renal arteries, the main renal veins, and the suprarenal and infrarenal portions of the aorta and inferior vena cava (IVC). The donor's aorta and IVC are sewn shut just cephalad to the origin of the main renal vessels, and any lumbar vessels are ligated. The kidneys are usually placed extraperitoneally in the right lower quadrant. In these types of transplants, the donor's aorta is anastomosed end-to-side to the recipient's EIA, and the donor's IVC is also anastomosed end-to-side to the recipient's EIV. The donor ureters are both implanted into the recipient's bladder (Fig. 28-2). The protocol for imaging this type of transplant will be different from a single kidney transplant. Instead of imaging the renal artery, the donor's aorta will be evaluated obtaining Doppler signals from the anastomotic site (Fig. 28-3). Next, Doppler signals should be taken from each main renal artery at the level of the renal hilum. This is followed by taking intrarenal Doppler signals. For the venous aspect, a signal is obtained at each renal hilum and in the donor IVC at the anastomosis. Each kidney must be evaluated for any pathology such as hydronephrosis or fluid collections (Fig. 28-4). The grafts will grow and will reach adult size within months after transplantation.

Although surgical practice varies nationwide, placement of an external drain next to the kidney is believed to decrease the incidence of lymphocele formation, a relatively common postsurgical complication that can cause graft dysfunction by compressing the renal parenchyma or vascular/ureteral anastomoses. Superinfection may also occur. Ureteral stents from the intrarenal collecting system into the bladder are commonly placed to reduce the likelihood of ureteral scarring

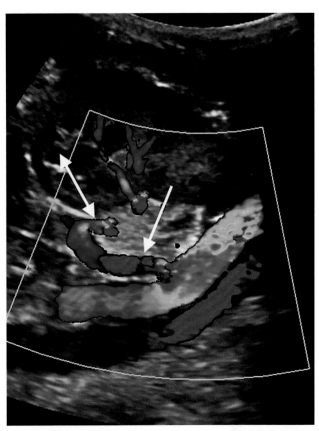

**FIGURE 28-3** The arrow is pointing to the donor aorta that is anastomosed to the external iliac artery. The double-headed arrow is pointing to the renal artery of the superior placed kidney.

or necrosis as well as extravasation of urine, which may lead to the development of urinomas. In most patients, the native kidneys are left in place.

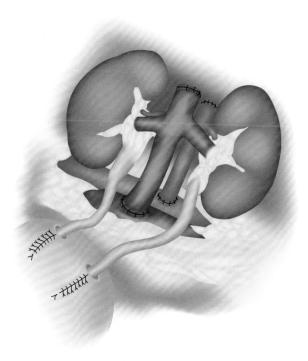

**FIGURE 28-2** En bloc pediatric kidney transplant. The aorta and IVC are used as opposed to the main renal artery and vein to connect to the iliac vessels. Both kidneys must be evaluated. (From Graham SD, Keane TE. *Glenn's Urologic Surgery*. 8th ed. Philadelphia, PA: Wolters Kluwer; 2015; Figure 13-14.)

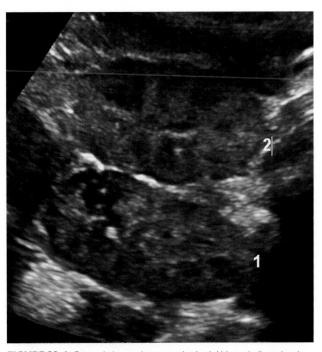

**FIGURE 28-4** Grayscale image demonstrating both kidneys indicated as 1 and 2 in this en bloc transplant.

## SONOGRAPHIC EXAMINATION TECHNIQUES

### Patient Preparation

Typically, no patient preparation is needed to evaluate a renal transplant. It may be helpful for the patient to have some urine in their bladder. It is important for the sonographer to review the surgical notes or speak to the surgeon before the initial or baseline US is obtained. The sonographer should know the following information at a minimum: location of the kidney, whether a single kidney or two pediatric kidneys were placed, which native vessels were used to anastomose with the donor main renal artery and vein, any vascular anomalies such as duplicated vessels, and any additional information that may affect the US examination. The sonographer should also review any recent studies, especially if pathology was present as well as to review the vascular anatomy and anastomotic sites. With the availability of electronic medical records, this information is now more easily available.

### Patient Positioning

The patient is examined in the supine position. If bowel or gas is obscuring part of the kidney, the patient may be turned into an oblique or a decubitus position to try and improve visualization of the kidney.

### Equipment

A 3 to 5 MHz curved linear array transducer can be used. This will provide an aperture to allow for insonation of the entire kidney. The transducer can be gently rocked to push bowel gas out of the way to improve visualization of the kidney. Varying the imaging depth will be necessary because of the superficial placement of most transplanted kidneys. In thin patients, a higher transducer frequency or harmonic imaging may improve resolution.

### Scanning Technique

Imaging protocols must be based on current accreditation guidelines and should be reviewed annually. These guidelines can be found at www.intersocietal.org/vascular and www.aium.org.

A baseline sonogram is usually obtained within 24 to 48 hours postoperatively. It is usually not necessary to evaluate the native kidneys, which are typically left in situ. The lie of the kidney will vary depending on the patient's anatomy. Usually, the kidney is superficial and runs with the axis of the incision site, with the hilum oriented inferiorly and posteriorly. The kidney will also be in a plane parallel to the skin surface, although, sometimes, the kidney will be tilted with either the upper or the lower pole closer to the skin and the other pole deeper in the body. This gives the appearance of the kidney almost being in a plane perpendicular to the skin surface. The length and width of the kidney should be accurately measured (Figs. 28-5 and 28-6). Some protocols may require a volume measurement of the kidney, which would require measuring the kidney

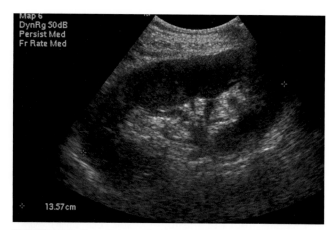

**FIGURE 28-5** Grayscale long-axis view of transplanted kidney (calipers). The renal cortex is relatively hypoechoic, homogeneous, and symmetric in thickness. Mild dilatation of the intrarenal collecting system within the echogenic central renal sinus is a normal finding.

in all three planes: length, width, and anterioposterior (AP) dimensions. The transplanted kidney will look like a normal kidney in shape and echotexture. A comparison view with the liver or the spleen cannot be obtained because the kidney is now located in the pelvis.

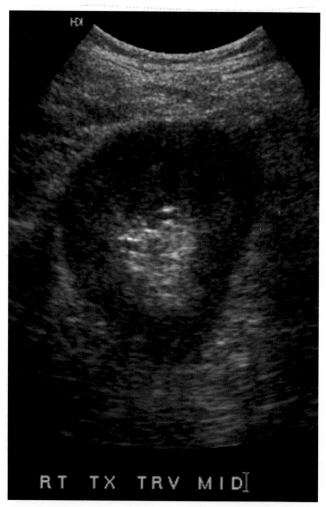

**FIGURE 28-6** Grayscale transverse view of transplanted kidney.

## Grayscale

Grayscale imaging should be performed first. Documented images should include views of the long axis of the kidney in the mid-plane to measure the length of the kidney as well as longitudinal views of the lateral and medial aspects of the kidney. Renal length is variable but is often slightly larger than the native kidney because the kidney will hypertrophy, usually reaching its maximal size by 6 months postop. Increase or decrease in renal length from one examination to the next is a nonspecific indicator of graft dysfunction. Next, views that are 90 degrees to the long axis of the kidney, that is, in the transverse plane, are obtained. Many laboratories obtain transverse views superior to the kidney, through the upper pole, mid pole with transverse and AP measurements, lower pole, and, finally, inferior to the kidney. The superior and inferior transverse views are used to evaluate for any perinephric fluid collections. However, a general survey should also be performed to look for fluid collections. Multiple longitudinal and transverse images of the bladder, or the bladder area if the patient has a Foley catheter in place, should be obtained. An oblique view showing the lower pole of the kidney and the bladder in the same image can also be recorded. This is a helpful image to evaluate for the presence of a urinoma. Any fluid collection seen near the bladder will require further investigation either by having the patient void or by instilling appropriate fluid through the patient's catheter to distend the bladder.

## Color and Spectral Doppler

After obtaining the requisite grayscale images, the sonographer should now perform the Doppler component of the examination. Color and spectral Doppler signals are obtained from the main renal artery, including angle-corrected peak systolic velocity measurements at the anastomosis and proximal and distal (hilar) segments (Figs. 28-7 and 28-8). A color image and spectral Doppler signal is also obtained from the EIA superior to the anastomosis. A color Doppler image of the main renal artery is essential to evaluate for kinking or torqueing. Color and spectral Doppler signals are obtained from the main renal vein, including the venous anastomosis with the EIV (Figs. 28-9 and 28-10). A color

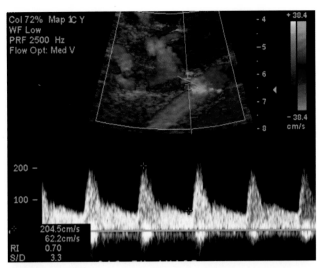

**FIGURE 28-8** Normal spectral Doppler tracing from the origin of the main renal artery. Note sharp systolic upstroke and continuous forward diastolic flow with an RI = 0.70. Mild elevation of the PSV in the main renal artery (204 cm/s) is common secondary to the acute angle of take off from the external iliac artery and increased blood flow through the single vessel. PSV, peak systolic velocity.

image and Doppler signal is also obtained from the EIV at the level of the anastomosis. Spectral tracings should be obtained from the intraparenchymal renal veins at the upper and lower poles. Note that the intraparenchymal renal veins will be found immediately adjacent to the intraparenchymal renal arteries. Color Doppler images demonstrating perfusion of the entire kidney should be obtained, with power Doppler images as needed (Fig. 28-11). Perfusion of the renal cortex should be symmetric and homogeneous throughout the transplant.

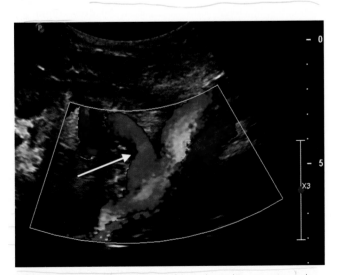

**FIGURE 28-7** Color Doppler image of the main renal artery anastomosis (arrow).

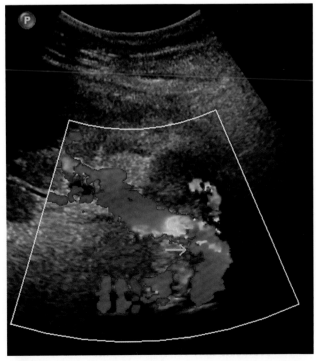

**FIGURE 28-9** Color Doppler image of the renal vein anastomosis (arrow).

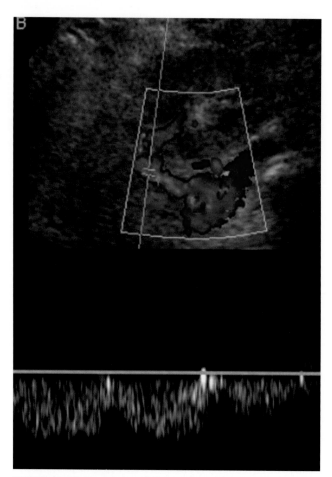

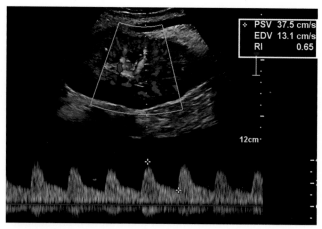

**FIGURE 28-12** Normal spectral Doppler tracing from an interlobar renal artery. Note sharp systolic upstroke and continuous forward diastolic flow. The amount of diastolic flow should equal approximately 25% of systolic flow with a RI < 0.70.

**FIGURE 28-10** Normal spectral Doppler tracing from the origin of the main renal vein. Note slight respiratory phasicity. Pulsatility of the venous tracing is caused by close proximity to the main renal artery.

Spectral Doppler signals from the segmental and interlobar arteries are obtained from the upper, mid, and lower poles, with angle-corrected peak systolic velocity measurements and calculation of the resistive index (RI). Some laboratories require sampling of the arcuate arteries as well. The normal arterial waveform has a low-resistance pattern characterized by continuous forward diastolic flow, an RI less than 0.7, and a sharp systolic upstroke with an acceleration time less than 70 to 80 ms (Fig. 28-12). The RI is a ratio that compares the amount of systolic and diastolic flow. The RI is angle independent so angle correction is not needed. The formula is as follows:

$$\text{(Peak systolic velocity} - \text{end-diastolic velocity)/peak systolic velocity}$$

In order to calculate the RI, it is critical to accurately measure end-diastolic velocity, which should be measured at the end of diastole right before the next systolic upstroke. It is important that the sonographer not mistake overlying venous flow, flow because of mirror artifact, or noise in the signal for true diastolic flow. By observing the amount of color in the interlobar arteries during diastole, the sonographer can subjectively estimate the RI. If the artery minimally diminishes, then there is good diastolic flow, and the RI will be <0.7. However, if there is hardly any signal left by the end of diastole, then the RI will likely be >0.8. If the color is flashy and pulsatile, and the artery completely disappears during end diastole, then there is no end-diastolic flow, and the RI will be 1.0. A normal RI is between 0.6 and 0.8. In general, end-diastolic velocity should equal at least 25% of peak systolic velocity.

## Technical Considerations

Typically, a curved linear array transducer is used with a frequency range of 3 to 5 MHz. If improvement in image quality is needed, harmonics and/or compound imaging may improve image quality and resolution as well as reduce artifacts. A proper color Doppler velocity scale should be chosen to allow for proper vessel fill-in. The scale may need to be adjusted as needed when changing from evaluating the arterial and venous signals. The color gain should be

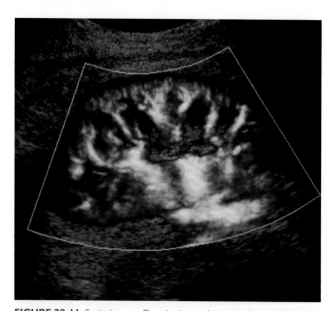

**FIGURE 28-11** Sagittal power Doppler image demonstrating normal cortical perfusion of the transplanted kidney. Note homogeneous perfusion of the renal cortex from the small interlobular arteries arising from the arcuate arteries coursing behind the renal pyramids parallel to the renal capsule.

increased until color speckles appear in the background of the image and then reduced until the color speckles are erased. The color box should be kept to a size that allows for a good frame rate.

The spectral Doppler baseline should be adjusted such that flow above as well as below the baseline can be assessed. Because the intraparenchymal renal arteries and veins are so small and close together, arterial and venous waveforms may both be displayed on the same image. The spectral Doppler scale should be adjusted such that the waveform fills the entire area available for the tracing. This will allow for better evaluation and measurement of the waveform. The Doppler spectral speed should be adjusted to allow visualization of three to five cardiac cycles. The Doppler gain should be increased until noise or speckle artifact appears in the background behind the Doppler waveform and then reduced until the speckles are gone.

## Pitfalls

A variety of Doppler settings may be required to demonstrate the presence of vascular pathology. For example, owing to the high velocity within an arteriovenous fistula (AVF) (see below), the color velocity scale will need to be greatly increased to reduce color aliasing and blooming so that only the area of the AVF is seen. Conversely, before thrombosis of a vessel is diagnosed, Doppler settings should be maximized for the detection of low-velocity blood flow.

# DIAGNOSIS

After the baseline US examination, subsequent renal transplant duplex Doppler US examinations are ordered to evaluate for potential causes of graft dysfunction. Patients with graft dysfunction most commonly present with nonspecific signs and symptoms such as renal failure, pain, or evidence of infection. The goal of the US examination is to differentiate between causes of graft failure that are best managed medically, such as ATN, pyelonephritis, drug toxicity, or rejection, from etiologies that require intervention such as hydronephrosis, symptomatic fluid collections, and vascular thrombosis or stenosis. Unfortunately, many of the grayscale US findings in such patients, such as increase in renal length, loss of or increase of corticomedullary differentiation, striation of the uroepithelium, and increased RI, are also nonspecific findings of graft dysfunction, and diagnosis may ultimately require US-guided renal biopsy. However, Doppler criteria are highly specific for most vascular complications following renal transplantation.

## Transplant Rejection

Rejection is one of the most common causes of graft loss and is the result of attack by the immune system on the transplanted organ just as the immune system would combat any foreign object or virus. There are three types of renal transplant rejection: hyperacute that occurs immediately postop because of the presence of preformed antibodies to the allograft; acute that usually begins approximately 2 weeks posttransplantation, with most cases occurring in the first 3 months; and chronic. Fortunately, adjusting the immunosuppression protocol can effectively treat most episodes of rejection.

Rejection is suspected when one or more of the following clinical signs are detected: sudden cessation of urine output called anuria, decreased urine output called oliguria, increase serum creatinine, protein or lymphocytes in the urine, hypertension, or swelling or tenderness of the graft. One of the earliest signs of rejection is oliguria, with an associated rise in serum creatinine and blood urea nitrogen (BUN). Serum creatinine and BUN determine how well the kidney is functioning because these waste products are normally removed from the blood by the kidneys. However, a rise in creatinine is a nonspecific finding and may indicate a variety of underlying renal pathologies. A biopsy should be performed in patients with a high level of creatinine that persists or continues to increase.

## Acute Tubular Necrosis

Another common cause of graft dysfunction is ATN. ATN is caused by ischemia and is more common in DD transplants than in LD. Risk factors for the development of ATN include prolonged ischemic time, hypotension or blood loss during surgery, prolonged intensive care unit time or severe illness of the donor, and harvest from a non–heart beating donor. ATN occurs in the early postoperative period, usually beginning day 2 or 3, and may be a cause for delayed function of the renal transplant. The patient may require dialysis until the kidney starts to function properly.[11,12] Some investigators have used diminished diastolic flow in the segmental arteries as an indicator of ATN. However, most clinicians use renal biopsy as the definitive diagnosis for ATN.[13,14] With recent relaxation of donor criteria and acceptance for transplantation of kidneys harvested from donors who are sicker and who have been ill for longer, ATN now often presents earlier and is more severe than previously.

## Fluid Collections

The most common perinephric fluid collections found postrenal transplantation are hematomas, urinomas, and lymphoceles. The size and location of the collection should be documented on each US examination.

Hematomas are found immediately postoperatively or after the biopsy. Their size, echotexture, and location will vary. Postoperative hematomas may be located anywhere surrounding the transplant. Hematomas that develop after the biopsy are typically found near the biopsy site, usually at the lower pole. Acutely, hematomas will be echogenic becoming more heterogeneous and complex with anechoic liquefied areas (Figs. 28-13 to 28-15). These collections should be followed to ensure that they are decreasing in size.

Urinomas form when urine leaks from either the ureteral anastomosis or a focal area of ureteral necrosis. These are usually discovered in the first few weeks posttransplant. Clinically, suspicion is raised when urine output decreases, especially in the absence of renal failure, or if there is leakage of urine from the surgical incision. US will demonstrate a fluid collection, usually located between the kidney and the bladder. Urinomas are typically anechoic unless superinfection has occurred, but some may contain septations (Fig. 28-16).

Lymphoceles occur when there is surgical disruption of the lymphatic chain. These collections usually appear 4

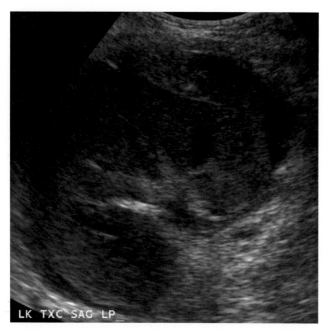

**FIGURE 28-13** Postoperative perinephric hematoma. Grayscale sagittal image demonstrating a heterogeneous hypoechoic fluid collection surrounding the kidney. The cortex of the lower pole appears compressed by this collection. The echogenicity of perinephric hematomas is variable, depending upon the time since hemorrhage occurred.

to 8 weeks postoperatively. Typically, these collections are discovered incidentally. However, lymphoceles can compress the ureter causing obstruction of the collecting system or become superinfected, both of which require percutaneous drainage or surgical marsupialization. On US, lymphoceles

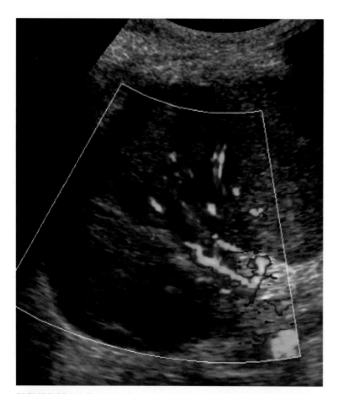

**FIGURE 28-14** Postoperative perinephric hematoma (same patient as in Fig. 28-13). Color Doppler image demonstrating decreased cortical perfusion because of pressure from the surrounding fluid hematoma.

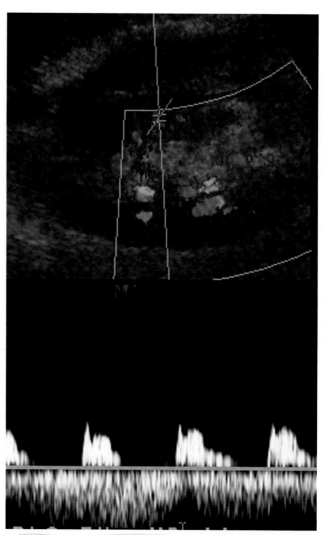

**FIGURE 28-15** Postoperative perinephric hematoma (same patient as in Figs. 28-13 and 12-14). Duplex Doppler image with a waveform obtained from an interlobular artery demonstrating no diastolic flow (RI = 1.0) because of increased peripheral vascular resistance from compression of the renal cortex by the surrounding hematoma, the so-called "Page Kidney" physiology. Note venous flow below the baseline.

are well-defined, anechoic fluid collections which may demonstrate multiple thin septations (Fig. 28-17). It is important not to confuse a urinoma with a lymphocele. Remember that urinomas will occur within the first few weeks posttransplant, whereas lymphoceles will be seen in a later time frame, after the first month.

## Hydronephrosis

Mild pelvocaliectasis (hydronephrosis) is a normal finding postrenal transplantation because the denervated kidney loses its autonomic tone, allowing the intrarenal collecting system to dilate. Patients are typically asymptomatic. However, true hydronephrosis may develop secondary to ureteral stricture from postsurgical scarring, ischemia or rejection, a blood clot in the ureter, bladder distension, decreased ureteric tone, or compression from surrounding lymphoceles or other fluid collections and posttransplant lymphoproliferative disorder. The sonographer should attempt to discover the cause and the level of the obstruction.

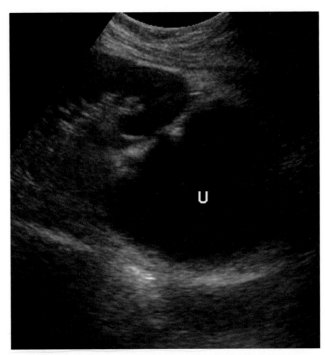

**FIGURE 28-16** Urinoma. Grayscale image demonstrating an anechoic large fluid collection (U) at the lower pole of the kidney between the transplanted kidney and the bladder (not visualized on this image).

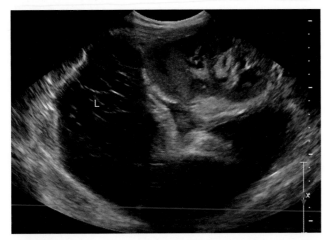

**FIGURE 28-17** Lymphocele. Grayscale longitudinal image demonstrating an anechoic fluid collection (L) with several fine septations extending superior and posterior to the kidney.

## Vascular Complications

Vascular complications may occur immediately postoperatively or have a delayed presentation. In the immediate postoperative period, venous or arterial thrombosis is suspected when there is sudden anuria or acute inset of pain in the region of the transplant. This is an emergent situation, and the diagnosis must be made quickly to allow appropriate percutaneous or surgical intervention to salvage the kidney.

### Arterial Thrombosis

Predisposing risk factors for renal artery thrombosis (RAT) include hypercoagulable states, hypotension, intraoperative trauma, mismatch of vessel size, and vascular kinking. Severe acute rejection and rarely emboli may result in occlusion or

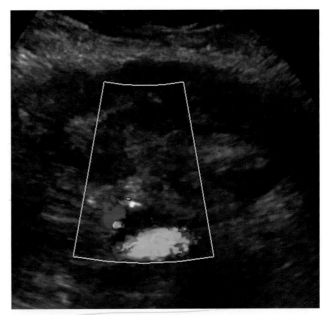

**FIGURE 28-18** Renal artery thrombosis. Color Doppler image of a newly transplanted kidney demonstrating complete absence of both venous and arterial flow in the kidney.

thrombosis of the intraparenchymal renal arteries. Intrarenal arterial thrombus may propagate to involve the main renal artery. RAT is estimated to occur in less than 1% of patients. RAT is more common in pediatric transplant, likely secondary to the small size of the recipient vessels. Sonographic findings of RAT include intraluminal echoes and absence of arterial and venous flow on color, power, or spectral Doppler interrogation of the intrarenal or main renal arteries and veins (Figs. 28-18 and 28-19). The sonographer should ensure that

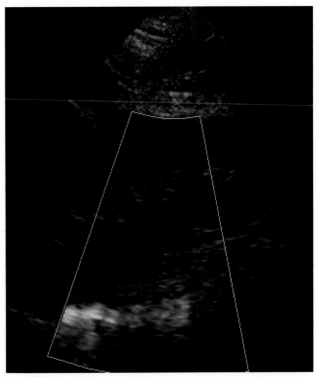

**FIGURE 28-19** Another patient with renal artery thrombosis using power Doppler to confirm the lack of flow. An arterial thrombosis from a hyperacute rejection was diagnosed at surgery.

all color Doppler controls, such as color velocity scale, color gain, color wall filter, and output power, are optimized for the detection of slow flow before making the diagnosis of RAT.

## Venous Thrombosis

Renal vein thrombosis (RVT) is also a rare event, occurring in less than 4% of renal transplants. RVT most commonly occurs within the first 24 to 48 hours postop. Patients with RVT may complain of pain or discomfort over the transplant caused by kidney swelling. Causes of RVT include surgical complications, compression by lymphocele or other pelvic fluid collection, propagation of an iliac vein thrombus, hypotension, hypercoagulable states, or torqueing of the vascular pedicle. Sonographic findings include enlargement of the kidney, decreased renal cortical echogenicity, an enlarged main renal vein that may or may not contain low-level echoes, and absence of flow on color, power, or spectral Doppler interrogation of the main renal vein. A very helpful finding confirming this diagnosis is the presence of reversed diastolic flow in the renal arteries, resulting in a biphasic waveform (Fig. 28-20). However, reversed diastolic flow in the main renal artery is not a specific finding of RVT and may be seen in other clinical scenarios (see Table 28-1). However, in these other clinical situations, flow in the main renal vein will be observed.

## Renal Artery Stenosis

RAS is the most common vascular complication following renal transplantation, occurring in approximately 10% of patients. Patients typically present within 6 to 12 months following transplantation with severe uncontrolled hypertension. Causes of RAS include postsurgical scarring or dissection, intimal hyperplasia, progressive atherosclerosis, or rejection. Vessel diameter mismatch or complex arterial reconstructions are predisposing risk factors. RAS occurs more commonly in LD and pediatric renal transplantation than following DD renal transplantation. RAS may also occur secondary to twisting

| TABLE 28-1 | Causes for Reversed Diastolic Arterial Flow in Renal Transplants |
|---|---|

Renal vein thrombosis
Severe acute tubular necrosis (ATN)
Hyperacute rejection
Page kidney (compression by surrounding fluid collection)

or kinking of the main renal artery. Excessive length of the renovascular pedicle predisposes to vascular torsion.

To diagnose RAS on US examination, the entire length of the main renal artery and the anastomotic site must be carefully evaluated. Color Doppler should be optimized for assessing relatively high arterial velocities. The sonographer should use color Doppler to look for areas of aliasing with possible narrowing along the course of the main renal artery as well as looking for sharp bends or kinking of the artery. Any area of narrowing or aliasing should be sampled with spectral Doppler with an angle <60 degrees and a sample volume just large enough to encompass the width of the renal artery. Doppler criteria for the diagnosis of RAS greater than 50% to 60% in a renal transplant include elevated peak systolic velocities > 250 cm/s, renal artery to EIA ratio > 2.0 to 3.0 as well as poststenotic turbulence. In some patients, the distal arterial signal from the intraparenchymal renal arteries may have a tardus-parvus waveform pattern (Figs. 28-21 to 28-24). Several recent studies suggest that PSVs > 300 cm/s in the immediate postoperative state may be within normal limits and the presence of a tardus parvus waveform substantially increases the specificity of an increase in PSV for RAS.

## PostBiopsy Vascular Complications

Patients who have had a renal biopsy may develop either an AVF or a pseudoaneurysm (PSA). An AVF is an abnormal connection between an artery and a vein. This causes the

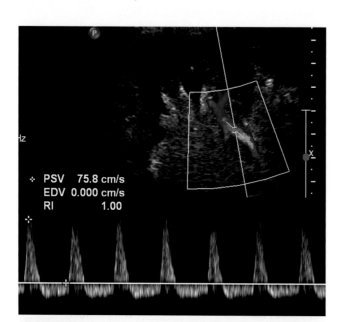

**FIGURE 28-20** Renal vein thrombosis. Spectral Doppler waveform from a segmental renal artery in the renal sinus ademonstrating reversed diastolic flow in this patient who presented with abrupt anuria 3 hours postsurgery. Thrombosis of the main renal vein was found at surgery.

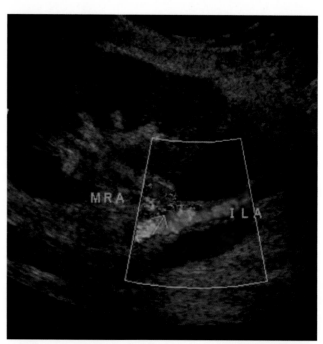

**FIGURE 28-21** Renal artery stenosis. Color Doppler image of the renal artery anastomosis demonstrating focal color aliasing and a soft tissue color bruit (*arrow*). ILA, internal iliac artery.

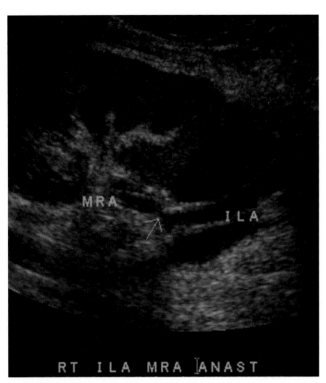

**FIGURE 28-22** Renal artery stenosis (same patient as in Fig. 28-21). Grayscale image demonstrating narrowing (arrow) of the main renal artery (MRA) above the anastomosis which was caused by kinking of the vessel. Excessive length of the donor MRA predisposes to kinking of the vascular pedicle.

arterial blood to empty directly into the vein, thus bypassing the capillary bed and creating a low-resistance gradient. Color Doppler will detect the presence of an AVF by demonstrating an area of color aliasing as well as a soft tissue color bruit (Fig. 28-25). A color bruit is caused by vibration of the surrounding soft tissue that reflects back toward the transducer with a low-velocity signal. The Doppler signal of the artery feeding the AVF will have high velocity in both peak systole and end diastole, whereas the draining vein will demonstrate a pulsatile relatively high-velocity waveform that may even resemble an arterial signal close to the AVF (Fig. 28-26).

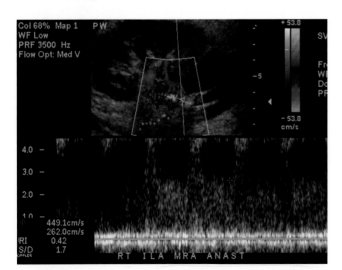

**FIGURE 28-23** Renal artery stenosis (same patient as in Figs. 28-21 and 28-22). Pulsed Doppler tracing obtained at the area of narrowing demonstrating increased PSV > 440 m/s.

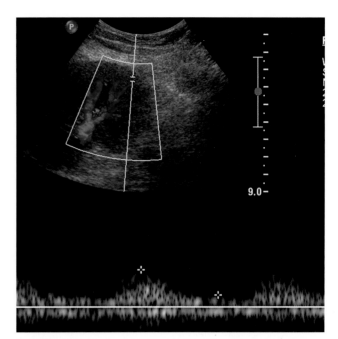

**FIGURE 28-24** A patient with severe kinking of the main renal artery demonstrating the downstream effect causing a marked tardus parvus waveform pattern.

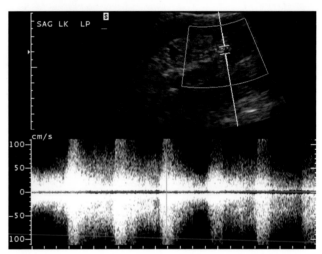

**FIGURE 28-25** Arteriovenous fistula (AVF). Duplex Doppler image from a patient status post renal biopsy demonstrating a soft tissue color bruit, increased systolic and diastolic flow as well as turbulence from an AVF at the lower pole of the transplanted kidney.

A PSA will be visualized on grayscale imaging as an anechoic rounded area within the renal parenchyma, which will fill-in with color in swirling pattern, termed the "yin-yang" sign (Figs. 28-27 to 28-29). A Doppler tracing obtained from the neck of the PSA where it joins the native artery will display a typical "to-and-fro" Doppler pattern, with flow heading toward the PSA during systole and away from the PSA during diastole. If the neck is wide, more random, bizarre waveform patterns may be observed.

Most AVFs or PSAs are incidental benign findings and can be safely followed by sonography until they resolve. If they affect renal function, are larger than 2 cm, expanding or extrarenal in location, the patient is referred to Interventional Radiology to have the AVF or PSA treated with either embolization or stent exclusion.

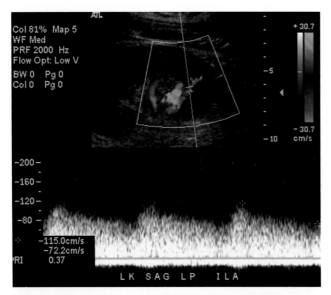

**FIGURE 28-26**  Arteriovenous fistula (AVF). Duplex Doppler image from another patient status post renal biopsy demonstrating an enlarged feeding artery in the renal sinus, color aliasing in an interlobar artery at the lower pole, and increased systolic and diastolic flow, resulting in an abnormally low RI = 0.37.

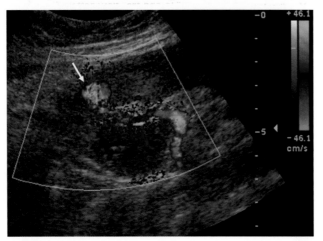

**FIGURE 28-27**  Pseudoaneurysm (PSA). Color Doppler image from a patient status post renal biopsy demonstrating a soft tissue color bruit and large round area of color flow in a "yin-yang" pattern compatible with a PSA (*arrow*) in the cortex of the upper pole of the transplanted kidney. Note significantly decreased flow in the surrounding renal cortex.

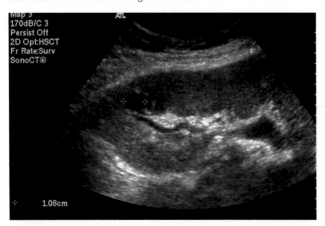

**FIGURE 28-28**  Pseudoaneurysm (PSA) (same patient as in Fig. 28-27). Grayscale image demonstrating and anechoic cystic area (calipers) in the upper pole cortex corresponding to the area that fills in with color in Figure 28-27 proving that this is a PSA and not a renal cyst.

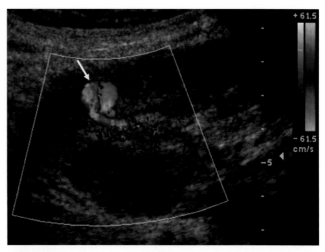

**FIGURE 28-29**  Pseudoaneurysm (PSA) (same patient as in Figs. 28-27 and 28-28). Color Doppler image of the PSA (*arrow*) with the color velocity scale increased demonstrating the "yin-yang" color-flow pattern typical of a PSA. This patient was taken to Interventional Radiology to have the PSA coiled because it was shunting blood away from the rest of the kidney.

Pathology Box 28-1 summarizes the vascular complications in renal transplant patients. The pathology along with the US appearance is described.

## LIVER TRANSPLANTATION

The first successful liver transplant was performed by Dr. Thomas Starzl in 1967. Since then, the liver has become the second most common organ to be transplanted after the kidney. Approximately 151,895 liver transplants have been performed in the United States since 1988. DD transplants account for the vast majority (145,693 patients), whereas 6,202 liver transplants from LD have been performed.[8] In 2016, 7,496 DD and 345 LD liver transplants were performed. As of June 2017, there were 14,309 patients on the liver transplant waiting list in the United States.[8]

For patients with either acute or chronic end-stage liver failure who are unresponsive to medical therapy, liver transplantation is the only available option. For such patients, organ availability is the rate-limiting factor. US is the initial imaging modality of choice for the evaluation of complications following liver transplantation. US is portable, readily available, without risk or contraindications and is a very sensitive test for the detection of vascular complications, postop fluid collections, and biliary complications. However, US is also extremely user dependent and requires an in-depth knowledge of the principles of vascular technology, abdominal anatomy, and general liver transplant physiology. Liver transplant US is performed bed side in the immediate peri/postoperative phases for routine surveillance or when there are clinical indications of suspected graft failure or vascular complications.

There are several conditions which can lead to liver failure and subsequently liver transplantation. Table 28-2 lists the most common indications for liver transplantation.

Patients with life-threatening liver disease are only placed on the transplant waiting list if they meet the established MELD criteria or have a high Child-Pugh score. MELD is the acronym of the Model for End-Stage Liver Disease, and the Child-Pugh score is used routinely by gastroenterologists to assess liver disease. These criteria are used to rank patients

**PATHOLOGY BOX 28-1**
*Vascular Complications in Renal Transplant Recipients*

| Pathology | Sonographic Appearance | | |
|---|---|---|---|
| | **Grayscale** | **Color Doppler** | **Spectral Doppler** |
| Renal artery thrombosis (RAT) | Intraluminal echoes Hypoechoic, swollen kidney Loss of corticomedullary differentiation | Absence of color flow | Absence of spectral Doppler signal in main renal artery and vein as well as in the intraparenchymal renal arteries and veins |
| Renal stenosis (RS) | Narrowing of vessel Poststenotic dilatation | Narrowing of vessel Focal color aliasing | ↑ PSV > 250 cm/s PSV ratio >2.0–3.0 Tardus-parvus waveform in intraparenchymal renal arteries AT > 70–80 ms |
| Renal vein thrombosis (RVT) | Intraluminal echoes Hypoechoic, swollen kidney Loss of corticomedullary differentiation | Absence of color flow Color void if thrombus is nonocclusive | No spectral Doppler signal in main or intraparechymal renal veins Reversed diastolic flow in renal arteries |
| Renal vein stenosis (PVS) | Focal Narrowing Poststenotic dilatation | Narrowing Focal color aliasing | ↑ velocity at site of stenosis Clinical significance likely if 3-4x increase in velocity in comparison to proximal renal vein or EIV |
| Pseudoaneurysm (PSA) | New anechoic round area in hepatic parenchyma Outpouching from main artery | "Yin-Yang" color pattern ± intraluminal thrombus Color aliasing in neck Color bruit | "To-and-fro" flow pattern in neck of PSA—if narrow A more disorganized flow pattern will be seen in wider necks |
| Arteriovenous fistula (AVF) | Tangle of tubular anechoic channels Draining vein may focally dilate and mimic PSA Normal | Spectrum of findings from tangle of vessels to rounder area of color flowand dilated feeding artery Soft tissue color bruit Focal color aliasing | ↑ PSV and ↑ end-diastolic velocity (EDV) in feeding artery Pulsatile, high-velocity flow in draining vein |

on the waiting list for liver transplants based on the severity of illness and eligibility of a patient. The criteria evaluate critical markers such as; serum bilirubin, which indicates how well the liver excretes bile; INR clotting time, which assesses adequacy of liver function; creatinine, which assesses kidney function; and mental function. There are a few pathologies for which the MELD criteria do not apply, including hepatocellular carcinoma, hepatopulmonary syndrome, familial amyloidosis, and primary oxaluria. In the event that a patient's medical urgency does not fall under the MELD score, one can apply for a MELD exception.[1]

There are criteria used to exclude patients from liver transplantation. Table 28-3 lists several of the contraindications for liver transplantation.

## The Operation

Most commonly, the liver transplant recipient receives a whole liver from a DD. This is referred to as an orthotopic liver transplant (OLT), which means that an organ is transplanted into its normal anatomic position in the recipient. Owing to organ shortage, partial liver transplants from an LD are now increasingly performed. Usually, the right lobe is transplanted. Occasionally, a liver from a DD is divided

**TABLE 28-2  Most Common Indications for Liver Transplantation**

Hepatitis C
Alcoholic liver disease
Cryptogenic cirrhosis
Primary biliary cirrhosis
Primary biliary sclerosing cholangitis
Budd–Chiari's syndrome
Hemochromatosis
Wilson's disease
Autoimmune hepatitis
Acute or fulminant liver failure
Hepatocellular carcinoma (early stage)

**TABLE 28-3  Contraindications or Exclusion Criteria for Liver Transplantation**

Extrahepatic malignancy
Untreated infection
Anatomic abnormality
Hepatocellular carcinoma that has metastasized or is larger than 5 cm
Advanced cardiopulmonary disease
Active substance abuse
End-stage Hepatitis B
Advanced age
Cholangiocarcinoma

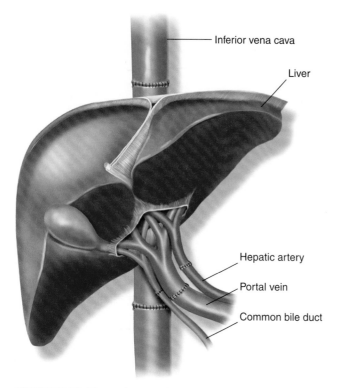

**FIGURE 28-30** Diagram demonstrating the most common surgical anatomy following orthotopic liver transplantation with an interposition IVC graft.

between two recipients, one receiving the right lobe and the other the left lobe. Children, in particular, often undergo partial or split liver transplantation.

The precise vascular and biliary anastomoses created depend upon the type of transplant as well as the donor and recipient anatomy (Fig. 28-30). Congenital anomalies of the hepatic vasculature and biliary tree are relatively common. Hence, there is wide variation in postsurgical anatomy. Most vessels and the common bile duct (CBD) in an OLT are anastomosed in an end-to-end fashion. During the OLT, once it is decided that the liver is suitable for donation, the organ procurement team will harvest the whole liver from a DD, including the extrahepatic vessels and CBD. The liver is transported to the recipient on ice in a preservative solution. The implantation team then removes the recipient's native liver and gallbladder, called the anhepatic phase. The donor's CBD is preferentially anastomosed to the recipient's common hepatic duct in an end-to-end fashion. If the recipient's common hepatic duct is deformed or diseased, a choledochojejunostomy will be created, whereby the biliary system will drain directly into the jejunum. The choledochojejunostomy is usually made by the Roux-en-Y, end-to-side, surgical method.

The arterial anastomosis is usually made between the donor's common hepatic artery or celiac artery and the recipient's common hepatic artery where it branches into the right and left hepatic arteries or the common hepatic artery at the level of the gastroduodenal artery. The hepatic arterial anastomosis is created with a "fish mouth" technique, whereby the smaller vessel's walls are split and sewn over the larger, usually the donor, vessel. This technique helps prevent the development of postsurgical stenosis at

the hepatic artery anastomosis. If the donor or recipient vessels are diseased, the surgeon may use the donor's iliac vessels to patch or bypass part of a stenotic vessel. When evaluating the vessels, one should remember that there are several anatomic variations of the hepatic arterial system, and the course that the artery takes may not necessarily be the expected one. Complete evaluation of the hepatic artery may require a great deal of scanning and numerous acoustic windows.

The portal vein is typically anastomosed in an end-to-end fashion between the donor and recipient main portal vein. If the donor's portal vein is scarred or thrombosed, a venous "jump" graft will have to be created to bypass the thrombus. The IVC may be "interposed" following resection of the donor IVC requiring both a supra and an infra hepatic end-to-end IVC anastomosis. However, in many centers, a "piggyback" technique is now preferred that leaves the recipient's IVC in place attaching the suprahepatic donor IVC to the recipient's hepatic venous confluence (Figs. 28-31 and 28-32).

Single-lobe LD transplants have become more common in recent years. The donor usually heals easily because the liver is one of the few organs that can regenerate quickly. The adult donor provides the right portion of his or her liver to an adult recipient or the left portion to a child. The donated right liver will have a right hepatic vein, a right portal vein, a right hepatic artery, and the right hepatic bile duct. This is obviously reversed if the left lobe is donated (Figs. 28-33 and 28-34). The middle hepatic vein may travel with the donated liver or remain with the donor depending upon the surgical plane and whether or not the medial segment of the left lobe is also harvested. The pediatric patient will often have a choledochojejunostomy and no gallbladder.

Because patients undergoing liver transplantation are extremely ill and because the surgery is complicated,

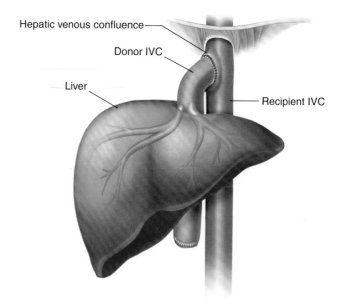

**FIGURE 28-31** Diagram demonstrating the piggyback technique for performing the IVC anastomosis. (Reprinted with permission from Pellerito JS, Polak JF, eds. *Introduction to Vascular Ultrasonography.* 6th ed. Philadelphia, PA: Elsevier Saunders; 2012.)

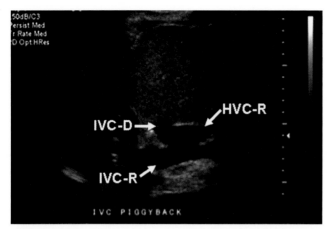

**FIGURE 28-32** Grayscale ultrasound of a piggyback IVC anastomosis. HVC-R, recipient hepatic vein confluence IVC-D, donor IVC; IVC-R, recipient IVC.

perioperative morbidity is relatively high. OPTN reports a 1-year graft survival rate of 86% for DD liver transplants and 90% for LD transplants. The 5-year graft survival rate is 72% and 78% for DD and LD transplants, respectively.[8]

## SONOGRAPHIC EXAMINATION TECHNIQUES

Proper patient positioning and optimizing the controls are essential for proper evaluation of the patient with a liver transplant. It is important for the sonographer to review operative notes so that they know what type of transplant the patient received and to understand all the various anastomotic sites as previously described. It can be very helpful for the US staff to have a drawing of the liver and the various connections, especially with single-lobe transplants or unusual hook-ups. This drawing can be scanned into the

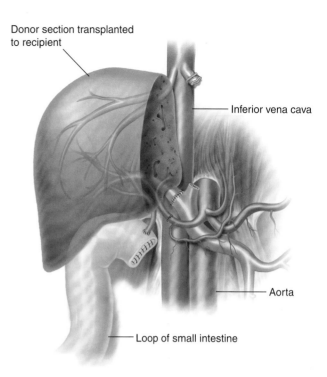

**FIGURE 28-34** Diagram demonstrating the surgical placement of a partial liver transplant in the recipient.

electronic records of the patient for future reference. Any prior studies should also be reviewed.

### Patient Preparation

An overnight fast may help minimize intestinal gas. A fasting state may also be needed to evaluate the size of the bile ducts.

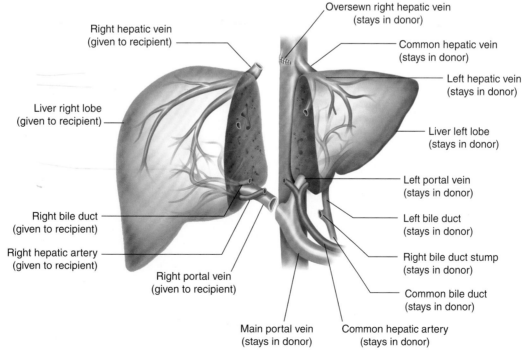

**FIGURE 28-33** Diagram demonstrating the surgical technique for dividing the liver for a partial or split liver transplantation.

## Patient Positioning

The patient is usually positioned supine. The transplanted liver may also be examined in the left lateral decubitus position.

## Equipment

A curved linear array transducer with lower frequencies such as a 5-1 MHz can be used to adequately insonate the transplanted liver. A transducer with a small footprint is also helpful. If intercostal scanning is needed, the sonographer may consider using a phased array transducer because this will allow better access between the ribs. Harmonic imaging may be used to help improve resolution and reduce artifacts. Varying imaging and Doppler frequencies can be helpful depending on the depth and position of the transplant's vessels.

## Scanning Technique

Before performing the study, the sonographer must consult the surgeon or surgical report to determine whether a full liver was transplanted or just a single lobe. In addition, any vascular anomalies should be determined, such as a piggyback IVC or unusual anastomosis of the hepatic artery or portal vein. The most common causes of transplant loss are graft failure/rejection followed by biliary complications. Some complications are related to surgical technique or the amount of time the liver was handled before transplant. Vascular complications are reportedly the third most common cause of transplant failure. After the initial postoperative baseline scan, physicians can use liver function tests to determine whether there are any abnormalities or signs of failure. Serial US examinations may be performed to ensure that there are no early signs of failure that are being overlooked. There are some complications related to rejection that often may not surface for years. Patients may present with abnormal liver function tests, ascites, pleural effusions, varices, sepsis, fever, biliary obstruction, leakage, infection, or splenomegaly. Because symptoms are so varied and nonspecific, imaging plays a critical role in the evaluation of the symptomatic liver transplant patient, especially in the immediate postoperative period. Biliary tract pathology, however, is often associated with hepatic artery stenosis (HAS) or occlusion, because the hepatic artery is the sole supply of blood flow to the biliary tree in the transplanted liver.[15,16]

### Grayscale

Standard scanning techniques are used to assess the transplanted liver. All portions of the transplant should be examined. The normal transplant is usually homogeneous in appearance and appropriately sized depending on the type of transplant. There should be a normal-appearing biliary tree that is free of dilatation, but the duct walls can appear thickened if biliary stents are in place. Remember that the CBD may not be in the usual place and may be difficult to visualize unless dilated. There is now constant drainage because the sphincter of Oddi no longer controls the flow of bile in the CBD into the duodenum. It is often possible to see surgical drains or stents that have been surgically placed to drain fluids from the peritoneal cavity. A small amount of perihepatic fluid is normal in the early postoperative period.

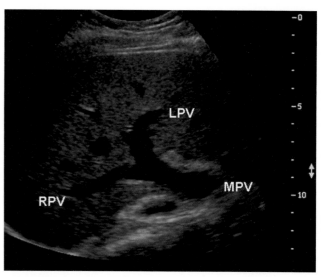

**FIGURE 28-35** Grayscale image of a normal orthotopic (deceased donor, complete) liver transplant. LPV, left portal vein; RPV, right portal vein; MPV, main portal vein.

A right-sided pleural effusion may also be present. These fluid collections should resolve within days (Fig. 28-35).

### Color and Spectral Doppler

Doppler examination of the transplant patient may be requested immediately postop depending on how challenging the surgery was. The basic liver transplant duplex US consists of grayscale images and angle-corrected velocity measurements of the intrahepatic main, right, and left hepatic arteries (Fig. 28-36). The main, right, and left portal veins with the anastomotic site are interrogated with color and spectral Doppler as well as waveforms of the IVC, and all three branches of the hepatic veins are recorded (Figs. 28-37 and 28-38). If vascular complications are detected intrahepatically, the recipient's native vessels may additionally be assessed with color and spectral Doppler to determine the level of dysfunction. The peak velocity should be measured in the portal veins, and the peak systolic velocity, as well as the RI should be measured in the hepatic arteries.

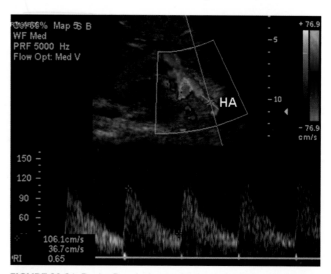

**FIGURE 28-36** Duplex Doppler image of the normal main hepatic artery (HA). Note sharp systolic upstroke and continuous forward diastolic flow with the RI = 0.65.

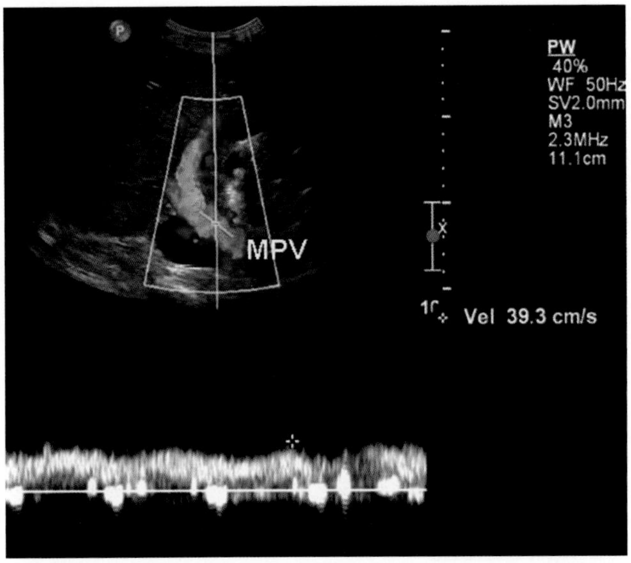

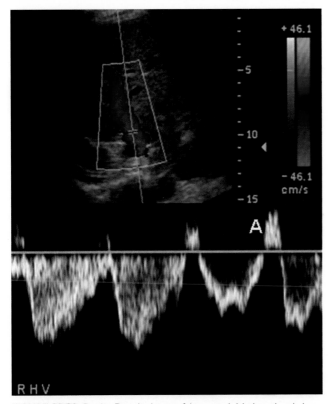

**FIGURE 28-37** Duplex Doppler image of the normal main portal vein (MPV). Note hepatopetal flow with slight respiratory variation.

**FIGURE 28-38** Duplex Doppler image of the normal right hepatic vein in a patient with a right lobe transplant. Flow is hepatofugal, heading away from the liver capsule. The pulsatility of the waveform reflects right heart pressure. The transient reversal of flow, labeled the "A" wave, is produced by the contraction of the right atrium.

## Technical Considerations

Owing to the limitations described earlier, perhaps, all of the Doppler measurements and images will have to be taken from the intercostal approach. This is actually an ideal method for evaluating the portal system, because the natural angle of the portal vein courses toward the transducer from this window, and will greatly enhance the Doppler shift and color fill-in.

## Pitfalls

One pitfall is the presence of a high-resistance signal in the hepatic arteries in the immediate postoperative period. This is thought to be caused by the liver being swollen causing an increase in the interstitial intrahepatic pressure as well as because of increased peripheral vascular resistance. In these patients, the RI may need to be calculated multiple times a day, depending on the patient's condition. This is done to look for an increase or a decrease in the amount of diastolic flow with the hope of catching the artery before it thromboses. Once the diastolic flow starts to increase, follow-up USs can be performed less frequently until the RI reaches a normal value (Figs. 28-39 to 28-41).

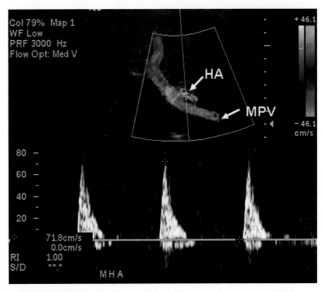

**FIGURE 28-39** Duplex Doppler image of the main hepatic artery (HA) immediately posttransplantation demonstrating complete absence of diastolic flow and with a RI = 1.0. This high-resistance waveform pattern is likely secondary to increased peripheral vascular resistance secondary to edema of the hepatic parenchyma. Within 48 hours posttransplantation, such a waveform pattern is not indicative of impending HA thrombosis

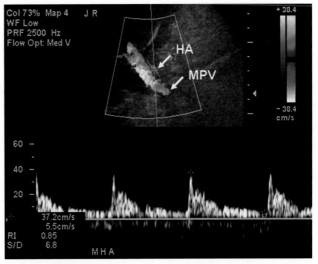

**FIGURE 28-40** Spectral Doppler tracing of the main hepatic artery (HA) 2 days later from the same patient as in Figure 28-39 demonstrating an increase in the amount of diastolic flow. The RI has dropped to 0.85.

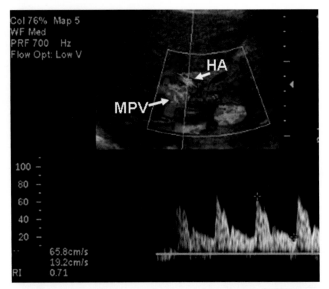

**FIGURE 28-41** Spectral Doppler tracing of the main hepatic artery (HA) from the same patient as in Figures 28-39 and 28-40 now 4 days postop demonstrating a normal waveform pattern with normal diastolic flow. The RI is now 0.71.

The postoperative abdominal scan may be very challenging because it will likely be a portable examination, and the scanning environment suboptimal. In addition, the patient will likely be using an automated breathing apparatus, have multiple lines, and a completely bandaged abdomen. Often, vacuum-assisted closure devices with foam centers are used for very large body cavity openings. An intercostal scanning technique may be the only method for sonographically evaluating the transplant. Occasionally, there will be residual air in the peritoneal cavity from the surgery adding to the difficult nature of seeing the abdominal structures from a midline approach.

## DIAGNOSIS

Vascular complications are easily detected by the presence, direction, and quantitative measurement of the blood flow to and from the allograft. Table 28-4 lists normal findings for the liver transplant. US examination has an important role in evaluating the patient with suspected graft dysfunction. Although there is no role for US in the diagnosis of rejection following liver transplantation, US is the procedure of choice for the initial evaluation of potential fluid collections, abnormalities of the biliary tree, and vascular complications.

## Nonvascular Postoperative Complications

There are several nonvascular posttransplant complications that can occur. Table 28-5 lists the most common complications. There are several postoperative complications that are nonvascular in nature that must be documented. One type is a biloma, which is leakage of bile from the biliary anastomotic site (Fig. 28-42). The standard grayscale US evaluation includes sagittal and transverse images with appropriate measurements of the pancreas, right kidney, biliary tree, and liver parenchyma. Any pathology such as free abdominal fluid, periadrenal collections, and hematomas are also documented. Indirect sonographic signs of vascular complications may be seen in the liver parenchyma. These are frequently infarcts caused by vascular insufficiency.

## Common Postoperative Vascular Complications

Table 28-6 lists the common vascular complications following liver transplantation. Using duplex US techniques, one may see color-filling defects when thrombus is present, color aliasing and spectral broadening with stenosis, or a complete

| TABLE 28-5   Common Nonvascular Postoperative Liver Transplantation Complications |
| --- |
| Bile duct obstruction |
| Anastomotic bile duct obstruction |
| Anastomotic stenosis/stricture |
| Stone formation |
| Bile leak/biloma |
| Biliary necrosis |
| Cholangitis |
| Postoperative bleeding |
| Hematoma |
| Abscess |
| Infection |
| Recurrent hepatitis |
| Splenic infarct |
| Recurrent malignancy |
| Lymphoproliferative disorder |

| TABLE 28-4   Normal Doppler Findings After Liver Transplantation[15,16] | | |
| --- | --- | --- |
| **Vessel** | **Direction/Color** | **Normal Doppler Values** |
| Main portal vein | Hepatopetal/above baseline/red | >125 cm/s = stenosis, respiratory variations |
| Right portal vein | Hepatofugal/below baseline/blue | Forward, continuous flow |
| Left portal vein | Hepatopetal/above baseline/red | Forward continuous flow |
| Main hepatic Artery | Hepatopetal/above baseline/red | RI > 0.50 and <0.80, AT < 80 ms, Velocity < 200 cm/s |
| Right hepatic Artery | Hepatofugal/below baseline/blue | Same |
| Left hepatic Artery | Hepatopetal/above baseline/red | Same |
| Inferior vena cava | Can be bidirectional/pulsatile | Velocity not measured |
| Hepatic veins | Hepatofugal/below baseline/blue | Velocity not measured |
| | (can also be slightly pulsatile because of proximity of heart) | |

AT, acceleration time.

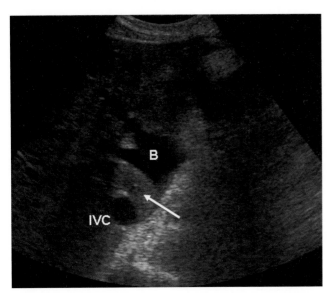

**FIGURE 28-42** Biloma (B). Note anechoic fluid collection anterior to the IVC and caudate lobe (*arrow*). Percutaneous aspiration proved this to be a biloma. This result should prompt immediate evaluation of the integrity of the biliary tree as well as evaluation of the hepatic artery to rule out thrombosis or stenosis.

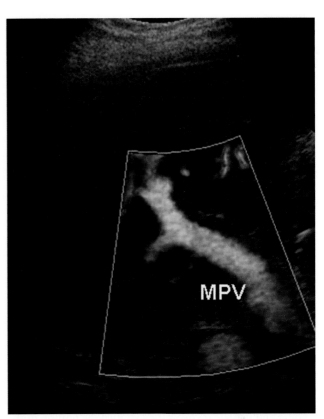

**FIGURE 28-43** Hepatic artery thrombosis. Power Doppler image at the porta hepatis demonstrating normal flow in the main portal vein (MPV). However, the hepatic artery is not visualized. Power Doppler should always be used to confirm absence of flow in a vessel because it is more sensitive to slow flow than color Doppler and is less angle dependent.

or partial absence of flow with thrombi. The presence of vascular findings on US may precipitate further imaging studies such as angiography, computerized tomography, and subsequent interventional procedures. Hepatic artery complications are cause for immediate surgical intervention because the hepatic artery is the sole blood supply to the bile ducts after transplantation, and lack of flow will lead to biliary necrosis and loss of the transplant.

### Hepatic Artery Thrombosis

Hepatic artery thrombosis (HAT) is the most common vascular complication of the OLT. It occurs in 2% to 12% of liver transplants.[15] The risk factors for developing HAT include rejection, prolonged transport time of organ, and end-to-end surgical technique for the hepatic artery anastomosis. Usually, the US examination will reveal absent or weak hepatic arterial flow. Postsurgical, a completely patent artery may be difficult to visualize because of vasospasm or parenchymal swelling (Figs. 28-43 and 28-44). Because of the impact on patient care, HAT usually requires imaging with other modalities.

### Hepatic Artery Stenosis

HAS occurs in up to 11% of the OLT patients.[16] The clinical symptoms are poor liver function tests or biliary ischemia. HAS is usually seen at the anastomotic site, and it is caused by surgical technique, clamp injuries, perfusion catheter

| TABLE 28-6 **Common Vascular Postoperative Liver Transplantation Complications** |
|---|
| Hepatic artery thrombosis |
| Hepatic artery stenosis |
| Pseudoaneurysm |
| Portal vein thrombosis |
| Portal vein stenosis |
| Inferior vena cava thrombosis |
| Inferior vena cava stenosis |
| Hepatic vein thrombosis |
| Hepatic vein stenosis |
| Biliary ischemia caused by hepatic artery stenosis |

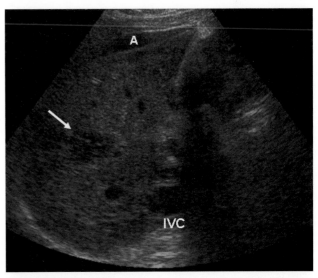

**FIGURE 28-44** Hepatic artery thrombosis (same patient as in Fig. 28-43). Grayscale image of the liver demonstrating a peripheral wedge shaped hypoechoic area (*arrow*) compatible with infarct as a result of hepatic artery thrombosis. Note peri-hepatic ascites (A).

injuries to the intimal lining, and interruption of the vasa vasorum. Areas of narrowing will display higher velocities and disturbed color flow. Lower RIs may be present as well as tardus-parvus waveforms in the intraparenchymal hepatic arteries, reflecting a prolonged acceleration time. If an interparenchymal tardus-parvus waveform is seen, it is likely because of HAS versus HAT (Figs. 28-45 to 28-48).

## Hepatic Artery Pseudoaneurysm

The PSA is an abnormal dilatation or ballooning of the hepatic artery that is either within the liver or extrahepatic. PSAs can also be caused by complete rupture or extravasation of blood surrounded by compressed normal tissues. Extrahepatic PSAs are caused by disruption of the intimal lining of the artery causing weakening and dilatation of the arterial wall that can easily rupture. Intrahepatic PSAs are generally thought to be caused by core needle biopsy or infections that can damage the integrity of the vessel wall. Extrahepatic PSAs are a rare finding and are more commonly seen at anastomotic sites. The patient usually presents with fever, biliary colic, or signs of hemorrhage. The Doppler waveform is often disorganized. There is a high risk of hemorrhage and resulting organ failure, so an interventional procedure must be performed to correct the PSA.

## Portal Vein Thrombosis

Portal vein thrombosis (PVT) is also another relatively rare finding and usually involves the extrahepatic portion of the

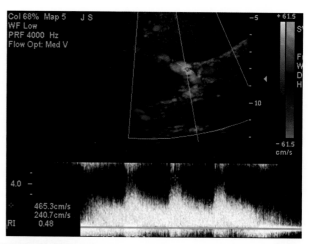

**FIGURE 28-46** Hepatic artery stenosis (same patient as in Fig. 28-45). Spectral Doppler tracing demonstrating increased PSV = 465 cm/s and turbulent flow. Notice the use of the color aliasing to guide placement of the Doppler cursor.

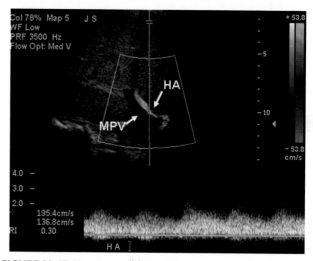

**FIGURE 28-47** Hepatic artery (HA) stenosis (same patient as in Figs. 28-45 and 28-46). Spectral Doppler waveform from the distal main HA demonstrating poststenotic turbulence. Note that there is no color fill-in of the portal vein (MPV). However, the absence of flow in the portal vein is artifactual because of the high color velocity scale used to eliminate the color aliasing where velocity is increased at the site of the HA stenosis.

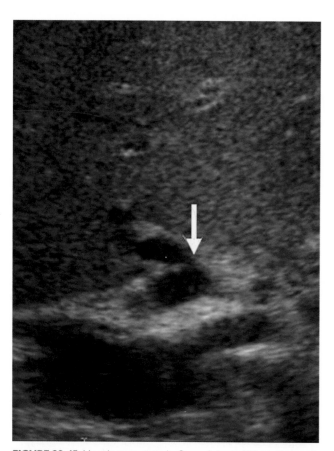

**FIGURE 28-45** Hepatic artery stenosis. Grayscale image of the porta hepatis demonstrating narrowing of the hepatic artery (arrow). This was believed to be because of poor surgical technique.

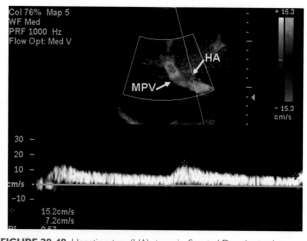

**FIGURE 28-48** Hepatic artery (HA) stenosis. Spectral Doppler tracing demonstrating a tardus-parvus waveform pattern distal to the proximal HA stenosis in another patient. MPV, main portal vein.

portal vein. Clinically, the patient may have early liver failure and signs of portal hypertension. The causes can be surgical injury, vessel length, or hypercoagulable states. PVT will display complete or partial flow voids with Color Doppler, and echogenic thrombus can be seen inside the lumen of the portal vein. A low velocity scale setting must be used to ensure that failure to see color inside the portal vein is not technical in nature. Power Doppler should also be used to verify absence of flow. Intervention is required to save the transplant. Due to the frequency of false positive US diagnoses of PVT due to low velocity flow, confirmation with other imaging studies such as magnetic resonance or computed tomography is often recommended before intervention.

## Portal Vein Stenosis

Portal vein stenosis (PVS) is an uncommon vascular injury occurring most frequently at the anastomotic site and is most often related to surgical injury and fibrosis or scarring. The patient may present with signs of worsening hepatic function that correlates with the degree of stenosis. On color and spectral Doppler, an area of narrowing is easily identified in this large vessel. Peak velocity at the area of greatest stenosis is usually ≥125 cm/s or an anastomotic to preanastomotic velocity ratio of 3:1. Angioplasty or stent placement will be required if the patient is symptomatic.

## IVC Thrombosis/Stenosis

Although rare, thrombosis or stenosis of the IVC is also a finding that is particularly relevant to the surgical technique used to connect the recipient/donor IVC. This finding is also associated with mechanical compression from fluid collections, hypercoagulability, vessel length, and retransplantation. The patient will often present with hepatic failure or lower extremity edema. It is helpful to know the surgical technique used so that all portions of the IVC can be sampled. Thrombus can be seen inside the lumen as well as visible signs of narrowing and velocity changes.

Pathology Box 28-2 summarizes the vascular complications in liver transplant patients. The pathology along with the US appearance is described.

## PATHOLOGY BOX 28-2
### Vascular Pathology in Liver Transplant Recipients

| Pathology | Sonographic Appearance | | |
| --- | --- | --- | --- |
| | Grayscale | Color Doppler | Spectral Doppler |
| Hepatic artery thrombosis (HAT) | Intraluminal echoes | No flow in main or intraparenchymal hepatic arteries | No spectral Doppler signal in main or intraparenchymal hepatic arteries |
| Hepatic artery stenosis (HAS) | Narrowing of main HA<br>May be obscured by overlying bowel gas | Focal narrowing and color aliasing at stenosis<br>Poststenotic dilatation | PSV > 200 cm/s at stenosis<br>Tardus-parvus waveform in intraparenchymal HAs<br>AT > 80 ms<br>RI < 0.5 to 0.6 |
| Portal vein thrombosis (PVT) | Intraluminal echoes<br>Distension of PV | No color flow—if occlusive<br>Focal color void with peripheral flow—if nonocclusive | Absence of Doppler signal—if occlusive<br>↑ velocity and tortuosity of main HA |
| Portal vein stenosis (PVS) | Narrowing of main PV<br>Poststenotic dilatation | Narrowing of PV<br>Focal color aliasing | ↑ velocity at narrowed segment<br>Vel >125 cm/s<br>May be clinically significant if velocity increased 3–4 times |
| Inferior vena cava (IVC) thrombosis | Intraluminal echoes<br>May extend into HVs<br>Distension of IVC | No color flow—if occlusive<br>Focal color void—if nonocclusive<br>May involve HVs | Absence of Doppler signal—if occlusive.<br>↑ velocity if small residual lumen<br>Flat waveforms in proximal HVs |
| IVC Stenosis | Narrowing of IVC | Narrowing of IVC<br>Focal color aliasing | ↑ velocity relative to proximal IVC<br>May be clinically significant if velocity increased 3–4 times |
| Pseudoaneurysm (PSA) | New anechoic round area in hepatic parenchyma<br>Outpouching from main HA | "Yin-Yang" color fill-in<br>± intraluminal thrombus<br>Color aliasing in neck | "To-and-fro" flow in neck—if narrow.<br>A more disorganized flow pattern seen in wider necks |
| Arteriovenous fistula (AVF) | Tangle of tubular anechoic channels<br>Focal dilatation of draining vein mimicking PSA | Spectrum of findings from tangle of vessels to rounder area of color fill-in<br>Focal color aliasing | ↑ PSV and ↑ EDV in feeding artery<br>Pulsatile, high-velocity flow in draining vein |

## SUMMARY

- US is the imaging modality of choice for evaluation of renal and hepatic transplants because it does not require the use of contrast agents that can affect renal function, uses no ionizing radiation, and can be performed portably at the bedside or in the operating room.
- Before starting the US examination, the sonographer should review the operative notes or talk to the transplant team to see how the vascular system and ureter were connected.
- Imaging protocols need to be based on accreditation standards with additional images obtained as needed to answer clinical questions.
- The arterial and venous anastomoses should be carefully examined with grayscale, color Doppler, and spectral Doppler.
- RIs are obtained from various intrarenal vessels as required by protocol.
- Rejection is one of the most common causes of renal transplant and is suspected in patients presenting with anuria, oliguria, or an increase in creatinine or BUN.
- The most common fluid collection in the immediate postoperative period is a hematoma.
- Urinomas occur when there is a leakage at the ureteral anastomosis, and is most commonly located between the kidney and the bladder.
- Fluid collections that contain multiple, thin septations usually are lymphoceles. Lymphoceles are uncommon before 4 to 6 weeks postoperatively.
- When hydronephrosis is discovered, a postvoid image needs to be obtained, and the sonographer should search for a cause such as blood clot in the ureter or a fluid collection compressing the ureter.
- Acute thrombosis of the main renal artery or vein can occur in the immediate postop period. Clinical signs include a rapid decrease or total cessation of urine output. This is a true emergency, and the sonographer needs to urgently rush to the recovery room and quickly verify the absence of flow.
- Reversed flow in the renal arteries is very suggestive of RVT but is a non-specific finding.
- Renal arterial stenosis (RAS) may be caused by a severe bend or kink in the main renal artery in the immediate postoperative period. Delayed RAS is most often caused by infiltration of the arterial wall by leukocytes (in the setting of chronic rejection), fibrosis, or atherosclerosis.
- When scanning a patient with a history of a renal transplant biopsy, the sonographer should pay close attention to the color Doppler findings to look for PSAs or AVFs.
- Before performing a liver transplant US, the sonographer must know whether the patient received a full or partial transplant, if there is a piggyback IVC anastomosis, and any unusual vascular or biliary anastomoses.
- Immediately postop, the RI of the main hepatic artery may be very elevated because of increased hepatic pressure usually secondary to edema. The RI should be followed as needed to look for improvement of diastolic flow.
- Extrahepatic fluid collections include hematoma and biloma.
- The biliary system receives blood only from the hepatic artery. Therefore, lack of arterial blood flow will lead to biliary necrosis. The sonographer needs to look for flow in not only the main hepatic artery but also in the main intrahepatic branches.
- The most common vascular complication following liver transplantation is HAT.
- Hepatic arterial stenosis is detected at the anastomosic site and is typically as a result of arterial injury during surgery. A tardus-parvus waveform in the intrahepatic vessels may be a clue.
- PVS is more commonly seen than PVT. The stenosis will be seen at the surgical anastomosic site and is typically a result of injury during surgery.
- With interposition placement of the IVC, there are two anastomotic sites, and it is important to evaluate both the suprahepatic and the infrahepatic IVC anastomoses to evaluate for IVC stenosis.
- For optimal transplant evaluation, good communication is needed between the surgeon, sonographer, and interpreting physician.
- For all transplants, the sonographer may need to use various patient positions, various transducer types and frequencies, and continually optimize the grayscale and Doppler settings.

## CRITICAL THINKING QUESTIONS

1. The transplant surgeon calls down requesting an emergency US on their patient who now has decreased urinary output. Is this really an emergency and why or why not?
2. A patient returns to US for a follow-up renal transplant sonogram. The patient informs you that he had a renal transplant biopsy 2 days ago. What should the sonographer be looking for as they obtain their images?
3. What is the significance of an elevated RI in a renal transplant?
4. Why is it important for the sonographer to review the operative notes before performing an examination of any transplanted organ?
5. Why is it normal to have an elevated RI in the hepatic artery in the immediate postop liver transplant?
6. What would be some unusual vascular findings of the portal vein in a patient with a liver transplant as opposed to a nontransplanted liver?

## MEDIA MENU

Student Resources available on thePoint® include:
- Audio glossary
- Interactive question bank
- Videos
- Internet resources

## REFERENCES

1. Hricik D. *Primer on Transplantation*. 3rd ed. Hoboken, NJ: Wiley-Blackwell; 2011.
2. Stanford.edu. Kidney Transplantation: Past, Present and Future. History. Available at: http://www.stanford.edu/dept/HPS/transplant/html/history.html. Accessed June 11, 2011.
3. Vollmer WM, Wahl PW, Blagg CR. Survival with dialysis and transplantation in patients with end-stage renal disease. *N Engl J Med*. 1983;308:1553–1558.
4. Cecka JM. The OPTN/UNOS renal transplant registry. *Clin Transpl*. 2005:1–16.
5. Rao PS, Merion RM, Ashby VB, et al. Renal transplantation in elderly patients older than 70 years of age: results from the Scientific Registry of Transplant Recipients. *Transplantation*. 2007;83:1069–1074.
6. United Network for Organ Sharing. https://www.unos.org/data/transplant-trends/#transplants_by_organ_type + year + 2016. Accessed May, 17, 2017.
7. United Network for Organ Sharing. Available at: https://www.unos.org/donation/kidney-paired-donation/. Accessed April 22, 2016.
8. The Organ Procurement and Transplantation Network. U.S. Department of Health & Human Services. Available at: http://optn.transplant.hrsa.gov/. Accessed June 25, 2017.
9. Hafner-Giessauf H, Mauric A, Muller H, et al. Long-term outcome of en bloc pediatric kidney transplantation in adult recipients—up to 22 years of center experience. *Ann Transplant*. 2013;18:100–106.
10. Memel DS, Dodd III GD, Shah AN, et al. Imaging of en bloc renal transplants: normal and abnormal postoperative findings. *AJR Am J Roentgenol*. 1993;160:75–81.
11. Irshad A, Ackerman SJ, Campbell AS, et al. An overview of renal transplantation: current practice and use of ultrasound. *Semin Ultrasound CT and MR*. 2009;30:298–314.
12. Umphrey HR, Lockhart ME, Robbin ML. Transplant ultrasound of the kidney, liver and pancreas. *Ultrasound Clin*. 2008;3(1):49–65.
13. Cosgrove D, Chan K. Renal transplants; what ultrasound can and cannot do. *Ultrasound Q*. 2008;24:77–87.
14. Kolonko A, Chudek J, Wicek A. Prediction of the severity and outcome of acute tubular necrosis based on continuity of Doppler spectrum in the early period after kidney transplantation. *Nephrol Dial Transplant*. 2009;24:1631–1635.
15. Singh AK, Nachiappan AC, Verma HA, et al. Postoperative imaging in liver transplantation: what radiologists should know. *RadioGraphics*. 2010;30:339–351.
16. Crossin JD, Muradali D, Wilson SR. US of liver transplants: normal and abnormal. *Radiographics*. 2003;23:1093–1114

## SUGGESTED READINGS

1. Busuttil RW, Klintmalm GB. *Transplantation of the Liver*. 3rd ed. Philadelphia, PA: Elsevier Saunders; 2015.
2. Danovitch G. *Handbook of Kidney Transplantation*. 5th ed. Baltimore, MD: Lippincott Williams & Wilkins; 2010.
3. Morris PM, Knechtle SJ. *Kidney Transplantation—Principles and Practice*. 7th ed. Philadelphia, PA: Elsevier Saunders; 2014.
4. Pellerito JS, Polak JF. *Introduction to Vascular Sonography*. 6th ed. Philadelphia, PA: Elsevier Saunders; 2012.
5. Rumack CM, Wilson SR, Charboneau JW, Levine D. *Diagnostic Ultrasound*. 4th ed. Philadelphia, PA: Elsevier Mosby; 2010.
6. Size GP, Lozanski L, Russo T. *Inside Ultrasound Vascular Reference Guide*. 1st ed. Pasadena, CA: Davies Publishing, Inc.; 2013.

# PART SEVEN

# MISCELLANEOUS

# Intraoperative Duplex Ultrasound

STEVEN A. LEERS

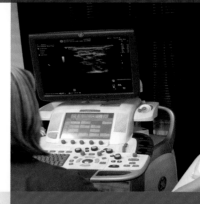

## CHAPTER 29

## OBJECTIVES

- List the types of vascular reconstructions where intraoperative ultrasound is helpful
- Describe the setup and preparation of the ultrasound equipment and transducer for use during an operative procedure
- Define the duplex ultrasound criteria applied to intraoperative data

## KEY TERMS

**endarterectomy**

**infrainguinal reconstruction**

**intraoperative**

**sterile technique**

## GLOSSARY

**autologous/autogenous** Self-produced, or from the same organism. In the case of bypass, using the patient's own tissue (i.e., saphenous vein)

**endarterectomy** Removal of plaque, intima, and part of media of an artery to restore normal flow through the diseased segment

**infrainguinal** Below the inguinal level. In the case of bypass, procedures done from the groin down (outflow procedures)

**prosthetic** A device replacing an absent or damaged part. In the case of bypass, a man-made tube used for the bypass procedure. Dacron and polytetrafluoroethylene are the examples

**revascularization** Restoration of blood flow to an organ or area by way of bypass, endarterectomy, or angioplasty and stenting

**sterile technique** Means by which a surgical field is isolated from nonsterile or contaminated materials

**surveillance** Keeping a watch over. In the case of revascularizations, it suggests periodically monitoring patency and functioning by some means

**visceral** Pertaining to the viscera; in this case, intestines or kidneys

Vascular surgery is unique in its requirement for intraoperative documentation of the technical success of revascularizations. In most surgical specialties, visual inspection and palpation are adequate to demonstrate this, but the meticulous nature of vascular surgery and the devastating result of technical errors demand more from the vascular surgeon. For decades, the necessity of documenting technical results has been acknowledged by vascular surgeons. Especially in lower extremity bypass but also in carotid endarterectomy, this has led to the suggestion of routine angiography at the completion of the procedure, before closing the wound and leaving the operating room. Color duplex ultrasound scanning is the natural extension of this routine, avoiding contrast exposure and offering the advantage of anatomic and physiologic information not provided by angiography. This chapter reviews current applications of duplex ultrasound scanning in the operating room and the results of such an approach.

# SONOGRAPHIC EXAMINATION TECHNIQUES

Vascular reconstructions which lend themselves to intraoperative application of duplex ultrasound scanning include carotid endarterectomy, infrainguinal, and visceral bypass. Especially in endovascular venous procedures, intravascular ultrasound (IVUS) also plays an increasingly important role. Lower extremity bypass results are plagued by problems related to inflow, outflow, and conduit. Duplex ultrasound bypass surveillance has been shown to enhance patency and limb salvage, and beginning surveillance in the operating room is a natural extension of that policy. Results of carotid endarterectomy are already consistently excellent so improvements are likely to be in small increments. Renal and visceral bypass patency depends on technical excellence, which is easily assessed with duplex ultrasound scanning. Table 29-1 summarizes the common vascular applications for intraoperative ultrasound and abnormalities that can be encountered.

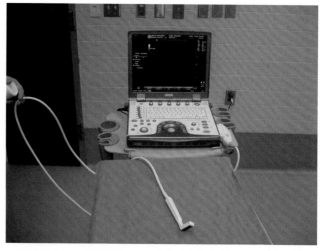

**FIGURE 29-1** Portable color duplex ultrasound system with "hockey stick" probe.

## Scanning Technique

At this author's institution, a GE Logiq e portable duplex ultrasound system with an i12L-RS, 4 to 10 MHz broadband multifrequency linear array transducer designed specifically for vascular applications is used. This transducer has a 10 × 29 mm footprint to allow access into small areas. A sterile sheath with a latex tip is filled with gel and used to isolate the transducer, being careful to remove any bubbles from the probe cover. The length of the probe cover allows a significant length of transducer and cord to be brought onto the sterile field. The wound is filled with saline, the overhead lights in the operating room are extinguished to make viewing of the image easier, and the scan is begun (Figs. 29-1 to 29-4). The scanning protocol is simple with the surgeon holding the transducer and the sonographer or vascular technologist optimizing the image and controlling the other components on the ultrasound console. In general, long-axis imaging alone is utilized. Grayscale

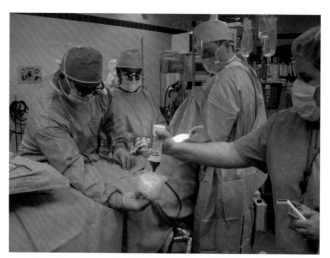

**FIGURE 29-2** Sterile sheath filled with gel, prior to placement of the ultrasound transducer.

| TABLE 29-1 | **Common Applications for Intraoperative Vascular Ultrasound** | |
|---|---|---|
| **Surgical Procedure** | **Anatomy Examined** | **Potential Complications** |
| Carotid endarterectomy | Common carotid artery | Intimal flap |
| | Internal carotid artery | Residual plaque |
| | External carotid artery | Platelet aggregate |
| | | Suture line abnormalities |
| | | Dissection |
| Infrainguinal revascularization | Inflow artery | Retained valves |
| | Outflow artery | AV fistulae |
| | Anastomotic regions | Platelet aggregate |
| | Entire conduit | Anastomotic or suture line abnormalities |
| Renal and mesenteric artery bypass | Anastomotic regions | Residual plaque |
| | Renal artery | Platelet aggregate |
| | Celiac artery | Dissection |
| | Mesenteric artery | Anastomotic or suture line abnormalities |

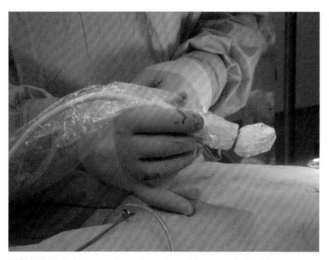

**FIGURE 29-3** Ultrasound transducer brought onto surgical field.

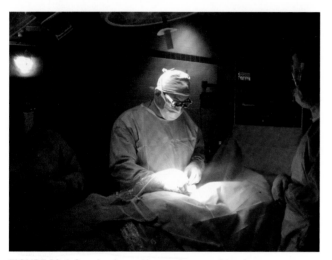

**FIGURE 29-4** Scanning done with operating room lights down.

images are first obtained to best visualize small defects not well seen with color scanning. Color is added to facilitate placement of the pulsed spectral Doppler gate. Images and waveforms are stored in cine loops as well as still images to allow careful interpretation. If an abnormality is identified which prompts revision, the scan process is repeated after revision. In infrainguinal revascularization, instillation of papaverine into the bypass is helpful in minimizing the effects of vasospasm frequently seen in these procedures.

### Technical Considerations

Intraoperative assessment during vascular reconstructions requires a team that is comfortable with the techniques described as well as the equipment necessary for the procedure. Modern color duplex ultrasound scanners are available in many shapes and forms, with many new easily portable machines enclosed in a simple laptop computer configuration. As noted in the preceding section, specific ultrasound transducers for intraoperative use have been developed for vascular applications in multiple anatomic areas. Operating rooms with extensive experience with this

technology frequently have dedicated ultrasound machines kept in the operating room at all times.

The vascular surgeon must be adept not only with the interpretation of vascular sonograms but also with the application of the transducer to maximize image acquisition. In procedures where a prosthetic material is used, this can be challenging because many such materials absorb air in their interstices that makes obtaining a meaningful image a challenge. In the case of prosthetic bypasses, this renders intraoperative scanning virtually impossible, but prosthetic patches on carotid endarterectomy usually allow adequate imaging by "working around" the patch. It is critical that the surgeon is directly involved in the scanning process along with the sonographer or vascular technologist to ensure accurate and dependable information.

The sonographer or vascular technologist is key to a successful intraoperative sonography program. Familiarity with operating room sterile technique is critical to the safe application of duplex ultrasound scanning, allowing the "nonsterile" sonographer to interact with the sterile team and field. Once the probe is sheathed and dispensed to the sterile field, the sonographer must work with the surgeon from a distance to maximize image acquisition as well as coordinate pulsed spectral analysis, color imaging, and grayscale imaging.

## CAROTID ENDARTERECTOMY

More than six decades after its introduction, carotid endarterectomy remains one of the most frequent operations performed by vascular surgeons, and admirable stroke rates below 3% are expected. With such excellent results, one would expect that intraoperative assessment would not be particularly fruitful. On the contrary, early large reviews using a variety of techniques identified residual defects in between 5% and 43% of examined arteries. While the majority of defects were found in the blindly endarterectomized external carotid artery, 6.5% of the collected cases had abnormalities in the internal carotid artery, usually at the distal end of the endarterectomy.[1]

Routine intraoperative angiography offers the advantage of visualizing the intracranial carotid artery as well as the cervical area. Lesions proximal in the common carotid artery (CCA) are usually not assessed however, and no physiologic data is identified. In an early study using routine completion angiography, Donaldson found 71 defects in a series of 410 carotid endarterectomies, warranting correction in 16% of cases. These corrections did not add to morbidity because the stroke rate remained below 2%.[2] Zannetti evaluated 1,305 carotid endarterectomies with completion angiography in 77% and identified 9% defects, 4% which were revised. There was an increased stroke rate in this group despite revision. Nevertheless, the overall stroke rate was less than 1%; this raises questions regarding the advantage of routine imaging.[3] Westerland reported a 19% incidence of defects requiring repair, with no postoperative occlusions in this group.[4]

### Current Intraoperative Evaluation

Currently, continuous wave Doppler interrogation alone is probably the most commonly used assessment during carotid endarterectomy. This method has been shown to be quite sensitive, but not specific, identifying abnormalities in 4.3% in early studies.[5] Although this modality is simple and fairly reliable in experienced hands, it usually requires a confirmatory study such as angiography to justify reexploration. B-mode ultrasound has also been utilized in completion studies to determine which findings signal the need for revision. Again, the incidence of complications is so low that it is difficult to make recommendations based on these smaller studies.[6]

Bandyk applied pulse Doppler spectral analysis to carotid endarterectomy sites and reported on 250 procedures using this technique.[7] In a follow-up study of 461 endarterectomies studied with duplex ultrasound scanning, less than 6% required intraoperative revision, and the permanent stroke rate was 1.3%. Patients with normal scans had a lower incidence of late postoperative stroke.[8] The Mayo clinic reported results in 87 patients using routine duplex ultrasound scanning. In this study, 9% had significant findings requiring immediate revision. Stroke rates were 1.9% and equal between normal and repaired groups. Two of three patients with significant common carotid lesions that were not addressed suffered strokes. These data suggest the safety and efficacy of routine duplex ultrasound scanning.[9] Numerous other small studies have shown similar advantages of intraoperative duplex sonography.[10–13]

Although completion duplex ultrasonography is intuitively beneficial, caution must be exercised in interpreting the results of these studies. Excellent results with endarterectomy without any monitoring have been established, and the possibility that reexploration carries risk to the patient is real. In fact, a review of a large database of New York state carotid endarterectomies failed to demonstrate difference in outcomes, regardless of type of intraoperative monitoring used.[14]

Still, the ease of application, lack of risk, and benefit of a normal intraoperative duplex ultrasound study argues for some application of this modality. How to interpret and react to abnormal studies remains controversial.

Intraoperative duplex ultrasound scanning after carotid endarterectomy still remains routine for some but not all surgeons. Scanning protocols include examination of the entire portion of the common, external, and internal carotid arteries that are accessible to the ultrasound transducer. Velocities are recorded from all the vessels, and the B-mode image is closely examined for any wall irregularities. Those surgeons utilizing the technique are comfortable with the scanning process and are reassured by the findings of a normal intraoperative study (Figs. 29-5 to 29-8).

## Diagnosis

Diagnostic criteria used may vary between institutions and are often simplified versions of normally applied standards. In fact, many of the abnormalities noted are in the common or external carotid arteries, where criteria are poorly established. Still, the abnormalities found in these vessels are usually so compelling that there is little disagreement about how to handle them. Abnormalities on the B-mode image can include residual plaque or a "shelf" lesion. Plaque remaining in the proximal CCA or distal internal carotid artery that appears as an abrupt edge

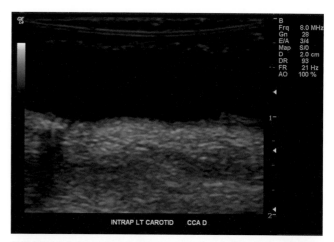

**FIGURE 29-5** Normal grayscale image of common carotid artery (CCA).

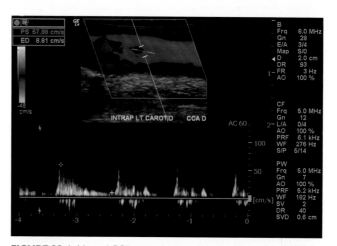

**FIGURE 29-6** Normal CCA spectral analysis. Note components of low-resistance ICA and high-resistance ECA in waveform. ECA, external carotid artery; ICA, internal carotid artery.

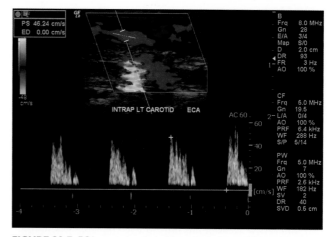

**FIGURE 29-7** ECA spectral analysis. Normal velocity and high-resistance waveform.

or outcropping is often referred to as a shelf lesion. If this residual plaque is greater than 2 mm thick, a revision may be performed. A piece of residual plaque can sometimes appear mobile, moving within the blood stream and necessitates a prompt revision. An intimal flap is another complication which may be apparent. If a flap is above

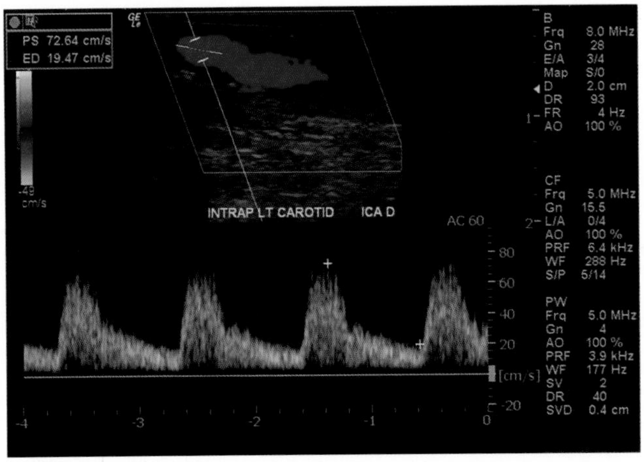

**FIGURE 29-8** Normal ICA spectral analysis. Note normal diastolic flow.

2 mm, revision is usually performed. Less commonly, a dissection occurring as a result of a vascular clamp injury may be present and require attention. The most common technical defects involve the external carotid artery, but many authors have avoided revision with no increased stroke risks.[15]

A focal peak systolic velocity (PSV) increase in the internal carotid artery can identify a significant complication. Reexamination or revision of the surgical site is warranted if the PSV exceeds 180 cm/s or the internal carotid to common carotid PSV ratio is greater than 2.5. In some patients, this may be associated with a fresh platelet aggregate which is often unable to be identified on the B-mode image because of its anechoic nature. Pathology Box 29-1 describes the ultrasound characteristics of common pathology observed during intraoperative ultrasound examinations.

Figures 29-9 to 29-13 demonstrate an abnormal finding in the CCA, the intraoperative findings, and the repeat scan following revision. This is an excellent example of the benefit of direct clinical application of this policy.

Outcome analysis has offered new insight into the commonly held beliefs and prejudices using large databases to answer specific questions. The large numbers of subjects allows statistically significant conclusions, but the data is so general that interpretation must be carefully balanced. The Vascular Study Group of New England (VSGNE) has prospectively collected data from a broad variety of surgeons and hospitals in New England, allowing careful evaluation of specific questions. In a 2011 study, they reviewed 6,115 carotid endarterectomies and found that 51% of surgeons rarely performed completion duplex ultrasound, 22% selectively, and 27% routinely. In most studies, a much smaller percentage routinely use completion imaging. In this study, there was no evidence that routine duplex ultrasound improved the incidence of stroke, although there was a slight decrease in 1 year re-stenosis in selective imagers. There was a significant increase in cerebrovascular accident (CVA) in patients whose arteries were reexplored on the basis of imaging, underlining the implications of false positive studies. The findings suggest that more work is needed to better define the place of completion imaging in preventing stroke, occlusion, or restenosis after carotid endarterectomy.[16]

---

### PATHOLOGY BOX 29-1
### *Common Intraoperative Sonographic Abnormalities*

| Pathology Observed | Ultrasound Characteristics |
|---|---|
| "Shelf" lesion/residual lesion | • Hyperechoic plaque projecting into the vessel lumen<br>• May display an abrupt edge |
| Intimal flap | • Small projection into vessel lumen usually less than 1 cm<br>• Disturbed flow or aliasing may be present |
| Dissection | • Linear object seen extending for several centimeters<br>• Parallel to vessel walls<br>• Turbulent or disturbed flow present |
| Platelet aggregate | • Hypo- or anechoic material adjacent to vessel wall<br>• Focal elevation in PSV<br>• Increased $V_r$ |
| Stenosis: carotid or lower extremity bypass graft | • PSV > 180 cm/s<br>• $V_r$ > 2.5 |
| Stenosis: renal or celiac artery | • PSV > 200 cm/s |
| Stenosis: superior mesenteric artery | • PSV > 275 cm/s |
| Arteriovenous fistula | • Patent branch may be seen arising from an in situ bypass<br>• Turbulence and aliasing present in area of side branch<br>• Elevated diastolic velocities in bypass graft proximal to side branch |
| Retained valve | • Hyperechoic structure protruding into lumen of vein bypass graft; may be associated with slight dilation of valve sinus<br>• Turbulence or aliasing may be present |
| Suture line/anastomotic problem | • Turbulence or aliasing may be present<br>• Kink or wall irregularity may be present |

PSV, peak systolic velocity; $V_r$, velocity ratio.

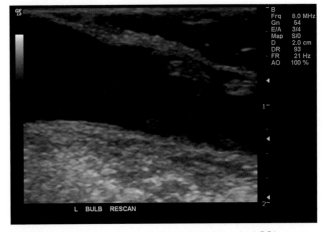

**FIGURE 29-9** Grayscale image of residual plaque in proximal CCA.

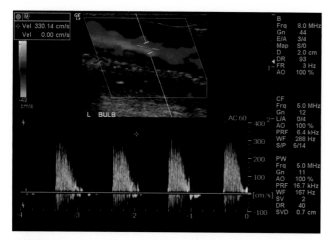

**FIGURE 29-10** Elevated velocity CCA consistent with severe stenosis.

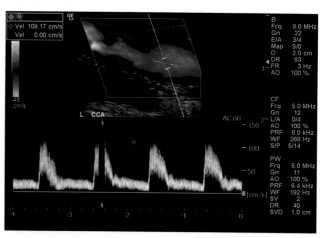

**FIGURE 29-13** Normal spectral analysis of CCA after revision.

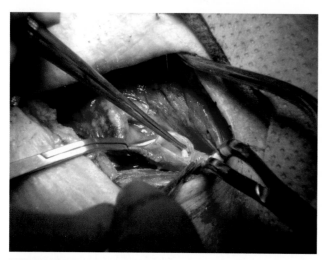

**FIGURE 29-11** Dissected plaque being removed from CCA.

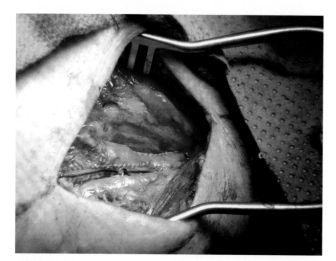

**FIGURE 29-12** Carotid bifurcation after endarterectomy and revision.

# INFRAINGUINAL REVASCULARIZATION

Infrainguinal revascularization can be performed for claudication or critical limb ischemia (CLI) and can be performed via percutaneous endovascular means or open surgical bypass using either autogenous (vein) or prosthetic (Dacron or polytetrafluoroethylene) material. Although carotid endarterectomy is a fairly standardized procedure, there are almost infinite variations in the performance of an infrainguinal reconstruction. Issues abound assessing and obtaining adequate arterial inflow, choice of an appropriate conduit for bypass depending on the level of the bypass and available autogenous material, and choice of adequacy of an outflow target. Any or all of these issues can result in success or failure of the procedure, and the number of steps in these often tedious operations creates many opportunities for failure. Despite these significant obstacles to success, the results in terms of patency and limb salvage continue to be quite admirable.

Early in the experience with infrainguinal revascularization, the superiority of autologous material over prosthetic in terms of bypass patency was demonstrated.[17] Adopting an all-autologous approach has introduced utilizing arm veins, small saphenous veins, deep veins, and even radial arteries. These "alternative" veins are more prone to abnormalities that can result in failure. Concomitantly, imaging advances and surgical techniques have allowed bypass to very distal arteries. This combination has compounded the already significant obstacles to success in the surgical treatment of infrainguinal occlusive disease.

## Current Intraoperative Evaluation

Surveillance of infrainguinal bypass has been well established as a means of enhancing autogenous bypass patency and resulting limb salvage.[18,19] Given the myriad of intraoperative issues previously described, it is intuitive that surveillance most appropriately should begin in the operating room. The methods of assessing bypasses in the operating room include palpation, continuous wave Doppler, angiography, angioscopy, and duplex ultrasound scanning. Although the "gold standard" was arteriography, there are many drawbacks to the technique, including inability to assess inflow, difficulty in visualizing the entire length of the conduit, and lack of physiologic information provided. Still, completion angiography has been liberally used, demonstrating between 6% and 12% defects requiring immediate revision.[20]

Duplex ultrasound scanning during lower extremity bypass offers unique advantages. The evaluation may begin with the imaging of the donor artery with pulsed spectral analysis, which allows characterization of adequate inflow. The entire length of the bypass conduit along with the anastomotic regions can be interrogated to identify retained valves, scarred areas, arteriovenous fistulae, or platelet aggregation. Technical adequacy of the often miniscule distal anastomosis can be assured. Abnormally low graft velocities may identify problems with poor outflow vessels. Thus, the entire circuit from inflow artery, through the conduit and distally into the outflow vessel, should be examined. Repeated scanning after repair of defects adds no risk.

## Diagnosis

Compared to carotid endarterectomy and renal bypass, infrainguinal bypass has the highest incidence of defects identified by duplex ultrasound scanning, 10% to 15%. Some institutions have championed the application of duplex ultrasound scanning in the operating room at the time of bypass. Furthermore, a normal duplex ultrasound scan was predictive of success, and unrepaired defects were strong predictors of failure.[21,22] Findings which prompted revision included a PSV > 180 cm/s and a velocity ratio ($V_r$) > 2.5. In areas of elevated velocities, retained valves may sometimes be apparent on the ultrasound image. Occasionally, platelet aggregate may form at the site of vessel wall injury. This is usually anechoic in nature but will demonstrate an increased velocity shift. In a small conduit vein graft, a PSV of 150 to 200 cm/s may be recorded as a result of hyperemic bypass flows rather than a focal stenosis. The $V_r$ in these small caliber grafts will remain less than 2.0. Lastly, arteriovenous fistulae may be identified within in situ grafts. Turbulent flow will be present in the region of the fistula with elevated diastolic flow velocities proximal to the fistula.

It should be noted that the technique of scanning in these instances is more complex and requires more time than scans done during carotid endarterectomy. Again, the interaction of the surgeon and sonographer or vascular technologist is of paramount importance in making such a system successful.

Prospectively collected patient information for large databases has again provided a statistically powerful tool to answer questions regarding completion imaging. The Vascular Quality Initiative (VQI) supported by the Society for Vascular Surgery is one of these databases, and has allowed researchers to evaluate the result of completion imaging. In 1,457 bypasses from this database, completion imaging was performed, including 20% duplex ultrasound scanning, 77% angiography, and 3.7% both modalities. Bypass patency at discharge and 1 year postoperatively was unaffected by completion imaging compared to no imaging, regardless of the modality used.[23] In a study from the VS-GNE, completion imaging was evaluated, lumping together duplex ultrasound scanning and angiography. Of 2,032 lower extremity bypasses, 67% had completion imaging by either duplex ultrasound scanning or angiography. Again, graft patency at discharge and 1 year was not affected by routine or selected use of completion imaging. The variety of bypass types and imaging strategies makes generalization challenging, but the findings certainly bring into question on commonly held beliefs.[24]

## INTRAABDOMINAL REVASCULARIZATION

Aortoiliac reconstructions involve vessels much larger than carotid or lower extremity procedures, so small technical defects that threaten graft patency are much less common. Assessment is usually by palpation or continuous wave Doppler. In the case of visceral (renal or mesenteric) revascularizations, however, minor technical defects can result in graft failure with catastrophic consequences. As a result, routine arteriography or duplex ultrasound scanning has been liberally applied. In this case, duplex sonography has distinct advantages because these small anastomoses are deeply located and more easily accessible with small intraoperative probes. In addition, renal bypass is frequently performed for salvage of renal function, and contrast exposure is avoided if possible. Evaluation of the proximal anastomosis by angiography would require large volumes of contrast under high-flow rates, another reason to adopt sonography.

Large studies have documented the feasibility and advantages of intraoperative visceral duplex ultrasound scanning. Hansen and associates applied sonography to 800 renal bypasses, using a velocity of 200 cm/s as indication to revise. Sensitivity was 86% and specificity was 100%.[25,26] Some degree of renal insufficiency was present in 75% of these reconstructions, underlining the advantages of avoiding contrast material. The consequences of failure in mesenteric revascularization are so catastrophic that intraoperative assessment is a natural adjunct to the procedure. In a study from the Mayo clinic, 68 visceral reconstructions were monitored with intraoperative duplex ultrasound scanning. A normal ultrasound was predictive of long-term patency, and an abnormal study was associated with early reintervention, graft failure, and death.[27] Their normal criteria includes a PSV < 200 cm/s for the celiac artery, a PSV < 275 cm/s for the superior mesenteric artery, a $V_r$ 2.0, and no technical defects (such as vessel narrowing, thrombus, dissection, or intimal flap). Studies are limited, and criteria for postop duplex ultrasound scanning after visceral bypass is just being described. No predictor for bypass failure has been validated.[28]

## PROCEDURES FOR VENOUS DISEASE

Although arterial reconstructions have received great attention in regard to operative monitoring with duplex sonography, venous interventions are done much more commonly, and duplex ultrasound scanning is no less useful in this important area. Along with mapping of varicose or incompetent veins, sonography is used for monitoring during Endo-Venous Laser Therapy (EVLT). Sonographic localization for central venous catheterization has also become the standard of care. These applications of ultrasound with venous procedures are reviewed in other chapters of this book.

IVUS is an evolving technology using an ultrasound probe mounted on an intravascular catheter. Intraluminal imaging offers a unique perspective and has been increasingly applied to endovascular treatment of acute and chronic venous occlusive disease. Increasing application and reviews suggest that IVUS may become the standard for intraoperative guidance of endovenous interventions.[29,30]

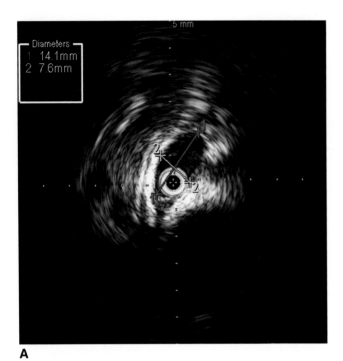

**A**

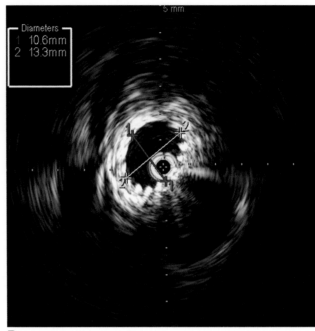

**B**

**FIGURE 29-14  A:** IVUS of a renal vein prior to stent placement. **B:** IVUS of renal vein after stent placement.

Figure 29-14 displays IVUS images before and after placement for a renal vein stent.

In some cases, endovascular treatment of stenotic lesions in anteriovenous fistulae, PAD, and cerebrovascular occlusive disease has been has been performed without contrast and radiographic control. In these cases, duplex sonography has been used as the sole imaging control during the procedure for angioplasty or stent placement. The advantages in terms of radiation and contrast exposure are obvious, but such a procedure does require a sophisticated imaging setup and has not been widely adopted. Still, excellent results have been reported using duplex ultrasound in these circumstances.[31]

## SUMMARY

- Success in vascular reconstructions is dependent on excellent preoperative imaging, careful operative planning, technical perfection in the operating room, and careful surveillance and follow-up.
- Intraoperative duplex sonography offers a unique opportunity to maximize the technical outcomes of surgical revascularization.
- It requires a commitment to excellence and a team approach which relies heavily on the interaction of surgeon and sonographer or vascular technologist.
- Adaption of these techniques has been intermittent, and the results are not well validated, but the simplicity, low cost, and avoidance of catastrophic complications make this a very attractive approach to help improve outcomes in complex vascular patients.

## CRITICAL THINKING QUESTIONS

1. You are asked to bring equipment down to the operating room to assist with an intraoperative ultrasound on a patient undergoing a carotid endarterectomy. You have multiple ultrasound systems in your department. Which one would you select and why?
2. In the operating room, the surgeon has the ultrasound transducer directly over the site of a completed carotid endarterectomy. In one area, there is a strong acoustic shadow and no image of the vessel. The surgeon moves the transducer slightly distally, and a normal carotid artery image is obtained. What is a likely explanation of this artifact?

## MEDIA MENU

Student Resources available on the**Point**° include:
- Audio glossary
- Interactive question bank
- Videos
- Internet resource

## REFERENCES

1. Barnes RW, Nix ML, Wingo JP, et al. Recurrent versus residual carotid stenosis. Incidence detected by Doppler ultrasound. *Ann Surg.* 1986;203:652–660.
2. Donaldson MC, Ivarsson BL, Mannick JA, et al. Impact of completion angiography on operative conduct and results of carotid endarterectomy. *Ann Surg.* 1993;217:682–687.
3. Zannetti S, Cao P, DeRango P, et al. Intraoperative assessment of technical perfection in carotid endarterectomy: a prospective analysis of 1305 completion procedures. *Eur J Vasc Endovasc Surg.* 1999;18:52–58.
4. Westerband A, Mill JL, Berman SS, et al. The influence of routine completion arteriography on outcome following carotid endarterectomy. *Ann Vasc Surg.* 1997;11:14–19.
5. Seifert KB, Blackshear WM Jr. Continuous-wave Doppler in the intraoperative assessment of carotid endarterectomy. *J Vasc Surg.* 1985;2:817–820.
6. Sawchuk AP, Flanigan DP, Machi J, et al. The fate of unrepaired minor technical defects detected by intraoperative ultrasonography during carotid endarterectomy. *J Vasc Surg.* 1989;9:671–676.
7. Bandyk DF, Kaebnick HW, Adams MB, et al. Turbulence occurring after carotid bifurcation endarterectomy: a harbinger of residual and recurrent carotid stenosis. *J Vasc Surg.* 1988;7:261–274.
8. Kinney EV, Seabrook GR, Kinney LY, et al. The importance of intraoperative detection of residual flow abnormalities after carotid artery endarterectomy. *J Vasc Surg.* 1993;17:912–923.
9. Panneton JM, Berger MW, Lewis BD, et al. Intraoperative duplex ultrasound during carotid endarterectomy. *Vasc Surg.* 2001;35:1–9.
10. Steinmetz OK, MacKenzie K, Nault P, et al. Intraoperative duplex scanning for carotid endarterectomy. *Eur J Vasc Endovasc Surg.* 1998;16:153–158.
11. Mays BW, Towne JZB, Seabrook GR, et al. Intraoperative carotid evaluation. *Arch Surg.* 2000;135:525–529.
12. Mullenix PS, Tollefson DF, Olsen SB, et al. Intraoperative duplex ultrasonography as an adjunct to technical excellence in 100 consecutive carotid endarterectomies. *Am J Surg.* 2003;185:445–449.
13. Schanzer A, Hoel A, Conte MS, et al. Restenosis after carotid endarterectomy performed with routine intraoperative duplex ultrasonography and arterial patch closure: a contemporary series. *Vasc Endovasc Surg.* 2007;41(3):200–205.
14. Rockman CB, Haim EA. Intraoperative imaging: does it really improve perioperative outcomes of carotid endarterectomy? *Semin Vasc Surg.* 2007;20:236–243.
15. Ascher E, Markevich N, Kallakuri S, et al. Intraoperative carotid artery duplex scanning in a modern series of 650 consecutive primary endarterectomy procedures. *J Vasc Surg.* 2004;39:416–420.
16. Wallaert JE, Goodney PP, Cronewett JL, et al. Completion imaging after carotid endarterectomy in the Vascular Study Group of New England. *J Vasc Surg.* 2011;54:376–385.
17. Veith FJ, Gupta SK, Ascer E, et al. Six-year prospective randomized comparison of autologous saphenous vein and expanded polytetrafluoroethylene grafts in infrainguinal reconstructions. *J Vasc Surg.* 1986;3:104–114.
18. Mills JL Sr. Is duplex surveillance of value after leg vein bypass grafting? Principal results of the vein graft surveillance randomized trial. *Perspect Vasc Surg Endovasc Ther.* 2006;18:194–196.
19. Lundell A, Lingblad B, Bergqvist D, et al. Femoropopliteal-crural graft patency is improved by an intensive surveillance program: a prospective randomized study. *J Vasc Surg.* 1995;21:26–34.
20. Mills JL, Fujitani RM, Taylor SM. Contribution of routine intraoperative completion arteriography to early infrainguinal bypass patency. *Am J Surg.* 1992;164:506–511.
21. Bandyk DF, Mills JL, Gahtan V, et al. Intraoperative duplex scanning of arterial reconstructions: fate of repaired and unrepaired defects. *J Vasc Surg.* 1994;20:426–433.
22. Johnson BL, Bandyk DF, Back MR, et al. Intraoperative duplex monitoring of infrainguinal bypass procedures. *J Vasc Surg.* 2000;31:678–690.
23. Woo K, Palmer OP, Fred E, et al. Outcomes of completion imaging for lower extremity bypass in the Vascular Quality Initiative. *J Vasc Surg.* 2015;62:412–416.
24. Tan TW, Rybin D, Cronenwett JL, et al. Routine use of completion imaging after infrainguinal bypass is not associated with higher bypass graft patency. *J Vasc Surg.* 2014;60:678–685.
25. Hansen KJ, Reavis SW, Dean RH. Duplex scanning in renovascular disease. *Geriatr Nephrol Urol.* 1996;6:89–97.
26. Hansen KJ, O'Neil EA, Reavis SW, et al. Intraoperative duplex sonography during renal artery reconstruction. *J Vasc Surg.* 1991;14:364–374.
27. Oderich GS, Panneton JM, Macedo TA, et al. Intraoperative duplex ultrasound of visceral revascularizations: optimizing technical success and outcome. *J Vasc Surg.* 2003;38:684–691.
28. Liem DK, Segal JA, Moneta GL, et al. Duplex scan characteristics of bypass grafts to the mesenteric arteries. *J Vasc Surg.* 2007;45:922–928.
29. Forauer AR, Gemmele JJ, Dasika NL, et al. Intravascular ultrasound in the diagnosis and treatment of iliac vein compression (May-Thurner) syndrome. *J Vasc Interv Radiol.* 2002;13:523–527.
30. Raja S. Best management options for chronic iliac vein stenosis and occlusion. *J Vasc Surg.* 2013;57:1163–1169.
31. Ascher E, Marks NA, Hingorani AP, et al. Duplex-guided endovascular treatment for occlusive and stenotic lesions of the femoral-popliteal arterial segment: a comparative study in the first 253 cases. *J Vasc Surg.* 2006;44:1230–1238.

# Hemodialysis Access Grafts and Fistulae

MICHAEL J. SINGH | AMY STEINMETZ | KARIM SALEM

**CHAPTER 30**

## OBJECTIVES

- Describe the difference between an arteriovenous fistula and graft
- Identify the duplex ultrasound findings of a normal arteriovenous fistula
- Define normal venous and arterial anatomy in the upper extremity
- Describe the venous Doppler findings in an occluded axillary vein
- Demonstrate proper probe positioning for imaging of a radiocephalic fistula
- Differentiate a forearm graft from a brachiocephalic fistula
- Quantify the degrees of stenosis based on Doppler findings

## KEY TERMS

**arteriovenous fistula**

**arteriovenous graft**

**hemodialysis access**

## GLOSSARY

**arteriovenous fistula** Any connection between an artery and a vein. This may be congenital, traumatic, or acquired. One type of acquired arteriovenous fistula is surgically created to allow for hemodialysis

**arteriovenous graft** A type of hemodialysis access which uses a prosthetic conduit to connect an artery to a vein to allow for dialysis

**hemodialysis access** Also known as vascular access, is a surgically created connection between an artery and a vein to allow for the removal of toxic byproducts from the blood via hemodialysis

Owing to various factors, the incidence of chronic kidney disease and end-stage renal disease is becoming more prevalent in the United States. In 2005, the Renal Data System determined that more than 106,000 patients began hemodialysis, and the total number of people undergoing hemodialysis had reached 341,000. The National Kidney Foundation-Kidney Dialysis Outcomes Quality Initiative was published in 1997 and recommended that 50% of future hemodialysis access be constructed with autogenous arteriovenous (AV) access. In 2005, the Centers for Medicare and Medicaid Services promoted the Fistula First Breakthrough Initiative. The goal of this was to expand the creation of new autogenous access to 66% by 2009.[1] As of December 2015, 63% of patients are using autogenous access.

The goal of AV fistula or graft creation is to provide a long-term hemodialysis access in addition to maintaining a low frequency of reinterventions and low complication rates. The tenet of hemodialysis access is creating an autogenous fistula distally as possible in the nondominant arm. This technique preserves the proximal vessels for future access options and allows the individual to carry out normal daily activities without restriction. Autogenous access is the preferred first line of therapy because of its superior patency rates and lower rate of complication compared to prosthetic grafts.[2] Upper extremity access is preferential because it maintains a lower infection rate and promotes easier access for hemodialysis. A native AV fistula is a surgically created anastomosis between any artery and vein. When fistula creation is not possible, a prosthetic graft may be used to connect the two vessels. These prosthetic grafts can be polytetrafluoroethylene (PTFE), Dacron, CryoGraft, or xenograft and typically tunneled in the subcutaneous tissue.

Failure of an AV fistula to mature and/or fistula thrombosis are not infrequent indications for reintervention. AV fistulae have expected 2-year primary patency rates of 40% to 69%. In comparison, 2-year primary patency rates for prosthetic grafts range from 18% to 30%. Secondary patency rates for fistulae are an acceptable 62% to 75% at 2 years. For prosthetic grafts, secondary patency rates remain in the range of 40% to 60%. The tradeoff for higher long-term AV fistula patency rates is an expected lower rate of maturation and higher potential for early thrombosis. More often, fistula maturation failure is caused by the obligatory use of small or suboptimal veins when attempting to create a fistula.[2]

## PREOPERATIVE EVALUATION

### Sonographic Examination Technique

Given the importance of finding a suitable conduit, preoperative evaluation of both arterial and venous systems is a necessity for successful creation of long-term access and fistula maturation. Vascular Professional Performance Guidelines have been established by The Society for Vascular Ultrasound.[3] Preoperative vein mapping is performed to determine suitability of the superficial veins of the upper extremity for the placement of dialysis access (Fig. 30-1). The upper extremity arterial system is also evaluated patency, size, and the presence of any pathology (Fig. 30-2). This may be performed on patients who have yet to start hemodialysis or in those who have undergone previous access procedures and require a secondary intervention or access creation.

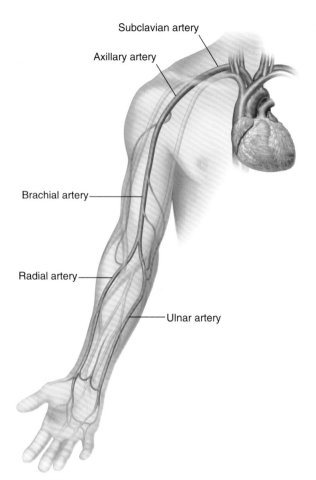

**FIGURE 30-2** Diagram of the normal arterial anatomy of the upper extremity.

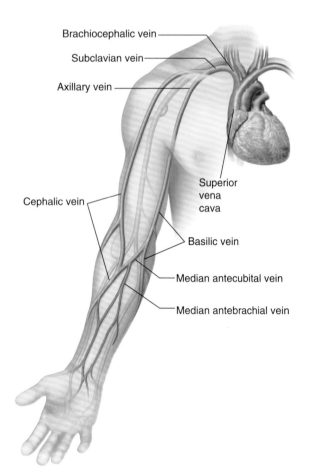

**FIGURE 30-1** Diagram of the normal venous anatomy of the upper extremity.

### Patient Preparation

The vascular technologist should introduce himself or herself and explain to the patient what and why vein mapping is being performed. An explanation of the technique and duration of study is essential. Questions and concerns from the patient should be addressed before initiating the study. The room should be comfortably warm to avoid vasospasm.

### Patient Assessment

The patient assessment must be complete prior to initiating the procedure. A comprehensive history should document the patient's ability to tolerate the imaging study and determination of any contraindications to the procedure. Obtaining a current medical history is essential. This includes all previous access procedures, medical, surgical and trauma history, medications, and arm dominance. Specifically, inquire about risk factors that may preclude fistula creation (i.e., central venous occlusion, tunneled catheters, pacemakers, defibrillators, or prior mastectomy with lymph node dissection). The focused physical examination should include bilateral arm blood pressure measurements; a qualitative examination of the brachial, radial, and ulnar artery pulses; an Allen test to demonstrate an intact palmar arch; and assessment of the superficial venous system using tourniquets. Findings suggestive of a central venous stenosis or occlusion include arm edema, prominent chest wall veins, or arm collaterals.

## Patient Positioning

Optimal patient positioning may be either in the supine or sitting position. The objective is to promote venodilation, and thus placing the arms in gravity-dependent position is beneficial.

## Scanning Techniques

During the procedure, sonographic characteristics of vessels, tissue, and blood flow must be observed and analyzed in order to ensure that appropriate data is documented for the interpreting physician. The assessment of the upper extremity venous system includes direct imaging of the superficial and deep systems with appropriate instrumentation. Spectral analysis with or without color Doppler imaging should be performed using a high-resolution linear transducer of at least 5 to 10 MHz. These frequencies are ideal for imaging relatively superficial structures. Following a standard protocol, start with the arterial system in the nondominant arm. If the arteries have acceptable size of >25 mm, proceed to imaging the venous system. If an abnormality is discovered in either the arteries or veins in the nondominant arm, consider imaging the contralateral arm.

The preoperative assessment of the arterial system includes direct imaging with ultrasound and in select situations indirect evaluation with physiologic testing. (Chapter 11 discusses the indirect evaluation of the upper extremity arterial system.) Studies are routinely performed only in the nondominant arm unless otherwise indicated by the referring physician.

B-mode grayscale imaging is used to assess the diameters of the ulnar and radial arteries. Measurements can be obtained at several locations along both vessels, but often a proximal and distal diameter measurement is adequate. Many laboratories also include a diameter measurement of the brachial artery in the event a more proximal fistula placement is planned. Arteries should also be assessed for calcification, intimal thickness, stenosis, and compliance (Fig. 30-3). Studies have shown that the quality of the arterial wall determines the capacity of the artery to dilate and accommodate the increased flow. In cases where an atherosclerotic vessel is present, the vessel is unable to compensatorily dilate, and thus increased flow is entirely dependent on the native arterial diameter. Generally, atherosclerosis in the upper extremities is most often observed in the subclavian artery. However, diabetic patients and those with chronic renal disease, the brachial, radial, and ulnar arteries often possess atherosclerotic disease.

B-mode grayscale imaging is used to assess the superficial arm veins and their spatial relationships. This begins in the transverse plane with evaluation of the cephalic, basilic, and median cubital veins starting at the wrist and moving proximally. B-mode imaging should confirm that the vein walls are compressible, free of thrombus, webbing, and calcium (Fig. 30-4). Transverse compression of the vein should be performed every 2 cm, and the diameter of the veins is recorded along their entire length (Fig. 30-5). Close attention should be paid to the antecubital fossa and areas of prior needle puncture. Documentation of vessel characteristics should include patency, depth, wall thickness, calcification, and location of thrombus or fibrosis.

A tourniquet may be used to restrict venous outflow allowing the vein to fully dilate. The tourniquet is placed just below the antecubital fossa to measure the diameter of the forearm veins and at the axillary region to measure the diameter of the veins of the upper arm.

Spectral Doppler analysis is performed in a sagittal plane. All Doppler studies are performed at an angle of 60 degrees or less with respect to the direction of flow. The actual venous velocity is not import; however, by using an angle of insonation of 60 degrees or less, an adequate Doppler

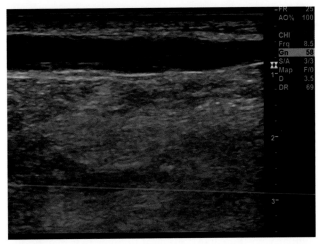

**FIGURE 30-4** Sagittal image of an arm vein with wall thickening and webbing present.

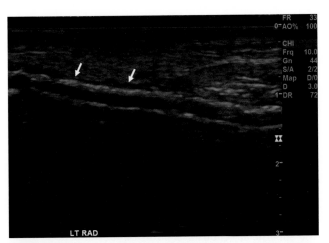

**FIGURE 30-3** Ultrasound image of a calcified radial artery. Note the bright white reflectors (*arrows*) along the vessel wall with acoustic shadowing.

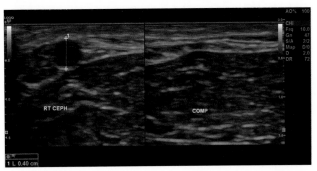

**FIGURE 30-5** Noncompressed and compressed images confirming patency in this cephalic vein. Vein diameter is also measured as 0.40 cm.

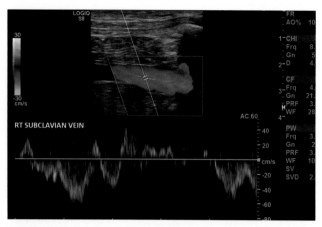

**FIGURE 30-6** Doppler imaging of the mid-subclavian vein showing respiratory phasicity.

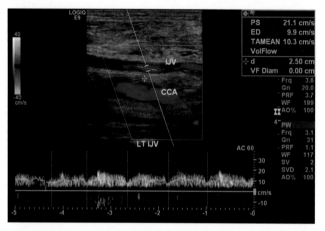

**FIGURE 30-7** Image of left internal jugular vein (IJV) with retrograde flow demonstrated in both the color-image and spectral waveforms. This indicates more central venous disease.

signal will be obtained. To complete the venous examination, spectral waveforms are performed while compressing the limb proximally or distally to demonstrate augmentation of venous flow. Patency of the proximal deep veins (brachial, axillary, and subclavian) should be confirmed. Spectral Doppler waveforms, including phasicity and flow direction, should be checked in the mid-subclavian vein and internal jugular vein (Fig. 30-6). Atypical findings that may be life threatening (central vein thrombosis) should immediately be conveyed to a health care provider (Fig. 30-7).

### Technical Considerations

Upon completion of the examination, preliminary results should be documented by the vascular technologist. A worksheet and brief summary will aid the interpreting physician who reviews the diagnostic images and report. Proper documentation is essential and includes examination date, indications for the procedure, technologists name, arm studied, and the patient's identification information. Any deviation from the protocol should be documented and explained on the worksheet.

The routine unilateral upper extremity vein mapping examination should expect to require 30 to 40 minutes. The goals are to provide an accurate high-quality examination,

and thus appropriate time should be allotted for the completion of this examination.

### Pitfalls

There are very few contraindications to this ultrasound-guided assessment. Some contraindications include local infections, obtrusive dressings, open wounds, and restricted patient positioning. Attempts should be made to adapt by using various approaches and scanning orientations to work around some of these obstacles.

## Diagnosis

For the assessment of the radial, ulnar, and brachial arteries, an arterial diameter of greater than 25 mm is expected for fistula creation and maturation. An artery at the antecubital fossa that is smaller than expected or the presence of two arteries at this site can indicate an anomalous takeoff of radial artery. The anomalous takeoff of the radial artery has been suggested to occur at the frequency of 5% to 10%. If an anomalous radial artery is present, the origin of the bifurcation should be documented because it may impact surgical planning. The grayscale image should demonstrate smooth walled vessels that are free of disease. Calcification will appear as bright white echoes along or within the vessel walls. Hypoechoic plaque may be difficult to demonstrate on a grayscale image and better delineated using color Doppler to demonstrate incomplete filling of the vessel lumen. The normal arterial spectral Doppler waveform should be high resistive with a rapid upstroke, sharp peak, and low-diastolic flow (Fig. 30-8).

Venous criteria for acceptable conduit diameter vary between physicians. Although there is no consensus, a favorable vessel diameter for creation of AV access is greater than 2.5 mm. Using this diameter as a minimum, it has been shown that high early maturation rates as well as an 83% 1 year patency rate can be obtained.[4] Vein walls should be completely compressible with light transducer pressure. A partially compressible or noncompressible vein suggests the presence of an occluding thrombus within the vein lumen, making it unusable as an autogenous conduit. In some instances, large tributaries may drain superficial forearm veins into complimentary or deep veins which can aid in maturation despite small or thrombosed upper arm veins.

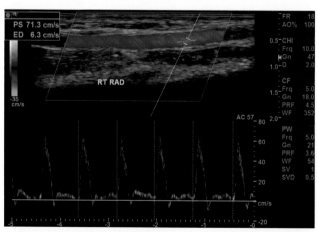

**FIGURE 30-8** Normal spectral waveform in the radial artery.

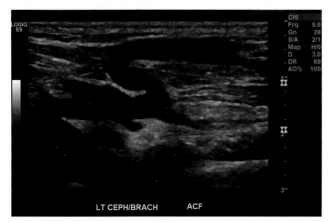

**FIGURE 30-9** Cephalic vein with large draining vein at the antecubital fossa.

For example, a suitable forearm cephalic vein may still be used if there is an adequate antecubital vein which drains the cephalic vein into the brachial or basilic vein, even in the presence of a small or thrombosed upper arm cephalic vein (Fig. 30-9). These tributaries should be noted to aid in operative planning. Venous Doppler signals from the central veins should display respiratory phasicity, cardiac pulsatility, and augmentation. These characteristics should be used to indirectly confirm patency of the central venous system.

## HEMODIALYSIS ACCESS EVALUATION

The goal of hemodialysis access is to provide a durable site for cannulation which is placed distally in the limb. This strategy allows the option for creation of a more proximal access should the distal AV fistula fail. There are numerous types of autogenous forearm AV access. Table 30-1 summarizes the various types of upper extremity AV access. A Brescia-Cimino fistula is frequently performed and involves mobilizing the distal cephalic vein at the wrist and

| TABLE 30-1 | **Types of Autogenous Arteriovenous Access** |
|---|---|
| **FOREARM** | |
| • Posterior radial artery to cephalic vein (snuffbox fistula) | |
| • Radial artery to cephalic vein (Brescia-Cimino fistula) | |
| • Radial artery to cephalic forearm vein transposition | |
| • Brachial artery to cephalic forearm vein-looped transposition | |
| • Radial artery to basilic forearm vein transposition | |
| • Ulnar artery to basilic forearm vein transposition | |
| • Brachial artery to basilic forearm vein-looped transposition | |
| **UPPER ARM** | |
| • Brachial artery to cephalic vein fistula | |
| • Brachial artery to basilic vein transposition | |
| • Brachial artery to brachial vein transposition | |

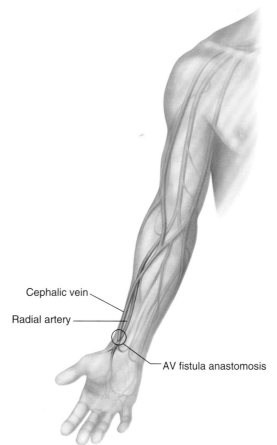

Cephalic vein

Radial artery

AV fistula anastomosis

**FIGURE 30-10** Diagram illustrating a radiocephalic fistula.

anastomosing it to the distal radial artery in an end-to-side configuration (Fig. 30-10). This type of fistula is ideal owing to its distal location and need for minimal dissection and vessel mobilization (Fig. 30-11). Occasionally, a "snuffbox fistula" may be created by connecting the posterior branch of the radial artery to the cephalic vein. In situations where the cephalic vein is suboptimal, the basilic vein is preferred. The medial location of the forearm basilic vein requires that it be transposed and juxtaposed to a distal artery (radial or ulnar) in order to create an AV fistula.

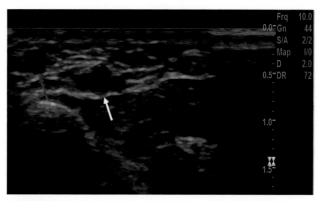

**FIGURE 30-11** Grayscale image of distal radial artery (*white arrow*) and distal cephalic vein (*blue arrow*) at the level of a planned radiocephalic (Brescia-Cimino) fistula.

Upper arm (proximal to the antecubital fossa) autogenous access is necessary when distal access options are not suitable or have failed. The most common upper arm access is a brachial artery to cephalic vein fistula which is created at the antecubital fossa (Fig. 30-12). For those patients with suboptimal cephalic veins, the upper arm basilic vein can be used, but because of its deep location, transposition of this vein is necessary (Fig. 30-13). Possible sites for arterial inflow include the brachial, radial, and ulnar arteries.

If the upper extremity is not suitable for access creation, the lower extremity may be used. A hemodialysis access can be created using the common femoral or superficial femoral arteries for inflow and transposed great saphenous or femoral veins. These types of lower extremity access are less frequently used for various reasons.

Approximately 8 to 12 weeks after the creation of an autogenous fistula, it should be mature and ready for needle cannulation. Fistula maturation is defined as a dilated, palpable, fistula that is suitable for hemodialysis with flow rates of >350 mL/min.[5] For those that failed to mature, it should be closely interrogated with ultrasound imaging. Low maturation rates correspond to the use of small or suboptimal veins for fistula creation.[2] Berman and Gentile were able to demonstrate a 10% improvement in autogenous access use with close follow-up and early secondary interventions.[6] This includes open revision, tributary ligation, or coil embolization (Fig. 30-14), as well as endovascular intervention and vein superficialization.

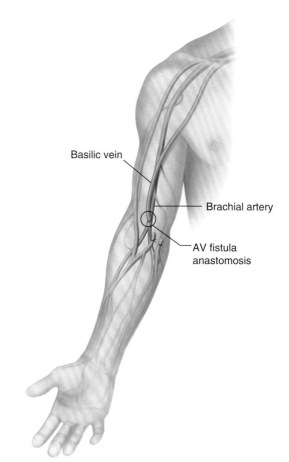

**FIGURE 30-13** Diagram illustrating a basilic transposition fistula.

Long-term follow-up of fistulae and grafts (Fig. 30-15) is essential for improved patency. Frequently, outflow vein segments, anastomoses, and vein to graft anastomoses develop a stenosis secondary to intimal hyperplasia (Fig. 30-16). Other indications for routine follow-up include pseudoaneurysm formation (Figs. 30-17 and 30-18), midgraft stenosis, and arterial stenosis. Vascular Professional Performance Guidelines have been established by The Society for Vascular Ultrasound,[7] and indications for evaluation include pseudoaneurysm formation, pulsatile mass, decreased thrill with pulsatile or absent flow, difficult cannulation, elevated recirculation time (>12%), elevated venous pressure during dialysis (>200 mm Hg), low-urea reduction rate (<60%), excessive bleeding following dialysis, arm edema, infection, and arterial steal symptoms. The same preoperative vein mapping contraindications are applied here.

## Sonographic Examination Technique

### Patient Preparation

As mentioned in the preceding section on preoperative scanning, the technologist should introduce himself or herself and explain why the dialysis access evaluation is being performed. An introduction and explanation of the technique, including the duration of study, is an essential component to all testing. During this time, any questions and concerns from the patient can be addressed. The room should be comfortably warm to avoid vasospasm.

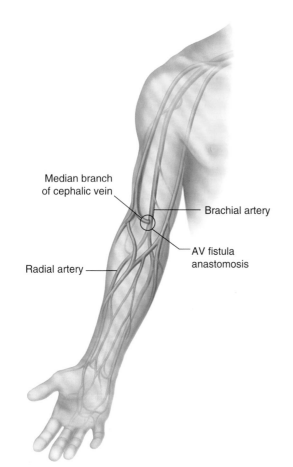

**FIGURE 30-12** Diagram illustrating a brachiocephalic fistula.

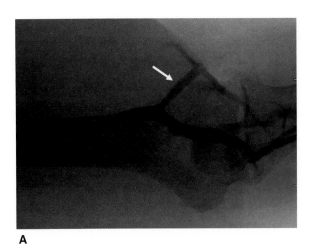

A

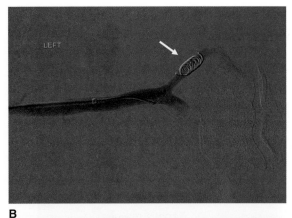

B

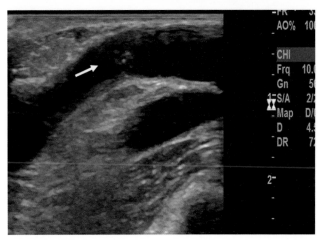

C

**FIGURE 30-14** **A:** Fistulogram indicating a large venous tributary (*arrow*). **B:** Placement of coil into tributary (*arrow*). **C:** Color ultrasound image of coil (*arrow*) in venous tributary.

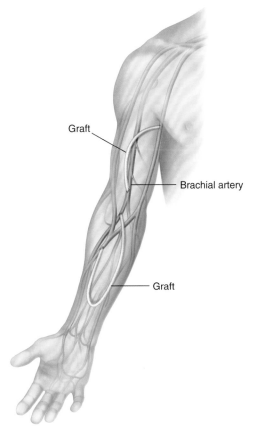

Graft

Brachial artery

Graft

**FIGURE 30-15** Diagram illustrating a forearm loop AV graft and upper arm AV graft.

**FIGURE 30-16** An AV fistula stenosis (*arrow*).

## Patient Assessment

The patient assessment is similar to that used for the preoperative testing and should be completed prior to initiating the procedure. A comprehensive medical and surgical history should be documented, including the patient's ability to tolerate the imaging study. Any potential contraindications should be determined. The history should include all previous access procedures, trauma history, medications, and arm dominance. If available, reviewing access diagrams or operative notes will clarify the access type and location. Specifically, inquire about any risk factors that may preclude fistula maturation or use, such as central venous thrombosis,

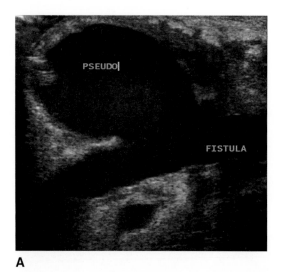
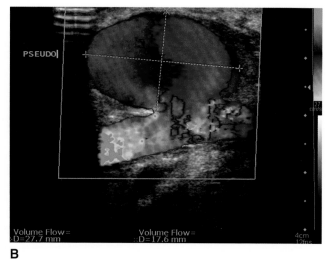

**FIGURE 30-17** **A:** Grayscale image of a pseudoaneurysm. **B:** Same pseudoaneurysm with color-flow imaging demonstrating the "yin-yang" appearance in the color pattern.

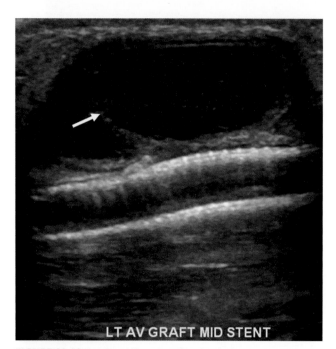

**FIGURE 30-18** A patient with a covered stent graft placed within an AV access to exclude a pseudoaneurysm (**arrow**).

placement of central venous catheters, pacemakers, or defibrillators. The focused physical examination should include a quantitative examination of the fistula or graft. Assessment of the presence of a thrill and the quality of the thrill throughout the entire access is important. Visual inspection of the arm and access site is necessary to assess for edema, redness, presence of collateral veins, rotation of access sites, and focal dilations.

## Patient Positioning

Optimal patient positioning may be either in the supine or sitting position with the arm extended and relaxed. Depending on the exact placement of the dialysis access site, the arm position may need to be adjusted during the course of the examination.

## Scanning Techniques

The patient and arm are placed in a comfortable position. Use minimal pressure and abundant ultrasound gel to optimize imaging. Characteristics of vessels, tissue, and blood flow must be observed and analyzed in order to ensure that appropriate data is documented for the interpreting physician. Appropriate labeling of structures and orientation is important because of the often confusing nature of a dialysis access. Spectral analysis with or without color Doppler imaging should be performed using a carrier frequency of at least 7 to 12 MHz. System presets should be adjusted to the high-flow settings, and decreasing color gain will minimize tissue bruit. Use B-mode to assess for various abnormalities such as perigraft masses, pseudoaneurysm, stenotic valves, and intimal flaps. Perigraft fluid collections and pseudoaneurysm can be differentiated using B-mode, color-flow imaging, and Doppler imaging. The fistula diameter should be measured along its length. Scanning the fistula in a transverse view will locate side branch tributary veins which can limit fistula maturation. Measure these tributary vein diameters and document their locations.

Doppler evaluation is used to document patency of the fistula and identify areas of stenosis. Doppler spectral analysis is performed in the sagittal plane. All Doppler samples must be performed at an angle of 60 degrees or less with respect to the direction of flow. Doppler cursor alignment should be parallel to the direction of flow. When a stenosis is found, velocities should be measured proximal, distal, and within the area of interest. Arterial inflow is first assessed with duplex imaging (Fig. 30-19). The inflow artery supplying a dialysis access should demonstrate a low-resistance waveform with constant antegrade flow throughout the cardiac cycle. Peak systolic velocities (PSV) should be recorded in the native artery proximal to the anastomosis, at the anastomosis, throughout the body of the fistula, and along the venous outflow. Scanning throughout the entire fistula or graft, obtaining spectral signals, and paying close attention to the needle puncture sites are essential. The examination must include the venous outflow and in some cases may extend into the chest for the assessment of the central veins. Color-flow imaging is helpful in this location.

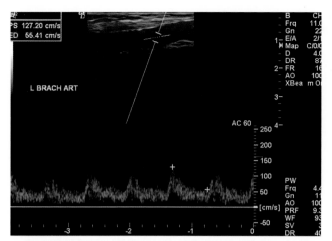

**FIGURE 30-19** Brachial artery inflow to dialysis access. Note the low-resistance waveform with constant antegrade flow throughout the cardiac cycle.

Volume flow measurements are useful when evaluating access function and are best accomplished with a wide-open sample gate. Volume flow calculations should be made in the midgraft or fistula at a site of normal flow, free of stenosis, tortuosity, and focal dilatation. The volumetric flow (mL/min) is calculated as: flow = time average velocity × area × 60. The area is calculated based on (½ diameter)$^2$ π. Most modern ultrasound systems are capable of measuring this automatically. The technologist manually measures the diameter which the ultrasound system then uses to calculate the area. A Doppler spectrum is recorded from which the system calculates the time average velocity. The time average velocity should be measured over three to four cardiac cycles to obtain an accurate calculation (Fig. 30-20). Some laboratories choose to obtain triplicate measurements of volume flow and average these three values to improve accuracy. Recently, some have also chosen to measure volume flow at an additional location within the inflow artery.

## Technical Considerations

Documentation should include the examination date, indications for the procedure, technologists name, arm studied, and the patient's identification information. Vessel characteristics, including patency, wall thickness, calcification, and

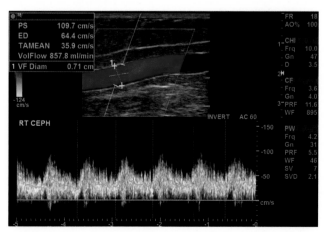

**FIGURE 30-20** A duplex ultrasound of a fistula with volume flow calculated.

thrombus content, should be recorded. Documentation of native vessel or fistula stenosis or thrombosis, anastomotic lesions, PSVs, poststenotic turbulence, or reversal of flow in arterial segments distal to the anastomosis is necessary. Any deviation from the protocol must be documented and explained. Similar to preoperative vein mapping for dialysis access, a thorough surveillance imaging of a fistula or graft with direct and indirect components will routinely require 35 to 45 minutes.

### Pitfalls

The examination of a fistula or graft presents a few unique challenges. It is a very superficial structure, and as such, it is possible to inadvertently partially compress it if too much transducer pressure is applied by the technologist or sonographer. This transducer pressure can result in elevated velocities recorded during the examination. Care should be taken to avoid excess transducer pressure. Another factor related to the position of the fistula or graft involves scanning mature access sites. As both fistulae and grafts age, they dilate, can become aneurysmal, can develop pseudoaneurysms, and can become tortuous (Fig. 30-21). All of these conditions make for an irregular scanning surface on the arm. The surface irregularities may require larger amounts of gel to maintain proper skin contact. Large pseudoaneurysms may require scanning from various approaches to fully document all findings. Occasionally, patients present with contraindications to scanning, including dressings, open wounds, or possibly decreased mobility leading to poor patient positioning.

## Diagnosis

The grayscale image should reveal an access free of thrombus or calcifications. Thrombus may appear hypoechoic or anechoic depending on its age (Fig. 30-22). Calcifications will appear as bright white reflectors with the vessel walls. In a fistula, the valves within the vein should not be evident and typically are adhered to the vessel wall. An incompetent valve projecting into the vessel lumen potentially could be a site for intimal hyperplasia formation.

Velocities through a fistula can vary greatly depending of vessel diameter, flow volume, and maturity of the fistula. A well-functioning fistula will have a PSV between 150 and 300 cm/s and end-diastolic velocities (EDV) of 60 to 200 cm/s (Fig. 30-23).[8] An anastomotic stenosis of >50% is suggested by a PSV ratio (anastomosis/2 cm upstream artery) of greater than 3:1. A venous outflow stenosis of >50% is represented by a PSV ratio (stenosis/vein 2 cm upstream) of greater than 2:1 (Fig. 30-24). A stenosis may also be present within fistula or the inflow/outflow vessels if the PSV of the fistula is <50 cm/s.[9] Marked spectral broadening, continuous forward diastolic flow, and a high velocity are expected to be seen throughout the fistula. The inflow artery will have a low-resistance flow, and increased PSV (30 to 100 cm/s) with pulsatility will be noted in the outflow vein.

## Disorders

Anastomotic and vein stenoses account for the majority (80%) of access complications. Multiple stenoses are not infrequently found in AV grafts. Outflow vein stenoses are represented by echogenic intraluminal lesions

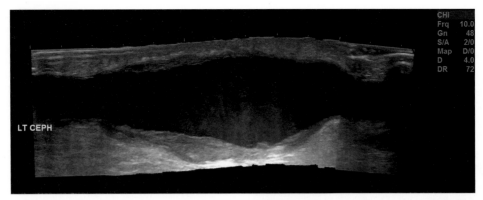

**FIGURE 30-21** Aneurysmal dilatation of an AV fistula.

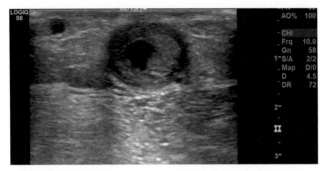

**FIGURE 30-22** Transverse image of an AV fistula with thrombus.

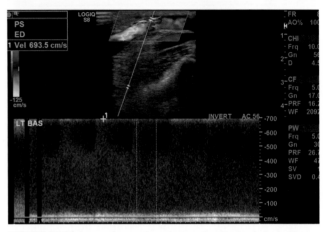

**FIGURE 30-24** Image of an anastomotic stenosis with elevated velocities.

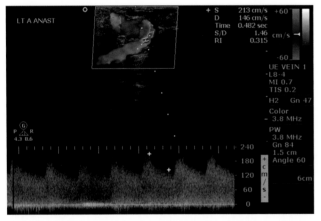

**FIGURE 30-23** Color-flow imaging and spectral Doppler of a normally functioning fistula.

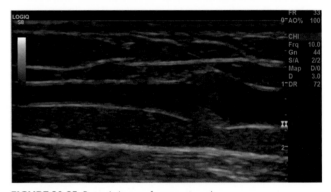

**FIGURE 30-25** B-mode image of venous stenosis.

which have luminal flow reduction on B-mode imaging (Fig. 30-25). A fistula or graft occlusion is represented by a high-resistance signal, absent flow lumen, and intraluminal echogenic thrombus (Fig. 30-26). Pathology Box 30-1 summarizes ultrasound findings of both normal and abnormal AV fistulae.

A normal flow volume should be >800 mL/min. A mild to moderate stenosis will decrease the volume of flow to 500 to 800 mL/min. If a severe stenosis is represented, the expected flow volume will be <500 mL/min.[9] When evaluating a new fistula or graft that has had adequate time to mature, a flow volume of <800 mL/min should prompt a careful interrogation for the cause of the reduction. This may include stenosis of the inflow artery, anastomosis, or outflow vein, central venous stenosis or occlusion, or large competing venous tributaries.

Retrograde flow in the artery distal to a fistula or graft anastomosis is a relatively common finding and is known as steal phenomenon that occurs in 75% to 90% of patients after access creation. Based on fluid dynamics, the low-resistance outflow vein draws antegrade flow from the inflow artery and in addition "steals" retrograde flow from the distal artery often through the intact palmer arch. The majority (95% to 98%) of the patients with steal phenomenon are asymptomatic. Patients with a symptomatic steal syndrome present with pain during hemodialysis or rest pain, and if advanced, tissue loss (i.e., ulcerations or gangrene). Defining the cause of

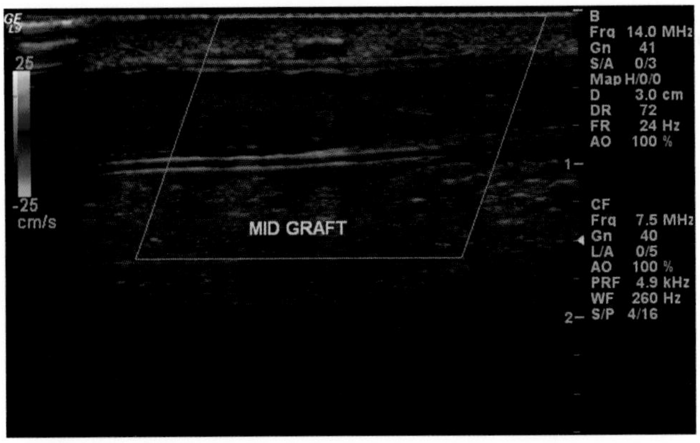

**FIGURE 30-26** Occluded AV graft with no color filling and thrombus presence within the graft.

steal syndrome is beyond the scope of this chapter but simplistically can be described as a problem with high flow through the fistula, insufficient distal collateral circulation, inflow arterial stenosis, or a combination. The diagnosis of steal syndrome is primarily a clinical diagnosis; however, noninvasive physiologic testing can confirm the diagnosis by measuring pressure and flow distal to the fistula which provides supportive evidence. A digital pressure of <40 mm Hg or a digital-brachial pressure index of <0.6 both describe patients with significant steal syndrome.

## PATHOLOGY BOX 30-1
### Arteriovenous Fistula Ultrasound Findings

| | B-Mode | Color Flow | Doppler |
|---|---|---|---|
| Normal AV fistula | Anechoic flow lumen free of intraluminal echoes | Lumen fills wall to wall with color flow | Low-resistive pulsatile flow without focal velocity elevation |
| Stenotic AV fistula | Intraluminal echoes, thickened walls | Reduced flow lumen, disturbed color-flow patterns | Elevated velocities in region of stenosis $V_r > 2$ in feeding artery or outflow vein $V_r > 3$ at anastomosis |
| Occluded AV fistula | Intraluminal echogenicity, loss of flow lumen | No flow | Absent Doppler signal |

$V_r$, volume ratio.

## SUMMARY

- Ultrasound imaging when used in conjunction with clinical examination has proven to be an extremely powerful tool for evaluation and management of hemodialysis access.
- Ultrasound is a highly sensitive noninvasive technique that complements the physical examination.
- Preoperative imaging of both the arterial and venous systems should routinely be performed to guide the physician when determining the ideal hemodialysis access site.
- Ultrasound imaging has proven to improve fistula maturation and have become the standard of care for preoperative access assessment.
- In addition, ultrasonography has shown to be extremely beneficial for access surveillance that appears to prolong access patency.

## CRITICAL THINKING QUESTIONS

1. B-mode imaging reveals a small (1.75 mm) calcified radial artery. What is the next step in the evaluation of this patient?

2. Dilated chest wall veins are found during the examination of a patient with a pacemaker and nonmaturing AV fistula. What noninvasive imaging study is recommended?
3. One week after creation of a radiocephalic fistula, a patient returns with a patent fistula and cool painful hand. What is the expected direction of flow in the distal native radial artery?
4. To assess fistula function, volumetric flow calculations are best measured in what part of the AV fistula?
5. A patient presents with a pulsatile mass superficial to an AV graft. A to-and-fro waveform pattern is seen at the base of the pulsatile mass. What is the diagnosis?

## MEDIA MENU

Student Resources available on thePoint® include:
- Audio glossary
- Interactive question bank
- Videos
- Internet resource

## REFERENCES

1. Sidawy AN. Arteriovenous hemodialysis access: The Society for Vascular Surgery practice guidelines. *J Vasc Surg*. 2008;48:1S–80S.
2. Macsata RA, Sidawy AN. Hemodialysis access: general considerations. In: *Rutherford's Vascular Surgery*. 7th ed. Philadelphia, PA: Saunders Elsevier; 2010:1104–1114.
3. Society for Vascular Ultrasound. Upper Extremity Vein Mapping for Placement of a Dialysis Access or Peripheral Bypass Graft. Vascular Technology Professional Performance Guidelines. Available at: http://connect.svunet.org/communities1/community-home/librarydocuments/viewdocument?DocumentKey=010e5be5-60a0-45a9-bf06-c3525440d498. Accessed September, 2016.
4. Silva MB, Hobson RW, Pappas PJ, et al. A strategy for increasing use of autogenous hemodialysis access procedures: impact of preoperative noninvasive evaluation. *J Vasc Surg*. 1998;27:302–308.
5. Miller PE, Tolwani A, Luscy CP, et al. Predictors of adequacy of arteriovenous fistulas in hemodialysis patients. *Kidney Int*. 1999;56(1):275–288.

6. Berman SS, Gentile AT. Impact of secondary procedures in autogenous arteriovenous fistula maturation and maintenance. *J Vasc Surg*. 2001;34:866–871.

7. Society for Vascular Ultrasound. Evaluation of Dialysis Access. Vascular Technology Professional Performance Guidelines. Available at: http://connect.svunet.org/communities1/community-home/librarydocuments/viewdocument?DocumentKey=a0784c6d-e522-4e3f-b5a1-718eefcde939. Accessed September, 2016.

8. Robbin ML, Lockhart ME. Ultrasound evaluation before and after hemodialysis access. In: Zweibel WJ, ed. *Introduction to Vascular Ultrasonography*. 5th ed. Philadelphia, PA: Elsevier Saunders; 2005:325–340.

9. Wellen J, Shenoy S. Ultrasound in vascular access. In: Wilson SE, ed. *Vascular Access Principles and Practice*. 1st ed. Philadelphia, PA: Lippincott Williams & Wilkins; 2010:232–240.

# Evaluation of Penile Blood Flow

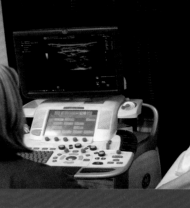

VICKI M. GATZ | SCOTT G. ERPELDING | SHUBHAM GUPTA

**CHAPTER 31**

## OBJECTIVES

- List the indications for a penile ultrasound examination
- Define the blood vessels examined during a penile ultrasound
- Explain the techniques used to measure a penile-brachial index
- Describe the diagnostic criteria used for penile examinations

## KEY TERMS

**cavernosal artery**

**corpora cavernosa**

**erectile dysfunction**

**penile-brachial index**

**Peyronie's disease**

**tunica albuginea**

## GLOSSARY

**cavernosal artery** One of three terminal branches of the common penile artery. It supplies blood flow to the corpora cavernosa

**corpora cavernosa** Two paired areas of spongy erectile tissue

**erectile dysfunction** The persistent inability to achieve or maintain an erection suitable for sexual intercourse; also known as impotence

**penile-brachial index** The ratio of penile systolic pressure and brachial systolic pressure

**Peyronie's disease** An acquired penile deformity caused by fibrosis of the tunica albuginea resulting in plaque formation

**priapism** Full or partial erection that continues more than 4 hours beyond sexual stimulation and orgasm or is unrelated to sexual stimulation

**tunica albuginea** The tough fibrous layer of connective tissue that surrounds the corpora cavernosa of the penis

Duplex Doppler ultrasound of the penis is an important tool in the evaluation and treatment for urologic diseases, specifically Peyronie's disease (PD) and erectile dysfunction (ED). In fact, the American Urologic Association (AUA) recognizes duplex Doppler ultrasound as an important tool to consider prior to proceeding with invasive treatments.[1] Duplex ultrasound of the penis and the cavernosal arteries was first described by Lue and colleagues in 1985.[2] The combination of high-resolution imaging and Doppler waveform analysis provides valuable information in the evaluation of penile abnormalities.

## ANATOMY

The arterial vascular supply to the penis originates from the internal iliac that branches into the internal pudendal that subsequently branches into the common penile artery.

The common penile artery has three branches (cavernous, bulbourethral, and dorsal). The cavernous branch supplies the corpora cavernosa. The corpora cavernosa are two masses of erectile tissue that are composed of multiple sinusoidal chambers. The tunica albuginea is a dense fibrous sheath that surrounds the sinusoids. The bulbourethral artery supplies the corpus spongiosum that contains the urethra. The dorsal artery courses along the dorsal aspect of the penis and supplies the glans and other nonerectile tissue (Fig. 31-1). As with all vasculature, variants exist and commonly come from the external iliac, obturator, and femoral arteries.[3] Venous drainage of the corporal bodies originates from venules below the tunica albuginea; this perforates the tunica through emissary veins. Dorsally, the circumflex and deep dorsal veins drain into the internal iliac or internal pudendal vein through the periprostatic plexus (Fig. 31-2). Ventrally, the bulbourethral, bulbar, crural, and cavernous

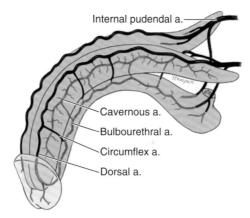

**FIGURE 31-1** The arterial vasculature of the penis. (Adapted with permission from Wein AJ, Kavoussi LR, Partin AW, et al. *Campbell-Walsh Urology.* 11th ed. Philadelphia, PA: Elsevier; 2016.)

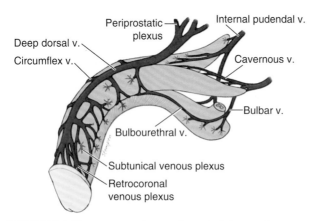

**FIGURE 31-2** The venous vasculature of the penis. (Adapted with permission from Wein AJ, Kavoussi LR, Partin AW, et al. *Campbell-Walsh Urology.* 11th ed. Philadelphia, PA: Elsevier; 2016.)

veins drain directly into the internal pudendal vein or branch into the periprostatic plexus.

## INDICATIONS

There are several indications for the ultrasound examination of the penis, including trauma, penile fracture, masses, or cancer. The evaluation of penile blood flow is performed in patients with PD and in those with ED.

## Peyronie's Disease

PD is an acquired penile deformity caused by fibrosis of the tunica albuginea, resulting in plaque formation. Fibrotic plaques in PD are thought to be caused by buckling of the penile shaft in an erect or a semi-erect state. This repetitive trauma causes microvascular tears in the penile shaft that results in changes in collagen deposition within the tunica with subsequent plaque formation, resulting in penile curvature.[4]

PD affects 0.5% to 20% of men depending on which patient population is being sampled. Dibenedetti et al.[5] reported that 0.5% of men per year were formally diagnosed with PD, whereas other studies reported prevalence rates between 3% and 5%.[6] PD can be accompanied by pain, deformity, emotional distress, and ED. Other causes of penile deformity distinguished from PD include congenital causes such as congenital curvature, corporal body disproportion, and chordee. Acquired causes of penile deformity include PD as well as iatrogenic chordee secondary to penile surgery.

The AUA recommends that all patients with PD have an intracavernosal injection (ICI) with or without duplex Doppler ultrasound prior to performing invasive treatments. The objectives of ICI with penile Doppler are to assess plaque size and characteristics such as the presence of calcifications because this can alter treatment modalities. Ultrasound is vital in assessing the blood flow to the corporal bodies. Physical examination objectives are to study penile curvature as well as other characteristics such as whether the curvature is monoplanar, biplanar, or multiplanar or if an hourglass deformity is appreciated.

ICI with penile Doppler should be performed when any invasive procedure is being planned such as prior to plaque excision and grafting or penile prosthesis placement, especially in patients with baseline ED because this would help direct treatment options. For example, the presence of dense calcification or curvature greater than 90 degrees would suggest that treatments such as intralesional plaque injections may be ineffective. Furthermore, in patients with marginal erectile function, or evidence of arterial insufficiency on penile Doppler, plaque excision and grafting holds a risk of worsening erectile function, which may render a patient impotent.

## Erectile Dysfunction

The physiologic process of an erection requires an increase in arterial inflow, smooth muscle relaxation in the corpora cavernosa, and an increase in venous resistance. During an erection, the arterial flow into the penis increases as the cavernosal artery dilates. The smooth muscle in the walls of the cavernosal sinusoids relaxes, which allows the sinusoids to expand and fill with blood. As the sinusoids fill, the corpora cavernosa expand, and the draining veins are pushed against the walls of the rigid tunica albuginea, resulting in veno-occlusion. These series of coordinated events rely heavily on the presence of a normal vascular system.

ED is a common problem in an aging male population with some studies estimating ED affecting over 30% to 50% of men aged 40 to 70 years.[7] Approximately 80% of ED is attributed to vascular disease.[8] There is a clear relationship between ED and PD; however, the extent of the relationship is debated. Some authorities believe that ED is integral in the development of PD. Patients with ED are thought to be more likely to have penile buckling during sexual activity, and therefore to have trauma, resulting in plaque formation. In general, most clinicians believe that penile deformity, emotional distress, and pain all contribute to ED, with the most common thread being vascular abnormalities.[9] Patients with ED may have hemodynamic abnormalities with arterial insufficiency, venous incompetence, or both. Arterial insufficiency can result from stenosis or occlusion in arteries which feed into the penile artery. Arterial causes of ED are more common in patients with diabetes, hypertension, hypercholesterolemia, and a smoking history.

## Priapism

Priapism is a persistent unwanted erection. Most priapism episodes are related to pathologically impaired drainage of blood from the penile bodies causing stasis of deoxygenated blood and a compartment syndrome within the penis—also called ischemic priapism or "low-flow" priapism. These are typically seen as a side effect of ED medications such as phosphodiesterase inhibitors, ICIs, and occasionally with other medication/substance use like trazodone, cocaine, and marijuana. A small subset of priapism episodes can be because of an abnormal communication between the penile arterial system and the cavernosal sinusoids. This is called "nonischemic" or "high-flow" priapism, and is mostly related to trauma. The treatments for low-flow and high-flow priapism are completely different, and therefore this distinction is essential. Doppler ultrasound can be used for differentiation between these two priapism categories, and can help guide further management. Specifically, in a case of high-flow, nonischemic priapism, intact or mildly increased resting flow is noted in the cavernosal arteries, and occasionally, the fistulous connection can be demonstrated as well. In most cases, the distinction between low-flow and high-flow priapism can be made on the basis of penile blood gas measurements, and color Doppler is not frequently utilized for this indication.

## NONIMAGING EXAMINATION TECHNIQUES

Penile-brachial pressure index or penile-brachial pressure (PBI) refers to measuring the arterial pressure of the penis divided by the brachial systolic blood pressure. Just as the ankle-brachial index (ABI) is a noninvasive tool to assess for peripheral vascular disease, the PBI is a noninvasive way to assess for penile vascular health.

### Patient Preparation and Positioning

There is no specific patient preparation required for this examination. The procedure should be explained to patient, and any questions should be answered. The patient is asked to undress from the waist down and provided a cover sheet or drape. The examination is performed with the patient supine.

### Equipment

Physiologic equipment is used to inflate cuffs for systolic pressure determinations. A continuous wave (CW) Doppler transducer is used to record waveforms and insonate arteries. A photoplethysmograph (PPG) may also be used to obtain pressures and waveforms. Because the vessels are relatively superficial, an 8-MHz CW Doppler transducer is usually sufficient.

Various sized blood pressure cuffs should be available. The measurement of brachial and ankle pressures usually require a 10-cm wide cuff, but this may vary depending on body habitus. For penile pressures, the cuff size can be 2.5 × 12.5 cm or 2.5 × 9 cm.

## Examination Technique

Most laboratory protocols include the measurement of an ABI in addition to the PBI. Appropriately sized cuffs are placed around each upper arm and at the each ankle. The brachial artery is insonated with the CW Doppler transducer. While listening to the brachial artery Doppler signal, the cuff on the upper arm is inflated until the signal is no longer heard. The pressure in the cuff is slowly deflated until the signal returns, marking the systolic blood pressure. This pressure determination is repeated for the contralateral arm. Ankle pressures are then recorded in the same manner insonating the posterior tibial and dorsalis pedis arteries bilaterally. The ABI is calculated by dividing the highest ankle pressure for each ankle by the highest brachial pressure. Most physiologic equipment performs this calculation automatically.

Some protocols also include obtaining a common femoral artery waveform. A CW Doppler held at approximately a 45-degree angle is used to insonate the common femoral artery, and a waveform is recorded.

Next, the PBI is obtained by placing a 2.5 cm digital cuff around the base of the flaccid penis. Either a PPG or CW Doppler may be used to measure the penile pressure. A PPG sensor is attached with double stick tape to the side of the penis, and a waveform is obtained. Pressure in the cuff is then inflated to 20 to 30 mm Hg above the pressure at which the obliteration of signal occurs. Normal penile systolic pressure is less than brachial systolic pressure so care should be taken to not overinflate the cuff pressure. The pressure in the cuff is then slowly deflated. The penile systolic pressure is noted at the point of the return of the PPG waveform. PPG is moved to contralateral side and repeated. PPG is then applied to dorsum of the penis and measurement repeated. A CW Doppler can be used in place of the PPG. The CW Doppler is placed just proximal to the glans, and the dorsal artery is located. The same inflation techniques are used.

## Pitfalls

This indirect technique does not provide specific anatomic information on the arterial or venous systems and does not provide additional anatomic information such as the presence of plaques. This technique does not assess physiologic changes that occur within the vasculature during an erection. Therefore, some have found the PBI of limited value in determining vascular causes for ED.[10,11]

## DIAGNOSIS

A multiphasic femoral arterial CW waveform is normal. Standard waveform criteria should be applied to the femoral waveforms with appropriate grading criteria (see Chapter 11). An ABI greater than 1.0 is normal. ABI values less than 1.0 indicate the presence of arterial disease which, depending on the level of disease, may impact blood flow to the penile arteries. The ABI may also be graded using appropriate criteria (see Chapter 11).

A PBI greater than 0.7 is considered normal. A PBI of between 0.6 and 0.7 is often reported as borderline abnormal. A PBI less than 0.6 is abnormal and consistent with vasculogenic impotence.[12] Table 31-1 summarizes the PBI criteria.

| TABLE 31-1 | Penile-Brachial Index Criteria |
|---|---|
| **PBI Value** | **Interpretation** |
| 0.7–1.0 | Normal |
| 0.6–0.7 | Borderline abnormal |
| <0.6 | Abnormal |

## SONOGRAPHIC EXAMINATION TECHNIQUES

### Patient Preparation and Positioning

There is no preparation needed for the ultrasound examination. The procedure should be explained to patient, and any questions should be answered. The patient is asked to undress from the waist down and provided a cover sheet or drape. The examination is performed with the patient supine. The flaccid penis is positioned in its anatomic position along the abdominal wall.

### Equipment

A duplex ultrasound system equipped with a high-frequency transducer is used for a penile ultrasound examination. The imaging frequency should be 7.5 MHz or higher. A small footprint transducer such as a hockey stick transducer is helpful for this examination. The image should be optimized for proper visualization given the depth of the structures in view. Proper Doppler angle correction of 60 degrees to the vessel wall should be used for spectral analysis. Lower angles are acceptable if 60 degrees is not possible. Angles greater than 60 degrees should never be used. Color Doppler can be used to assist in vessel localization and should also be optimized.

### Scanning Technique

The ultrasound transducer should be positioned on the ventral surface at the base of the penis. Scan the entire penis in both transverse and longitudinal planes from the glans to the base. The corpora cavernosa should be identified. The entire tissue should be evaluated for any pathology, especially the presence of plaques. Documentation is obtained with multiple images in the various scanning planes. The plaque location and length are recorded.

The cavernosal arteries are found near the central and medial aspects of the corpora cavernosa (Fig. 31-3). Although they can be identified within the grayscale image, color imaging is used to aid in their rapid visualization. Preinjection measurements are obtained and include a diameter measurement of the cavernosal arteries as well as a peak systolic velocity (PSV) and end-diastolic velocity (EDV) (Fig. 31-4).

A physician performs the injection into the cavernosa. A single injection will act upon both corpora cavernosa. The injection consists of a vasoactive pharmacologic agent or agents that will induce and maintain an erection. Alprostadil (prostaglandin E1) is available for ICI as Edex or Caverject,

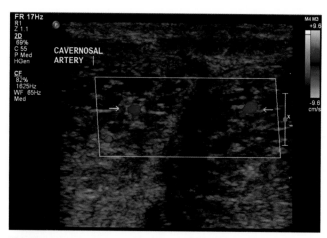

**FIGURE 31-3** Coronal view of the cavernosal artery (at *arrows*) and vein. The corpora cavernosa are the slightly circular homogeneous structures containing the blood vessels.

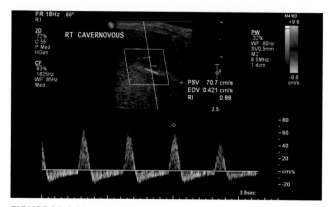

**FIGURE 31-4** Normal preinjection waveform of the cavernosal artery.

and can be used for the study. When used by itself, 10 to 20 mcg of alprostadil can be used for the study. Alternatively, a mixture of two to four different vasoactive agents can be prepared by a compounding pharmacy and stored in the refrigerator for several weeks. This author prefers a mixture of three vasoactive agents (Trimix)—alprostadil (20 mcg/mL), phentolamine (1 mg/mL), and papaverine (30 mg/mL). An injection of 0.25 mL of this solution is used. The procedural team then leaves the room, and the patient is given some privacy. Access to erogenous literature is not necessary, but may be considered.

After 15 minutes, the examination resumes, and postinjection measurements are conducted. Penile length in the erect state is measured. Estimation of penile curvature is documented. This can be done cognitively, or in certain cases using a goniometer if more precise measurement of the angle is needed. The diameter of the cavernosal artery is again measured. Arterial signals from both the cavernosal arteries are obtained by recording PSV and EDV. A preferred location to image the cavernosal arteries is at the penoscrotal junction on the ventral aspect of the penis, lateral to the urethra. This provides a relatively unobscured window to image the arteries. A representative waveforms and velocity are measured from the deep dorsal vein.

Some laboratories prefer to obtain serial spectral waveforms at intervals of 5, 10, 15, and 20 minutes following injection. The exact timing of these postinjection measurements varies somewhat between laboratories. Several measurements are often needed to obtain the highest velocity.

## Pitfalls

An ICI may be contraindicated in the patient who is sensitive to the medications used in the injection. If the patient is anticoagulated, this may also be a contraindication to the injection. Priapism, a prolonged erection persisting without stimulation, can be another potential complication.

## DIAGNOSIS

### Grayscale Characteristics

The corpora cavernosa normally appear as two circular structures with a homogeneous echo texture. Plaques will appear as a thickening of the tunica with increased echogenicity. They consist of a dense fibrous scar and often are associated with calcification. The calcification will produce an acoustic shadow (Fig. 31-5). Plaques within the tunica correspond anatomically to the fulcrum of the curvature on the penis. For instance, in a patient with a 90-degree dorsal curvature with the fulcrum at the mid penile shaft, the plaque will be noted on the dorsal aspect of the penis, at the point of maximum concavity.

Normal diameter for the cavernosal artery is 0.3 to 0.7 mm in diameter. During an erection, the artery dilates to approximately 1.0 mm in diameter.[13] The diameter of these small arteries can be difficult to adequately measure, and as such, the diameter is not a key diagnostic feature.

### Spectral Doppler Characteristics

The primary diagnostic tool is the evaluation of velocity changes. Initially, in the flaccid state, the cavernosal

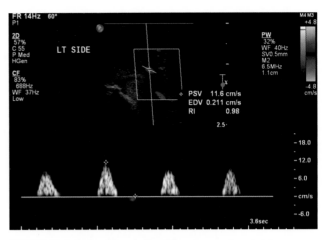

**FIGURE 31-6** Peak systolic velocity <25 cm/s, suggesting arterial insufficiency.

arteries demonstrate a relatively low PSV with the absence of a reverse flow component. The PSV is usually greater than 13 cm/s.[14] Following the injection, the PSV increases, and there is little or no diastolic flow. A PSV >35 cm/s is considered normal.[15]

Arterial insufficiency is associated with a postinjection PSV <25 cm/s (Fig. 31-6). A PSV <10 cm/s denotes severe arterial insufficiency. An EDV >5 cm/s during peak erection is consistent with veno-occlusive dysfunction (Fig. 31-7). A PSV between 25 and 35 cm/s may be associated with mild disease, but is interpreted after assessing clinical history, erection firmness, and other parameters.

Following the injection, the velocity in the deep dorsal vein should not increase. A normal value is <3 cm/s. A velocity of 10 to 20 cm/s is considered to be moderately increased. A velocity >20 cm/s is noted to be markedly increased. A venous velocity increase above 4 cm/s is considered to be associated with a venous leak.

Figure 31-8 represents a flowchart of the penile ultrasound procedure and interpretative criteria for velocity measurements. The procedure outlined may vary slightly between laboratories, particularly with the timing of the data collection.

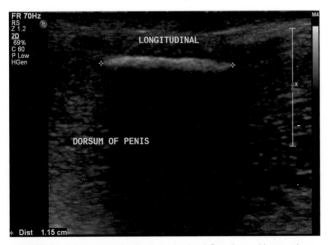

**FIGURE 31-5** Dorsal penile plaque measuring 1.5 cm long with acoustic shadowing.

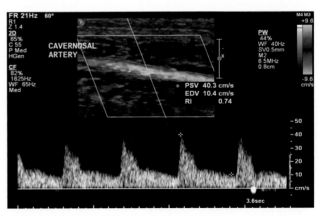

**FIGURE 31-7** Elevated EDV consistent with veno-occlusive dysfunction.

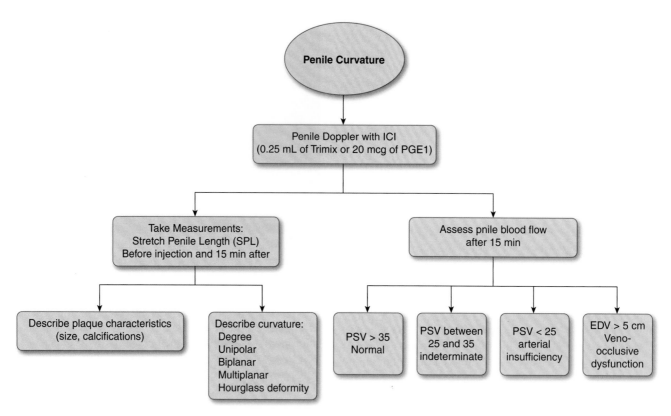

**FIGURE 31-8** Flowchart of penile ultrasound procedure and velocity criteria.

## SUMMARY

- Penile duplex ultrasound is considered an important component in assessing patients with ED or PD, especially if an intervention is planned.
- PBI measurements can also be performed to identify impairments in penile arterial inflow.
- Ultrasound can detect plaques along the tunica albuginea, which can be associated with PD.
- Blood flow changes are measured post-ICI.
- Velocity criteria for the cavernosal artery have been established to aid in the diagnosis of vasculogenic impotence.

## CRITICAL THINKING QUESTIONS

1. A patient with suspected ED presents for a PBI study. The patient has an allergy to adhesive tape. Can you still perform the test and how?

2. When performing a penile ultrasound examination, you have the choice of multiple ultrasound transducers. Which transducer would be preferred and why?

## MEDIA MENU

Student Resources available on thePoint° include:
- Audio glossary
- Interactive question bank
- Videos
- Internet resource

## REFERENCES

1. Nehra A, Alterowitz R, Culkin DJ, et al. Peyronie's Disease: AUA Guidelines. 2015. Available at: https://www.auanet.org/education/guidelines/peyronies-disease.cfm. Accessed July 30, 2016.
2. Lue TF, Hricak H, Marich KW, et al. Vasculogenic impotence evaluated by high-resolution ultrasonography and pulsed Doppler spectrum analysis. *Radiology*. 1985;155:777–781.
3. Wein AJ, Kavoussi LR, Partin AW, et al. *Campbell-Walsh Urology*. 11th ed. Philadelphia, PA: Elsevier; 2016.
4. Devine CJ Jr, Somer KD, Ladaga LE. Peyronie's disease: pathophysiology. *Prog Clin Biol Res*. 1991;360:355–358.
5. Dibenedetti DB, Nguyen D, Zografos L, et al. A population-based study of Peyronie's disease: prevalence and treatment patters in the United States. *Adv Urol*. 2011:282503.
6. Rochelle JC, Levine LA. Survey of primary care physicians and urologist regarding Peyronie's disease. *J Urology*. 2005;173:254–255.
7. Feldman HA, Goldstein I, Hatzichristou DG, et al. Impotence and its medical and psychosocial correlates: results of the Massachusetts Male Aging Study. *J Urol*. 1994;151:54–61.
8. Kendirci M, Nowfar S, Gur S, et al. The relationship between the type of penile abnormality and penile vascular status in patients with Peyronie's disease. *J Urol*. 2005;174:632–635.

9. Kendirci M, Trost L, Sikka SC, et al. The effect of vascular risk factors on penile vascular studies in men with erectile dysfunction. *J Urol.* 2007;178:2516–2520.

10. Aitchison M, Aitchison J, Carter R. Is the penile brachial index a reproducible and useful measurement? *Br J Urol.* 1990;66:202–204.

11. Mueller SC, von Wallenberg-Pachaly H, Voges GE, et al. Comparison of selective internal iliac pharmaco-angiography, penile brachial index and duplex sonography with pulsed Doppler analysis for the evaluation of vasculogenic (arteriogenic) impotence. *J Urol.* 1990;143:928–932.

12. Chiu RCJ, Lidstone D, Blundell PE. Predictive power of penile/brachial index in diagnosing male sexual impotence. *J Vasc Surg.* 1986;4:251–256.

13. Wahl SI, Rubin MB, Bakal CW. Radiologic evaluation of penile arterial anatomy in arteriogenic impotence. *Int J Impot Res.* 1997;9:93–97.

14. Corona G, Fagioli G, Mannucci E, et al. Penile Doppler ultrasound in patients with erectile dysfunction (ED): role of peak systolic velocity measured in the flaccid state in predicting arteriogenic ED and silent coronary artery disease. *J Sex Med.* 2008;5:2623–2634.

15. Herbener TE, Seftel AD, Nehra A, et al. Penile ultrasound. *Semin Urol.* 1994;12:320–332.

# Vascular Applications of Ultrasound Contrast Agents

DANIEL A. MERTON

**CHAPTER 32**

## OBJECTIVES

- Describe the basic characteristics of ultrasound contrast agents
- Describe how ultrasound contrast agents enhance ultrasound images
- List the most important characteristics of ultrasound contrast agents
- Describe the basic concepts of contrast-specific ultrasound imaging technology
- List the most common vascular applications of contrast-enhanced sonography

## KEY TERMS

**contrast-enhanced sonography**

**microbubbles**

**ultrasound contrast agent**

## GLOSSARY

**contrast-enhanced sonography** The use of medical ultrasound imaging after administration of an ultrasound contrast agent

**microbubbles** Encapsulated gas-containing structures that are typically smaller than 8 microns in size

**ultrasound contrast agent** Compositions that, after administration, alter the acoustic properties of body tissues (including blood) typically resulting in higher ultrasound signal reflectivity; also known as ultrasound contrast medium

The use of ultrasound contrast agents in the United States is currently limited to echocardiographic and liver applications. However, in other parts of the world, the use of contrast-enhanced sonography (CES) has been established as a valuable imaging procedure for a wide number of applications. The use of ultrasound contrast agents (UCAs) that are administered intravenously (IV) has been shown to improve the evaluation of blood flow through both large and small vessels and the cardiac chambers. CES has been shown to reduce or eliminate some of the current limitations of ultrasound imaging (US). These limitations include contrast resolution on grayscale (B-mode) US, as well as the detection of slow blood flow and flow in very small vessels using color-flow imaging (CFI) or pulsed Doppler with spectral analysis. Advances in US equipment technology have resulted in "contrast-specific" imaging modes that, when combined with UCAs, markedly improve the capabilities of diagnostic sonography and expand its already impressive range of clinical applications.

## TYPES OF ULTRASOUND CONTRAST AGENTS

The concept of using contrast agents to enhance the diagnostic potential of US dates back to 1968 when Gramiak and Shah injected agitated saline directly into the ascending aorta and cardiac chambers during echocardiographic examinations.[1] These and subsequent investigations revealed that microbubbles formed by agitation of saline resulted in strong reflections of the ultrasound beam arising from within the normally echo-free lumen of the aorta and chambers of the heart. Currently, IV administered agitated saline is utilized for the so-called "bubble study" echocardiography examinations, including the assessment of patients with suspected pulmonary hypertension or intracardiac shunts (Fig. 32-1).[2,3] However, microbubbles produced by simple agitation of saline are nonuniform in size, relatively large, and unstable. After peripheral venous administration, microbubbles within agitated saline do not persist through

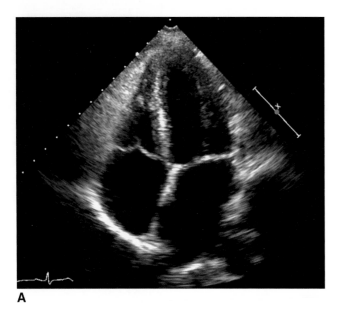
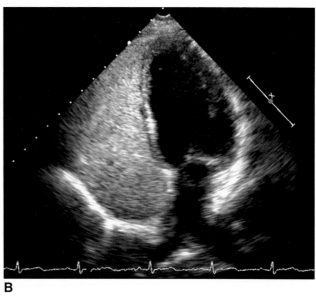

**A**                                                        **B**

**FIGURE 32-1** Use of agitated saline as an ultrasound contrast agent. The patient previously had a stroke, and an echocardiogram was ordered to rule out a patent foramen ovale (PFO). On the grayscale examination (**A**), no obvious PFO was visualized. After intravenous injection of 10 mL of agitated sterile saline (**B**), bubbles can be seen filling in the right heart, but no bubbles were visualized on the left side of the heart. No PFO was identified. (Image courtesy of Kara Lopresti, RDCS, Thomas Jefferson University Hospital, Philadelphia, PA.)

passage of the pulmonary and cardiac circulations, which makes this technique unsuitable for sonographic evaluations of the left heart and systemic circulation.

Numerous attempts have been made to encapsulate gas in order to make a more suitable microbubble-based UCA that can be administered IV for CES examinations. For an UCA to be clinically useful, it should be nontoxic, have microbubbles or microparticles that are small enough to traverse the pulmonary capillary beds (i.e., less than 8 microns in size) but large enough to reflect US signals, and be stable enough to provide multiple recirculations. A number of agents possess these desirable traits and are commercially available worldwide. Table 32-1 summarizes some of the current clinically available UCAs.

## Ultrasound Contrast Agent Administration

Typically, contrast is administered in small (<3 mL) IV bolus injections via an upper extremity vein which, depending on the agent administered and patient characteristics, typically provide several minutes of enhancement. When necessary, a second administration of contrast can be performed. Ultrasound contrast media can also be administered via slow IV infusion to provide prolonged enhancement. Albrecht and

colleagues found that the infusion of contrast provided enhancement lasting as much as 12 minutes or more compared to just over 2 minutes with a bolus injection.[4] The additional enhancement time provided by the infusion of contrast is useful for difficult and time-consuming evaluations of vessels such as the renal arteries. Infusion of contrast has also been investigated as a means to assess limb perfusion and perfusion deficits, which could prove useful for evaluation of patients who have peripheral artery disease (PAD).[5]

## Tissue-Specific and Targeted Agents

The kinetics of UCA microbubbles following IV injection is complex, and each agent has its own unique characteristics.[6] In general, after IV administration, blood-pool UCAs are contained exclusively in the body's vascular spaces. When a vascular agent's microbubbles rupture, their shell products are metabolized or eliminated by the body, and the gas is exhaled.

Tissue-specific UCAs differ from vascular agents in that the microbubbles of these agents are removed from the blood pool and taken up by, or have an affinity toward, specific tissues, for example, thrombus or the reticuloendothelial system in the liver and spleen. Thus, tissue-specific agents possess two unique characteristics: an affinity for

| TABLE 32-1 | Ultrasound Contrast Agents | | |
|---|---|---|---|
| **Contrast Agent** | **Manufacturer** | **Microbubble Shell** | **Microbubble Gas** |
| Optison | GE Healthcare, Princeton, NJ | Human serum albumin | Octafluoropropane ($C_3F_8$) |
| Definity | Lantheus Medical Imaging, N. Billerica, MA | Lipid | Octafluoropropane ($C_3F_8$) |
| SonoVue Marketed as Lumason in the United States | Bracco Imaging SpA, Milan, Italy | Phospholipid | Sulfur hexafluoride ($SF_6$) |

the targeted tissue and the ability to alter that tissue's sonographic detectability. By changing the signal impedance (or other acoustic characteristics) of normal and abnormal tissues, these agents improve the detection of abnormalities and can permit more specific sonographic diagnoses. Like blood-pool agents, tissue-specific UCAs are typically administered by IV injection. Some tissue-specific UCAs also enhance the sonographic detection of blood flow so that they can be used to improve the detection of flow as well as enhance targeted tissue. Because tissue-specific UCAs target specific types of tissues and their behavior is predictable, they are considered molecular imaging agents.[7]

One type of tissue-specific UCA that is of particular interest for vascular applications is thrombus-specific agents.[8] Although the administration of a blood-pool UCA can be used to better delineate the functional lumen of both arteries and veins, blood-pool agents do not directly enhance the sonographic appearance of thrombi. However, research is ongoing to develop UCAs attached to fibrin, platelets, or other components of blood clots to enhance their sonographic detection.[9]

## Therapeutic Agents

Investigations are ongoing in the development of UCAs that can be used for a variety of therapeutic applications.[10] Typically, therapeutic UCAs have a specific ligand or other binding moiety attached to their shell that has an affinity for a particular receptor (target). Researchers have investigated the ability to enhance thrombolysis using acoustic energy with and without nontargeted UCA microbubbles. A significant amount of additional research has been performed using thrombus-targeting UCAs that, when insonated, enhance thrombolysis (referred to as "sonothrombolysis").[11-13] This concept, if applied to the intracranial vessels, offers a potential noninvasive therapy for patients who suffer from embolic stoke.

## CONTRAST-SPECIFIC EQUIPMENT MODIFICATIONS

Although microbubble-based UCAs can be used with conventional grayscale US, color-flow modes, and spectral Doppler to enhance the detection of blood flow, the clinical utility of UCAs is vastly improved by the use of contrast-specific imaging software. Numerous investigations have been performed to better understand the complex interactions between acoustic energy (i.e., the US beam) and UCA microbubbles which has, in turn, resulted in modifications to US instrumentation that is specifically designed to exploit these interactions, as described below.

## Harmonic Imaging

Harmonic imaging (HI) can be performed with the same transducers used for conventional US. In HI mode, the US system is configured to receive only echoes at the second harmonic frequency which is twice the transmit frequency (e.g., 6.0 MHz for a 3.0 MHz transducer).[14,15] When subjected to the acoustic energy present in the US field, UCA microbubbles oscillate in size (i.e., they get larger and smaller). The reflected echoes from the oscillating microbubbles

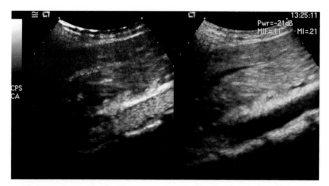

**FIGURE 32-2** Combined conventional and contrast-specific imaging display. This dual-image display of a normal aorta demonstrates the conventional grayscale ultrasound image on the right and the low-MI contrast-specific (pulse-inversion) mode on the left. The combination of contrast with contrast-specific imaging provides the ability to visualize blood flow within the aorta with a higher frame rate and better spatial resolution than is provided by contrast-enhanced color Doppler imaging.

contain energy components at the fundamental frequency as well as at higher and lower harmonics.[16] In HI mode, the echoes from the oscillating microbubbles have a higher signal-to-noise ratio than would be provided by using conventional US so that regions with microbubbles are more easily appreciated visually. Thus, contrast-specific HI provides a means to visualize contrast-enhanced blood flow and contrast-containing tissue using B-mode imaging. These modes obviate the need to use Doppler (which is susceptible to artifacts and other limitations) for the detection of blood flow. Many US equipment manufacturers offer contrast-specific imaging modes, including simultaneous dual displays of the contrast-enhanced image and the conventional US image in real time (Fig. 32-2).

## Low-Mechanical Index Imaging and Intermittent Imaging

During CES examinations, the energy present within the ultrasound beam can have a detrimental effect on contrast microbubbles.[17] Contrast-specific imaging modes are designed to utilize low acoustic output power (as defined by the mechanical index [MI]) to avoid or minimize microbubble destruction.

Intermittent imaging is an additional approach used to reduce microbubble destruction during CES examinations. Intermittent imaging mode captures images at user-defined pulsing intervals based on a period of time (e.g., 2 seconds) or triggered by a point in the cardiac cycle (e.g., the R wave of an electrocardiogram). This reduces the exposure of contrast microbubbles to the acoustic energy and allows additional microbubbles to enter the field between image captures. The additional microbubbles then contribute to an even greater increase in reflectivity of the contrast-containing vessel or tissue than is possible by continuous real-time imaging.

In some situations, it is desirable to rapidly destroy contrast microbubbles in an organ or vessels and observe the reperfusion of contrast-containing blood flow into the region of interest. An intermittent mode developed for this purpose—often referred to as "flash echo"—briefly increases the transmitted acoustic power to intentionally destroy the microbubbles of contrast. After the microbubbles are destroyed, a low-MI imaging mode is used to observe reperfusion of blood into the region over time.

## CLINICAL APPLICATIONS

The use of CES has been investigated for virtually all clinical applications of sonography.[18-24] CES has been found to be beneficial for diverse applications such as transcranial Doppler (TCD) evaluations, enhancing assessment of abdominal trauma and improving detection of vesicoureteral reflux in children.[25-27] Contrast agents have proven particularly valuable for echocardiographic examinations and are routinely utilized as a rescue tool to salvage otherwise nondiagnostic examinations. Thus, echocardiography remains the most common application of UCAs, and their use for evaluation of the heart is considered indispensable as a means to improve the delineation of endocardial borders, to assess regional wall motion, and for the detection of intracavitary thrombus.[28,29]

The second most common application of UCAs (after echocardiography) is for evaluations of liver lesion detection and characterization.[30-38] The sensitivity of CES for the detection and characterization of focal liver lesions has been reported to be comparable to that of more expensive modalities, including contrast-enhanced computed tomography (CT) or magnetic resonance imaging.[39]

CES offers several benefits over many other imaging modalities; it does not require the use of ionizing radiation, UCAs have a good safety profile and CES has good patient acceptance. It is cost-effective. These traits are becoming more important in today's health care environment and will likely contribute to continued advances in the use of UCAs for screening, diagnosis, and therapy of a wide range of abnormalities.

Vascular applications of CES include evaluation of peripheral vessels, the cerebrovascular system, as well as the abdominal and retroperitoneal vasculature.[40-42] Qualitative assessments (i.e., detection of blood flow or areas that lack blood flow) can be performed using conventional CFI modes

or, more commonly, contrast-specific imaging modes. When necessary, improved characterization of blood flow can be accomplished using spectral Doppler analysis.

### Peripheral Applications

Limitations to sonographic assessment of peripheral arteries and veins include poor visualization of deeply located and/or small vessels and low-velocity or low-volume blood flow (Fig. 32-3). The use of CES has been found to facilitate and improve assessments of the peripheral vasculature, including evaluations of patients before and after bypass surgery and increase the diagnostic confidence level of examination interpretations.

#### Peripheral Arterial Applications

Signal attenuation resulting from atherosclerotic plaque which, in severe situations causes acoustic shadowing, can limit visualization of arterial walls as well as blood flow detection and characterization. The addition of UCAs has been found to overcome some of these limitations. Even in cases where the vessel lumen is obscured by shadowing, CES has been found to be helpful to detect flow in a vessel segment distal to the shadowed area so that a tight stenosis can be differentiated from complete occlusion.

The ability of UCAs to function as a rescue tool for nondiagnostic conventional Doppler evaluations was confirmed in a study by Langholz et al.[43] These investigators studied 33 patients with iliac or lower extremity arterial disease. All of the CES examinations were considered adequate in answering the diagnostic question for the patients studied. The group particularly remarked on the improvement of visualization of flow in the iliac artery, which could be seen after contrast despite the presence of overlying bowel gas.

Several recent reports have described the use of CES for assessment of PAD.[44-48] A report by Duerschmied et al. described the use of CES to evaluate calf muscle perfusion and vascular collateralization in patients with PAD. The authors concluded that CES could be used to detect perfusion

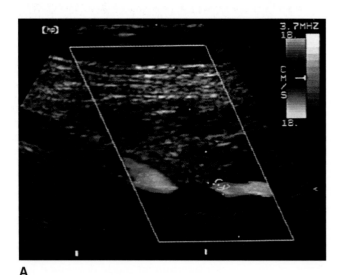
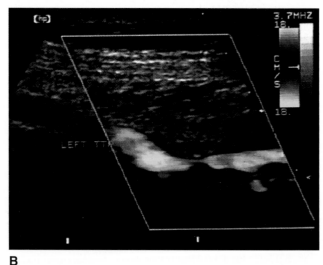

A                                                    B

**FIGURE 32-3** Contrast-enhanced color Doppler imaging of calf vessel flow. The baseline image (**A**) demonstrates a vessel segment that does not contain detectable blood flow. After injection of contrast (**B**), there is continuity of flow through the vessel, and a stenosis is seen. (Adapted by permission from Goldberg BB, Raichlen JS, Forsberg F, eds. *Ultrasound Contrast Agents.* 2nd ed. London, UK: Informa Healthcare; 2001.)

deficits as well as the degree of arterial collateralization in patients with symptomatic PAD.

### Peripheral Venous Applications

The use of conventional compression sonography has been proven effective for evaluation of patients with suspected venous thromboses. Thus, UCAs have not been widely utilized for peripheral venous applications.

In 1999, Puls et al. described their results using Levovist (administered via an upper extremity IV access site) in 31 patients who had suspected deep vein thrombosis (DVT) and at least one vein segment that was inadequately imaged with color Doppler imaging.[49] All patients had a venogram for comparison. Baseline CDI was inadequate in 43 of 279 vessel segments, and contrast enhancement was seen in 40 of these 43 segments. Of the 27 vein segments that were confirmed to have DVT, 18 were detected on baseline imaging, while CES identified 25. Five of the seven additional DVTs detected with CES were below the knee. Three iliac vein thromboses were identified with CES, but only one was detected at baseline. The overall diagnostic accuracy increased from 60% (26 of 43 vein segments) at baseline to 86% (37 of 43 vein segments) after contrast administration.

## Cerebrovascular Applications

The use of CES for evaluations of the cerebrovascular system includes assessments of both the intra- and extracranial vasculature. Color-flow–guided duplex Doppler sonography has become a mainstay for the evaluation of the carotid and vertebral arteries, and in some cases, it is the only imaging examination performed before endarterectomy. The use of CES for carotid and other relatively large vessel evaluations has the potential to permit direct assessments of the functional lumen and plaque morphology in a similar manner as other imaging modalities (Fig. 32-4). If CES were to be used routinely, it has the potential to reduce the need for additional, more expensive diagnostic imaging studies.

### Extracranial Applications

The use of UCAs for evaluation of the carotid arteries has been found to enhance Doppler signals and improve visualization of blood flow using contrast-specific imaging modes, resulting in improved delineation of the residual lumen. CES can also be used to differentiate tight stenoses from carotid artery occlusion (Fig. 32-5).

A published study by Pfister et al. described the use of conventional Doppler US, 3D US (with and without an UCA and contrast-enhanced B-flow imaging (GE Healthcare, Waukesha, WI)) for presurgical evaluations of the extent of internal carotid artery (ICA) stenosis in 25 patients.[50] The authors found that contrast-enhanced 3D B-flow had the highest correlation (93%) with surgical findings. They also reported that the use of 3D CES was particularly valuable in cases of circular calcifications with severe stenoses, and that CES facilitated assessment of the morphology of ICA plaque.

The use of CES to differentiate ICA stenoses from occlusions was the focus of a report by Hammond et al.[51] They compared the diagnostic accuracy of CES, time-of-flight magnetic resonance angiography (MRA), and contrast-enhanced MRA (CE-MRA) using digital subtraction angiography as a reference standard in 31 patients with suspected carotid occlusion on conventional US. The authors concluded that in cases where occlusion is confirmed by either CES or CE-MRA, no additional imaging is required.

### Intracranial Applications

Sonographic assessments of the intracranial vasculature are often limited by insufficient acoustic windows, low-velocity flow, and signal attenuation through the calvarium. The use of CES for evaluation of the intracranial circulation can overcome many problems related to vessel visualization and expand the clinical utility of transcranial US examinations. The addition of UCAs has been found to improve the ability to evaluate intracranial blood flow, leading to fewer nondiagnostic studies and higher diagnostic confidence levels (Fig. 32-6).

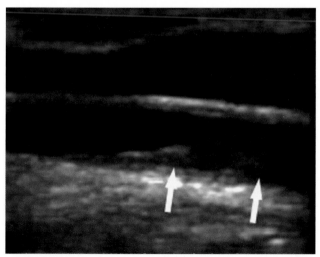

**A**

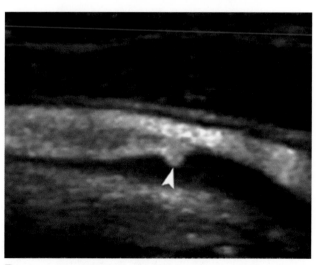

**B**

**FIGURE 32-4** Improved delineation of plaque ulceration. The baseline scan (**A**) demonstrates an area of plaque along the deep wall of the common carotid artery (*arrows*). After injection of contrast (**B**), the functional lumen fills with contrast-containing blood and an area of ulceration (*arrowhead*) in the plaque is identified. Unlike Doppler sonography, CES provides the ability to directly assess the functional lumen and plaque morphology in a manner similar to conventional angiography and CT angiography. (Image courtesy of Steven Feinstein, MD, Rush University Medical Center, Chicago, IL.)

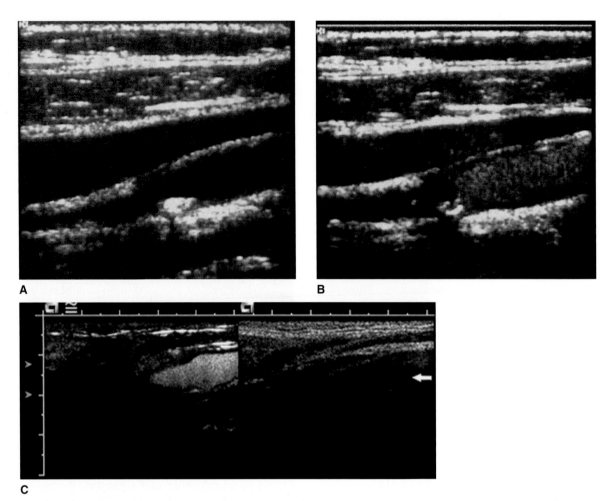

**A**    **B**    **C**

**FIGURE 32-5**  Carotid artery occlusion. Baseline imaging of the carotid bulb (**A**) demonstrates an echogenic plaque. After injection of contrast (**B**), contrast-enhancement of flow is identified in the functional lumen of the common carotid artery, but no enhanced flow is seen distal to the plaque. A carotid occlusion was confirmed with digital subtraction angiography. In a different patient (**C**), CES using a dual-image display with low-MI contrast-specific imaging on the left and conventional US on the right demonstrates blood flow up to the location of an occlusion. Note that the presence of contrast causes acoustic shadowing on the conventional image (*arrow*). (**A** and **B**: Adapted by permission from Goldberg BB, Raichlen JS, Forsberg F, eds. *Ultrasound Contrast Agents*. 2nd ed. London, UK: Informa Healthcare; 2001. **C**: Courtesy of David Cosgrove, FRCR, Hammersmith Hospital, London, UK.)

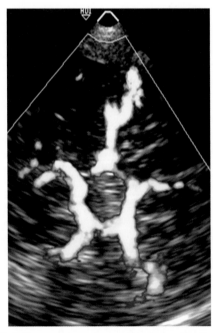

**FIGURE 32-6**  Contrast-enhanced power Doppler imaging of intracranial vessels. (Image courtesy of Jeff Powers, PhD, Philips Ultrasound, Bothell, WA.)

Droste et al. used CFI and pulsed Doppler with spectral analysis to evaluate 47 patients with insufficient acoustic windows before and after administration of Sonovue.[52] A total of 67 temporal windows provided insufficient acoustic access (both temporal windows in 20 patients and 27 unilateral studies). Contrast-enhanced TCD significantly improved the number of intracranial vessel segments that could be evaluated by pulsed Doppler and allowed color-flow detection of flow in longer vessel segments. Only 26 middle cerebral arteries could be evaluated using noncontrast TCD compared to 65 with CES.

Specific indications for transcranial CES include assessments of patients with arterial occlusions and stenoses, venous thrombosis, and the detection of blood flow in solid brain tumors.[53-55] The use of CES to assess intracranial hemodynamic effects of extracranial carotid artery stenoses and occlusions has been reported.[56] CES has also been used intraoperatively to improve the localization of the feeding arteries and draining veins of arteriovenous malformations.[57]

### Evaluation of Carotid Artery Vasa Vasorum and Plaque Neovascularity

The use of CES to evaluate blood flow in the vasa vasorum and carotid artery plaque neovascularization is a new and intriguing area of investigation.[58-63] Some investigators have

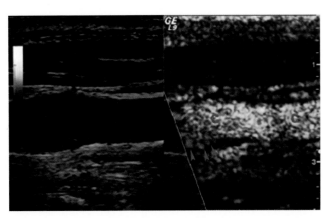

**FIGURE 32-7** Neovascularization of the carotid artery vasa vasorum. This dual-image display shows the conventional US image on the left and the low-MI contrast-specific image on the right. Contrast-enhanced blood flow is seen within the functional lumen of the carotid artery (C) and tiny vessels within the adventitial vasa vasorum (*arrowheads*) consistent with neovascularity. (Image courtesy of Steven Feinstein, MD, Rush University Medical Center, Chicago, IL.)

equated atherosclerotic plaque with a tumor because, like tumors, plaque requires a nutrient-rich blood supply in order to grow. Studies have shown that plaque neovascularization is predominantly derived from the arterial wall vasa vasorum with changes to the vascular morphology preceding the development of obvious plaque and luminal narrowing. These early vascular changes can be identified using CES (Fig. 32-7).

Furthermore, the density of vessels in atherosclerotic plaques has been found to correlate with the degree of inflammation and other processes that contribute to plaque destabilization and rupture. Contrast-enhanced intravascular ultrasound has been used for high-resolution imaging of flow in vasa vasorum and plaque inflammation.[64] In the future, the use of CES for evaluation of the carotid artery vasa vasorum and plaque neovascularization may prove to be a valuable, noninvasive method to identify patients who have vulnerable plaques and better determine a patient's risk of cardiovascular events. The use of CES for this application could also complement sonographic measurements of the intima-media thickness as a means to monitor the response to antiatherosclerotic therapies.

## Abdominal and Retroperitoneal Applications

Abdominal vascular applications of sonography include the evaluation of the aorta and its branches, veins of the systemic, as well as portal venous system and blood flow in abdominal organs. The use of CES has been investigated for all of these applications and has been found to be highly beneficial in many. The use of CES has also improved the use of sonography for evaluations of organ perfusion and tumor characterizations.

### Hepatic Applications

UCAs have shown the potential to improve the accuracy of hepatic sonography, including enhanced detection and characterization of hepatic masses and improved detection of intra- and extrahepatic blood flow. In April 2016, Lumason became the first UCA to gain approval by the US Food and

Drug Administration (FDA) for liver lesion characterization. CES has been shown to improve the detection of hepatic blood flow in normal subjects as well as patients with liver disease and portal hypertension.[65–67] CES has also been used effectively for assessment of flow through transjugular intrahepatic portosystemic shunts (TIPS) (Fig. 32-8).[68,69]

There are several phases of contrast enhancement within the liver when using CES. The timing and degree of contrast enhancement is highly dependent on a number of variables, including the patient's physiologic status, manner of UCA administration, and MI values used during the CE US examination. Table 32-2 summarizes these phases of contrast enhancement.

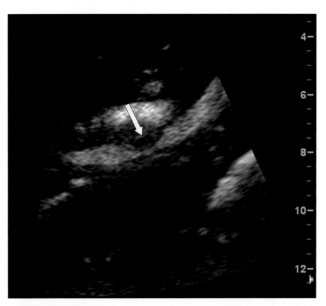

**FIGURE 32-8** CES of a transjugular intrahepatic portosystemic shunt (TIPS). A stenosis (*arrow*) is identified in this TIPS using contrast-specific grayscale CES. (Image courtesy of Antonio Sergio Marcelino, MD, Sirio-Libanes Hospital and Cancer Institute of University of Sao Paulo, Sao Paulo, Brazil.)

**TABLE 32-2 Hepatic Phases of Contrast Enhancement as Demonstrated Using CES**

**PHASE 1**

After a peripheral intravenous injection of a blood-pool UCA, the first phase of enhancement (*arterial phase*) occurs when contrast arrives in the hepatic artery. This phase typically begins 10–20 s postinjection and continues for 30–45 s postinjection. The arterial phase is used to determine the degree and pattern of the arterial blood supply to a tumor or region of interest.

**PHASE 2**

The *portal venous phase* occurs next when contrast arrives in the intrahepatic portal veins and typically lasts for approximately 2 min postinjection. This phase is used to determine the contribution of the portal venous system to the tumor's blood supply.

**PHASE 3**

The *late phase* occurs when contrast enters the hepatic microvasculature and is identified by an increase in the echogenicity of the liver parenchyma. This phase lasts until the UCA is no longer present in the vascular spaces and is generally limited to about 4–6 min after UCA administration. The late phase provides information regarding the washout of contrast-containing blood from the tumor or region of interest.

## Renal Applications

The sonographic evaluation of the main renal arteries and intrarenal vessels in patients with suspected renal artery stenosis (RAS) is limited by factors, including the deep location of the vessels, overlying bowel, and patient obesity. Furthermore, there may be limited sonographic windows to view the renal arteries, and these windows may not be in optimal locations from which to obtain adequate Doppler angles. A significant number of patients have anatomic variations of the renal vasculature, including duplicate or accessory renal arteries, and these variations can be very difficult to identify with conventional US. Thus, sonographic examinations for RAS are extremely operator dependent and often time consuming.

By improving the signal intensity of Doppler flow signals and increasing the likelihood of obtaining adequate Doppler flow information, UCAs have been found to be helpful during examinations of patients with suspected RAS (Fig. 32-9).[70,71] Thus, in cases where the renal arteries are not well visualized or the spectral waveforms are of poor quality, administration of an UCA can potentially reduce the number of technically inadequate or otherwise nondiagnostic examinations as well as reduce examination time.

Diagnostic US is generally a reliable method of evaluating patients with renal masses, particularly in the differentiation of cystic from solid lesions. Sonography is usually accurate in identifying large (>2 cm) renal cell carcinomas and tumor thrombi in the renal veins and inferior vena cava. However, in some cases, sonography cannot identify small neoplasms or differentiate solid renal lesions from normal anatomic variations, such as a prominent column of Bertin or persistent fetal lobulation. In these cases, other imaging studies such as contrast-enhanced CT, CE-MRI, or needle biopsy may be required for a definitive diagnosis.

The use of CES has been shown to improve the ability to detect flow in the intrarenal vessels and to allow more accurate differentiation of renal masses and other entities. Furthermore, CES provides a means of identifying differences in contrast uptake (i.e., differences in vascularity) between tumors and normal renal parenchyma. Because UCAs are not nephrotoxic, the use of CES for renal applications may be particularly beneficial when a CE-MRI examination is contraindicated.

## Organ Transplants

Sonography is routinely used to evaluate renal, hepatic, and pancreatic transplants. The modality is often employed as a first-line examination in the immediate postsurgical period as well as for serial studies to assess organ viability. After organ transplantation sonography is used to detect postsurgical fluid collections,

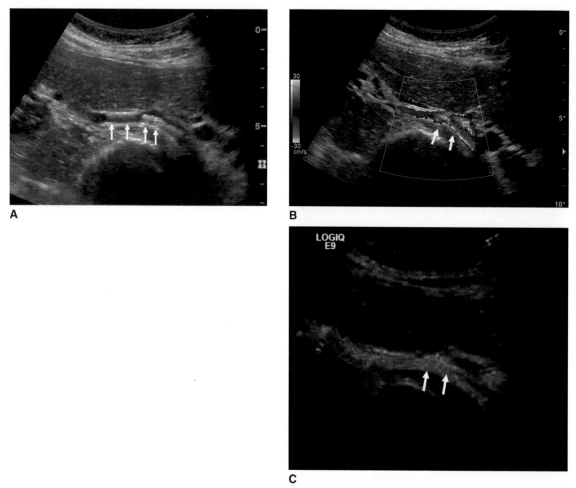

**FIGURE 32-9** Renal artery stent evaluation in a patient with fibromuscular dysplasia. A precontrast grayscale image (**A**) demonstrates two echogenic stents (*arrows*) within the patient's right renal artery. Evaluation of blood flow through the stented vessel segment using color Doppler imaging (**B**) suggested the presence of disturbed flow; however, the CES evaluation (**C**) indicated no flow abnormality. (Images courtesy of Hans-Peter Weskott, MD, Klinikum Region Hannover, Hannover, Germany.)

identify urinary or bile obstructions, and to assess blood flow to and from the transplanted organ. Conventional sonography is also useful in the evaluation of blood flow within the organ, but does not have an adequate level of sensitivity to detect flow at the microvascular level (i.e., tissue perfusion). When a vascular abnormality is suspected, angiography or contrast-enhanced CT may be necessary to obtain a definitive diagnosis.[72] However, angiography is invasive, CT requires ionizing radiation, and administration of contrast media required for these exams may be contraindicated in renal compromised patients.

The enhanced detection of blood flow provided by CES improves the assessment of blood flow in the arteries and veins that supply the transplant, the host vessels to which these vessels are anastomosed, as well as the parenchyma of transplanted organs (Fig. 32-10). CES has also been found to improve the ability to detect ischemic regions within native and transplanted organs.[73-75]

Several published reports have described the use of CES for evaluation of liver transplant recipients.[76,77] Sindhu et al. reported on the use of CES to examine 31 liver transplant patients with suspected hepatic artery thrombosis and compared the results to arteriography or follow-up US. They reported that in approximately 63% of studies, CES could have obviated the need for arteriography.

## Aortic Graft and Stent Surveillance

The use of CES is gaining attention as a viable alternative to other diagnostic imaging examinations used to evaluate patients after endovascular repair (EVAR) of abdominal aortic aneurysms.[78-81] Endoleaks with persistent perigraft flow within the aneurysm sac are common complications of EVAR procedures. Thus, strict postprocedure surveillance of these patients is required to enable early detection of endoleaks. Although computed tomographic angiography (CTA) is commonly utilized as a surveillance method, the use of CT contrast is contraindicated in some patients (e.g., those with chronic renal insufficiency), and repeated CTA examinations cause high levels of radiation exposure. Because of the safety of UCAs and lack of potentially harmful ionizing radiation, CES offers a viable alternative to conventional angiography and CTA, particularly when CTA is contraindicated and for serial studies. Furthermore, the ability to assess blood flow in real time using CES has been found to improve characterization of endoleaks (Fig. 32-11).

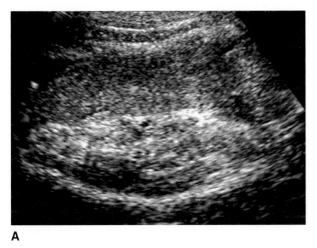

**A**

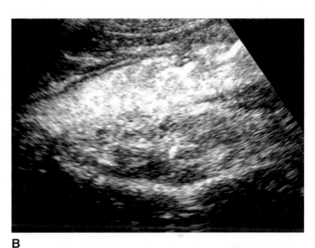

**B**

**FIGURE 32-10** Pancreatic transplant evaluation. Baseline (**A**) and postcontrast (**B**) images of a transplanted pancreas. The homogeneous enhancement seen with the addition of contrast confirms normal vascularity in the gland. (Image courtesy of Antonio Sergio Marcelino, MD, Sirio-Libanes Hospital and Cancer Institute of University of Sao Paulo, Sao Paulo, Brazil.)

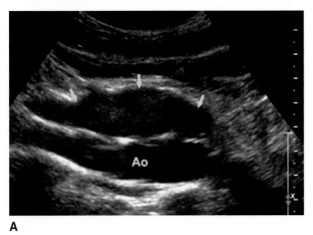

**A**

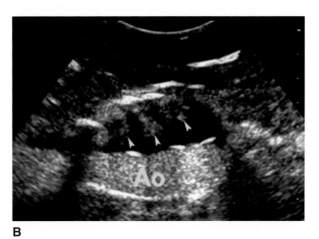

**B**

**FIGURE 32-11** Aortic endograft evaluation. Using conventional grayscale US (**A**), a fluid-filled region (*arrows*) anterior to the aorta (Ao) was identified, but it was difficult to determine the nature of this fluid. A CES study (**B**) demonstrated flow within the functional lumen and small amounts of contrast-containing blood (*arrowheads*) within the fluid pocket consistent with a small leak of the graft. (Image courtesy of Carlos Ventura, MD, Ultrasound Division, Albert Einstein Hospital and Radiology Institute of University of Sao Paulo, Sao Paulo Brazil.)

Pfister et al. reported their experience using CES for surveillance of aortic stent grafts. Thirty patients were serially evaluated with CES, and their results were compared to either CTA or MRA as the gold standard. All CTA/MRA detected endoleaks using CES, yielding a 100% sensitivity.

## Other Abdominal Applications

Other common abdominal/retroperitoneal applications of US include assessment of flow in the mesenteric arteries for mesenteric ischemia, the aorta and iliac arteries to evaluate suspected aneurysms, stenoses, or dissections, and the inferior vena cava for evaluation of filters or thromboses (Fig. 32-12). Often, these examinations are limited by the presence of overlying bowel and bowel gas, or the affects of signal attenuation over vessel depth. The addition of an UCA is clinically valuable for assessment of the abdominal vasculature and can reduce the need for additional imaging examinations.[82] CES performed well compared to CTA when used to assess endovascular stents in visceral artery aneurysms.[83]

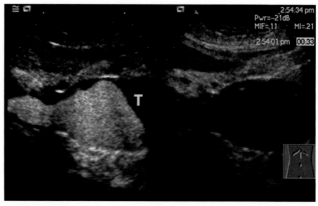

**FIGURE 32-12** CES of an abdominal aortic aneurysm (AAA). The image on the left, obtained using low-MI contrast-specific imaging, demonstrates an area within the AAA that does not contain flow (T) consistent with intraluminal thrombus. The thrombus is not well seen on the conventional US image (shown at right). (Image courtesy of David Cosgrove, FRCR, Hammersmith Hospital, London, UK.)

## SUMMARY

- Three UCAs are currently being marketed in the United States: Definity, Lumason, and Optison.
- As of this writing, all three agents are FDA approved for echocardiographic applications, and Lumason is also indicated for characterization of focal liver lesions in adult and pediatric patients.
- In the future, additional agents and/or clinical applications of existing agents are likely to become available.
- UCAs have been shown to improve the detection of blood flow in large and small vessels throughout the body as well as to improve the sonographic detection and characterization of tumors, inflammation, and other abnormalities in many body regions.
- The enhancement capabilities of UCAs have been shown to have the ability to salvage nondiagnostic US examinations and render them diagnostic.
- The use of UCAs has also resulted in new applications of the modality that were not possible without their use.
- Improvements in US technology that exploit the acoustic behavior of contrast microbubbles are further improving the clinical capabilities of CES.
- The use of CES is expected to increase because sonography becomes more omnipresent throughout medical disciplines.

## CRITICAL THINKING QUESTIONS

1. A hypertensive patient is referred to the noninvasive vascular laboratory to rule out RAS. During the examination, the main renal arteries are not well visualized using color Doppler imaging, and the sonographer is having difficulty obtaining adequate spectral Doppler waveforms. How could the administration of an UCA help in this examination?

2. A patient who received an aortic endograft presents to the emergency department 3 weeks postsurgery with a sudden onset of abdominal pain and an abdominal bruit. The emergency medicine physician is concerned that the patient's symptoms may be related to a complication from the recent aortic repair. A sonography performed in the emergency department demonstrates a fluid collection with what appears to be color-flow signals immediately adjacent to the aorta. However, the sonographer is having difficulty determining if the color signals are the result of flash artifacts from the pulsatile aorta or true flow in the collection. How could the administration of an UCA help in this important differentiation?

## MEDIA MENU

Student Resources available on thePoint° include:
- Audio glossary
- Interactive question bank
- Videos
- Internet resource

## REFERENCES

1. Gramiak R, Shah PM. Echocardiography of the aortic root. *Invest Radiol.* 1968;3:356–366.
2. Lopes LR, Loureiro MJ, Miranda R, et al. The usefulness of contrast during exercise echocardiography for the assessment of systolic pulmonary pressure. *Cardiovasc Ultrasound.* 2008;6:51.
3. Harrah JD, O'Boyle PS, Piantadosi CA. Underutilization of echocardiography for patent foramen ovale in divers with serious decompression sickness. *Undersea Hyperb Med.* 2008;35(3):207–211.
4. Albrecht T, Urbank A, Mahler M, et al. Prolongation and optimization of Doppler enhancement with a microbubble US contrast agent by using continuous infusion: preliminary experience. *Radiology.* 1998;207:339–347.

5. Naehle CP, Steinberg VA, Schild H, et al. Assessment of peripheral skeletal muscle microperfusion in a porcine model of peripheral arterial stenosis by steady-state contrast-enhanced ultrasound and Doppler flow measurement. *J Vasc Surg.* 2015;61(5):1312–1320.

6. Blomley MJK, Harvey CJ, Eckersley RJ, et al. Contrast kinetics and Doppler intensitometry. In: Goldberg BB, Raichlen JR, Forsberg F, eds. *Ultrasound Contrast Agents: Basic Principles and Clinical Applications.* 2nd ed. London, UK: Martin Dunitz Ltd.; 2001:81–89.

7. Miller JC, Thrall JH, Commission of Molecular Imaging. Clinical molecular imaging. *J Am Coll Radiol.* 2004;1:4–23.

8. Unger EC, Wu Q, McCreery T, et al. In: Goldberg BB, Raichlen JS, Forsberg F, eds. Thrombus-specific contrast agents for imaging and thrombolysis. *Ultrasound Contrast Agents.* 2nd ed. London, UK: Martin Dunitz Ltd.; 2001:337–345.

9. Takeuchi M, Ogunyankin K, Pandian NG, et al. Enhanced visualization of intravascular and left atrial appendage thrombus with the use of a thrombus-targeting ultrasonographic contrast agent (MRX-408A1); in vivo experimental echocardiographic studies. *J Am Soc Echocardiogr.* 1999;12:1015–1021.

10. Khokhlova TD, Haider Y, Hwang JH. Therapeutic potential of ultrasound microbubbles in gastrointestinal oncology: recent advances and future prospects. *Therap Adv Gastroenterol.* 2015;8(6):384–394.

11. Laing ST, McPherson DD. Cardiovascular therapeutic uses of targeted ultrasound contrast agents. *Cardiovasc Res.* 2009;83(4):626–635.

12. Molina CA, Barreto AD, Tsivgoulis G, et al. Transcranial ultrasound in clinical sonothrombolysis (TUCSON) trial. *Ann Neurol.* 2009;66(1):28–38.

13. Ebben HP, Nederhoed JH, Slikkerveer J, et al. Therapeutic application of contrast-enhanced ultrasound and low-dose urokinase for thrombolysis in a porcine model of acute peripheral arterial occlusion. *J Vasc Surg.* 2015;62(2):477–485.

14. Forsberg F, Liu JB, Rawool NM, et al. Gray-scale and color Doppler flow harmonic imaging with proteinaceous microspheres. *Radiology.* 1995;197(P):403.

15. Kono Y, Mattrey RT. Harmonic imaging with contrast microbubbles. In: Goldberg BB, Raichlen JS, Forsberg F, eds. *Ultrasound Contrast Agents.* 2nd ed. London, UK: Martin Dunitz Ltd.; 2001:37–46.

16. Forsberg F, Picolli CW, Merton DA, et al. Breast lesions: imaging with contrast-enhanced sub-harmonic US: initial experiences. *Radiology.* 2007;244(3):718–726.

17. Harvey CJ, Blomley MJK, Cosgrove DO. Acoustic emission imaging. In: Goldberg BB, Raichlen JR, Forsberg F, eds. *Ultrasound Contrast Agents: Basic Principles and Clinical Applications.* 2nd ed. London, UK: Martin Dunitz Ltd.; 2001:71–80.

18. Lencioni R, ed. *Enhancing the Role of Ultrasound with Contrast Agents.* Milan, Italy: Springer-Verlag; 2006.

19. Quaia E, ed. *Contrast Media in Ultrasonography: Basic Principles and Clinical Applications.* Berlin, Germany: Springer-Verlag; 2005.

20. Zamorano JL, Fernandez MA. *Contrast Echocardiography in Clinical Practice.* Milan, Italy: Springer-Verlag; 2004.

21. Albrecht T, Thorelius L, Solbiati L, et al. *Contrast-Enhanced Ultrasound in Clinical Practice: Liver, Prostate, Pancreas, Kidney and Lymph Nodes.* Milan, Italy: Springer-Verlag; 2005.

22. Liu JB, Merton DA, Goldberg BB, Ultrasound contrast agents. In: McGahan JP, Forsberg F, Goldberg BB. eds. *Diagnostic Ultrasound: A Logical Approach.* 2nd ed. New York, NY: Informa Healthcare; 2008.

23. Merton DA. Abdominal applications of ultrasound contrast agents. In: Hagen-Ansert SL, ed. *Textbook of Diagnostic Ultrasonography.* 6th ed. Philadelphia, PA: Mosby Elsevier Inc.; 2006.

24. Abramowicz JS. Ultrasound contrast media: has the time come in obstetrics and gynecology? *J Ultrasound Med.* 2005;24:517–531.

25. Llompart-Pou JA, Abadal JM, Velasco J, et al. Contrast-enhanced transcranial color sonography in the diagnosis of cerebral circulatory arrest. *Transplant Proc.* 2009;41:1466–1468.

26. Valentino M, Serra C, Zironi G, et al. Blunt abdominal trauma: emergency contrast-enhanced sonography for detection of solid organ injuries. *AJR Am J Roentgenol.* 2006;186:1361–1367.

27. Papadopoulou F, Anthopoulou A, Siomou E, et al. Harmonic voiding urosonography with a second-generation contrast agent for the diagnosis of vesicoureteral reflux. *Pediatr Radiol.* 2009;39:239–244.

28. Grayburn PA, Raichlen JS. Evaluation of the heart at rest. In: Goldberg BB, Raichlen JR, Forsberg F, eds. *Ultrasound Contrast Agents: Basic Principles and Clinical Applications.* 2nd ed. London, UK: Martin Dunitz Ltd.; 2001:143–154.

29. Nathan S, Feinstein SB. Evaluation of the heart during exercise and pharmacologic stress. In: Goldberg BB, Raichlen JR, Forsberg F,

eds. *Ultrasound Contrast Agents: Basic Principles and Clinical Applications.* 2nd ed. London, UK: Martin Dunitz Ltd.; 2001:155–164.

30. Luo W, Numata K, Morimoto M, et al. Role of Sonazoid-enhanced three-dimensional ultrasonography in the evaluation of percutaneous radiofrequency ablation of hepatocellular carcinoma. *Eur J Radiol.* 2010;75:91–97.

31. EFSUMB Study Group. Guidelines and Good Clinical Practice Recommendations for Contrast Enhanced Ultrasound (CE-US)—Update 2008. *Ultrasound Med.* 2008;29:28–44.

32. Burns P, Wilson S. Focal liver masses: enhancement patterns on contrast-enhanced images—concordance of US scans with CT scans and MR images. *Radiology.* 2007;242:162–174.

33. Strobel D, Raeker S, Martus P, et al. Phase inversion harmonic imaging versus contrast-enhanced power Doppler ultrasound for the characterization of focal liver lesions. *Int J Colorectal Dis.* 2003;18(1):63–72.

34. Catala V, Nicolau C, Vilana R, et al. Characterization of focal liver lesions: comparative study of contrast-enhanced ultrasound versus spiral computed tomography. *Eur Radiol.* 2007;17(4):1066–1073.

35. Maruyama H, Sekimoto T, Yokosuka O. Role of contrast-enhanced ultrasonography with Sonazoid for hepatocellular carcinoma: evidence from a 10-year experience. *J Gastroenterol.* 2016;51(5):421–433.

36. Kim TK, Khalili K, Jang HJ. Local ablation therapy with contrast-enhanced ultrasonography for hepatocellular carcinoma: a practical review. *Ultrasonography.* 2015;34(4):235–245.

37. D'Onofrio M, Crosara S, De Robertis R, et al. Contrast-enhanced ultrasound of focal liver lesions. *AJR Am J Roentgenol.* 2015;205(1):W56–W66.

38. Cantisani V, Wilson SR. CEUS: where are we in 2015? *Eur J Radiol.* 2015;84(9):1621–1622.

39. Trillaud H, Bruel JM, Valette PJ, et al. Characterization of focal liver lesions with SonoVue® enhanced sonography: international multicenter-study in comparison to CT and MRI. *World J Gastroenterol.* 2009;15(30):3748–3756.

40. Needleman L, Merton DA. Imaging of peripheral vascular pathology. In: Goldberg BB, Raichlen JR, Forsberg F, eds. Ultrasound Contrast Agents: Basic Principles and Clinical Applications. 2nd ed. London, UK: Martin Dunitz Ltd.; 2001:267–275.

41. Robbin ML. The utility of contrast in the extra-cranial carotid ultrasound examination. In: Goldberg BB, Raichlen JR, Forsberg F, eds. *Ultrasound Contrast Agents: Basic Principles and Clinical Applications.* 2nd ed. London, UK: Martin Dunitz Ltd.; 2001:239–252.

42. Pfister K, Rennert J, Uller W, et al. Contrast harmonic imaging ultrasound and perfusion imaging for surveillance after endovascular abdominal aneurysm repair regarding detection and characterization of suspected endoleaks. *Clin Hemorheol Microcirc.* 2009;43:119–128.

43. Langholz J, Scliel R, Schurman R, et al. Contrast enhancement in leg vessels. *Clin Radiol.* 1996;51:31–34.

44. Lindner JR, Womack L, Barrett EJ, et al. Limb stress-rest perfusion imaging with contrast ultrasound for the assessment of peripheral arterial disease severity. *JACC Cardiovasc Imaging.* 2008;1(3):343–350.

45. Duerschmied D, Zhou Q, Rink E, et al. Simplified contrast ultrasound accurately reveals muscle perfusion deficits and reflects collateralization in PAD. *Atherosclerosis.* 2009;202(2):505–512.

46. Seol SH, Davidson BP, Belcik JT, et al. Real-time contrast ultrasound muscle perfusion imaging with intermediate-power imaging coupled with acoustically durable microbubbles. *J Am Soc Echocardiogr.* 2015;28(6):718–726.

47. Thomas KN, Cotter JD, Lucas SJ, et al. Reliability of contrast-enhanced ultrasound for the assessment of muscle perfusion in health and peripheral arterial disease. *Ultrasound Med Biol.* 2015;41(1):26–34.

48. Aschwanden M, Partovi S, Jacobi B, et al. Assessing the end-organ in peripheral arterial occlusive disease-from contrast-enhanced ultrasound to blood-oxygen-level-dependent MR imaging. *Cardiovasc Diagn Ther.* 2014;4(2):165–172.

49. Puls R, Hosten N, Bock JS, et al. Signal-enhanced color Doppler sonography of deep venous thrombosis in the lower limbs and pelvis. *J Ultrasound Med.* 1999;18:185–190.

50. Pfister K, Rennert J, Greiner B, et al. Pre-surgical evaluation of ICA-stenosis using 3D power Doppler, 3D color coded Doppler sonography, 3D B-flow and contrast enhanced B-flow in correlation to CTA/MRA: first clinical results. *Clin Hemorheol Microcirc.* 2009;41(2):103–116.

51. Hammond CJ, McPherson SJ, Patel JV, et al. Assessment of apparent internal carotid occlusion on ultrasound: prospective comparison

of contrast-enhanced ultrasound, magnetic resonance angiography and digital subtraction angiography. *Eur J Vasc Endovasc Surg.* 2008;35(4):405–412.

52. Droste DW, Boehm T, Ritter MA, et al. Benefit of echocontrast-enhanced transcranial arterial color-coded duplex ultrasound. *Cerebrovasc Dis.* 2005;20(5):332–336.

53. Kunz A, Hahn G, Mucha D, et al. Echo-enhanced transcranial color-coded duplex sonography in the diagnosis of cerebrovascular events: a validation study. *AJNR Am J Neuroradiol.* 2006;27:2122–2127.

54. Bogdahn U, Holscher T, Schlachetzki F. Transcranial color-coded duplex sonography (TCCS). In: Goldberg BB, Raichlen JR, Forsberg F, eds. *Ultrasound Contrast Agents: Basic Principles and Clinical Applications.* 2nd ed. London, UK: Martin Dunitz Ltd.; 2001:253–265.

55. Droste DW. Clinical utility of contrast-enhanced ultrasound in neurosonology. *Eur Neurol.* 2008;59(Suppl 1):2–8.

56. Gómez-Choco M, Schreiber SJ, Weih M, et al. Delayed transcranial echo-contrast bolus arrival in unilateral internal carotid artery stenosis and occlusion. *Ultrasound Med Biol.* 2015;41(7):1827–1834.

57. Wang Y, Wang Y, Wang Y, et al. Intraoperative real-time contrast-enhanced ultrasound angiography: a new adjunct in the surgical treatment of arteriovenous malformations. *Neurosurgery.* 2007;107:959–964.

58. Shah F, Balan P, Weinberg M, et al. Contrast-enhanced ultrasound imaging of atherosclerotic carotid plaque neovascularization: a new surrogate marker of atherosclerosis? *Vasc Med.* 2007;12(4):291–297.

59. Magnoni M, Coli S, Marrocco-Trischitta MM, et al. Contrast-enhanced ultrasound imaging of periadventitial vasa vasorum in human carotid arteries. *Eur J Echocardiogr.* 2009;10:260–264.

60. Coli S, Magnoni M, Sangiorgi G, et al. Contrast-enhanced ultrasound imaging of intraplaque neovascularization in carotid arteries: correlation with histology and plaque echogenicity. *J Am Coll Cardiol.* 2008;52(3):223–230.

61. Staub D, Patel MB, Tibrewala A, et al. Vasa vasorum and plaque neovascularization on contrast-enhanced carotid ultrasound imaging correlates with cardiovascular disease and past cardiovascular events. *Stroke.* 2010;4(1):41–47.

62. Song ZZ, Zhang YM. Contrast-enhanced ultrasound imaging of the vasa vasorum of carotid artery plaque. *World J Radiol.* 2015;7(6):131–133.

63. Vavuranakis M, Sigala F, Vrachatis DA, et al. Quantitative analysis of carotid plaque vasa vasorum by CEUS and correlation with histology after endarterectomy. *Vasa.* 2013;42(3):184–195.

64. Ruiz EM, Papaioannou TG, Vavuranakis M, et al. Analysis of contrast-enhanced intravascular ultrasound images for the assessment of coronary plaque neoangiogenesis: another step closer to the identification of the vulnerable plaque. *Curr Pharm Des.* 2012;18(15):2207–2213.

65. Albrecht T, Blomley MJ, Cosgrove DO, et al. Non-invasive diagnosis of hepatic cirrhosis by transit-time analysis of an ultrasound contrast agent. *Lancet.* 1999;353:1579–1583.

66. Lee KH, Choi BI, Kim KW, et al. Contrast-enhanced dynamic ultrasonography of the liver: optimization of hepatic arterial phase in normal volunteers. *Abdom Imaging.* 2003;28(5):652–656.

67. Sellars ME, Sidhu PS, Heneghan M, et al. Infusions of microbubbles are more cost-effective than bolus injections in Doppler studies of the portal vein: a quantitative comparison of normal volunteers and patients with cirrhosis. *Radiology.* 2000;217(P):396.

68. Skjoldbye B, Weislander S, Struckmann J, et al. Doppler ultrasound assessment of TIPS patency and function—the need for echo enhancers. *Acta Radiol.* 1998;39:675–679.

69. Uggowitzer MM, Kugler C, Machan L, et al. Value of echo-enhanced Doppler sonography in evaluation of transjugular intrahepatic portosystemic shunts. *Am J Roentgenol.* 1998;170(4):1041–1046.

70. Missouris CG, Allen CM, Balen FG, et al. Non-invasive screening for renal artery stenosis with ultrasound contrast enhancement. *J Hypertens.* 1996;14(4):519–524.

71. Needleman L. Review of a new ultrasound contrast agent—EchoGen emulsion. *Appl Radiol.* 1997;26(S):8–12.

72. Karamehic J, Scoutt LM, Tabakovic M, et al. Ultrasonography in organs transplantation. *Med Arh.* 2004;58(1 Suppl 2):107–108.

73. Benozzi L, Cappelli G, Granito M, et al. Contrast-enhanced sonography in early kidney graft dysfunction. *Transplant Proc.* 2009;41(4):1214–1215.

74. Boggi U, Morelli L, Amorese G, et al. Contribution of contrast-enhanced ultrasonography to nonoperative management of segmental ischemia of the head of a pancreas graft. *Am J Transplant.* 2009;9(2):413–418.

75. Faccioli N, Crippa S, Bassi C, et al. Contrast-enhanced ultrasonography of the Pancreas. *Pancreatology.* 2009;49(5):560–566.

76. Leutoff UC, Scharf J, Richter GM, et al. Use of ultrasound contrast medium Levovist in after-care of liver transplant patients: improved vascular imaging in color Doppler ultrasound. *Radiology.* 1998;38:399–404.

77. Sidhu PS, Shaw AS, Ellis SM, et al. Microbubble ultrasound contrast in the assessment of hepatic artery patency following liver transplantation: role in reducing frequency of hepatic artery arteriography. *Eur Radiol.* 2004;14(1):21–30.

78. Giannoni MF, Palombo G, Sbarigia E, et al. Contrast-enhanced ultrasound for aortic stent-graft surveillance. *J Endovasc Ther.* 2003;10(2):208–217.

79. Iezzi R, Cotroneo AR, Basilico R, et al. Endoleaks after endovascular repair of abdominal aortic aneurysm: value of CEUS. *Abdom Imaging.* 2010;35(1):106–114.

80. Pfister K, Rennert J, Uller W, et al. Contrast harmonic imaging ultrasound and perfusion imaging for surveillance after endovascular abdominal aneurysm repair regarding detection and characterization of suspected endoleaks. *Clin Hemorheol Microcirc.* 2009;43(1):119–128.

81. Partovi S, Kaspar M, Aschwanden M, et al. Contrast-enhanced ultrasound after endovascular aortic repair-current status and future perspectives. *Cardiovasc Diagn Ther.* 2015;5(6):454–463.

82. Oka MA, Rubens DJ, Strang JG. Ultrasound contrast agent in evaluation of abdominal vessels. *J Ultrasound Med.* 2001;20:S84.

83. Castagno C, Varetto G, Benintende E, et al. Contrast-enhanced sonographic follow-up after stenting of visceral artery aneurysms. *J Ultrasound Med.* 2016;35(3):637–641.

# Complementary Vascular Imaging

BRIAN BURKE

## CHAPTER 33

## OBJECTIVES

- Name three alternate imaging modalities that can supplement duplex sonography for vascular diagnosis

- Recognize the clinical scenarios that favor the use of complementary vascular imaging techniques

- List important contraindications or limitations to the use of CT and MR

- State the main advantages and disadvantages of CT and MR relative to contrast angiography for vascular diagnosis

## GLOSSARY

**contrast** A pharmaceutic agent injected as part of an imaging test to distinguish vessels from nonvascular structures, and to highlight changes in size and shape of vessels

**enhancement** Increase in image brightness within a vascular lumen after contrast injection

**reformat/reconstruction** Alternate presentation of a digital image (i.e., three-dimensional volume rendered reconstruction)

**spatial resolution** Ability of an imaging test to discriminate fine detail

**subtraction** Electronic manipulation of an image leaving only the contrast-enhanced structures visible

## KEY TERMS

**computed tomography angiography (CTA)**

**contrast**

**digital subtraction angiography (DSA)**

**enhancement**

**magnetic resonance angiography (MRA)**

**maximum intensity projection (MIP)**

**reconstruction**

**radiation**

**reformat/reconstruction**

**spatial resolution**

**subtraction**

---

Imaging specialists have several modalities at their disposal for use in evaluation of blood vessels in the body. Contrast angiography, the traditional gold standard, has been advanced over the years by the use of digital technology, allowing reduced contrast loads and more rapid image acquisition. Doppler ultrasound imaging has been utilized for decades as a noninvasive alternative, especially for superficial vessels in the neck and extremities, which are readily accessible to sonographic interrogation. More recently, refinements in computed tomography (CT) and magnetic resonance (MR) hardware and image processing methods have led to the development of CT angiography (CTA) and MR angiography (MRA) as versatile and robust techniques with broad applications in vascular imaging.

This chapter reviews the basic methodology of these alternate imaging techniques, describes their clinical applications, and compares their diagnostic efficacy with that of Doppler ultrasound imaging.

## MODALITIES

### Digital Subtraction Angiography and Digital Subtraction Venography

#### Principles

Arteriography remains the gold standard for imaging evaluation of blood vessels. It is capable of higher spatial resolution than the other techniques, and can depict smaller and higher order branch vessels accurately. It has an additional advantage of facilitating guidance of therapeutic interventions by manipulating catheters and other devices within vessels using fluoroscopic guidance.

#### Technique

Angiography generates images of vascular lumina by filling them with iodinated contrast and exposing them to X-rays.

Modern angiography systems have replaced film with digital detectors, and the resolution of the resulting digital image is dependent on the size of the pixel matrix. The detector is coupled with an X-ray tube in a C-arm (Fig. 33-1) that surrounds the patient and can be rotated in two axes to demonstrate the desired anatomy. The patient table can be moved to enable runoff arteriography.

Digital subtraction is achieved by obtaining a "mask" image before injection of contrast. This mask is digitally subtracted from the postinjection images to yield new images which display contrast only (Fig. 33-2). Patient cooperation is required for success because motion or respiratory excursions result in mismatch between the mask and the postcontrast image. However, the technique has the advantage of permitting substantial reduction in contrast loads.

Contrast administration requires vascular access, meaning direct puncture of a vessel and placement of a catheter in the vessel of interest. Arterial access sites include the common femoral, brachial, and radial arteries. Venous access sites vary depending on the site of intervention, but frequently include the common femoral and brachial veins. The amount and rate of contrast injection depends on the size of the blood vessel and the rate of blood flow. Current trends favor the use of nonionic or low-osmolar iodinated contrast to minimize discomfort and adverse reactions associated with injection.

## Accuracy

As previously stated, contrast angiography remains the gold standard for vascular diagnosis, and its accuracy has been verified by surgical correlation. For example, in the carotid system, digital subtraction angiography (DSA) images of good diagnostic quality provide sensitivity of 95%, specificity of 99%, and accuracy of 97% in the diagnosis of luminal stenosis.[1] Similar results are achievable in the lower extremity arteries, although rates of vessel opacification may limit accuracies in the smaller vessels of the lower leg and foot.

DSA is a two-dimensional technique, and because arterial lesions tend to be eccentric, a single run may not demonstrate the full extent of luminal narrowing. Multiple projections are often necessary to best estimate the degree of stenosis.

## Limitations

DSA is more invasive than the other imaging techniques because of direct arterial access, so more complications can occur. Injury at the access site can cause bleeding complications, pseudoaneurysm, or arteriovenous fistula formation. Intravascular injuries can include intimal dissection, intramural hematoma, or plaque embolization.

Although incidence of allergic reactions to iodinated contrast is much less for arterial injection than for intravenous injection, this remains a relative contraindication and may require premedication. Poor renal function is also a relative

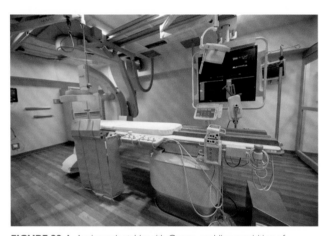

**FIGURE 33-1** Angiography table with C-arm, enabling acquisition of orthogonal and oblique angle image projections.

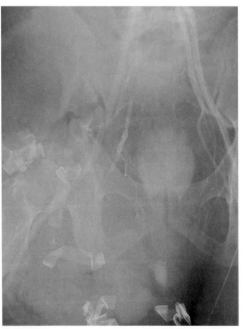

A

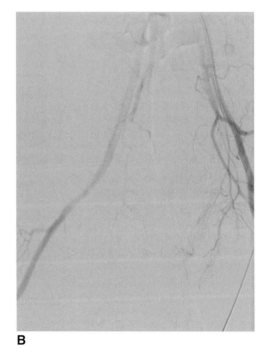

B

**FIGURE 33-2** Digital subtraction angiograms result when a precontrast "mask" is electronically subtracted from a contrast-enhanced image (**A**), leaving an image consisting solely of contrast in vessel lumens (**B**).

contraindication. The use of an alternate contrast agent, such as gadolinium or carbon dioxide, can be considered. The cost of DSA generally exceeds that of the competing imaging modalities.

## Computed Tomography Angiography/Computed Tomography Venography

### Principles

CTA, like DSA, utilizes X-rays to demonstrate contrast-enhanced blood vessels. As a cross-sectional technique, however, the image is acquired as an axial section through the body. The data can be digitally manipulated to present the image in alternate planes or as a three-dimensional reconstruction. In addition, because the contrast resolution of CT is considerably superior to projectional radiography, the vessel wall and surrounding soft tissue structures are visible to a much greater degree. The same high-contrast resolution permits adequate opacification of the vascular system with a peripheral venous injection.

### Technique

CT scanners are configured with an X-ray source emitting a fan-shaped beam, mounted on a rotating ring opposite to an arc of X-ray detectors (Fig. 33-3). The source rotates through a 360° circle as the patient moves on a table within the beam. Current scanners employ multiple detectors (64 or more) and a helical pattern of scanning such that a volume of data is acquired rather than serial discrete slices. The scan is acquired through the area of interest during a single breath hold, while contrast is injected at a rate of 3 to 5 mL/second.

Arrival of the contrast bolus in the vessel of interest must be accurately timed to maximize the contrast between the enhanced vessel lumen and the surrounding soft tissues. Bolus tracking software is incorporated into the scanner to detect the arrival of contrast within the volume of interest and allow initiation of scanning at the appropriate time (Fig. 33-4). Other scan parameters, including field of view, slice thickness, and pitch, are modified according to the need for anatomic coverage.

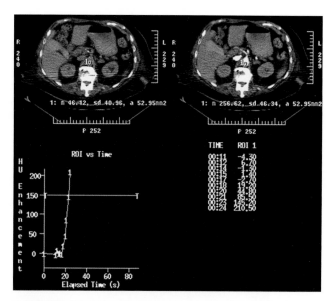

**FIGURE 33-4** Analyzing a time-enhancement curve after administering a test bolus of contrast accounts for individual variation in blood flow. The study can be performed with optimal scan delay to maximize enhancement in the vessels of interest.

Because the effective slice thickness is less than 1 mm, the data can be digitally manipulated such that an image of isotropic resolution can be displayed in any projection. Further data manipulation can render the image in a 3D format. The 3D images can be displayed with a maximum intensity projection (MIP) format where pixel density corresponds to luminal caliber, or in a shaded surface display format which emphasizes the intimal contour (Fig. 33-5). The 3D images can then be manipulated on a workstation into a variety of projections.

### Accuracy

Published studies have shown high efficacy for CTA in a variety of applications in comparison to DSA. For the diagnosis of >50% stenosis in the carotid bifurcation, CTA demonstrated a sensitivity of 89%, specificity of 91%, and accuracy of 90%.[2] CTA has essentially replaced ventilation/perfusion (V/Q) scanning for the diagnosis of pulmonary embolism on the basis of its ability to detect smaller emboli and the lack of recurrent thromboembolic disease in outcomes studies after negative CTA. For the peripheral circulation, CTA is essentially equivalent in accuracy to DSA for vessels larger than 1 mm in diameter. For the lower extremity arterial circulation in the diagnosis of >50% stenosis, Willmann and colleagues[3] found sensitivity of 96%, specificity of 96%, and accuracy of 96%.

### Limitations

The presence of extensive intimal calcification hinders visualization of the vascular lumen in smaller vessels, making it difficult to distinguish stenosis from occlusion. Artifact generated from nearby metallic objects (joint prostheses and surgical clips) can render a vessel segment uninterpretable.

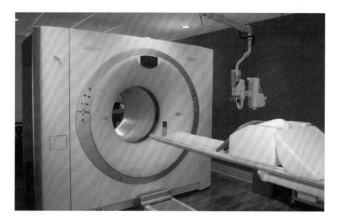

**FIGURE 33-3** Large patient volumes can be scanned with multidetector CT technology within a single breath hold, allowing the acquisition of images of long vascular segments during peak enhancement.

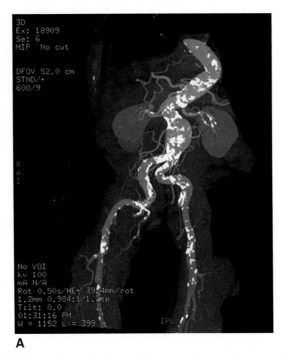
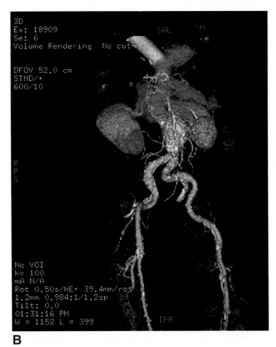

**FIGURE 33-5** The axial scan data from a CTA can be postprocessed to present the image in a form that is familiar to clinicians, and enhances perception of abnormalities, such as the MIP image (**A**), or the volume-rendered reconstruction (**B**).

Allergic reactions to contrast are more frequently encountered with the venous injections for CTA as compared to arterial contrast administration for DSA. A history of anaphylactic reaction to contrast may preclude the performance of the study. Poor renal function is also a relative contraindication to the use of iodinated contrast. Extravasation of contrast at the injection site can result in pain, swelling, and tissue damage.[4]

Because CT is so commonly performed in current medical practice, and because CTA incurs a higher exposure than most conventional CT studies, the long-term risk of radiation-induced cancers is a concern. Models estimate approximately 29,000 future cancers related to CT scans performed in the United States in 2007.[5] Dose reduction compatible with the As Low As Reasonably Achievable principle should be applied to every study.

## Magnetic Resonance Angiography/ Magnetic Resonance Venography

### Principles

The growth of vascular applications in magnetic resonance imaging (MRI) has ensued from the development of fast scan techniques and image processing software, enabling breath hold imaging of large body parts. MRA competes with CTA and Doppler techniques for evaluation of the cerebral, visceral, and peripheral arterial and venous circulation. Although slightly less robust than CTA in its sensitivity to motion artifact, in cooperative patients it allows accurate depiction of small vessels without exposure to ionizing radiation.

For MRI, a strong magnetic field is applied to the patient, causing protons within the body to align with the field (Fig. 33-6). This orientation is disturbed by further

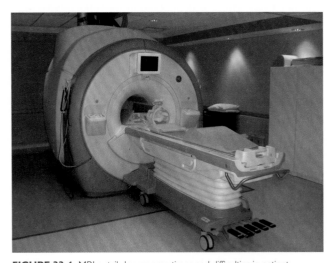

**FIGURE 33-6** MRI entails longer scan times and difficulties in patient monitoring compared to CT.

application of magnetic gradients and radiofrequency pulses. After the pulse subsides, the protons reorient themselves, in the process of which energy is emitted. This radiofrequency energy, which is dependent on the nature and density of the tissue of origin, forms the basis of the MR image.

### Technique

MRA can be performed with or without contrast administration. Noncontrast MRA utilizes the time-of-flight method. With this technique, protons within flowing blood entering a previously excited tissue volume generate a strong signal. This flow-related enhancement is strongest when the vessel is oriented perpendicular to the tissue slice. Selective arterial or venous time-of-flight studies can be achieved by presaturating the protons above or below the imaged tissue to suppress signal within the arteries or veins, respectively.

Contrast-enhanced MRA, like CTA, involves breath hold imaging of the area of interest while peak concentrations of contrast are present within the vessels. Imaging sequences with short acquisition times that have low-spatial resolution are utilized, but can be repeated quickly to create the appearance of a contrast angiogram.

Contrast agents for MRA are chelates of gadolinium, which has paramagnetic properties, resulting in strong increase in signal intensity in the enhanced vessel. This effect is transient, necessitating the use of bolus timing to capture peak enhancement. However, newer contrast agents remain within the blood pool for longer periods and enable delayed scanning, especially useful for venous applications. The use of a moving table makes it possible to follow a contrast bolus through the lower extremities for an arterial runoff study. Subtraction techniques can be employed, as with DSA, to maximize contrast between enhancing and nonenhancing pixels.

### Accuracy

State-of-the-art MRA offers high accuracies in a variety of applications, similar to those achieved with CTA. A recent meta-analysis evaluating contrast-enhanced MRA for disease in the internal carotid artery showed the following sensitivities and specificities: for moderate (50% to 69%) stenosis, 66% and 94%; for severe (70% to 99%) stenosis, 95% and 92%; and for occlusion, 99% and 99%.[6] A second study evaluating diagnostic performance in the lower extremities found sensitivity of 95% and specificity of 96% for contrast-enhanced MRA in the diagnosis of >50% stenosis.[7] Lesser accuracy is achieved for the deep visceral vessels where respiratory and peristaltic motion limits resolution.

### Limitations

General contraindications to MRI (certain implanted devices, metallic foreign bodies, and claustrophobia) apply to MRA as well. Patients who are unable to cooperate or breath hold are poor candidates for these studies. Stents, filters, and other vascular implants generate local artifacts that can render the study nondiagnostic.

Patients with poor renal function are at risk for the development of nephrogenic systemic fibrosis after exposure to gadolinium-based contrast agents. This risk is most significant for patients with an estimated glomerular filtration rate (GFR) of <30 mL/min/1.73 m².[8]

## APPLICATIONS

### Cerebrovascular Disease

DSA is the gold standard for evaluation of the carotid bifurcation and the intracranial vessels (Fig. 33-7). Major studies performed in the 1990s (North American Symptomatic Carotid Endarterectomy Trial and Asymptomatic Carotid Atherosclerosis Study) established methodology for quantifying carotid stenosis based on this method. However, in the current era with maturing of the noninvasive modalities, DSA has been largely replaced for diagnostic purposes. It still plays an important role for guidance of therapeutic interventions, such as carotid stent placement.

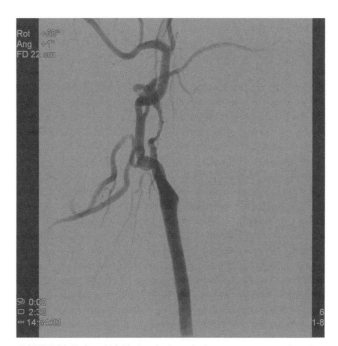

**FIGURE 33-7** Carotid DSA showing irregular long-segment narrowing of the proximal internal carotid artery with excellent spatial resolution.

There is long experience with the use of Doppler ultrasound in the diagnosis of disease in the extracranial carotid arteries. Well-established criteria exist for the detection and grading of stenosis and occlusion of the internal carotid artery. Limitations include heavily calcified lesions which inhibit interrogation of the entire lumen. In addition, the intrathoracic and intracranial segments of the carotid vessels are inaccessible.

Grading of stenoses by CTA or MRA is based on either visual estimation or caliper measurement, either from the source axial images or processed image reconstructions (MIP images) (Figs. 33-8 and 33-9). Spatial resolution for these

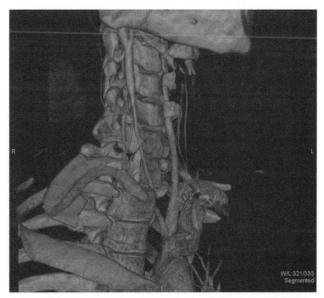

**FIGURE 33-8** Volume rendered reconstruction of a carotid CTA showing smooth, long-segment narrowing of both common carotid arteries in a patient with vasculitis.

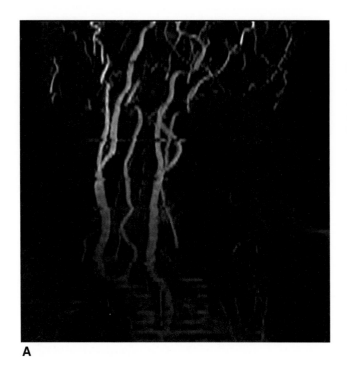

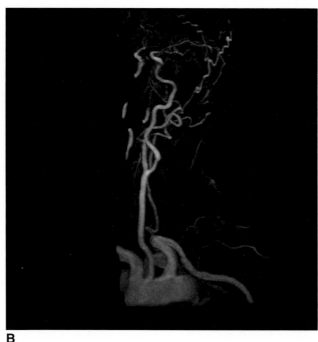

**A**                                                    **B**

**FIGURE 33-9** Time-of-flight (TOF) MRA (**A**) suffers from more artifacts and lesser spatial resolution than contrast-enhanced MRA (**B**). The proximal stenosis in the left internal carotid artery is better depicted in the latter image.

techniques is not as good as for DSA, but the cross-sectional nature of the image results in improved characterization of irregular/eccentric vessel narrowing than the projectional images with DSA.[9] In addition, the improved contrast resolution for CT and MR allows visualization and characterization of the vessel wall and intimal plaque, whereas DSA depicts only the vessel lumen. Calcified plaque appears as a signal void on MRA.[10]

The distinction between high-grade stenosis and occlusion has important treatment implications. All modalities have high levels of accuracy in making this distinction; it should be realized, although, that turbulent flow at the site of a critical stenosis may result in a focal signal void within the lumen on time-of-flight (noncontrast) MRA. Occasionally, a correlative study with another modality is helpful to resolve uncertainty.

Evaluation of the postoperative or poststented carotid system is best performed by ultrasound or CTA because surgical clips or stents cause local field inhomogeneity with image artifact obscuring the vessel.

## Peripheral Arterial Disease

Vascular diagnosis in the lower extremities involves distinguishing between focal lesions which are amenable to angioplasty or stenting, and multifocal or diffuse disease that would benefit from surgical bypass. Treatment planning requires evaluation of the distal runoff vessels because untreated distal disease increases likelihood of stent or graft failure. Initial evaluation of symptomatic patients is with Doppler measurement of ankle-brachial index (ABI), where an ABI <0.90 indicates flow-limiting disease. Determination of the anatomic site and extent of disease is performed using duplex sonography, CTA, or MRA. Contrast arteriography,

like in the carotid system, is principally used for guidance of endovascular interventions (Fig. 33-10).

CTA for peripheral arterial diagnosis includes evaluation of the abdominal aorta, the iliac arteries of the pelvis, and a lower extremity runoff arteriogram (Fig. 33-11). Precontrast imaging can be very helpful in patients with extensive vascular calcifications. Bolus tracking is necessary to ensure imaging at the time of peak luminal opacification, and

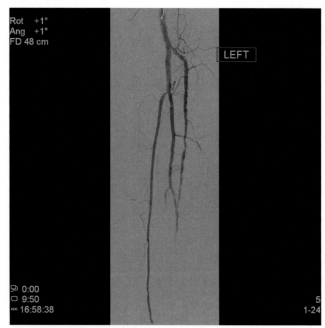

**FIGURE 33-10** DSA of the infrapopliteal circulation showing multifocal narrowing in the anterior tibial artery. This run preceded angioplasty and stent placement.

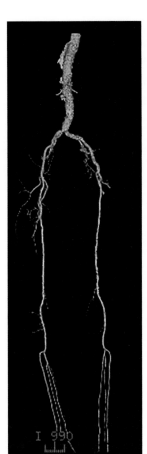

**FIGURE 33-11** CTA volume reconstructions facilitate surgical and endovascular treatment planning. These are reviewed along with the two-dimensional axial scans when interpreting the study.

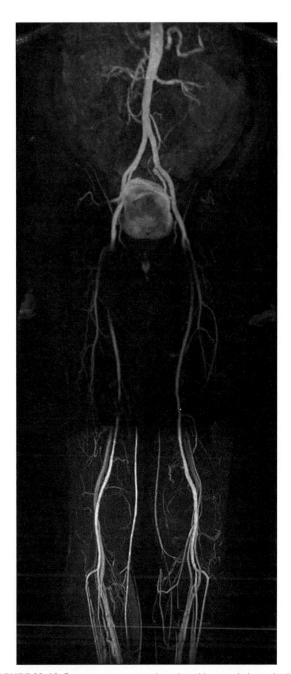

**FIGURE 33-12** Fast scan sequences and moving tables permit the evaluation of the abdominal aorta through the feet in a single MRA. Note the overlapping arteries and veins in the lower legs.

delayed imaging of the calves may be required when extensive disease results in delay in contrast reaching the feet.

In addition to identifying and grading sites of occlusion and stenosis, CTA can demonstrate vascular anomalies, pathways of collateral flow, and evidence of thromboembolic disease. Depiction of the soft tissues surrounding vessel lumina helps to characterize aneurysms and vascular malformations, and to identify postoperative fluid collections. Post-processing of the CT data to create 3D or volume-rendered reconstructions yields an image format that facilitates presurgical planning.[11]

Contrast-enhanced MRA provides similar anatomic coverage to CTA in the lower extremities (Fig. 33-12). The extent of calcified plaque is less well depicted; stents and surgical clips cause local artifacts that obscure luminal findings. However, rapid-sequence imaging in the calves with small contrast boluses (i.e., Time Resolved Imaging of Contrast Kinetics or "TRICKS" sequences) generate runoff arteriograms of high-spatial and temporal resolution.

Less cooperative patients who would benefit from rapid scan acquisition, and those with vascular stents or other metallic implants, should be imaged with CTA. On the other hand, patients with iodine allergies, and diabetics with extensive vascular calcifications, will be better served by MRA.[12]

## Peripheral Venous Disease

Duplex sonography is the first-line examination for venous thrombosis in the upper and lower extremities because of its low cost, high accuracy, and ability to perform serial exams with no radiation exposure. It is limited where there is no acoustic access.

Contrast venography is seldom performed any more for diagnosis, but is an essential component of therapeutic measures such as thrombolysis and venous stent placement, frequently as part of management of dialysis fistulas (Fig. 33-13).

CT venography (CTV) is sometimes performed in conjunction with pulmonary CTA in patients with suspected thromboembolic disease, allowing a complete workup with a single contrast injection. Imaging of the pelvis and lower extremities is delayed until the veins are opacified, and adequate imaging through the calf veins is frequently possible.

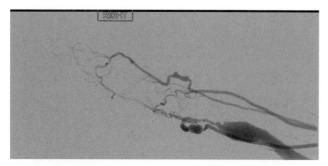

**FIGURE 33-13** DSA is frequently employed for diagnosis and treatment of complications of dialysis fistulae. In this radiocephalic AV fistula, there is narrowing of the fistula and the outflow vein. AV, arteriovenous.

CTV and MR venography (MRV) are especially useful centrally, where sonographic access is limited (Fig. 33-14). Thrombosis of the dural venous sinuses, superior and inferior vena cava, mesenteric and iliac veins is often best detected by these methods. Specific indications include thoracic outlet syndrome, May–Thurner syndrome, and ovarian vein thrombosis (Fig. 33-15). MRV in pregnant patients can be performed without contrast administration to avoid fetal exposure.[13]

The anatomy of complex venous malformations or arteriovenous malformations may be best depicted with these cross-sectional methods. Distinguishing between bland and tumor thrombus by contrast-enhanced MRV has been described. Finally, detection of usable venous access sites in chronic dialysis patients with multiple thrombosed veins is facilitated by use of MRV.

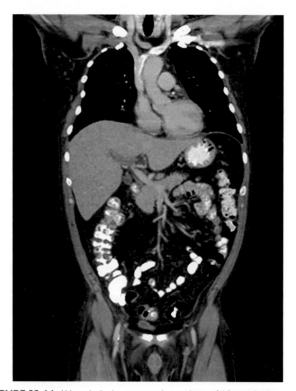

**FIGURE 33-14** Although duplex sonography can be useful for evaluation of the visceral vasculature, this coronally reconstructed CT venogram allows confident diagnosis of thrombosis of the main portal vein at the porta hepatis extending into the right portal vein.

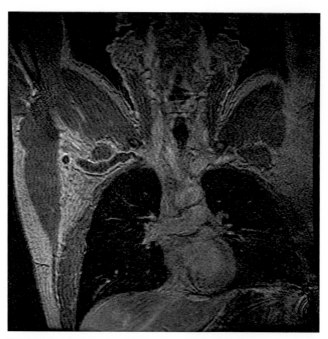

**FIGURE 33-15** Thoracic outlet syndrome. Coronal MRV with arms above the head showing right subclavian vein thrombosis with narrowing of the vein segment trapped between the clavicle and first rib.

## Abdominal Aorta

Contrast angiography is used as a road map prior to surgical treatment of aneurysm (Fig. 33-16). It is also considered the gold standard for evaluation of aortic dissection. However, it only visualizes the aortic lumen and does not assess the vessel wall, or thrombus within an aneurysm, so the full size and extent of aneurysm is not reliably evaluated.

CTA is very useful prior to aneurysm repair by showing the size of the aneurysm and its relationship to adjacent vessels. Accurate measurements of the vessel lumen are necessary to plan endograft placement. Follow-up after surgical or endovascular treatment is usually performed with CTA, although sonography reliably detects change in size of the aneurysmal sac and can demonstrate endoleak (Fig. 33-17).[14]

MRA is an acceptable alternative for evaluation of aneurysm and dissection. MRA is especially helpful when iodinated contrast is contraindicated (Fig. 33-18).

## Renovascular Disease

Multiple modalities have been applied to make the diagnosis of renal artery stenosis, often complicated by the desire to minimize iodinated contrast exposure to patients with renal insufficiency. DSA has high accuracy for estimating stenosis severity, and is reliable for detection of stenoses in branch vessels and for fibromuscular dysplasia (FMD) (Fig. 33-19). But, because of its invasive nature and the low incidence of the diagnosis in the hypertensive population, DSA is usually reserved for a confirmatory test and to guide stent placement.

Duplex sonography of the renal arteries is frequently employed for screening. However, it is technically demanding. High-accuracy rates are most often seen in labs with

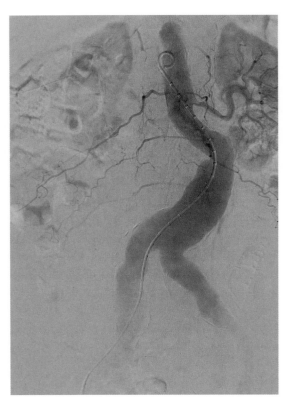

**FIGURE 33-16** Abdominal aortic aneurysm and bilateral common iliac aneurysms demonstrated by DSA. The vessel lumen is shown, but the wall and mural thrombus are not visualized.

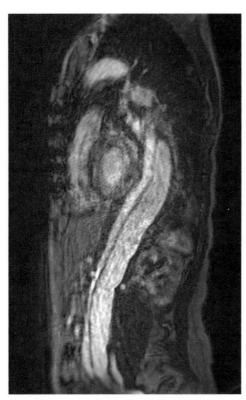

**FIGURE 33-18** Sagittal aortic MRA depicting the intimal flap of an aortic dissection extending from the thoracic aortic arch through the common iliac arteries.

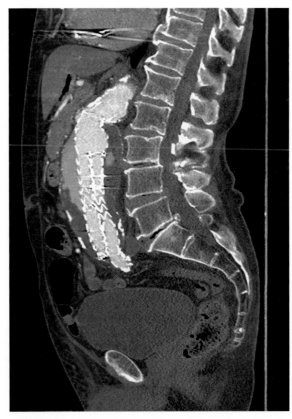

**FIGURE 33-17** Sagittal reconstruction of aortic CTA showing endovascular repair of aortic aneurysm by placement of a bifurcated stent graft. Presence of contrast within the excluded aneurysmal lumen is consistent with endoleak.

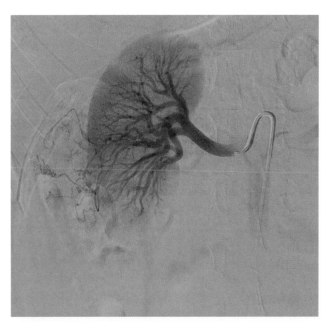

**FIGURE 33-19** The higher order branches of the right renal artery are well demonstrated on this selective DSA. The vascular mass arising from the lower pole of the kidney is an angiomyolipoma.

experienced sonographers and that maintain a high volume of studies.

CTA is highly accurate for proximal renal artery stenosis and can usually identify FMD (Fig. 33-20). It is more successful than ultrasound in identifying accessory renal arteries. Because it permits evaluation of the surrounding

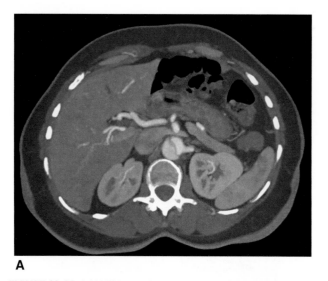

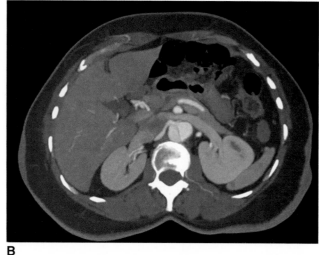

**A**

**B**

**FIGURE 33-20** Axial MIP images from a renal artery CTA showing the origin and proximal segments of the left (**A**) and right (**B**) renal arteries. Note the aortic dissection with both renal arteries arising from the true lumen.

soft tissues, it will pick up the occasional renal or adrenal tumor causing hypertension.

Contrast-enhanced MRA has slightly decreased spatial resolution compared to CTA, mostly because of tissue motion associated with the longer image acquisition times. Good accuracy is achievable in the proximal renal arteries, although overestimation of stenosis is possible where extensive atherosclerotic plaque is present (Fig. 33-21). MRA is not useful after renal artery stent placement.[15]

## Mesenteric Arteries

Chronic mesenteric ischemia because of arterial insufficiency usually ensues with occlusion or high-grade stenosis of at least two of the three major mesenteric arteries (celiac,

superior mesenteric, and inferior mesenteric arteries). DSA, CTA, and MRA are all sufficient to demonstrate the origin and proximal extent of these arteries and are highly accurate in making this diagnosis. In contrast, embolic disease and vasculitis more often present with narrowing or occlusion in the smaller branch vessels, for which contrast angiography is necessary to depict (Fig. 33-22). However, CTA and MRA are well suited to show bowel wall thickening and pneumatosis in cases of bowel ischemia, and can show thrombotic disease in the mesenteric veins (Figs. 33-23 and 33-24).[16,17]

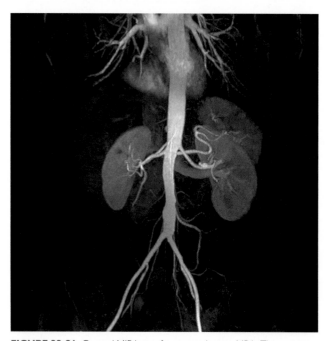

**FIGURE 33-21** Coronal MIP image from a renal artery MRA. The intraparenchymal branches are less well seen than with DSA.

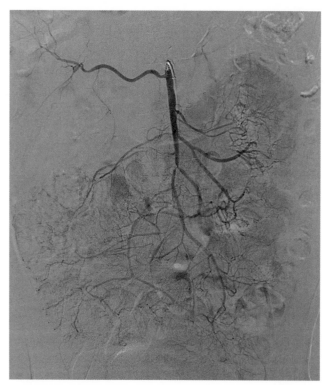

**FIGURE 33-22** Selective injection of the superior mesenteric artery from a mesenteric DSA. Peripheral stenoses seen at the origin of the ileal branches would be difficult to detect by CTA or MRA.

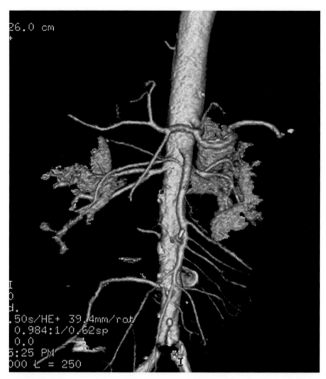

**FIGURE 33-23** 3D volume reconstruction of the abdominal CTA showing the branching pattern of the celiac and superior mesenteric artery in a coronal projection.

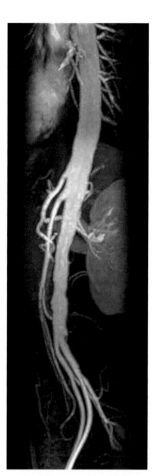

**FIGURE 33-24** Sagittal MIP projection from a mesenteric MRA showing the celiac artery and SMA. The IMA is mostly obscured in this view. IMA, inferior mesenteric artery; SMA, superior mesenteric artery.

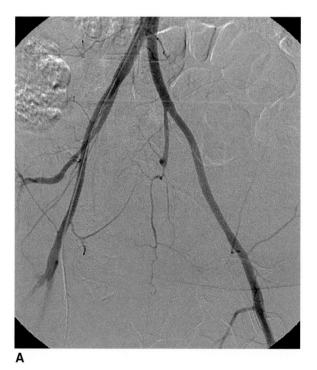

**A**

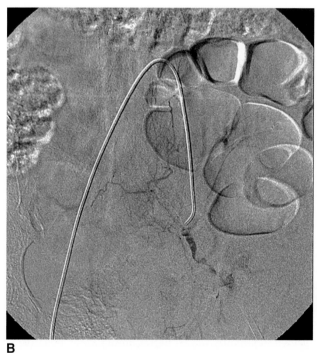

**B**

**FIGURE 33-25** Pelvic DSA following motor vehicle accident. Initial aortic injection (**A**) showing vasospasm of the left internal iliac artery. Subsequent selective injection (**B**) demonstrating contrast extravasation from the posterior division of the internal iliac artery consistent with active bleeding. Coil embolization of the artery successfully stopped the hemorrhage.

| TABLE 33-1 | **Comparison of Types of Angiography** | |
|---|---|---|
| **Modality** | **Advantages** | **Disadvantages** |
| DSA | • Gold standard<br>• High-spatial resolution<br>• High accuracy<br>• Facilitates guidance of interventions | • Uses X-rays<br>• Potential allergic reaction to iodinated contrast<br>• Requires arterial puncture<br>• Potential complications at access site<br>• 2D technique thus needs multiple projections |
| CTA | • 3D reconstructed images<br>• Provides vessel wall, plaque and surrounding tissue details<br>• Rapid image acquisition<br>• Less demanding for older/sicker patients | • Uses X-rays<br>• Allergic reaction to contrast<br>• Limited by intimal calcification<br>• Metal objects produce artifacts |
| MRA | • Can be performed without contrast<br>• No X-rays needed<br>• Safe in patients with iodine allergies<br>• Safe for pregnant patients | • Contraindicated with implanted devices<br>• Calcification will cause a signal void<br>• Gadolinium can be nephrotoxic<br>• Longer acquisition times |

## Vascular Trauma

In the setting of trauma, vascular injury can present with vasospasm, intimal injury with or without occlusion, vascular disruption, or pseudoaneurysm formation (Fig. 33-25). Because these patients often incur additional soft tissue injury, contrast CT is frequently the initial test performed. Contrast extravasation during the arterial phase of enhancement confirms and localizes the site of injury. Pseudoaneurysm is readily detected as well (Fig. 33-26). Directed arteriography can then be performed to guide endovascular treatment (embolization).

MRA is generally not considered a viable option in the setting of acute trauma because of the longer acquisition times and the difficulty in monitoring unstable patients inside the magnet. In the special case of iatrogenic femoral artery injury after catheterization, sonography is generally sufficient for diagnosis and guidance of therapeutic thrombin injection.

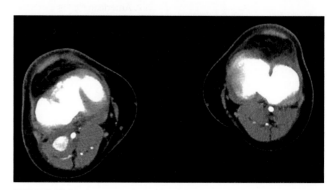

**FIGURE 33-26** Axial image from a lower extremity CTA after trauma. There is a pseudoaneurysm arising from the lateral aspect of the right popliteal artery via a thin neck.

### SUMMARY

- Noninvasive cross-sectional imaging techniques such as CTA and MRA are complementary to duplex sonography.
- The advantages of CTA and MRA in imaging of blood vessels overlap.
- CTA and MRA may be preferred for these applications depending on patient factors and institutional expertise.
- Diagnostic yield from these tests may be comparable to, if not superior to, that achievable with contrast arteriography.

### CRITICAL THINKING QUESTIONS

1. A patient presents with a suspected pulmonary embolus. A lower extremity ultrasound examination is negative for thrombus, but because of the patient's body habitus, the pelvic veins cannot be adequately visualized with ultrasound. Which type of imaging would be most appropriate?
2. In a patient with poor renal function and markedly decreased GFR, which type of angiography should be avoided?

### MEDIA MENU

Student Resources available on **thePoint** include:
- Audio glossary
- Interactive question bank
- Videos
- Internet resources

## REFERENCES

1. Croft RJ, Ellam LD, Harrison MJG. Accuracy of carotid angiography in the assessment of atheroma of the internal carotid artery. *Lancet*. 1980;315(8176):997–1000.
2. Herzig R, Burval S, Krupka B, et al. Comparison of ultrasonography, CT angiography, and digital subtraction angiography in severe carotid stenoses. *Eur J Neurol*. 2004;11(11):774–781.
3. Willmann JK, Baumert B, Schertler T, et al. Aortoiliac and lower extremity arteries assessed with 16-detector row CT angiography: prospective comparison with digital subtraction angiography. *Radiology*. 2005;236(3):1083–1093.
4. American College of Radiology. *Adverse Effects of Iodinated Contrast Media, in Manual on Contrast Media* Version 7. American College of Radiology; 2010:19–23.
5. Berrington de Gonzalez A, Mahesh M, Kim K, et al. Projected cancer risks from computed tomographic scans performed in the United States in 2007. *Arch Intern Med*. 2009;169: 2071–2077.
6. Nederkoorn PJ, van der Graaf Y, Hunink MGM. Duplex ultrasound and magnetic resonance angiography compared with digital subtraction angiography in carotid artery stenosis: a systematic review. *Stroke*. 2003;34:1324–1332.
7. Pollak AW, Norton PT, Kramer CM. Multimodality imaging of lower extremity peripheral arterial disease: current role and future directions. *Circ Cardiovasc Imaging*. 2012;5:797–807.
8. American College of Radiology. *Nephrogenic Systemic Fibrosis in Manual on Contrast Media Version 7*. American College of Radiology; 2010:49–55.
9. Anderson GB, Ashforth R, Steinke DE, et al. CT angiography for the detection and characterization of carotid artery bifurcation disease. *Stroke*. 2000;31:2168–2174.
10. Debrey SM, Yu H, Lynch JK, et al. Diagnostic accuracy of magnetic resonance angiography for internal carotid artery disease: a systematic review and meta-analysis. *Stroke*. 2008;39(8):2237–2248.
11. Fleischmann D, Hallett RL, Rubin GD. CT angiography of peripheral arterial disease. *J Vasc Interv Radiol*. 2006;17:3–26.
12. Collins R, Cranny G, Burch J, et al. A systematic review of duplex ultrasound, magnetic resonance angiography and computed tomography angiography for the diagnosis and assessment of symptomatic lower limb peripheral arterial disease. *Health Technol Assess*. 2007;11:1–184.
13. Krinsky G. Body MR venography: the new gold standard. *Appl Radiol*. 2004;33(2):26–33.
14. Moriwaki Y, Matsuda G, Karube N, et al. Usefulness of color Doppler ultrasonography (CDUS) and three-dimensional spiral computed tomographic angiography (3D-CT) for diagnosis of unruptured abdominal visceral aneurysm. *Hepatogastroenterology*. 2003;49:1728–1730.
15. Tan KT, van Beek EJR, Brown PWG, et al. Magnetic resonance angiography for the diagnosis of renal artery stenosis: a meta-analysis. *Clin Radiol*. 2002;57:617–624.
16. Aschoff AJ, Stuber G, Becker BW, et al. Evaluation of acute mesenteric ischemia: accuracy of biphasic mesenteric multi-detector CT angiography. *Abdom Imaging*. 2009;34:345–357.
17. Meaney JF, Prince MR, Nostrant TT, et al. Gadolinium-enhanced MR angiography of visceral arteries in patients with suspected chronic mesenteric ischemia. *J Magn Reson Imaging*. 1997;7:171–176.

# Quality Assurance

TERRENCE D. CASE | ANN MARIE KUPINSKI

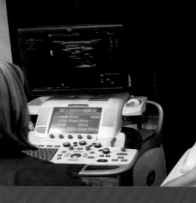

**CHAPTER 34**

## OBJECTIVES

- Define the term "gold standard"
- Describe the common statistical terms, including sensitivity, specificity, and accuracy
- Define other commonly used statistical parameters
- Calculate basic statistical values using a Chi-square test
- Describe the concept of peer review

## GLOSSARY

**accuracy** The overall percentage of correct results

**gold standard** A well-established and reliable testing parameter which for vascular disease is often angiography

**peer review** The evaluation of one's work by other experts in the same field

**sensitivity** It is the ability of a test to detect disease

**specificity** It is the ability of a test to correctly identify a normal result

## KEY TERMS

**accuracy**

**gold standard**

**negative predictive value**

**peer review**

**positive predictive value**

**sensitivity**

**specificity**

Ultrasound is a technology that is safe and reliable when used by well-trained sonographers in a department that is focused on quality assurance (QA). QA refers to a program for the systematic monitoring and evaluation of the various aspects of vascular testing to ensure that standards of quality are being met. It has taken years of research and development to convince physicians and other health care providers that ultrasound technology alone is accurate in the assessment of vascular disease. To achieve that confidence, the ultrasound profession relied on statistics to demonstrate the effectiveness of sonography and Doppler in the assessment of vascular disease.

## STATISTICS

Statistics is the science of making effective use of numerical data relating to groups of individuals or experiments. It deals with all aspects of the collection, analysis, and interpretation of such data. In addition, statistics is used in the planning of the collection of data, in terms of the design of surveys and experiments. This chapter briefly reviews some of the common terminology and methods used to determine the accuracy of vascular ultrasound reports or studies.

## Comparing Diagnostic Tests

### The "Gold Standard"

Medical science has borrowed the term "gold standard" to compare one form of a diagnostic test with another that is well established, reliable, and considered the reference standard. The "gold standard" is assumed to be the truth. The "gold standard" in vascular imaging typically refers to an angiogram (or in some cases a venogram). The angiogram has a long history of accuracy, and therefore all newer types of vascular imaging must be compared to it to determine the presence or absence of disease and the extent to which it presents. However, there are some risks with angiography, which may be as minimal as a hematoma at the insertion site to allergic reaction to the dye, which could end with either a stroke or even death. In medicine, the benefits must always outweigh the risks, and although ultrasound is considered safe and accurate now, it had to be first compared with the gold standard in order to establish accuracy. Ideally, a vascular ultrasound would match the gold standard 100% of the time, but this is often not the case. There are various common measurements employed to compare testing results to a gold standard.

461

## True Positive

True positives (TP) are the number of studies performed by ultrasound which state that disease is present and the gold standard agrees with the ultrasound findings. For example, an ultrasound shows a dilated noncompressible femoral vein with no flow, the venogram demonstrates an occluded femoral vein, and the physician's diagnosis is a deep venous thrombosis (DVT). Thus, all are in agreement that disease is present: a TP.

## True Negative

True negatives (TN) are the number of negative findings reported by ultrasound that were also reported negative by the gold standard. For example, the ultrasound indicates no evidence of echogenic plaque and normal flow velocities in the proximal internal carotid artery, an arteriogram does not identify any disease, and the physician's interpretation is no internal carotid artery disease. Thus, all are in agreement that no disease is present: a TN.

## False Positives

Unfortunately, there are some cases where the ultrasound and gold standard do not agree. When using arteriography as the gold standard, those findings in almost every case represent the correct findings. There may be a situation where the duplex ultrasound demonstrates velocity elevations consistent with a stenosis, but the arteriogram finds no disease. Another example may be a case where the sonographer fails to properly compress a vein, which is then interpreted as an occluded vein. Subsequent venography demonstrates a patent, thrombus-free vessel. Fortunately, disagreements are relatively rare, but statistics is necessary to help identify these inaccuracies. When these mismatches occur, studies can be carefully reviewed to determine the specific source of the error.

The examples in the preceding paragraph are false positive (FP) results. FP are studies that are reported positive, but found to be negative by the gold standard. Another variation of the FP result could occur when a carotid ultrasound study met the criteria for a 50% to 79% stenosis, but the arteriogram only detected a 40% stenosis. This is a FP; however, it is important here for both radiology and ultrasound to be clear about what a FP constitutes. A difference of 5% error in velocity measurement could put the findings in one category or another. While the categories are significantly different and could effect medical management, the actual difference is relatively small.

## False Negative

A false negative (FN) states that a study is normal when the gold standard identifies disease. An example of a FN would be, if a normal aortic diameter is reported by ultrasound but the arteriogram shows a tortuous aorta with a 3.0 cm abdominal aortic aneurysm. Some might argue that this may be a relatively minor error and have little clinical significance. But a report stating "No DVT in femoral vein" that turns out to be a FN, may be life threatening. Clearly, the sonographer wants to have a high degree of TP and TN with no or very few FN and FP.

## Accuracy

QA statistics utilize the calculations of TN, TP, FN, and FP in order to determine other indicators which describe the results of a test. Accuracy is one such indicator. Accuracy can be thought of as the degree of "closeness" of something to its actual value. For example, in the vascular laboratory, we gather imaging and Doppler data to identify carotid artery disease into a category such as 50% to 79% or 80% to 99% stenosis. We, typically, then compare our results (duplex findings) with the "gold standard" (arteriogram results) to see how "close" the ultrasound findings are to the actual value (degree stenosis). Accuracy is the percentage of correct results. Not only it is important to be accurate to identify disease when disease is present, but also to identify normal vessels when disease is absent. Accuracy is calculated as the total number of correct tests divided by the total number of all tests.

## Sensitivity

Sensitivity measures the proportion of actual positives studies, which are correctly identified. It is the ability to identify disease when disease is present. When positive ultrasound studies correlate closely with positive arteriogram findings, then the test is said to have good sensitivity. Ultrasound is very good at determining if DVT is present in the lower extremities, but of no use in detecting pneumonia in the lungs. Here one might say that ultrasound is very sensitive for DVT, but has no sensitivity for detecting pneumonia.

If a condition is potentially fatal and a treatment exists, one would want to maximize the sensitivity of a test. In vascular testing, one might want to maximize the sensitivity in detecting a high-grade carotid stenosis or an abdominal aortic aneurysm. Both of these conditions could be potentially fatal but are easily treated.

Sensitivity is calculated by taking the TP results and dividing these by the all positive results as determined by the gold standard.

## Specificity

As sonographers, we know it is not only important to identify disease when it is present but to be certain that when we fail to find disease, no disease truly exists. Physicians rely heavily on the ultrasound reports and more often than not, manage the patient based on the sonographer's findings alone. However, in the early 1980s when duplex ultrasound was first utilized to assess the presence or absence of DVT, ultrasound studies were in almost every case, followed up by a venogram. After time, the consistency in accuracy and reliability of duplex ultrasound to identify or rule out DVT, eventually led to the virtual end of venograms performed for the detection lower extremity DVT. Using duplex ultrasound to rule out DVT is said to have good specificity. Specificity is the ability of a test to identify something as normal or the absence of disease.

When a confirmatory test is expensive or invasive, then one would want to maximize specificity of the ultrasound examination. This would avoid further unnecessary in normal patients.

Specificity is calculated by dividing the number of TN results by all the negative results as identified by the gold standard.

## Reliability

Reliability is the consistency of obtaining similar results under similar circumstances. In a sense, it is accuracy over a period of time. A laboratory or ultrasound department is reliable when the results of the tests produced are consistently accurate. Once the medical community determines that a department produces reliable results on a consistent basis, confidence in the department is ensured.

## Positive Predictive Value

The positive predictive value (PPV) is the proportion of patients with positive test results that are correctly identified. It is an important measure of a diagnostic method, such as ultrasound, that provides the probability that a positive test reflects the underlying disease for which the test is being conducted. In other words, of all the positive venous studies in a department, the PPV is the percentage which correctly predicted a DVT based on the gold standard. This is calculated as the number of TP studies divided by all the positive studies (TP plus FP).

## Negative Predictive Value

The negative predictive value (NPV) is the proportion of negative test results when there is no underlying disease present. It is an important measure of a diagnostic method, such as ultrasound, that provides the probability that a negative test reflects the absence of disease. If this test states there is no arterial obstruction of the arteries in the lower extremity, one can be confident that there is no disease is present if the NPV is high.[1]

## THE CHI-SQUARE TEST

The Chi-square (pronounced "kye" as in sky) is a statistical test that in sum compares the difference between what one "expects" and what one actually "observes."[2] If ultrasound velocities meet a criteria of 50% to 79%, that is what is expected to be seen on the arteriogram. What is observed in this example is the arteriogram results which either agree or disagree with the expected results as seen on the ultrasound.

The more tests that are performed that agree with the "gold standard," or the narrower the difference between what is expected and what is observed, the greater the accuracy of the studies. On the other hand, the more disagreements identified or the wider the difference between what is expected and observed, the lesser the accuracy of the studies.

The simplified Chi-square is a table containing four letters (A through D). Each letter represents the results of what was expected and what was observed. For the purpose of evaluating ultrasounds, the duplex ultrasound results typically are defined as what is expected. The angiogram represents the gold standard or what was observed.

## Chi-Square Exercise

Before attempting to calculate some data using the Chi-square, try this simple exercise. With a blank sheet of paper, draw a blank Chi-square (a box containing four equal squares). Write in the correct identifiers for the vertical axis, Duplex ultrasound and for the horizontal axis, angiography (Fig. 34-1). Next, identify and write in A (TP), B (FP), C (FN), and D (TN) in the appropriate boxes, as shown in Figure 34-1.

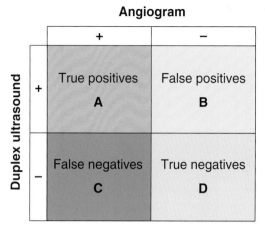

**FIGURE 34-1** Basic design of a Chi-square table comparing observed results (angiography) with expected results (duplex ultrasound). The cells of the Chi-square are identified, indicating the appropriate placement of TP, FP, TN, and FN data.

Now, take your finger and sweep it across boxes A and B (Fig. 34-2). These boxes represent all the studies (both duplex ultrasound and angiogram) that were reported as positive. Here we want many TP and as few FP as possible. These numbers will be used to calculate the PPV. Next, sweep your finger across C and D. The sum of these two boxes represents all the studies that were reported as negative. Here we want to have as many TN and as few FN as possible. These numbers will be used to determine the NPV.

Now, sweep your finger down boxes A and C (Fig. 34-3). The numbers in these two boxes will be used to calculate the sensitivity of the study. Again, the fewer the FN, the better the sensitivity. Lastly, draw your finger down boxes B and D. These numbers are used to calculate the specificity of the test. As with the previous calculations, specificity is improved by high large number of TN and low number of FP.

Finally, sweep your finger diagonally down the Chi-square from right to left (Fig. 34-4). Here you will intersect the box containing the TP (A) and the TN (D) whose total will be divided by the sum of all four squares (A + B + C + D). This is the calculation of overall accuracy.[3,4]

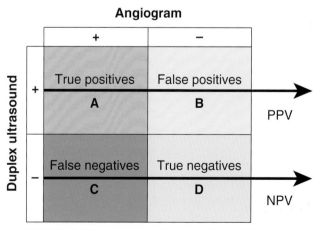

**FIGURE 34-2** A Chi-square table to calculate positive predictive value (PPV) and negative predictive value (NPV).

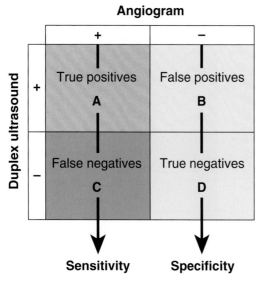

FIGURE 34-3 A Chi-square table to calculate sensitivity and specificity.

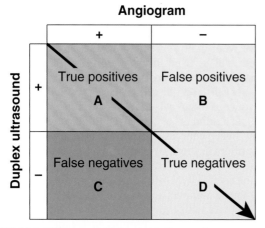

FIGURE 34-4 A Chi-square table to calculate the overall accuracy.

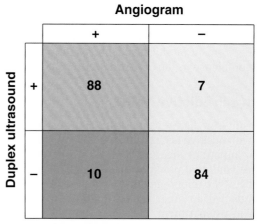

**FIGURE 34-5** A Chi-square table with sample data filled in comparing results of duplex ultrasound to angiography.

Table 34-1 provides a summary of the statistical parameters of sensitivity, specificity, PPV, NPV, and accuracy. All of these parameters can be calculated from the Chi-square.

By examining these calculations, it can be seen that the accuracy is both related to the ability to correctly find disease and correctly identify the absence of disease.[5] Thus, the absolute value for accuracy must be between the values of sensitivity and specificity. The accuracy must also be between the NPV and PPV.

## Statistics Quiz

Applying the formulas already provided to the data presented in Figure 34-5, solve for the following questions:

1. What is the sensitivity of this study?
   A) 95%          B) 90%
   C) 60%          D) 85%

| TABLE 34-1 | Statistical Parameters Calculated Using a Chi Square Table | |
|---|---|---|
| **Statistical Parameter** | **Chi-Square Table Variable** | **Actual Measurement** |
| Sensitivity | $\dfrac{A}{A+C}$ | $\dfrac{TP}{TP+FN}$ |
| Specificity | $\dfrac{D}{D+B}$ | $\dfrac{TN}{TN+FP}$ |
| PPV | $\dfrac{A}{A+B}$ | $\dfrac{TP}{TP+FP}$ |
| NPV | $\dfrac{D}{C+D}$ | $\dfrac{TN}{FN+TN}$ |
| Accuracy | $\dfrac{A+D}{A+B+C+D}$ | $\dfrac{TP+TN}{TP+FP+FN+TN}$ |

Key: A, B, C, D refer to cell values of the Chi-square table, refer to Figure 34-1.
TP: true positives, TN: true negatives, FP: false positives, FN: False negatives.

2. What is the specificity of this study?
   A) 92%                B) 96%
   C) 60%                D) 85%
3. What is the positive predictive value?
   A) 93%                B) 96%
   C) 60%                D) 85%
4. What is the negative predictive value?
   A) 33%                B) 96%
   C) 60%                D) 89%
5. What is the accuracy?
   A) 76%                B) 96%
   C) 91%                D) 85%

## PEER REVIEW

The utilization of invasive vascular testing such as angiography and venography has declined over the past years because the accuracy of vasular ultrasound has been more thoroughly validated. This welcome change in practice has also reduced the ability to verify the quality of vascular ultrasound results by comparisons with angiographic gold standards. This trend is particlarly evident for venous duplex ultrasounds because fewer venograms are routinely performed in the assessment of venous disease.

In light of this, the need for assessing the quality of vascular ultrasounds still exists. In fact, quality is even more important because patient care decisions are more likely being made soley on ultrasound results alone.

Peer review offers a well-established alternative method of QA. The concept of peer review is based on the work of one person being evaluated by an expert of the same field. The process of peer review is an ongoing program involving both physicians and sonographers. This collaberation allows feedback to be shared among colleagues in order to maintain and improve the accuracy of the testing provided.

A typical peer-review process will be conducted with a set number of cases that are randomly collected. The process can specify the collection interval and assortment of cases. Particular indicators which reflect the various aspects of the testing performed are critqued. Examples of these specific quality indicators are as follows:
- Test appropriateness
- Adherance to criteria
- Technical quality
- Adherance to protocol
- Completeness
- Timeliness

In some laboratories, physicians may be responsible for the diagnostic review, including the adherance to criteria. Technical staff may evaluate completeness of the study and adherance to established protocols. The data can be collected onto forms, summarized, and discussed at QA meetings. Inaccuracies and deficiencies can be identified, and action plans to improve results can be formulated.

---

### SUMMARY

- Statistical values are an integral part of a QA program.
- Periodic review of ultrasound data and comparison to gold standards will enable a vascular laboratory or ultrasound department to ensure reliable data.
- It is important for the vascular technologist or sonographer to understand the calculation and meaning of common statistical parameters.
- Peer-review data can be a useful adjunct to statistical analysis with correlative imaging. Peer-review data, in some cases, may be the only source of QA data available.

- These QA statistics and peer-review data will serve to identify potential discrepancies which in turn can be used to adjust everyday work practices. This will maximize the quality of duplex utlrasound testing results.

### MEDIA MENU

Student Resources available on thePoint® include:
- Audio glossary
- Interactive question bank
- Videos
- Internet resources

### REFERENCES

1. Case T. *Primer of Non-invasive Vascular Technology*. 1st ed. Boston, MA: Little Brown; 1996.
2. Matthews DE, Farewell VT. *Using and Understanding Medical Statistics*, 5th ed, Basel, Switzerland; Karger; 2015.
3. Rumwell C, McPharlin M. *Vascular Technology: An illustrated Review*. 5th ed. Pasadena: Davies Publishing; 2014.
4. Baldi B, Moore DS. *The Practice of Statistics in the Life Sciences*. New York: Freeman & Company; 2009.
5. Ridgeway DP. *Introduction to Vascular Scanning*, 4th ed., Pasadena, CA: Davies Publishing; 2014.

# INDEX

Page numbers followed by *f*, *t*, and *b* indicate figures, tables, and boxes, respectively.

arteriovenous malformations, 454
arteritis, 105
  diagnosis, 106–107, 106f
  signs and symptoms, 105–106
  sonographic examination techniques, 106
artifacts, 449
  clutter, 22, 23f
  comet tail, 22, 22f
  enhancement, 22, 23f
  grating lobes, 22, 23f
  mirror-image, 22, 23f
  reverberation, 22, 22f
  shadowing, 22, 22f
As Low As Reasonably Achievable
  principle, 450
atherosclerosis, 189, 331, 339b
atherosclerotic stenosis, 190b, 339
ATN (acute tubular necrosis), 382, 387
ATV ( anterior tibial vein), 234–235
autogenous access, 420
autogenous arteriovenous access, types of,
  419, 419t
autogenous fistula, 420
automatic compression/decompression
  technique, 283
AVF. See arteriovenous fistula
awkward postures, WRMSDs, 28
axillary artery
  evaluation of, 185
  transitions, 182
axillary vein, 253
  transverse view, 253, 253f

**B**

balloon angioplasty, 359
Bandyk applied pulse Doppler spectral
  analysis, 408
basilic vein, 264, 264f, 265f, 269f
  sagittal image of, 305f
Bernoulli principle, 54, 54f
bilateral brachial artery, measurement of,
  189
biliary ducts, 365f
biloma, 399f
bioeffects, transducers, 15
bland thrombus, 454
bleeding, 306, 306b
  complications, 448
"blind" Doppler, 18, 18f
bloc pediatric kidney transplant, 383f
blood flow, within kidney, 342
blue toe syndrome, 310
blunt and penetrating trauma, 184
B-mode characteristics, 283, 326, 326f
  and color Doppler images of
    heterogeneous irregular plaque, 75f
  grayscale imaging, 417
  iatrogenic injury, 76, 78f
  image of carotid bifurcation, 76f
  intraluminal defects, 74–76, 77f
  plaque, 73–74, 75f
  ultrasound, 285, 408
B-mode controls
  focal zone, 21
  frequency, 21
  imaging depth, 21
  overall gain, 21
  spatial compounding, 21
  time gain compensation (TGC), 21
  tissue harmonic imaging (THI), 21
bolus tracking, 449, 449f, 452
bowel ischemia, 456
brachial arteries, 186, 188f
  duplicated, 182

inflow to dialysis access, 423f
brachial systolic pressures, 83
brachial vein, 253, 269f
brachiocephalic fistula, 419f, 420f
brachiocephalic veins, 251, 302f
  color image, 251f
  spectral Doppler waveform, 252, 252f
"bubble study" echocardiography
  examinations, 435
Budd-Chiari's syndrome, 364, 378–379,
  378–379f, 379b
Buerger's disease, 185
bypass grafts, 326–328, 327f

**C**

calcification, 271–272, 271b, 272f
calcified radial artery, 417f
calf muscle perfusion, 438
capillaries, 38–39
cardiac arrhythmias, 84
cardiac assist devices, 84
cardiac cirrhosis, 377–378, 378f
cardioembolic disease, 219, 221
  Doppler spectrum of patient, 221f
  scanning technique, 221, 222f
cardiogenic arterial embolism, 184
Cardiovascular Credentialing International
  (CCI), 292
carotid aneurysm
  diagnosis, 103
  signs and symptoms, 103
  sonographic examination techniques, 103
carotid arteries, 74f, 77f, 78, 78f, 79f, 85f,
  439f
  common carotid and external, 93–94
  duplex evaluation, 71f
  occlusion, 440f
  pathology, 74b
  plaque neovascularization, 440–441, 441f
  pseudoaneurysm, 78f
  systems, 88
  thrombosis, 76
  vasa vasorum, 440–441, 441f
carotid artery stenting (CAS), 113
  post-CAS diagnostic features, 116
    duplex ultrasound criteria, 120t
    duplex ultrasound velocity criteria for
     in-stent restenosis, 116–119, 118t
    stent fracture and migration, 119
    surveillance frequency, 119
  sonographic examination techniques,
    115–116, 117f
  techniques, 115
carotid bifurcation, 410f
carotid body tumor (CBT), 102
  signs and symptoms, 102
  sonographic examination techniques, 103
    color image, 103f
    diagnosis, 103
    technical considerations, 103
carotid endarterectomy (CEA), 406, 407,
  408, 411
  current intraoperative evaluation, 407–
    408, 408–409f
  diagnosis, 408–409, 409–410f
  eversion vs. traditional CEA, 110, 110f
  mean velocities and ratio and degree of
    restenosis, 114t
  patch closure, and, 109–110
  pathology associated with, 113b
  post-CEA diagnostic features, 112, 112f
    restenosis, 112–113
  PSVs, EDVs, and ICA/CCA ratios, 115t
  sonographic examination techniques

endarterectomy dacron patch, 111f
  patient positioning, 111
  patient preparation, 110–111
  pitfalls, 111–112
  scanning techniques, 111
  technical considerations, 111
carotid siphon (CS), 135–136, 137f
carotid system, 448
  arteritis. See arteritis
  carotid aneurysm. See carotid aneurysm
  CBT. See carotid body tumor
  dissections/intimal flaps, 99
    diagnosis, 100–101
    signs and symptoms, 99–100
    sonographic examination techniques,
     100, 100f
  false aneurysm. See pseudoaneurysm
  FMD. See fibromuscular dysplasia
  PA. See pseudoaneurysm
  pathology, 107b
  RIAI. See radiation-induced arterial injury
  tortuosity and kinking, 97–98
    diagnosis, 99
    signs and symptoms, 98
    sonographic examination techniques,
     98–99, 98–99f
    technical considerations, 99
CAS. See carotid artery stenting
CA stenosis by duplex scanning, 328t
catheter
  constant observation of, 296
  vessel and placement of, 448
caval fistulas, 356b
cavernosal arteries, 430
cavernous transformation, 377, 377f
CBD (common bile duct), 394
CBT. See carotid body tumor
CCA. See common carotid artery
CEA. See carotid endarterectomy
CEAP classification. See clinical, etiologic,
  anatomic, and pathophysiologic
  classification
celiac artery, 324, 324f, 330f
  causes of, 331
  occlusion, 332b
  pathology, 332b
celiac artery compression syndrome, 332b
celiac mesenteric artery, 457f
CE-MRA (contrast-enhanced MRA), 439
central VAD placement, 304
central vascular access device placement,
  302
  anatomy, 302, 302f, 303f
  central placement, 304
  implanted ports, 303, 303f
  longitudinal approach to, 305f
  nontunneled, 303
  peripheral placement, 303–304
  sonographic examination techniques,
    304, 304f
    air embolism, 306, 306b
    bleeding, 306, 306b
    cardiac arrhythmias, 306, 306b
    nontarget puncture, 306, 306b
    scanning technique, 304–305, 305f
    technical considerations, 306, 306b
    vein damage, 306, 306b
  tunneled, 303
central venous catheterization, sonographic
  localization for, 411
cephalic vein, 252, 264, 264f, 265f, 268,
  269f, 417f
  longitudinal view, 252f
  transverse view, 252f
cerebrovascular accident (CVA), 70, 409